Manual of
TRANSFUSION MEDICINE

Manual of
TRANSFUSION MEDICINE

Ramadas Nayak MBBS MD
Professor and Head
Department of Pathology
Yenepoya Medical College
Yenepoya (Deemed to be University)
Mangaluru, Karnataka, India

Formerly
Head, Department of Pathology
Kasturba Medical College, Mangaluru
Manipal Academy of Higher Education
Karnataka, India
askdr.nayak@gmail.com

Rakshatha Nayak MBBS MD DNB
Tutor
Department of Pathology
Yenepoya Medical College
Yenepoya (Deemed to be University)
Mangaluru, Karnataka, India

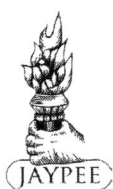

JAYPEE BROTHERS MEDICAL PUBLISHERS
The Health Sciences Publisher
New Delhi | London

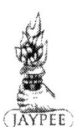 **Jaypee Brothers Medical Publishers (P) Ltd**

Headquarters
Jaypee Brothers Medical Publishers (P) Ltd
4838/24, Ansari Road, Daryaganj
New Delhi 110 002, India
Phone: +91-11-43574357
Fax: +91-11-43574314
Email: jaypee@jaypeebrothers.com

Overseas Office
J.P. Medical Ltd
83 Victoria Street, London
SW1H 0HW (UK)
Phone: +44 20 3170 8910
Fax: +44 (0)20 3008 6180
Email: info@jpmedpub.com

Website: www.jaypeebrothers.com
Website: www.jaypeedigital.com

© 2020, Jaypee Brothers Medical Publishers

The views and opinions expressed in this book are solely those of the original contributor(s)/author(s) and do not necessarily represent those of editor(s) of the book.

All rights reserved. No part of this publication may be reproduced, stored or transmitted in any form or by any means, electronic, mechanical, photocopying, recording or otherwise, without the prior permission in writing of the publishers.

All brand names and product names used in this book are trade names, service marks, trademarks or registered trademarks of their respective owners. The publisher is not associated with any product or vendor mentioned in this book.

Medical knowledge and practice change constantly. This book is designed to provide accurate, authoritative information about the subject matter in question. However, readers are advised to check the most current information available on procedures included and check information from the manufacturer of each product to be administered, to verify the recommended dose, formula, method and duration of administration, adverse effects and contraindications. It is the responsibility of the practitioner to take all appropriate safety precautions. Neither the publisher nor the author(s)/editor(s) assume any liability for any injury and/or damage to persons or property arising from or related to use of material in this book.

This book is sold on the understanding that the publisher is not engaged in providing professional medical services. If such advice or services are required, the services of a competent medical professional should be sought.

Every effort has been made where necessary to contact holders of copyright to obtain permission to reproduce copyright material. If any have been inadvertently overlooked, the publisher will be pleased to make the necessary arrangements at the first opportunity. The **CD/DVD-ROM** (if any) provided in the sealed envelope with this book is complimentary and free of cost. **Not meant for sale.**

Inquiries for bulk sales may be solicited at: jaypee@jaypeebrothers.com

Manual of Transfusion Medicine

First Edition: **2020**
ISBN: 978-93-88958-60-8
Printed in India

Dedicated to

Students who inspired us,
Patients who provided the knowledge,
Our parents and family members, who encouraged and supported us.

Ramadas Nayak
Rakshatha Nayak

Images Contribution

1. Dr Aravind P (MD Pathology), Associate Professor, Department of Pathology and Incharge Blood Bank Officer, AJ Institute of Medical Sciences and Research Centre, Mangaluru, Karnataka, India.
2. Mr PR Gopalkrishna [BSc (MLT), MSc (MLT)], Quality and Technical Manager, AJ Blood Bank and AJ Hospital and Research Centre, Mangaluru, Karnataka, India.
3. Mr Srinivas Shetty, Venus Diagnostics, Mangaluru, Karnataka, India.
4. Ms Suparna Laha (PhD), Faculty, Molecular Biology Division, Yenepoya Research Centre, Yenepoya University, Mangaluru, Karnataka, India.

Preface

The laboratory discipline of transfusion medicine (also known as immunohematology or blood banking) is the most fascinating and challenging field in clinical laboratory medicine. All postgraduates in Pathology as well as laboratory technicians involved in blood banking should know the basic knowledge of transfusion medicine. The terms Blood Center/Bank (Banking) and Transfusion Medicine are often used interchangeably, and with the present amendment the term blood bank is replaced by Blood Center. The term Blood Center (Bank) refers to a blood collection and processing center whereas completion of the associated tasks is known as Blood Banking. Transfusion service is the laboratory area responsible for pretransfusion testing and blood product distribution (usually located in the hospital).

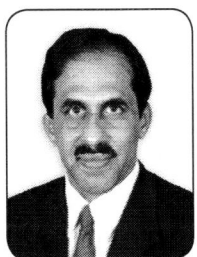

Ramadas Nayak

It intends to provide basic concepts of transfusion medicine required to be known by postgraduate students of medical laboratory technology and laboratory professionals and other health care professionals. There have been exciting advances in transfusion medicine and this book provides knowledge in a simple, lucid and reproducible format. It is accompanied by many illustrative figures, photographs, tables and boxes. It includes updates on the field of blood banking.

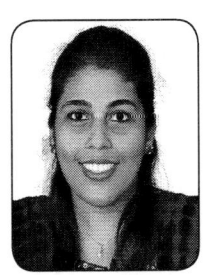

Rakshatha Nayak

Organization and Features of the Book

The content of this book is organized into 25 chapters, beginning with basic immunology related to blood group serology and interactions between antigens and antibodies. The successive chapters cover the most common blood groups, pretransfusion testing protocols, transfusion reactions, blood components, apheresis (one of the fastest growing and most promising methods of blood collection and component harvesting), hemolytic disease of the newborn, hemovigilance, quality assurance and regulatory issues. The book is written at a level adaptable for multiple categories of students. The important features of this book are:

- Each chapter begins with chapter outlines listing the important elements in the chapter
- Presented in a clear and concise manner and text in bullet form for easy review and recollection
- Written in a manner that is readable, interesting, and easily understood by students
- Key points are provided in bold words so that it will help the students to just brush through the entire book within few hours before the examination or viva voce
- Tables, illustrations, figures and boxes are incorporated into the chapters as appropriate to make it easier to understand the contents
- Summary of chapter for an overview of the chapter's important points
- Self-assessment exercises at the end of each chapter provide the questions frequently asked in the qualifying examinations
- Color plates have been added for better understanding.

Acknowledgments

Our sincere thanks to all our family members, especially Smt Rekha Nayak, Ms Rashmitha Nayak, Mr Ramnath Kini and Mr Ramnath Nayak, who have patiently accepted our long preoccupation with this work. A special thanks to Master Rishab Kini, who kept us agile throughout the preparation of this book.

We wish to express our gratitude to Mr Yenepoya Abdulla Kunhi, Honorable Chancellor, Yenepoya (Deemed to be University—Accredited by NAAC with "A" grade), Mangaluru, Karnataka, India, for giving us an opportunity to serve this prestigious institution. We are indebted to Mr Farhaad Yenepoya, Pro-Chancellor, Yenepoya (Deemed to be University), for the inspiration and encouragement. We are grateful to Dr M Vijaya Kumar (Vice-Chancellor) and Dr Ganghadhar Somayaji KS (Registrar), Yenepoya (Deemed to be University), for the encouragement.

We are thankful to all our friends who contributed fantastic images for this book. Our sincere thanks to Dr Aravind P (MD Pathology), Associate Professor, Department of Pathology and Incharge Blood Bank Officer, AJ Institute of Medical Sciences and Research Centre, Mangaluru; Mr PR Gopalkrishna [BSc (MLT), MSc (MLT)], Quality and Technical Manager, AJ Blood Bank and AJ Hospital and Research Centre, Mangaluru; Dr Sharada Rai (Professor and Head), Department of Pathology, Kasturba Medical College (Mangaluru), Manipal Academy of Higher Education (Manipal); Dr Shamee Shastry, Professor and Head, Department of Immunohematology and Blood Transfusion, Kasturba Medical College (a constituent of Manipal Academy of Higher Education) Manipal, Karnataka; Dr Chandrika Rao, Associate Professor and Incharge Blood Bank, Department of Pathology, KS Hegde Medical Academy (a constituent of Nitte Deemed to be University); Dr Karthick and Dr Vishnupriya, Tamil Nadu.

We would like to express our gratitude to all our friends, colleagues, undergraduate and postgraduate students (Department of Pathology, Yenepoya Medical College, Mangaluru) who helped us in the different stages of preparing the manuscript; to all those who provided support, talked things over, read, offered comments and assisted in the editing, proofreading and design.

A special thanks to Shri Jitendar P Vij (Group Chairman), Mr Ankit Vij (Manading Director), and Mr MS Mani (Group President) of M/s Jaypee Brothers Medical Publishers (P) Ltd, New Delhi, India, for publishing the book in the same format as wanted, well in time. We are grateful to Shri Jitendar P Vij for unmasking our talent as authors.

We would like to offer a huge appreciation to the wonderful work done by Dr Madhu Choudhary (Publishing Head–Education), Ms Pooja Bhandari (Production Head), Ms Sunita Katla (Executive Assistant to Group Chairman and Publishing Manager), Dr Priyanka Kumari (Development Editor), Ms Samina Khan (Executive Assistant to Publishing Head–Education), Mr Rajesh Sharma (Production Coordinator), Ms Seema Dogra (Cover Visualizer), Ms Neelam (Proofreader), Mr Rajesh Gurkundi (Graphic Designer), and Mr Om Prakesh (Typesetter) of M/s Jaypee Brothers Medical Publishers (P) Ltd, New Delhi, India.

We thank Mr Venugopal V (Bengaluru) and Mr Vasudev H (Mangaluru) of M/s Jaypee Brothers Medical Publishers (P) Ltd for taking this book to every corner of Karnataka.

Last but definitely not least, a thank you to our undergraduate and postgraduate students, without you, we would not write. You make all our books possible.

This book would not be possible without all of the people mentioned above and we are indebted to them for their friendship, support and assistance. There are many more people we could thank, but space and modesty compel us to stop here.

Contents

1. **Basic Immunology Related to Blood Group Serology**   1
   Immune System *2*
   Terminologies used in Immunology *2*
   Components of Immune System *4*
   Immunoglobulins *6*
   Immune Response *8*
   Immunohematology *10*
   Traditional Laboratory Testing Methods *17*
   Nontraditional Laboratory Testing Methods *19*
   Blood Group Antigens *19*
   Blood Group Alloantibodies and Autoantibodies *20*
   Complement System and Blood Banking *20*
   Historical Overview of Blood Banking/Blood Transfusion Service (BTS) *22*

2. **Blood Group Genetics**   25
   Chromosomes *25*
   Cell Division *27*
   Genetic Principles in Blood Banking *30*
   Population Genetics *33*
   Molecular Genetics *33*

3. **ABO Blood Group System**   38
   Red Blood Cell Groups *38*
   ABO and H Blood Group System Antigens *41*
   Secretors and Nonsecretors *47*
   Subgroups of A, AB and B *47*
   Null Phenotypes *51*
   Basic Genetic Features of ABO Group System *53*
   ABO/ABH Antibodies *55*

4. **ABO Blood Grouping: Methods and Discrepancies**   61
   Blood Banking Reagents *61*
   ABO Grouping/Typing *69*
   Methods of ABO Grouping *71*
   Alternative Methods to the Tube Test *76*
   Factors causing Discrepancies during ABO Testing *85*
   ABO Discrepancies, Problems Encountered and their Solutions *86*

5. **Rh Blood Group System**   98
   Introduction of Rh (D) System *98*
   Nomenclature *99*
   Rh Antigens *101*

Rh Antibodies *103*
Rh (D) Grouping/Typing *104*

6. Other Blood Group Systems — 112

Lewis Blood Group System (ISBT no. 007) *113*
MNS Blood Group System (ISBT no. 002) *115*
Kell and Kx Blood Group Systems (ISBT no. 006 and 019) *116*
Duffy Blood Group System (ISBT no. 008) *118*
Kidd (JK) Blood Group System (ISBT no. 009) *119*
Lutheran Blood Group System (ISBT no. 005) *120*
The P Blood Group: P1PK (ISBT no. 003), GLOB (028) and FORS Blood Group Systems (031) *122*
I Blood Group System (ISBT no. 027) *124*
Diego Blood Group System (ISBT no. 010) *125*
Cartwright (YT) Blood Group System (ISBT no. 011) *125*
XG Blood Group System (ISBT no. 012) *126*
Scianna Blood Group System (ISBT no. 013) *126*
Dombrock Blood Group System (ISBT no. 014) *127*
Colton Blood Group System (ISBT no. 015) *128*
Landsteiner-Wiener Blood Group System (ISBT no. 016) *129*
Chido/Rodgers Blood Group System (ISBT no. 017) *129*
Gerbich Blood Group System (ISBT no. 020) *130*
Cromer Blood Group System (ISBT no. 021) *130*
Knops Blood Group System (ISBT no. 022) *131*
Indian Blood Group System (ISBT no. 023) *132*
OK Blood Group System (ISBT no. 024) *133*
RAPH Blood Group System (ISBT no. 025) *133*
JMH Blood Group System (ISBT no. 026) *134*
GIL Blood Group System (ISBT no. 029) *134*
JR Blood Group System (ISBT no. 032) *135*
Lan Blood Group System (ISBT no. 033) *135*
Vel Blood Group System (ISBT no. 034) *135*
CD59 Blood Group System (ISBT no. 035) *136*
Applications of Other Blood Groups to Routine Blood Banking *136*

7. Donor Selection and Blood Collection — 138

Types of Donors and Donation *139*
Donor Selection *140*
Blood Collection *147*
Hemoglobin Estimation of Donor *156*
Processing of the Donor Blood *160*

8. Preservation, Storage and Transport of Blood — 162

Preservation of Blood *162*
Storage of Blood *166*
Changes in Stored Blood (Effects of Storage of Blood) *169*
Platelet Preservation *171*
Pathogen Reduction Technology *172*

9.	**Antihuman Globulin Test**	173

Antihuman Globulin Reagents *174*
Principles of the Antiglobulin Test *178*
Direct Antiglobulin Test *179*
Indirect Antiglobulin Test *181*
Alternative Methods to the Tube Test *183*
Sources of Error in Antiglobulin Test *185*
Quality Control for Antiglobulin Test *185*

10.	**Antibody Detection (Screening) and Identification**	188

Basic Concepts in Red Cell Antigen Expression *189*
Types of Antibodies in Transfusion Medicine *190*
Antibody Detection (Screening) *191*
Antibody Identification *198*
Interpretation (Evaluation) of Panel Results *203*
Complex Antibody Identification *216*
Considerations Following Antibody Identification *218*

11.	**Pretransfusion and Compatibility Testing**	220

Steps in Pretransfusion Testing *220*
Crossmatch Testing (Crossmatching) *225*
Pretransfusion Testing in Special Circumstances *234*

12.	**Blood Components and their Preparation**	242

Whole Blood *243*
Blood Components *245*
Preparation of Blood Components *246*
Red Blood Cell Components *247*
Platelet Components *254*
Plasma Components *260*
Granulocyte Concentrates *270*

13.	**Apheresis**	274

Methods of Apheresis *276*
Donor Cytapheresis *280*
Donor Plasmapheresis *285*
Therapeutic Apheresis *286*
Donor/Patient Complications Common to All Apheresis Procedures *292*

14.	**Adverse Effects of Blood Transfusion**	296

Hemolysis *296*
Adverse Transfusion Reactions *300*
Immediate/Acute Transfusion Reactions *302*
Delayed Transfusion Reactions *318*
Silent Transfusion-Related Adverse Events *326*
Transfusion-Related Adverse Events in Special Patient Scenarios *327*

15.	**Investigations in a Case of Transfusion Reaction**	330

Investigation (Work-Up) of Suspected Adverse Transfusion Reactions *330*

16. Transfusion-Transmitted Diseases — 346
Transfusion-Transmitted Diseases *346*
Screening Blood Donors for Transfusion-Transmitted Infections *357*
Prion Disease *366*
Safety Measures in Laboratory during Testing for HIV and Hepatitis *366*
Detection of Malaria in Blood Donors *367*

17. Nucleic Acid Amplification Test in Blood Banking — 369
Nucleic Acid Amplification Test *370*
Polymerase Chain Reaction (PCR and RT PCR) *372*
Transcription-based Amplification *377*

18. Hemolytic Disease of Newborn — 379
Etiopathogenesis of HDFN *380*
Rh (D) Hemolytic Disease of the Fetus and Newborn *383*
Prevention of Rh (D) HDFN *394*
ABO Hemolytic Disease of Fetus and Newborn (HDFN) *397*
Alloantibodies Causing Hemolytic Disease of the Fetus and Newborn Other than Anti-D *400*

19. Transfusion Therapy in Selected Patients and Blood Substitutes — 402
Transfusion Therapy in Selected Patients *402*
Autologous Blood Donation and Transfusion *411*
Alternatives to Transfusion *414*
Plasma Substitutes *419*

20. Automation and Recent Advances in Blood Bank — 422
Automation in Immunohematology *422*
Automated Testing in Transfusion Medicine *425*
Recent Advances in Blood Banking *425*
Virtual Blood Bank *429*
Recent Advances in Therapy *430*
Safe Blood Transfusion *430*
Protocols in Blood Bank *433*

21. Hemovigilance, National Blood Policy and Biomedical Waste — 436
Hemovigilance *436*
Recipient Hemovigilance *438*
National Blood Policy *441*
Medicolegal and Ethical Concerns in Blood Banking and Transfusion Services *442*
Problems Faced by the Blood Transfusion Services in India *444*
Biomedical Waste *444*

22. Quality Programs in Blood Banking and Transfusion Medicine — 450
Quality Program *451*
Quality Assurance *464*
Quality Control *466*
Quality Assurance in the Transfusion Laboratory *487*

23. Major Histocompatibility Complex Molecules — 492
Classification of HLA *494*
Techniques for Detection of HLA (HLA Typing) *498*
Donor-Recipient Crossmatch *507*
Techniques for Detection of HLA Antibodies *509*
Post-Transplant Immunological Monitoring *513*
HLA and Transplantation *514*

24. Hematopoietic Progenitor Cell Transplantation — 519
Hematopoietic Progenitor Cell (HPC) Collection *520*
Processing HPC Products *527*
Cryopreservation of Hematopoietic Grafts *529*
Transplanting the Recipient *530*
Complications of Hematopoietic Stem Cell Transplantation *533*
Transfusion Therapy for HPC Transplantation *535*
Ex Vivo Manipulation of Hematologic Cells *535*

25. Transfusion Regulation and Legislation — 538
Blood Bank Regulations and Legal Framework in India *538*
Licensing Procedure *583*
Evolution of Blood Safety Program in India *586*

Bibliography — *591*

Index — *593*

Color Plate 1

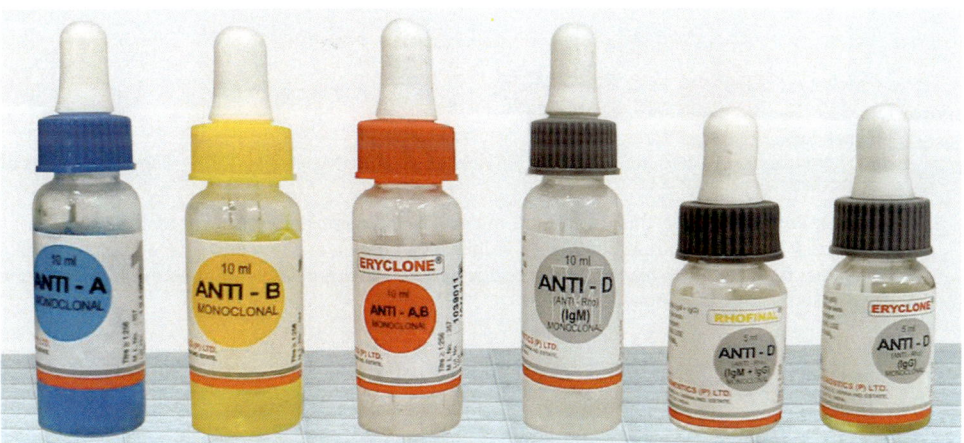

Fig. 4.1: Routine blood bank testing reagents (from left to right anti-A, anti-B, anti-A, B and anti-D [IgM, IgM+IgG and IgG]).

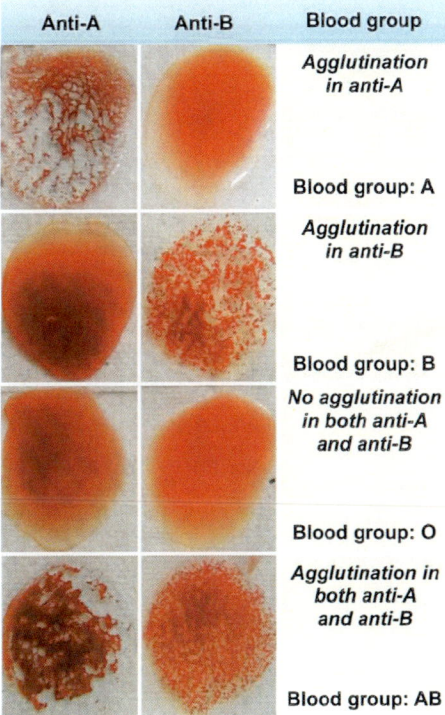

Fig. 4.7: Interpretation of blood group by slide method interpretation of blood group by slide method.

Color Plate 2

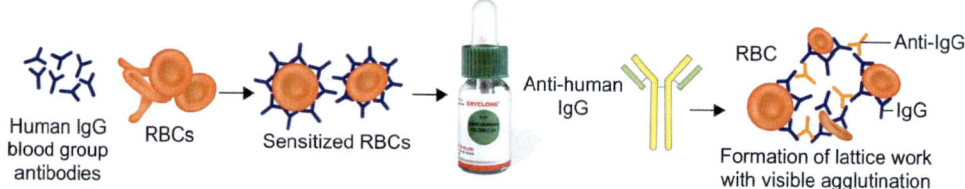

Fig. 9.4: *Antiglobulin test.* This detects IgG molecules and complement protein molecules that are attached (sensitized) to red cells but will produce a visible agglutination reaction only after adding AHG reagent. AHG antibodies present in AHG reagent form a bridge between adjacent RBCs sensitized by human immunoglobulin (IgG) or complement components.

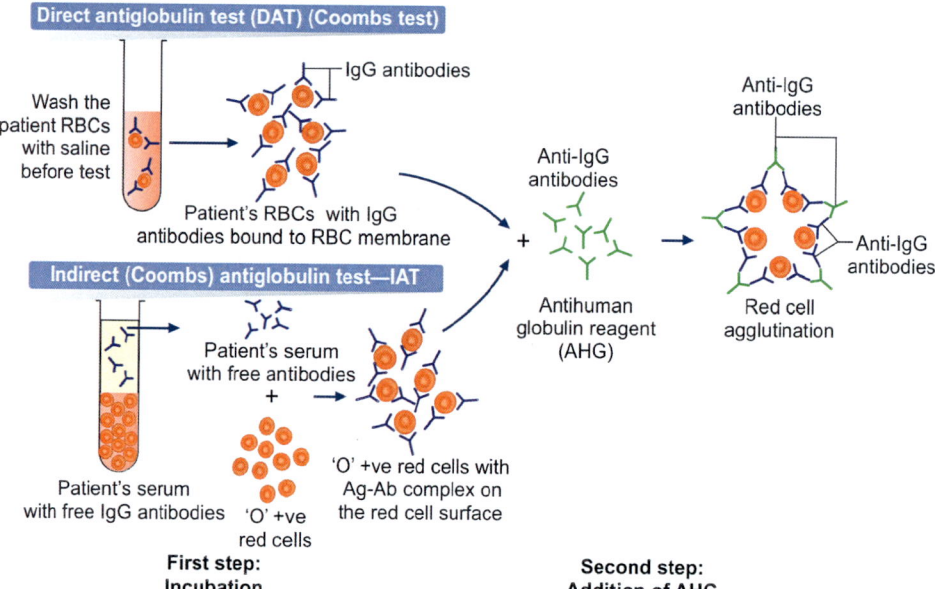

Fig. 9.5: Method of direct and indirect methods of antiglobulin test (Coombs test).

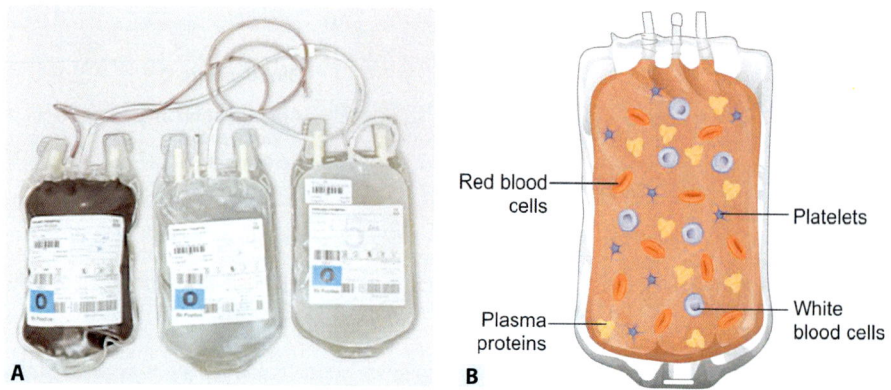

Figs. 12.2A and B: (A) Whole blood collected (first bag on the left) in a triple bag; (B) Various contents of whole blood (diagrammatic).

Color Plate 3

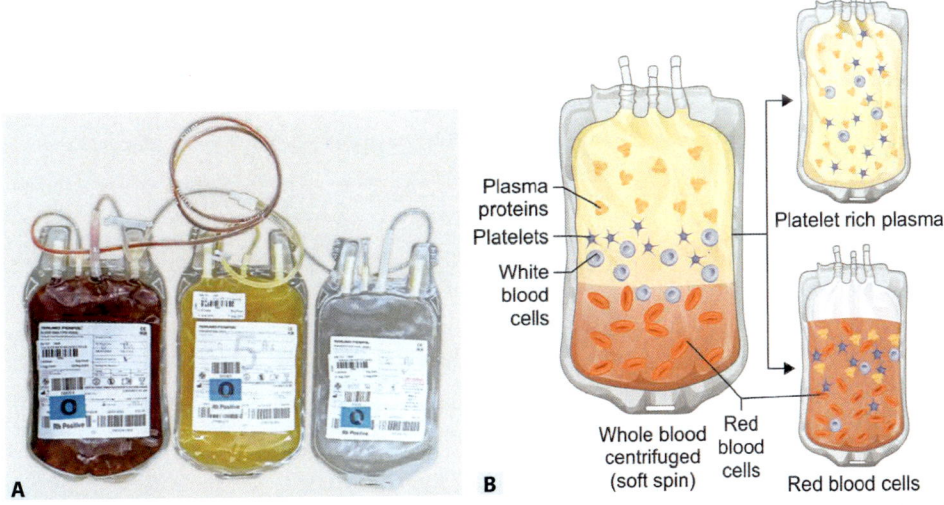

Figs. 12.9A and B: (A) Packed red cells in first bag (on left) and platelet rich plasma in second bag; (B) Platelet rich plasma produced from whole blood (diagrammatic).

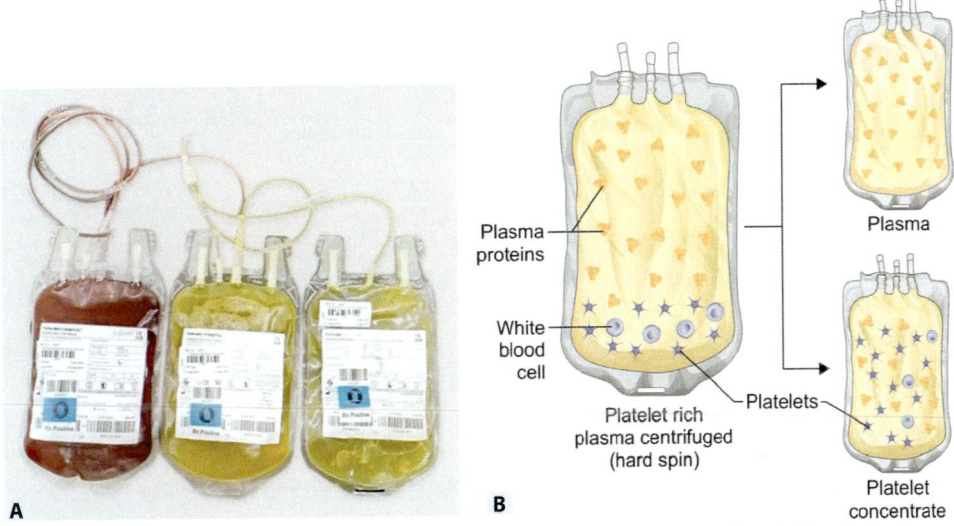

Figs. 12.10A and B: (A) Packed cells (first from left), platelet poor plasma (second from left) and platelet concentrate (third from left); (B) Production of platelet concentrates from platelet rich plasma (diagrammatic).

Color Plate 4

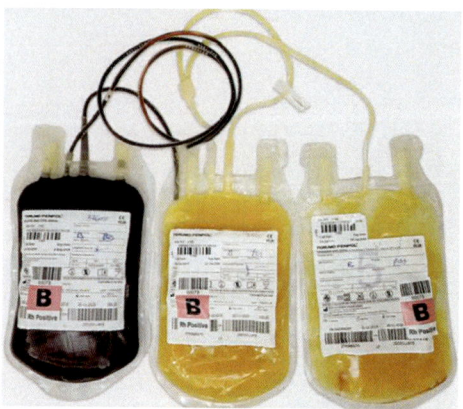

Fig. 12.12: From left to right-packed red cells, fresh frozen plasma (FFP) and platelets.

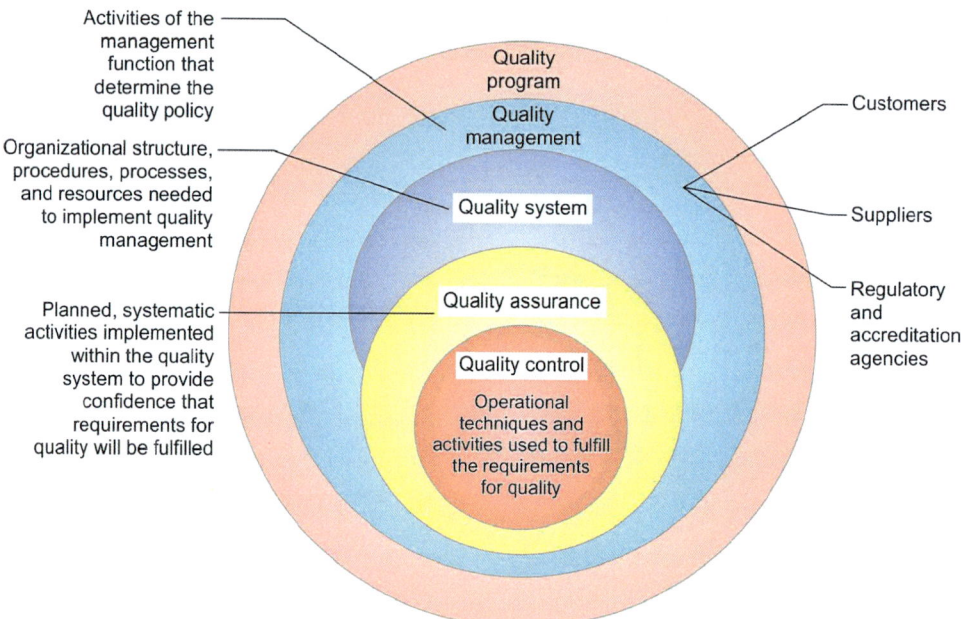

Fig. 22.1: Quality program activities with their interactions.

CHAPTER 1

Basic Immunology Related to Blood Group Serology

CHAPTER OUTLINE

- Immune system
- Terminologies used in immunology
- Components of immune system
- Immunoglobulins
- Immune response
- Immunohematology
- Traditional laboratory testing methods
- Nontraditional laboratory testing methods
- Blood group antigens
- Blood group alloantibodies and autoantibodies
- Complement system and blood banking
- Historical overview of blood banking/blood transfusion service (BTS)

INTRODUCTION

Immunity is defined as a resistance (defense mechanism) exhibited **by host against invasion by any foreign antigen**, including microorganisms. Immunology is the branch of medicine and biology concerned with immunity. Immunohematology is an integral part and plays an important role in transfusion medicine.

- **Immunohematology** deals with the serologic, genetic, biochemical and molecular study of antigens associated with membrane structures on the cellular constituents of blood (red blood cells [RBCs], white blood cells [WBCs], and platelets). It also deals with the immunologic properties and reactions of blood components and constituents.
- **Transfusion medicine** (Fig. 1.1) includes the transfusion of blood, its components, and derivatives.

Basic concepts of immunology: For understanding the principles of immunohematology,

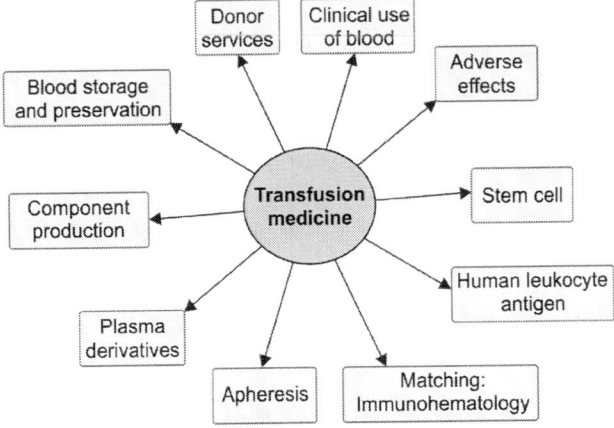

Fig. 1.1: Various components of transfusion medicine.

it is necessary to know the basic concepts of immunology. These include the antigens, antibodies, antigen-antibody reactions and complement affecting the antigen-antibody reaction. The application of immunohematology principles in the clinical laboratory is usually carried out in the blood bank or transfusion services department. Immunohematologists perform and interpret various serologic and molecular assays which help in the diagnosis, prevention, and management of immunization associated with transfusion, pregnancy, and organ transplantation.

IMMUNE SYSTEM

Role of Immune System

The immune system plays two main roles in the human body.
1. It provides the immune mechanism which protects the body against external foreign substances. The immune response is a highly evolved system and is necessary for survival. It rapidly responds to any foreign material or pathogens that invade the body and can initiate a series of events to eliminate this foreign material or pathogens.
2. It plays an important role in the identification and destruction of abnormal cells. These abnormal cells may be malignant cells, cells infected with microorganism or cells coated with antibodies. It has an ability to distinguish between self and nonself antigens.

Immune system is like a double-edged sword. Though immune system is protective in most of the situations, sometimes a hyperactive immune system may cause fatal diseases.

Types

The immune system consists of two lines of defense namely innate and adaptive immune response/immunity.

Innate (Natural/Native) Immune Response

Its salient features are:
- **First line of defense present by birth.**
- Provides **immediate initial protection** against an invading pathogen. It is triggered by substances which indicate potential danger to a host. These substances are common to many pathogens, such as bacterial lipopolysaccharide or viral nucleic acid.
- **Does not depend on the prior contact** with foreign antigen or microbes.
- **Lacks specificity, but highly effective.**
- **Triggers the adaptive immune response.**
- **No memory and no self/nonself recognition are seen.**
- **Innate immune cells:** These include monocyte-derived macrophages, neutrophils (polymorphonuclear neutrophils [PMNs] and dendritic cells [DCs]).

Adaptive Immune Response

If the innate immune system fails to provide effective protection against invading microbes, the adaptive immune system is activated. Thus, it is the second and more complex immune response that may follow the innate response. It specifically targets antigens present in the immunizing substance. It is characterized by the development of antigen-specific antibody and T cell responses. Three **characteristic features** are: (1) **specificity**, (2) **diversity** and (3) **memory**. Other salient features are:
- **Second line of defense** acquired during life.
- **Capable of recognizing both microbial and nonmicrobial substances.**
- **Takes more time** (days to weeks) **to develop** and is **more powerful than innate immunity.**
- **Long-lasting protection.**
- Prior exposure to antigen is present.
- **Adaptive immune cells:** T and B lymphocytes, and null cells.

TERMINOLOGIES USED IN IMMUNOLOGY

Transfusion medicine needs sound knowledge of antigens and antibodies. For understanding the immune system, it is essential to know some essential terms used in immunology.

Basic Immunology Related to Blood Group Serology

- **Antigen (Ag):** Any substance (usually foreign or a nonself) that is recognized as foreign by the body and capable of inducing immune response (antibody formation) in an immunocompetent individual. These antigens bind specifically to an antibody or cell-surface receptors of T lymphocytes. All antigens are not capable of eliciting an immune response. **Blood group antigens are present on the surface of RBCs.**
- **Immunogen:** It is a substance capable of provoking an antibody-mediated immune response when it is introduced into an immunocompetent host to whom it is foreign. The terms antigen and immunogen are often used synonymously. The immune response is initiated by the presentation of an **antigen** (initiates formation of and reacts with an antibody) or **immunogen** (initiates an immune response). The term antigen is more commonly used in blood banking because the primary testing is the detection of antibodies to blood group antigens.
- **Immunogenicity:** The ability of an antigen to elicit an immune response is known as its immunogenicity. The immunogenicity of an antigen is depends on:
  - **Characteristics of antigens:** These include degree of foreignness, molecular size and configuration, temperature, pH, and ionic environment and antigenic complexity (depends on the number of available epitopes or antigenic determinants).
  - **Host's genetically determined immune responsiveness.**
- **Antibody (Ab):** If a foreign antigen is introduced into an immunocompetent individual, a protein produced in response to it is called an **antibody**. Antibody is an immunoglobulin that is produced and secreted by activated B lymphocytes (**plasma cells** derived from B lymphocytes) after stimulation by a specific immunogen. Immunoglobulin proteins consist of two identical heavy chains and two identical light chains. The light chains recognize a particular **epitope** on an antigen and facilitate clearance of that antigen. While **all antibodies are immunoglobulins, not all immunoglobulins are antibodies.** Immunoglobulin molecules for which no complementary material or antigen has been recognized are simply called immunoglobulins, not antibodies.
  - **Alloantibodies:** They are formed in response to antigens from individuals of the same species. These are the type of antibodies involved in transfusion reactions.
  - **Heteroantibodies (xenoantibodies):** They are antibodies produced in response to antigens from another species.
  - **Autoantibodies:** They are made in response to the body's own antigens.
- **Antigen-presenting cell (APC):** APC is any cell that can process and present antigenic peptides in association with **class II major histocompatibility complex (MHC) molecules** and deliver a **costimulatory signal** necessary for T cell activation. The professional APCs include **macrophages, DCs, and B cells**. Nonprofessional APCs, which function in antigen presentation only for short periods include thymic epithelial cells and vascular endothelial cells.
- **Epitope (antigenic determinant):** It is a **portion/site of an immunogen/antigen** that is recognized and combines specifically with an antibody of B lymphocyte or antigen receptor of a T lymphocyte (T-cell receptor [TCR]-MHC combination or TCR ligand-CD1 complex).
- **Haptens:** They are well-defined molecules that are too small to be immunogenic (i.e. they cannot stimulate antibody production) by themselves but can induce an antibody response when attached to (coupled with) a carrier protein. The hapten molecules have a molecular weight (MW) less than 10,000 daltons (D). The carrier protein should have a MW greater than 10,000 D.
- **Immune system:** It is a collective term for all the cells and tissues involved in

immune activity (host defense system). Included in this system are the cells of the immune system, the thymus, lymph nodes, spleen, bone marrow, portions of the liver, gastrointestinal tract (GIT) and mucosa-associated lymphoid tissue.
- **Receptor:** It is a molecule or cell membrane protein molecule whose configuration allows it to form a tightly fitting complex with another molecule of complementary shape (**ligand** which is **molecule that binds to a receptor**).
- **Cytokine:** It is a low molecular weight protein secreted from an activated cell that affects the function or activity of other cells. Cytokines regulate the intensity and duration of the immune response by exerting a variety of effects on lymphocytes and other immune cells that express the appropriate receptor.
- **Clone:** It is a population of genetically identical cells derived from successive divisions of a single progenitor cell (a cell that originates from a stem cell and differentiates into a more specialized cell).

COMPONENTS OF IMMUNE SYSTEM

Immune system is made up of special cells, proteins, tissues and organs.

Organs Involved in Immune System

They may be central organs or peripheral organs.
- **Central organs:** Bone marrow, liver and thymus.
- **Peripheral organs:** Lymph nodes and spleen.

The mucosal-associated lymphoid tissues (i.e. GIT-associated and bronchus-associated lymphoid tissues) also play an important role by involving both central and peripheral functions.

Cells of the Immune System

Cells of immune responses (lymphocytes and other cells) migrate among lymphoid and other tissues and the vascular and lymphatic circulations.
1. Lymphocytes are the primary cells involved:
   a. Naïve lymphocytes
   b. T lymphocytes
   c. B lymphocytes
   d. Natural killer (NK) cells
2. Dendritic cells
3. Macrophages.

Naïve Lymphocytes

These are **mature lymphocytes which have not encountered the antigen** (immunologically inexperienced). After the lymphocytes are activated by recognition of antigens, they differentiate into:
- **Effector cells:** They **perform the function of eliminating microbes.**
- **Memory cells:** They **live in a state of heightened awareness** and are better able to combat the microbe in case it infects again.

T Lymphocytes

T (thymus-derived) lymphocytes develop from precursors in the thymus.

Distribution: Mature T cells are found in:
- **Peripheral blood** where it constitutes 60–70% of lymphocytes
- **T cell zones of peripheral lymphoid organs** namely paracortical region of lymph node and periarteriolar sheaths of spleen.

Subsets of T lymphocytes: Naïve T cells can differentiate into two major subtypes namely (1) **CD4** and (2) **CD8**.
1. **T helper cells:** These cells have a cell surface marker called CD4 and hence are also called **CD4+ cells**. They **help B cells in antibody formation**; constitute two-thirds of circulating T cells. They recognize antigen presented by class II human leukocyte antigen (HLA) molecules.
2. **T cytotoxic cells:** These cells have the surface marker CD8 and hence are called **CD8+ cells**. They constitute one-third of circulating T cells and recognize antigens in context of class I HLA molecules.

B Lymphocytes

B (bone marrow-derived) lymphocytes develop from precursors in the bone marrow.

Distribution
- **Peripheral blood:** Mature B cells constitute 10–20% of the circulating peripheral lymphocyte population.
- **Peripheral lymphoid tissues:** Lymph nodes (cortex), spleen (white pulp), and mucosa-associated lymphoid tissues (pharyngeal tonsils and Peyer's patches of GIT).

Functions of B cells: All the mature, naïve B cells express membrane-bound immunoglobulins on their surface that functions as B-cell receptors (BCRs) for antigen. B cells recognize antigen via these BCRs.
- **Production of antibodies:** The primary function of B cells is to **produce antibodies**. After stimulation by antigen and other signals, B cells develop into **plasma cells**. These cells secrete antibodies which are the mediators of humoral immunity.
- **Antigen-presenting cell:** B cells also serve as APCs and are very efficient at antigen processing.

Dendritic Cells

As the name suggests these cells have numerous fine cytoplasmic processes that resemble dendrites. These are important APCs in the body.

Macrophages

Macrophages are a part of the mononuclear phagocyte system.

Processing of antigen: In adaptive immune response, macrophages process the antigens present in the phagocytosed microbes and protein antigens. After processing, the antigen is presented to T cells and thus, they function as APCs in T cell activation.

Adaptive Immune Responses

It can be classified into two main divisions.
1. **Humoral immunity:** In this type, immunity is mediated by soluble protein products called antibodies produced by B lymphocytes and helper T cells. Antibody is capable of reacting with the specific antigen responsible for its production. Macrophages also participate in the effector phase of humoral immunity. Macrophages get activated by interferon-gamma (IFN-γ).
2. **Cell-mediated immunity (cellular immunity):** Cellular immunity is mediated T lymphocytes, macrophages and their soluble products called cytokines. It is localized reaction to organism, usually intracellular pathogens. Macrophages are main effector cells in certain types of cell-mediated immunity, the reaction that serves to eliminate intracellular microbes. In this type of response, T cells activate macrophages and increase their capability to kill ingested microbes. Macrophages efficiently phagocytose and destroy microbes which are opsonized (coated) by immunoglobulin G (IgG) or C3b through their respective receptors. Cell-mediated cytotoxicity is important in lysis of virus infected cells and rejection of allograft and tumor cells. Other cytotoxic cells involved in cell-mediated immune response are natural cells (NK). These NK cells are able to attack the target cells and kill them.

Components of Adaptive Immune Response

Natural Killer Cells
- Nonphagocytic **large** (little larger than small lymphocytes) **granular** (numerous cytoplasmic **azurophilic granules**) **lymphocytes**.
- Comprise about 5–15% of **human peripheral lymphoid cells**.

Function: Natural killer cells provide **defense against many viral infections** and other **intracellular pathogens** and also **has antitumor activity**, causing lysis of cells with which they react. Killing of the cells is performed without prior exposure to or activation by these microbes or tumors. Because of this ability, NK cells act an early line of defense against viral infections and few tumors.

Major histocompatibility complex molecules (Discussed in chapter 23).

IMMUNOGLOBULINS

The function of the immune system is to defend the body from externally derived agents and from potentially dangerous self-constituents. The main effector cells of specific immunity are lymphocytes. The lymphocytes possess receptors capable of discriminating one antigen from another (based on differences in their molecular configuration).

Immunoglobulins are a group of serum proteins.

Antibodies: Immunoglobulins for which a corresponding antigen can be identified are called antibodies.

Immunoglobulins: They lack corresponding antigen are simply called immunoglobulins and are not antibodies.

Types of Immunoglobulins

There are five classes of immunoglobulins designated as: (1) IgM, (2) IgG, (3) IgA, (4) IgD, and (5) IgE. Of these, IgM, IgG and IgA (rarely) antibodies are produced against RBC antigens and mainly involved in blood group serology.

Structure of Immunoglobulin Molecule (Fig. 1.2)

Immunoglobulin consists of amino acid molecules linked by peptide bonds forming amino acid chains.

Heavy and light chains: All immunoglobulins share the same basic structure consisting of four chain molecules. The basic immunoglobulin unit consists of two identical heavy chains and two identical light chains held together by disulfide bonds. Immunoglobulin molecules are proteins and therefore have two terminal regions namely (1) the **amino** ($-NH_2$) terminal and (2) the **carboxyl** (-COOH) terminal.

- **Light chains:** The light chains belong to two antigenetically different isotypes, i.e. (1) Kappa (K) and (2) Lambda (λ). In any immunoglobulin molecule, the two light chains are always identical, being either Kappa or Lambda.
- **Heavy chains:** The heavy chains are different for each class of immunoglobulins (Table 1.1).
- **Disulfide bond:** Each light chain is joined to one heavy chain by a disulfide bond. One or more disulfide bonds link the two heavy chains in an area of considerable flexibility called the hinge region. The four

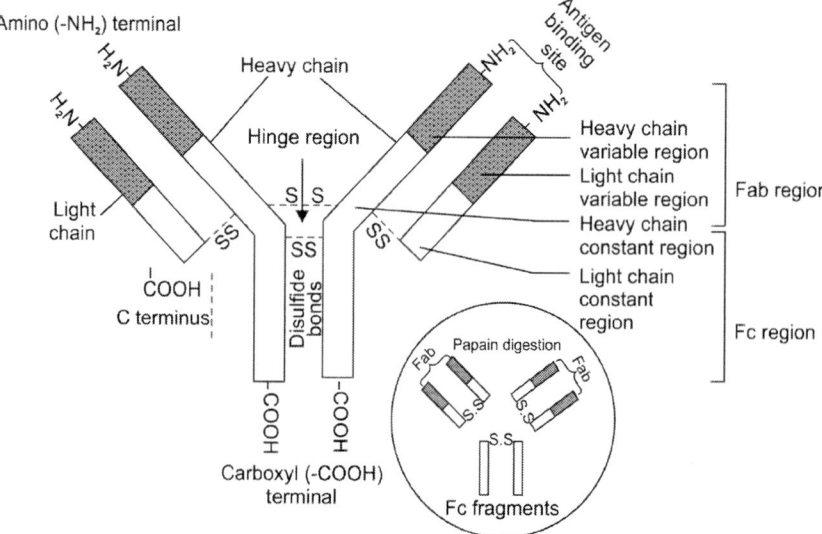

Fig. 1.2: Schematic representation of basic immunoglobulin (IgG) structure. The inset shows formation of antigen-binding fragment (Fab) and constant fragment (Fc) after enzymatic cleavage of the IgG molecule by papain.

Basic Immunology Related to Blood Group Serology

Table 1.1: Types of heavy chain in different immunoglobulin molecules.

Type of immunoglobulin	Type of heavy chain
IgA	Alpha (α)
IgG	Gamma (γ)
IgM	Mu (μ)
IgD	Delta (δ)
IgE	Epsilon (Σ)

chains bound by covalent (disulfide) and noncovalent bonds give "Y" configuration.

- **Variable region:** The portion near the amino terminus or N-terminus of both light and heavy chains of immunoglobulins is called variable region. The antigenic specificity of the immunoglobulin molecule lies in this portion. They are termed variable because they are structured according to the great variation in antibody specificity.
- **Constant portion:** The carboxyl region of all heavy chains and the light chains has a relatively constant amino acid sequence and is called as the constant region. The five isotypes of heavy chains and two of light chains are determined by the amino acid sequences of the constant portion.

Digestion of Immunoglobulins

Digestion of an immunoglobulin molecule with the proteolytic enzyme papain results in cleavage or splitting of the heavy chain at the hinge region. This produces three separate fragments namely: two Fab and one Fc fragments (Fig. 1.2 inset).

- **Two Fab fragments:** These fragments are identical and consist of one light chain linked to the N-terminal half of the heavy chain. These N-terminal fragments retain the specificity of the antibody and are called Fab fragments (fraction antigen binding). Structurally and functionally, the Fab fragments consist of the portions of the immunoglobulin from the hinge region to the amino terminal end and are the regions responsible for binding antigen.
- **One Fc fragment:** The Fc fragment is that portion of the immunoglobulin molecule from the carboxyl region to the hinge region (from both heavy chains) still joined to one another by the hinge region disulfide bonds. This is the nonantibody protein fragment capable of crystallization and is called Fc fragment. Fc fragments on IgG antibody is responsible for complement fixation, for placental transfer, monocyte binding by Fc receptors on cells and reaction with antihuman globulin (AHG).

Individual Immunoglobulin Classes

IgM Antibodies (Fig. 1.3)

These antibodies readily and **very strongly agglutinate the red cells carrying the corresponding antigens in saline**. Therefore, they are known as **complete antibodies**. IgM exists in serum as a **pentamer** and **cannot cross the placental barrier**. They **activate complement through the classic pathway** and markedly enhance the inflammatory and phagocytic defense mechanisms. The **optimal temperature is room temperature** (i.e. 20–24°C).

IgG Antibodies (Fig. 1.4)

Immunoglobulin G antibodies are also called **"incomplete antibody"**, because **they do not cause agglutination of red cells with corresponding antigen in saline**. They can **readily cross the placenta** and responsible for hemolytic disease of newborn (HDN). It tends to combine with and remain attached to cell surface antigens, where its presence can be detected in vitro by antiglobulin testing. In vivo, cells or particles coated with IgG undergo markedly enhanced interaction with cells that have receptors for the Fc portion of gamma chains, especially neutrophils and macrophages. The **optimum temperature for reaction of IgG is 37°C**. IgG antibodies **account for the majority of the clinically significant antibodies directed against blood**

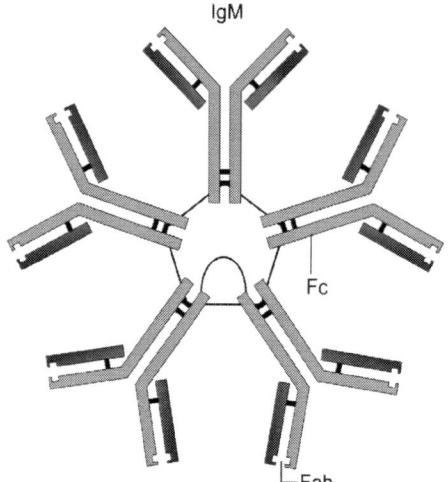

Fig. 1.3: IgM pentamer (polymer formed from five molecules of a monomer) immunoglobulin molecule (joined together).

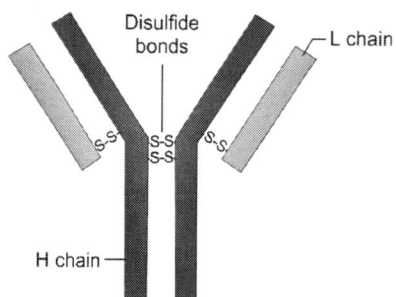

Fig. 1.4: Monomer containing only one immunoglobulin unit (e.g. IgG, IgD and IgE molecule).

group antigens. There are **four subclasses** of IgG: (1) IgG1, (2) IgG2, (3) IgG3, and (4) IgG4.
- Most IgG antibodies contain all four subclasses. However, some are predominantly or exclusively composed of a single subclass.
- The subclasses have different biologic properties.
  - All bind to the crystallizable fragment (Fc) receptors on macrophages. All can cross the placental barrier. All except IgG4 are capable of binding to complement through the classic pathway.
  - IgG1 and IgG3 bind complement much more efficiently than IgG2.

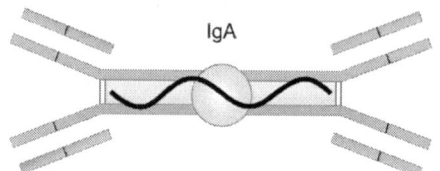

Fig. 1.5: IgA dimer composed of two identical simpler monomers (Ig) are joined together.

- IgG1 constitutes 65–70% of the total IgG found in serum.

IgA Antibodies (Fig. 1.5)

It serves **no physiologic function**. Most of the IgA mass and all of its physiologic significance exist in mucosal secretions. It is important to know that people deficient in IgA may have anti-IgA. **IgA antibodies against RBC antigens usually occur with IgG and IgM antibodies having the same specificity.** These IgA antibodies neither cross the placental barrier nor do they fix complement. IgA antibodies can cause agglutination in saline.

The location of cellular components, red cell antigen and antibody in a blood sample is depicted in Figure 1.6.

The salient features of antibodies (immunoglobulins) are presented in Table 1.2.

■ IMMUNE RESPONSE

Immune response after exposure to an antigen is influenced by the host's previous history with the foreign material. There are two types of immune responses: (1) primary and (2) secondary.

Primary immune response: It is the response of the body when an immunocompetent individual is exposed for first time to a foreign antigen (nonself antigen). In this, there is a lag period/phase, i.e. the time between exposure to the antigen and appearance of detectable antibody. It can vary from a few days to weeks or even months. It depends on factors like nature and quantity of the antigen, route of administration and protein synthesizing capacities of the host. The **antibody that appears in the blood after first contact with**

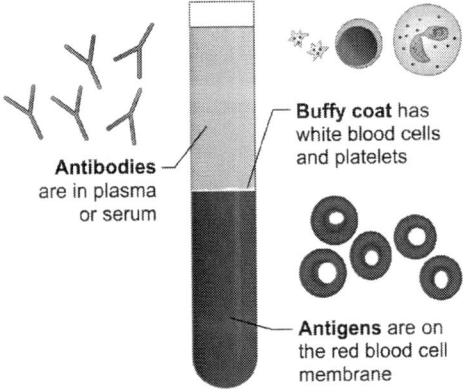

Fig. 1.6: Blood sample depicting the location of cellular components, red cell antigen and antibody. The serum or plasma contains the antibody, whereas the red cell membrane contains the antigen.

an antigen is always IgM type. After some days, IgG becomes detectable. If there is no further exposure to the antigen, the level of circulating IgM antibody peaks and then declines, while IgG antibody persists for longer time. Apart from immune responses, the primary immune response generates memory cells. These memory cells contribute to the immune response on second or subsequent exposure to the same antigen (i.e. secondary or anamnestic immune response).

Anamnestic or secondary immune response: Even if the antigen that caused the primary response disappears from the body, circulating T cells and memory B cells continue to persist. When there is a subsequent or second contact with the same antigen, memory B cells **respond far more rapidly** than unstimulated cells. There is **no lag period** and the dose of the antigen can be very small. The memory cells exhibit rapid proliferation of the IgG secreting progeny. This is called anamnestic or secondary response. Within a short time (within hours or a day), the level of circulating IgG antibody rises sharply. The IgG response may be as much as 100 times greater than the primary response. The affinity of antibody molecules for the antigens will also be greater than in primary response.

Antibody level and time of development of primary and secondary antibody responses are shown in Figure 1.7.

Table 1.2: Salient features of antibodies (immunoglobulins).

Features	IgM (millionaire's antibody)	IgG (subtypes: IgG1, IgG2, IgG3, IgG4)	IgA	IgE (reaginic/homocytotropic antibody)	IgD
Approximately % of total Ig	5%	80% (maximum)	15%	Trace	Trace
Molecular weight (Daltons [Da])	900,000 (maximum)	150,000	150,000 to 300,000	190,000	180,000
Type of heavy chain	μ	γ	α	ε	δ
Structure	Pentamer (maximum size)	Monomer	Dimer (in glandular secretions), monomer (in serum)	Monomer	Monomer
Complement activation	Yes (classical pathway)	Yes (classical pathway)	Activates alternate complement pathway	No	No
Transport across placenta	No	Yes	No	No	No
Half-life (days)	5	21	6	2	3
Main function	Primary immune response	Secondary immune response Functions as B-cell receptor	Mucosal immunity Highly effective at neutralizing toxins	Allergic diseases, defense against parasite infection and anaphylactic reaction	Unknown

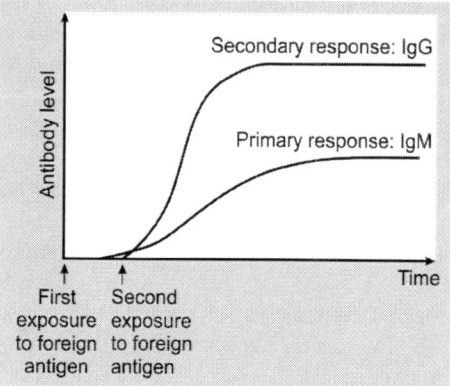

Fig. 1.7: Antibody level and time of development of primary and secondary antibody responses.

Differences between primary and secondary immune response are presented in Table 1.3.

■ IMMUNOHEMATOLOGY

Red Cell Antigen-Antibody Reactions in Vivo

Transfusion, Pregnancy and Immune Response

During transfusion and pregnancy, a patient is exposed to many potentially foreign antigens present on red cells, white cells, and platelets. These foreign antigens have immunogenic potentiality. These foreign antigens may activate the immune system of the patients or patient may be "sensitized", with the resultant production of circulating antibodies. The **antibodies produced in response to transfusion and pregnancies are** classified as **alloantibodies**.

Antibody screen test: It is performed on the recipient to detect any existing red cell alloantibodies before transfusion.
- **Detection of alloantibody:** If a red cell alloantibody is found, a test is done to identify the specificity of the antibody.
- **Specificity of alloantibody:** Once the specificity is identified, donor units lacking the red cell antigen are selected for transfusion.
- **Importance:** Detecting and identifying alloantibodies in the patient before transfusion are important to **avoid the formation of antigen-antibody complexes in vivo** (within the patient's body), which would reduce the survival of the transfused cells.

Immunization during pregnancy: Immunization may also occur during pregnancy due to entry of fetal blood cells into the maternal circulation at delivery. Alloantibody may develop as an immune response to RBC, WBC, or platelet antigens of fetal origin. Routinely females are screened during the first trimester of pregnancy for the presence of red cell alloantibodies. These red cell alloantibodies can destroy fetal red blood cells before or after delivery. The destruction of red cell may lead to clinical complications due to anemia and high levels of bilirubin in the fetus or newborn.

Red Cell Antigen-Antibody Reactions in Vitro

The combination of antibody with antigen produces a variety of observable results. Antigen-antibody reactions are important in immunohematology. In blood group serology

Table 1.3: Differences between primary and secondary immune response.

Features	Primary response	Secondary response
Cells that mediate the response	Circulating T lymphocytes	Memory B cells
Lag period	Long: Weeks to months Usually 5–10 days	Short: Hours to days Usually 1–3 days
Antibody isotype	IgM first; followed by IgG Usually IgM > IgG	IgG response and under certain situations IgA or IgE
Peak response	Smaller	Larger
Dose of antigen required to elicit response	Higher the dose faster the response	Even minute doses produce 100-fold increased response

(immunohematology), the most common reactions are as follows:
- Agglutination: Hemagglutination
- Hemolysis
- Neutralization
- Precipitation

Agglutination and Hemagglutination

Antigen-antibody reactions occurring in laboratory testing (in vitro) are detected by visible agglutination of the RBCs (hemagglutination) or development of hemolysis at the completion of testing (a positive result).

Hemagglutination: It produces the clumping of red cells that result when antibody molecules combine with antigenic determinants on adjacent red cells. This brings RBCs together and forms a visible aggregate.

- A **positive reaction** in immunohematologic testing is indicated by **agglutination**. A positive result **indicates that an antigen-antibody immune complex was formed**, and the specificity of the antibody matched the antigen in the test system.
- A **negative reaction** in immunohematologic testing is indicated by **no agglutination**. Negative result/reaction **suggests that there is no formation of antigen-antibody complex** and indicates that the antibody in the test system is not specific for the antigen.

Agglutination is the end point for most test involving red cells and blood group antibodies. It is the **primary and most common reaction observed in routine transfusion practice.**

Stages of agglutination

Agglutination occurs in two stages namely (1) sensitization and (2) visible agglutination (lattice formation).

Sensitization (or antibody binding/attachment to red cells): In the first stage of red cell agglutination, there is simple coating or binding of an antibody to an antigen on the red cell membrane. This stage needs an immunologic recognition between the antigen and antibody. During this recognition stage, the antigen-binding sites of the antibodies become closely associated with the antigenic determinants (epitopes) on the RBC membrane (Fig. 1.8). The **antibodies and antigens are held together loosely by noncovalent bonds**. This **does not produce clumping or visible agglutination of red cells in saline**. Since no visible agglutination is seen, an additional step is needed to produce visible agglutination or to otherwise measure the reaction by the use of albumin, proteolytic enzymes, or AHG reagent. This stage depends on factors such as the pH, temperature of the reaction, incubation time, and ionic strength of the suspension medium.

Visible agglutination (Lattice formation): After the red cells have been sensitized with antibody molecules, visible agglutination (Fig. 1.9) occurs when several RBCs are physically joined together by the union of antigen with antibody. This stage depends on factors such as distance between red cells, optimal concentrations of antigen and antibody, and time and speed of centrifugation.

- **Enhancement of contact:** The use of **proteolytic enzymes** (e.g. **papain** or **ficin**) can increase/enhance cell-to-cell contact of RBCs.
- **Adding antiserum:** RBCs sensitized by **incomplete antibodies** (antibodies that will not react in saline) agglutinate when **antiserum against human IgG** is added (antiglobulin/Coombs test).

Factors affecting agglutination

Agglutination is a reversible chemical reaction. Various factors can affect reactivity of antigen-antibody RBC agglutination reactions. These

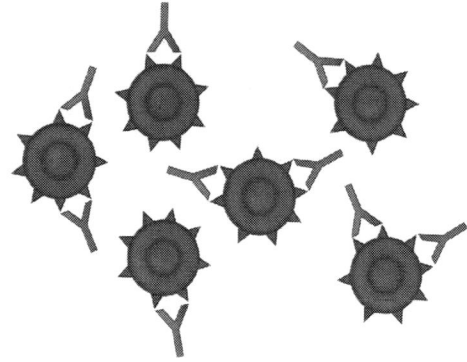

Fig. 1.8: Sensitization of RBCs with antibodies.

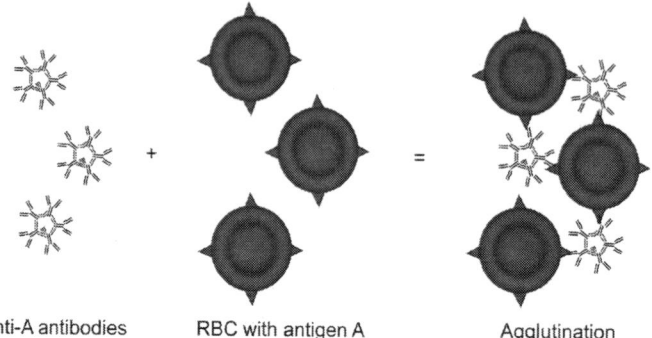

Fig. 1.9: Agglutination is the clumping of red cells together because of interactions with specific antibodies.

factors can be manipulated to enhance (or decrease) agglutination. Agglutination reactions are affected by the concentration of the reactants (antigen and antibody) and by factors such as pH, temperature, and ionic strength. The surface charge, antibody isotype, RBC antigen dosage, and the use of various enhancement media, AHG reagents, and enzymes are all important in antigen-antibody reactions. The most important factors are discussed in the following sections:

Antigen-Antibody ratio (cell-to-serum ratio) (Fig. 1.10)

Amount of available antigen and antibody affects hemagglutination.

- **Equivalence: For agglutination** reactions to occur, it is necessary to have optimal proportions of antigen and antibody, i.e. equal amount/proportions of antigen-antibody. Any deviation from this ratio decreases the efficiency of the reaction and a loss of the **zone of equivalence** between antigen and antibody ratio. Thus, adding equal volumes of serum and 2-5% suspension of red cells is sufficient and is recommended for all routine blood banking procedures. The recommended ratio in red cell serology is one drop of serum to one drop of 2-5% red cells (or 2 drops of serum to 1 drop of the RBC suspension). It gives the proper balance between antigen and antibody to allow sensitization and agglutination to occur. This ratio may be altered, depending on the test method used.
- **Prozone:** It **occurs when antibody molecules are in excess than that of available antigenic sites.** This **results in false-negative reactions**. When **antibody (immunoglobulin)** is present in the test system **in excess** (when compared to antigen concentration), false-negative reactions occur as a result of prozone.
- **Antigen excess (postzone):** When the antigen is in excess, false-negative reactions occur due to **postzone effect**. In both prozone and postzone effect, the agglutination may not occur. This can give rise to false-negative results.
- The antigen-antibody test systems can be manipulated to overcome the effects of excessive antigen or antibody. If this is suspected following steps will help to correct it.
  – **Excessive antibody:** If the problem is due to excessive antibody, the **plasma or serum may be diluted with the appropriate buffer.**
  – **Excessive antigen:** The problem of excessive antigen can be solved by **increasing the serum-to-cell ratio**, which increases the number of antibodies available to bind with each RBC.
  – **Weakly reactive antibody:** If the antibody is weakly reactive (weak expression of antigen on RBCs—**dosage effect**),

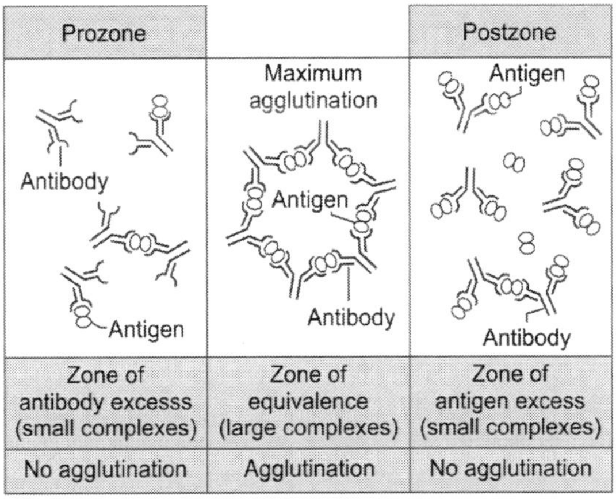

Basic Immunology Related to Blood Group Serology

Prozone		Postzone
	Maximum agglutination	Antigen
Antibody	Antigen	
	Antibody	Antibody
Zone of antibody excesss (small complexes)	Zone of equivalence (large complexes)	Zone of antigen excess (small complexes)
No agglutination	Agglutination	No agglutination

Fig. 1.10: Diagrammatic representation of the effects of varying concentrations of antigen and antibody on lattice formation.

increasing the antibodies present can increase the test's sensitivity. In such cases, the **serum-cell-ratio may be doubled** (2 drops serum and 1 drop 2–5% red cell). This provides more antibodies to react with the available antigens. While investigating adverse transfusion reactions, it may be desirable to increase the serum-cell-ratio by as much as 10- to 20-fold. This should be done only when enhancing media or potentiators have not been included in the test system.

Effect of pH

The ideal pH for antigen-antibody reactions in which most antibodies react best at a neutral pH. It ranges between 6.5 and 7.5, which is similar to the pH of normal plasma or serum. The pH values below 6 or above 8 reduce the reactivity. Stored saline has a pH of 5.0–6.0, hence buffered saline is preferred in serologic testing. However, some anti-M show enhanced reactivity at a pH of 6.5 and acidifying the test system may help in distinguishing anti-M from other antibodies.

Temperature and phase of reactivity

The optimal temperature at which an antibody reacts can provide useful clues to antibody identity. Depending on the thermal specificity, most antibodies form two broad categories:

1. Those **reactive at "cold" temperature** (e.g. 4–25°C). **IgM antibodies** react best at 4–25°C.
2. Those **reactive at "warm" temperature** (e.g. 30–37°C). **IgG antibodies** react best at 30–37°C.

Temperature of agglutination is determined by the nature of antigen and the type of reaction and not by the class of antibody. **Binding with carbohydrate antigens** (as with ABO antigen-antibody reactions) **occurs best at low temperatures**, while **bindings with protein antigens** (as with Rh antigen-antibody reaction) **occurs best at 37°C** due to the protein nature of the antigen. **Antibodies that react** in vitro only at temperature **below 30°C** rarely cause destruction of transfused antigen-positive red cells and are considered clinically insignificant. When performing pretransfusion compatibility testing, the focus is on **clinically significant** antibodies. They generally react at 37°C or with the anti-IgG in the AHG reagent.

Red cell ionic charge

Red blood cells have a negative charge at this surface which **makes RBCs to repel** each other. The negative charge is due to sialic acid molecules on the surface of RBCs. This natural repulsive force which holds the RBC apart is called **zeta potential**. This is protective and keeps RBCs from adhering to each other in the peripheral blood. The distance which keeps the RBCs apart is very small but sufficient to prevent the small IgG molecules to bridge the gap and agglutinate the red cells. However, large IgM molecules bridge the gap and bring the red cells together causing agglutination of RBCs.

Ionic strength

In normal saline, Na⁺ and Cl⁻ ions cluster around and partially neutralize opposite charges on antigens and antibody molecules. This interferes with the association of antibodies with antigen. A **decrease in the ionic strength of the medium of suspension, increases the association of Ab with Ag**. The use of **low ionic strength solutions** (LISS), or low salt media contains 0.2% sodium chloride and they decrease the ionic strength of medium.

Incubation time (length of incubation)

Incubation time is also important for antigen-antibody reactions. If incubation time is too little (less contact time), only few sensitized RBCs will be detected by routine methods. If the incubation time is allowed to continue for too long, bound antibody may begin to dissociate from the RBCs. **Incubation time is different for different blood group antibodies**. Incubation time also depends on temperature and medium in which the reaction takes place. Optimum **incubation time for most blood group reactions in saline environment is 30–60 minutes at 37°C**. Weak reactive antibodies may require longer time. Addition of **enhancement agents or potentiators may shorten the incubation time**. For example, enhancement agents like LISS or polyethylene glycol (PEG) can reduce the incubation time to 10–15 minutes at 37°C.

Freshness of serum and RBCs

Best antigen-antibody reaction occurs with fresh serum and freshly prepared red cells. If serum is not immediately used, it should be stored at –20°C or lower.

Enhancement media

Agglutination reactions for IgM antibodies and their corresponding RBC antigens are easily observed in saline medium and these antibodies usually do not need enhancement or modifications to react strongly with antigens. **IgG antibodies react best at 37°C and are generally responsible for hemolytic transfusion reactions and HDN**. Hence, detection of IgG antibodies is clinically more significant than IgM. Many enhancement techniques or potentiators are available to discover the presence of IgG antibodies. Many of the **enhancement media act by reducing the zeta potential of RBC membranes**. Reducing the zeta potential allows the more positively charged antibodies to get closer to the negatively charged RBCs. Thus, enhancement techniques or potentiators increase RBC agglutination by IgG molecules. Various methods for enhancement are:

- **Physical methods:** Centrifugation and agitation enhance antigen-antibody reaction.
  1. **Centrifugation:** It is an effective method to enhance agglutination reactions. It reduces the reaction time by increasing the gravitational forces on the reactants, brings the cells close together and increases the chance of association between antibody and antigen. During centrifugation, sensitized RBCs overcome their natural repulsive effect (zeta potential) for each other and agglutinate more efficiently. High-speed centrifugation is one of the most efficient methods used in blood banking. However, centrifugation should not cause packing of cells too tightly, which may lead to false-positive reactions.
  2. **Agitation:** Another method of enhancing antigen-antibody reaction often employed by the shakers used for rapid plasma reagin (RPR) and Western blot testing.
- **Chemical methods:**
  1. **Bovine albumin (22% or 30% concentration):** It increases the dielectric constant of the medium and reduces the zeta potential (i.e. reduce electric repulsion between cells). It also affects the surface tension between cells,

thus causing antibody-coated cells to agglutinate. Thus, by reducing zeta potential and surface tension, albumin **enhances antigen-antibody binding**. Bovine albumin does not cause agglutination of noncoated cells.

2. **Enzymes:** Papain is the proteolytic enzyme most commonly used in blood group serology. Others include bromelin, ficin, and trypsin. These enzymes act by:
   - **Lowering the zeta potential:** Sialic acid is the major contributor of the net negative change at the red cell surface which keeps cells separated from each other in an ionic suspending medium. Enzymes cleave sialic acid molecules and reduce the negative charge on RBCs.
   - Cleaving of protein also **increases the surface tension** between cells thus predisposing to agglutination.
   - They cause **spicule formation on the red cell**. This increases the potential number of contact points.

   Note: Certain red cell antigens can undergo denaturation by enzyme treatment, e.g. M, N, S, Fy^a, and Fy^b. Thus, it is important not to use enzyme treatment while detecting any of these antigens.

3. **Antihuman globulin (AHG) reagent:** AHG causes agglutination of sensitized/coated cells. AHG bridges the gap between the IgG molecules attached to the red cells and enhances their agglutination. This is the **most common as well most sensitive method used to detect antigen-antibody reaction in immunohematology**.

The direct AHG test is used to determine if RBCs are coated with antibody or complement or both.

Polyethylene glycol and polybrene are macromolecule additives used with LISS to enhance agglutination reactions. PEG is more effective than albumin, LISS, or polybrene for detection of weak antibodies. These reagents have been used in automated and manual testing systems.

Grading and scoring of hemagglutination are presented in Table 1.4.

Hemolysis

In immunohematology laboratory, apart from agglutination as an indicator of an antigen-antibody reaction, red cell hemolysis in the tube is also an indicator of the activity of an antigen and antibody (antigen-antibody reaction) in vitro.

- Hemolysis (Fig. 1.11) is the rupture or breakdown of red cells with release of intracellular hemoglobin. In vitro, hemolysis requires activation of complement cascade. Complement system gets activated when there is antigen-antibody complex (immune complex). Hemolysis does not

Table 1.4: Grading and scoring of hemagglutination.

Grade	Appearance	Score
4+	Red cell button—one solid aggregate with a clear background	10
3+	Several medium to large aggregates with a clear background	8
2+	Many small to medium aggregates with a clear background	5
1+	Many small aggregates with a turbid background with many free red cells	3
+ or w	Few small aggregates with many unagglutinated cells	2
±m or +m	Aggregates visible only under microscopic examination	1
0	Negative—absence of aggregates (no agglutination)	0
R	Rouleaux (nonspecific aggregation that appears like a stack of coins and disappears with addition of saline)	NA
H	Hemolysis—presence of free hemoglobin in the serum	10

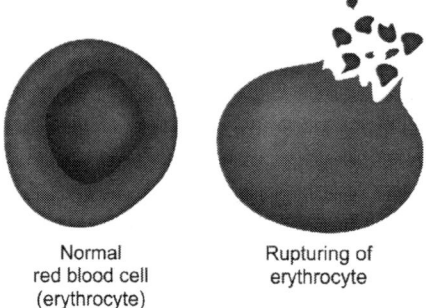

Fig. 1.11: Diagrammatic appearance of normal RBC and ruptured/hemolyzed RBC.

occur if the antigen-antibody reaction takes place in serum that lacks complement (stored blood) or in anticoagulant that chelates/binds to Ca^{++} and Mg^{++} (both Ca^{++} and Mg^{++} necessary for complement activation). Hence, for demonstration of hemolysis fresh serum samples (without anticoagulants) should be used.

- **Hemolysin:** Antibodies that have the capacity to activate complement on reacting with antigens on red cells and cause hemolysis are called hemolysins.
- Many blood group antibodies on reacting with the antigens on red cells activate the complement and produce membrane attack complex (MAC). MAC causes damage to RBC membrane leading to destruction of RBCs. This in turn releases the intracellular fluid in the RBCs into the serum.
- In the test system, hemolysis is identified by the pink or red coloration of the supernatant fluid after tubes are centrifuged. IgM antibodies predominantly activate complement while IgG rarely does so.
- Some red cell antibodies characteristically produce hemolysis in vitro, such as antibodies to the Lewis system antigens and anti-Vel.

Note: Testing for hemolysin is mandatory prior to release of the so-called universal red cells/whole blood of group "O" to a recipient with non-O (A, B, AB) group.

Neutralization (Inhibition)

Soluble form of blood group antigens can also combine with soluble blood group antibody. It will result in full or partial neutralization (inhibition) of antibody. There is **no formation of a visible precipitate**. In this reaction, if the strength of the antibody diminishes or if it disappears completely, an antigen-antibody reaction can be assumed to have taken place.

Missing or weak antigens/antibodies can often be detected with the help of neutralization reactions.

Precipitation (Fig. 1.12)

When soluble antibody reacts with soluble antigen and **forms an insoluble, usually visible complex**, the reaction is called as precipitation. Such complexes are seen in test tubes as a sediment or ring and in agar gels as a white line. Precipitation is the end point of procedures such as immunodiffusion and immunoelectrophoresis. Examples for precipitation reactions are venereal disease research laboratory (VDRL) and RPR tests performed in the blood bank to screen for syphilis.

- **Antigen and antibody should be present in optimal proportions** for the occurrence of precipitation. In an ideal reactive condition, an equivalent amount of antigen and antibody binds.

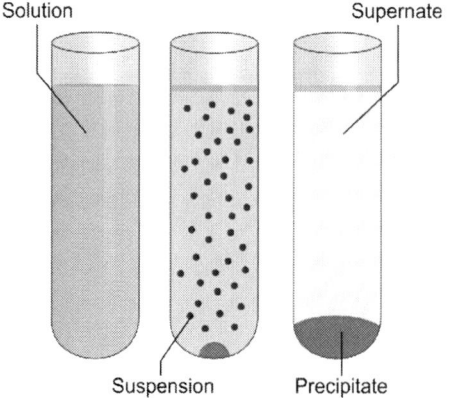

Fig. 1.12: Diagrammatic reorientation of appearances of solution, suspension and precipitate.

- **Prozone phenomenon (refer pages 12 and 13):** If there is excess of unbound Ab (immunoglobulin), there will be very few Ag sites to combine with the molecules and the lattice structure is not formed. Ag-Ab complexes are formed but do not accumulate sufficiently to form a visible lattice. An excess of leads of antibody leads to a phenomenon called a prozone. It is important to rule out prozone phenomenon while screening for atypical antibodies like anti-D in a woman giving a sample for indirect antiglobulin test, during antenatal checkup.
- A surplus of antigen leads to a **postzone effect** (refer page 13).

TRADITIONAL LABORATORY TESTING METHODS

These include hemagglutination (a special type of agglutination), precipitation, agglutination inhibition, and hemolysis.

Other techniques which are used to quantify antigen or antibody with the use of a radioisotope, enzyme, or fluorescent label—such as radioimmunoassay (RIA), enzyme-linked immunosorbent assay (ELISA) or enzyme immunoassay (EIA), Western blotting (WB), and immunofluorescence (IF).

In transfusion medicine, much laboratory testing involves detection and identification of antibodies in patient's plasma. These assays can be mainly divided into: (1) fluid-phase assays (agglutination-based methods) and (2) solid-phase assays.

Fluid-Phase Assays (Agglutination-Based Methods)

Uses of Agglutination-Based Tests in Blood Bank

Agglutination is used for:
- **Serologic cross-matching** (donor RBCs incubated with recipient plasma or serum)
- **Screening for unexpected antibodies** (reagent RBCs of known blood group antigen composition incubated with recipient plasma or serum)
- **Blood group antigen phenotyping** of the donor or recipient (test RBCs are incubated with monoclonal antibodies or reagent-quality antisera of known specificity).

Methods (Refer Pages 71-84 of Chapter 4)
- **Manual tube testing:** Agglutination detected by adhesion of RBCs to one another in post-centrifuge pellet.
- **Microtiter plate:** Agglutination visualized by spread pattern of RBCs in individual wells.
- **Column agglutination technique:**
  - **Gel-based testing:** After agglutination is allowed to take place, the reaction mixture is centrifuged through a gel-matrix (usually composed of dextran-acrylamide). Unagglutinated RBCs pass through the gel, whereas larger, agglutinated RBCs are retained at the top or within the matrix. Details are presented in chapter 4.
  - **Glass microbeads technology** (refer pages 78-82)

Agglutination reaction tests are sensitive and easy to perform. However, the formation of agglutination depends on antigen-antibody ratio (refer Fig. 1.10 on page 13).

Solid-Phase Assays

In these assays, a specific antigen or antibody is immobilized on a solid matrix, usually made of plastic. It can be used for either antigen detection or antibody detection. A solution containing antigen/antibody (depends on which has to be tested, i.e. if antigen in the testing sample to be tested then antibody and vice versa) is placed on the well; polystyrene (or other plastic used) directly absorbs antigen/antibody from the solution and irreversibly binds to antigen/antibody to the plastic. The well is washed, the analyte is added and incubated with the antigen/antibody-coated solid phase, and its adherence is measured.

Solid-Phase Assays for Phenotyping RBCs (Fig. 1.13)

Antibodies specific for a known blood group antigen are coated onto the round bottom

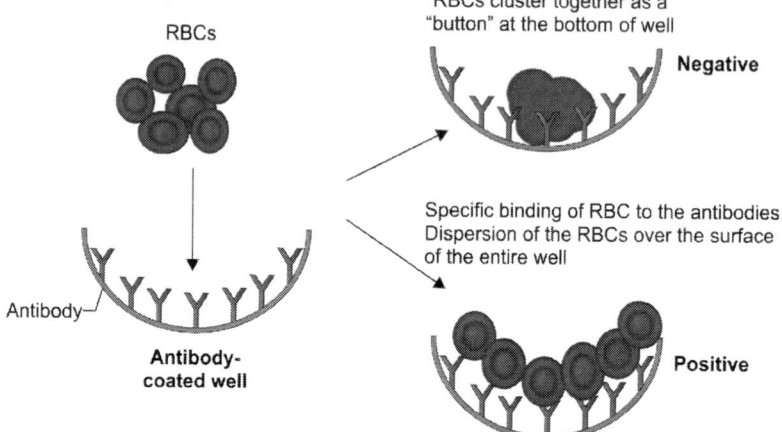

Fig. 1.13: Solid-phase assays for phenotyping RBCs.

of the microtiter plates. RBCs to be analyzed are added to the microplate wells, allowed to adhere and then the microplate is centrifuged.
- **Positive reaction:** Specific binding of RBC to the antibodies results in dispersion of the RBCs over the surface of the entire well. This indicated the presence of antigen on the RBCs.
- **Negative reaction:** No binding of RBC antigens to the antibodies on the well of microtiter plates. The red cells cluster together as a "button" at the bottom of well.

Solid-Phase Assays for Detecting Antibodies to RBC Antigens (Fig. 1.14)

In this test, antigen-coated RBCs (or red cell fragments) are coated onto the microtiter plate wells. Patient's serum to be tested is added. It is incubated and washed. If the patient serum contains antigen-specific antibodies, they will bind to antigen-coated red cells in the microtiter plate. Then indicator red cells (coated with antihuman IgG) are added.

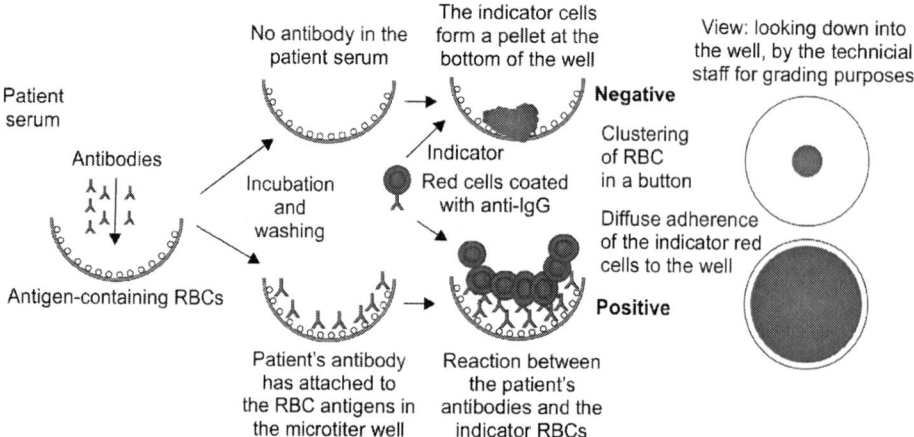

Fig. 1.14: Solid-phase assays for detecting antibodies to RBC antigens.

- **Positive reaction:** It is characterized by diffuse adherence of the indicator red cells to the well.
- **Negative reaction:** It is characterized by clustering of indicator red cells in a button.

Enzyme-Linked Immunosorbent Assay

Discussed on pages 359-63 of chapter 16.

NONTRADITIONAL LABORATORY TESTING METHODS

Western Blot

Discussed on pages 364-5 of chapter 16.

Flow Cytometry

Recent techniques to study immunologic reactions are fluorescence-assisted cell sorting (FACS) and flow cytometry. Flow cytometry has revolutionized the analysis of cell populations.

Principle: In flow cytometry, antibodies tagged with a fluorescent dye (i.e. fluorescent tag-labeled antibodies) against cell surface molecules are used. These antibodies are incubated with target population of cells. These "stained" cells are then passed through a flow cytometer. As the cells coated with fluorescent-labeled antibody travel in the flow cytometer, the cells are exposed to lasers which excite the fluorescent tags. This causes emission of a brightly fluorescent color of a specific wavelength that can be detected by sensors in the flow cytometer. Fluorescence is assessed on cell-by-cell basis. This allows visualization and quantification of minor population cells present in a complex mixture.

Suspension Array Technology

Suspension array technology (SAT) combines the specificity of solid-state antigen/antibody interaction (ELISA) with the sensitivity of flow cytometry. In transfusion medicine, it is used for identification of HLA-specific alloantibodies for screening platelet donors and blood group genotyping.

BLOOD GROUP ANTIGENS

The term **blood group** is not only used for genetically encoded **red cell antigens** but also to the immunologic diversity expressed by **other blood constituents, including leukocytes, platelets, and plasma.**

Location of gene and mode of inheritance: Most blood group genes (few exceptions) are located on the **autosomal chromosomes** and their inheritance follows Mendelian laws of inheritance. A majority of blood group alleles also demonstrate **codominance.** In codominance, the products of **both alleles of a gene pair exert** an observable **effect** and are thus equally dominant (e.g. the alleles A and B of the blood group system ABO; O is recessive to A and B). That means genetic heterozygotes at a particular locus will express both gene.

Many **membrane-associated structures** on blood cells **act as antigens** because they are capable of reacting with a complementary antibody or cell receptor. A majority of these antigens are capable of eliciting an antibody-mediated immunologic response and are thus are immunogenic (refer page 3). Each antigen can have a variety of different epitopes or specific antigenic determinants page 3. Epitopes are discrete, immunologically active regions of the antigen. The epitopes can interact with specific lymphocyte membrane receptors or secreted complementary antibody.

About a **dozen of antigen systems** are significant and are commonly important in the transfusion medicine. Individuals who lack certain antigens, when exposed to them may form antibodies. These antibodies may be detected on routine testing in the blood bank products.

Immunogenicity

An antigen capable of eliciting an immune response is called as *immunogenicity*. Blood group antigens greatly vary in their capability to elicit an immune response. The **most immunogenic are A, B, and RhD antigens**. Hence, all blood to be transfused must be matched for these antigens between the blood donor and the recipient. About 50-75% of D-negative individuals would produce anti-D if transfused with only one unit of D-positive blood. Apart from AB and D antigen, K followed by Fy^a antigens are also immunogenic.

BLOOD GROUP ALLOANTIBODIES AND AUTOANTIBODIES

Majority of clinically significant blood group antibodies are IgG or IgM type and occasionally an IgA type.

Classification of Blood Group Antibodies

Blood group antibodies can be classified as:

Alloantibody: This reacts with a foreign antigen not present on the patient's own RBC. Identification of alloantibodies and selection of compatible blood components are the most important functions of a transfusion medicine service.

- **Naturally occurring antibodies:** These antibodies that are present in our body in the absence of an apparent stimulus. Some alloantibodies to RBC antigens are called naturally occurring. The antigenic stimulus for this is unknown and these antibodies may appear regularly in the serum of persons who lack the corresponding antigen. For example in the ABO blood group system. These antibodies are commonly of IgM type and occur in serum without any specific red cell antigenic stimulus (e.g. anti-A, anti-B, anti-P).

  These antibodies are present in individuals who lack that particular antigen. They develop in infancy by 4-8 months and are maintained with little variation throughout the life. They again reduce in old age. Other naturally occurring antibodies are produced only in a small number of individuals.

- **Acquired antibodies:** Most blood group alloantibodies are produced as the result of immunization to foreign RBC antigens. The immunization may occur either during previous transfusion of blood components or following pregnancy. These antibodies are usually IgG type. Examples include Rh antibodies like anti-D and anti-Kell produced by external sensitization.

Autoantibody: It reacts with an antigen on the patient's own cells.

COMPLEMENT SYSTEM AND BLOOD BANKING

The complement system or complement, is a complex group of over 20 circulating serum and cell membrane proteins that play a number of biologic roles. They play most important role in immunohematology in that they are able to lyse the cell membranes of antibody-coated RBCs. They have a multiple function within the immune response. Their primary roles include immune adherence, phagocytosis, direct lysis of cells and bacteria, as well as assisting with opsonization to facilitate phagocytosis. Their peptide fragment split products play roles in inflammatory responses such as increased vascular permeability, smooth muscle contraction, chemotaxis, migration, and adherence. It is often involved in blood group reactions and immunological disorders. Complement plays an important role in the sensitization and destruction of transfused RBCs by alloantibody or the destruction of autologous RBCs by autoantibody. Complement is also important in immunohematologic testing. The complement components are unstable and heat liable. Hence, it is important for serum specimens to be fresh for blood bank testing.

The complement system is a group of plasma proteins synthesized in the liver, and are native precursor components. They are sequentially numbered from C1 to C9. The number refers to their discovery date, not to their activation sequence. The four unique serum proteins of the alternative pathway are designated by letters: factor B, factor D, factor P (properdin), and IF (initiating factor). Complement components circulate in inactive form as proenzymes, with the exception of factor D of the alternate pathway. The cleavage products of complement proteins are distinguished from parent molecules by adding suffixes from "a" to "e" as they are cleaved (e.g. C3a and C3b).

Pathways of Complement System Activation (Fig. 1.15)

The complement proteins may be activated in a **cascade** of events. The decisive step in complement activation is the proteolysis of the third component, C3. Cleavage of C3 can occur by any one of the three pathways: (1) the classical, (2) alternative, and (3) lectin pathways.

1. **Classical pathway:** It is activated by **antigen-antibody** (Ag-Ab) complexes. The antibodies involved are IgM, IgG1, or IgG3 antibody and get activated when the C1 component binds to the Fc portion (refer page 6) of the antibody molecule.

2. **Alternative pathway or properdin system:** It is triggered by microbial surface molecules (e.g. endotoxin, or lipopolysaccharides/LPS), complex polysaccharides, cobra venom, and other substances and does not require specific antibody for activation. Thus, they get activated **in the absence of antibody**.

3. **Lectin pathway:** It directly activates C1 when plasma mannose-binding lectin (MBL) binds to mannose on microbes. MBL in turn activates proteins of the classical pathway.

Role of Complement in RBC Destruction

The reactions that take place from C5 to C9 are termed the membrane attack complex and result in lesions on the RBC surface. These lesions allow the rapid passage of ions, and the cell lyses from osmotic pressure changes. When antibody binds to intrinsic (self) RBC

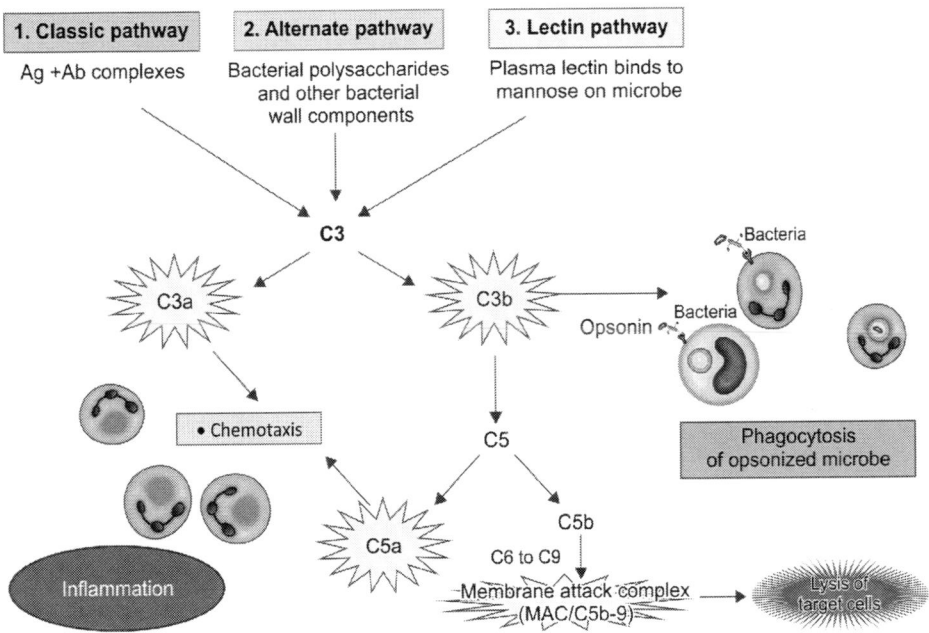

Fig. 1.15: Different pathways of activation and functions of the complement system. All pathways of activation lead to cleavage of C3.

antigens on the RBC membrane, it activates the complement by classic pathway. Complement may also be activated on RBCs when an **exogenous antigen** (nonself, e.g. drugs like penicillin which acts as hapten) **adsorbed to its cell surface**. For example, penicillin-coated RBCs and forms antipenicillin antibodies.

RBC-antibody complexes usually activate complement by the classical pathway. Antibody-coated RBCs are removed by cells of the mononuclear phagocyte system.

Intravascular Hemolysis (Fig. 1.16)

Intravascular RBC hemolysis is usually caused by antibodies directed against the ABO antigens. Rarely, hemolysis may be due to other IgM blood group antibodies or some complement-fixing IgG antibodies (e.g. anti-Kidd antibodies). Intravascular lysis occurs when large amounts of complement are rapidly activated. It results in complete activation of complement cascade and generation of the terminal membrane attack complex (C5-9). This complex polymerizes to form pores in the RBC membrane and the extracellular fluid enters the cell. The RBCs swell and burst by osmotic lysis.

Extravascular Hemolysis

Majority of extravascular hemolysis is due to IgG antibodies against RBC antigen. When IgG antibodies bind RBCs, it activates the complement and the complement-coated RBCs are removed from the circulation and are destroyed in the RE (reticuloendothelial) system.

HISTORICAL OVERVIEW OF BLOOD BANKING/BLOOD TRANSFUSION SERVICE (BTS)

- The first attempt for blood transfusion was made in 1492. During this, to save life of a Pope Innocent VIII (who was in coma), an attempt was made by orally administering blood from 3 healthy boys. However, it resulted in death of all of them.
- In 1628, English physician William Harvey discovered the circulation of blood.
- During 1665-1667, Dr Richard Lower (England) and Dr Jean-Baptiste Denys, an eminent physician of King Louis XIV of France recorded successful blood transfusion in animals and reported transfusions from lambs to humans. After this, transfusing the blood from animals to humans was prohibited by law, delaying the advances in transfusion medicine for about 150 years.
- In 1795, in Philadelphia, an American Physician, Philip Syng Physick, performed the first human blood transfusion, although he does not publish this information.
- In 1818, James Blundell, a British obstetrician transfused human blood to a female with postpartum hemorrhage. During 1825-1830, he performed ten transfusions, of which five were beneficial to the patients.
- In 1840, Samuel Armstrong Lane and Blundell, undertook first successful whole blood transfusion to treat a case of hemophilia.

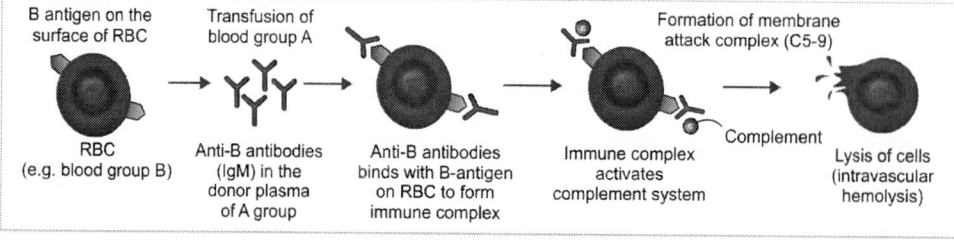

Fig. 1.16: Red cell lysis through membrane attack complex (MAC). Binding of IgG or IgM antibody to an antigen promotes complement fixation. Activation of complement leads to formation of MAC which causes cell lysis. Example—transfusion of A group blood to individual with B group.

- Clotting was the main obstacle for transfusion of blood. In 1869, Braxton Hicks recommended the use of sodium phosphate as a nontoxic anticoagulant.
- Karl Landsteiner (Australian physician) discovered the major milestone by identifying ABO group in 1901. He also explained the rational for blood incompatibility and hemolytic transfusion reaction. Landsteiner won the Nobel Prize for Medicine for this discovery in 1930. The discovery of the ABO blood group system marked the beginning of modern blood banking and transfusion medicine. Landsteiner noted the presence of agglutinating antibodies in the serum of individuals who lacked the corresponding ABO antigen.
- AB blood group was discovered in the year 1902 by A Decastello and A Sturli.
- In 1907, Hektoen suggested that the safety of transfusion can be improved by cross-matching.
- In 1912, Roger Lee (physician) from Massachusetts General Hospital coined the term "Universal Donor" and "Universal Recipient".
- The Rh blood group system was discovered by Karl Landsteiner, Alexander Wiener, Philip Levine and RE Stetson in 1940.
- Successful blood transfusion was achieved in 1914. Huston reported the use of sodium citrate and glucose as diluents and anticoagulant solution for transfusion.
- In 1915, sodium citrate was used by Richard Lewisohn to prevent clotting of blood. This has helped the process of collection of blood from donors and storage easier.
- In 1916, Rous and Turner introduced citrate-dextrose solution as anticoagulant for blood collection. This has resulted in more practical and safer transfusion of blood.
- MNS system was discovered in the year 1927. P blood group system was also discovered in the same year.
- Early in 1932, the first blood bank was established in Leningrad Hospital, Russia to combat blood loss in World War II.
- Dr Charles Drew first described the techniques in blood transfusion and establishment of blood bank.
- In 1930–1940 another major blood group Rh blood group system was discovered by Karl Landsteiner.
- In 1940, Edwin Cohn developed fractionation—plasma, albumin, protein.
- In 1943, P Beeson first published the transfusion-transmitted hepatitis.
- In 1945, Coombs, Mourant, and Race described the use of AHG (Coombs test) for detection of incomplete antibodies.
- Kell blood group was discovered in the year 1946. This blood group was named after Mrs Keller, the mother of first child to be affected with HDN. Kidd blood group was named after Mrs Kidd whose serum contained the antibody and antigen was named "JK" after woman's child John Kidd, who suffered HDN.
- In 1948, developed the plastic bag for blood collection.
- Duffy group was detected in 1950. Mr Duffy was a hemophilia patient.
- Bombay blood group was discovered by Dr YM Bhende and colleagues in the year 1952.
- In 1962, antihemophilic factor was discovered and use of component was understood.
- In 1964, plasmapheresis was introduced.
- In 1965, cryoprecipitate was first used.
- In 1971, HBsAg antigen detection test was introduced for safe blood transfusion.
- In 1981, reported the first case of acquired immunodeficiency syndrome (AIDS). The causative agent for AIDS was identified on 1983. In 1985, ELISA screening test for HIV antibodies was available.
- In 1985, donated blood screening for HIV was started.
- In 1998, it was made mandatory to test for hepatitis C for blood transfusion.
- Recent advances:
  - Nucleic acid amplification test for detecting genetic materials of viruses even before antibodies develop.

- Blood components are prepared and used for transfusion.
- Recombinant thrombopoietin available.
- Hemopoietic stem cell transplantation.
- Automation in blood banking and apheresis.

SUMMARY

- When the immune system comes across a foreign substance or antigen for the first time, the innate immune system responds quickly to get rid of the offending organism or toxin.
- The adaptive immune system also called as acquired immunity takes longer time to respond to antigen. The adaptive immune system has the additional feature of memory.
- Antigens are foreign molecules that combine with an antibody or immunoglobulin. Red cells, white cells, and platelets have numerous antigens and they can elicit an immune response after exposure from transfusions, pregnancy, and transplantation.
- Antibodies are immunoglobulins secreted by plasma cells. Immunoglobulins are a group of serum proteins. Immunoglobulins for which a corresponding antigen can be identified are called antibodies. There are five classes of immunoglobulins designated as: (1) IgM, (2) IgG, (3) IgA, (4) IgD, and (5) IgE.
- Traditional methods of detecting antigen-antibody reaction include agglutination, hemolysis and neutralization.
- Agglutination is a reaction between antigen and antibody and is a two-step process. The first step in characterized by initial binding of antibody with antigen and is also known as sensitization. During sensitization, antibody binds to antigen on a RBC membrane, but agglutination is not observable. Lattice formation is the second step of the agglutination process.
- Hemolysis is the destruction of RBCs with release of intracellular hemoglobin.
- Complements are components present in plasma which may be activated by classical, alternative or lectin pathway.

SELF-ASSESSMENT EXERCISE

Write short notes on:
- Immune system and its various components
- Immunohematology
- Traditional laboratory testing methods
- The complement system and blood banking

CHAPTER 2

Blood Group Genetics

CHAPTER OUTLINE

- Chromosomes
- Cell division
- Genetic principles in blood banking
- Population genetics
- Molecular genetics

INTRODUCTION

During mid-19th century, the Augustinian monk Gregor Mendel observed that certain features pass from parents to their children/offspring. A child usually looks like their parents and is due to inheritance of certain characteristics from parents. This **transmission of characteristics from parents to children is known as heredity**. The **basic unit of heredity is gene**, which **consists of portion** of deoxyribonucleic acid (**DNA molecules**).

Genetics: Genetics is the study which **deals with the science of genes**, heredity, and its variation in living organisms.

CHROMOSOMES

Genetic information is carried on double strands of DNA known as chromosomes. Chromosomes are structures within the nucleus that contain DNA. Chromosomes **appear as colored bodies** and **carry the hereditary material namely genes**. These chromosomes are arranged in two sets of 23 each per cell. One set is inherited from the father and the other from the mother. Humans have 23 pairs/sets of chromosomes have two types namely:

1. **Autosomal chromosomes (autosomes):** Each set of chromosomes have 22 autosomes and are **identified by numbers from 1 to 22**. The corresponding individual autosomes in each set are identical to one another in shape and size and are named as homologous pair.
2. **Sex chromosomes:** The **X and Y** chromosomes are known as the sex chromosomes because they determine sex. The human cells contain one pair of sex chromosomes. Females have two X chromosomes (46XX) and males have one X and one Y chromosome (46XY).

Through cell division, the genetic material in cells is replicated and identical chromosomes are transmitted to the daughter cells. This cell division occurs through a process called mitosis in somatic cells and through meiosis in gametes.

- Mitosis is the cell division in somatic cells that results in the same number of chromosomes.
- Meiosis is the cell division in gametes that results in half the number of chromosomes present in somatic cells.

Components of Chromosome (Fig. 2.1)

Chromosomes consist of:
- **Deoxyribonucleic acid (DNA):** It consists of chain of nucleotides. Each nucleotide (Box 2.1) is composed of
- Nitrogenous base.
  - Deoxyribose sugar
  - Phosphate molecule

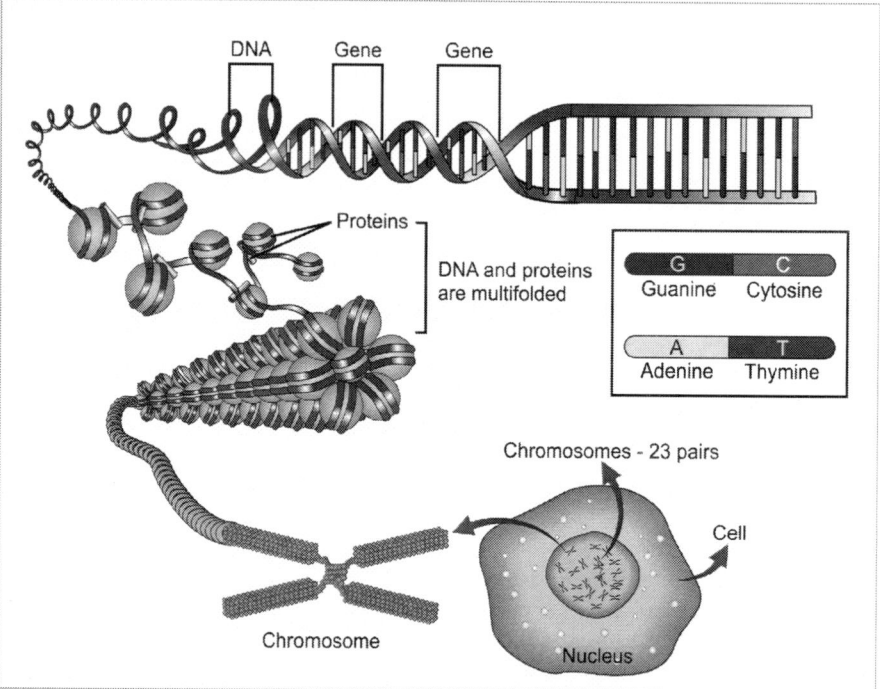

Fig. 2.1: Structure of chromosome, deoxyribonucleic acid (DNA), and gene. Strands of DNA are wound and packed tightly into chromosomes located within the nucleus of a cell. The basic units of heredity consist of segments of DNA called genes.

Box 2.1: Components of nucleotides.

- Nitrogenous base
- Sugar (deoxyribose in DNA and ribose in RNA)
- Phosphate molecule

- **Protein** which consists of approximately equal parts of:
  - Basic core protein namely **histone**
  - Acidic **nonhistone** protein
- **Small amount of ribonucleic acid (RNA)**.

Mixture of DNA and protein which forms a tightly packed complex is called **chromatin**.

Types of Nucleic Acids

Nucleic acids are of two types namely—DNA and RNA.

Deoxyribonucleic Acid

Location of DNA
- **Nuclear/chromosomal DNA:** Most of the DNA is inside the nucleus.
- **Mitochondrial DNA (mtDNA):** Mitochondria contains small amount of DNA.

Structure of DNA
The structure of DNA was first described by **James D Watson and Francis Crick** in 1953 for which they received Nobel Prize (1962). The majority of chromosomal **DNA is double-stranded helix** comparable to a twisted ladder. But it is **single-stranded at the end** of chromosomes, where it is called **telomere**.

Nucleotides

Each DNA (and also RNA) strand **consists of chain of nucleotides** (Fig. 2.2).

Structure of nucleotide unit: Each **nucleotide chain** is made up of **three main components** namely—nitrogenous base, deoxyribose (ribose in case of RNA) sugar and phosphate molecule.
1. **Nitrogenous base:** These bases are classified into two types.
   i. **Purines:** The purine bases are **adenine** (abbreviated A) and **guanine** (G).

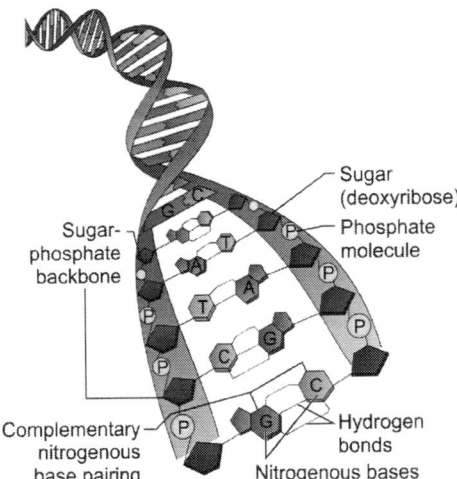

Fig. 2.2: Structure of nucleotide unit.

ii. **Pyrimidines:** The pyrimidine bases are **thymine** (T), **cytosine** (C) and **uracil** (U, which usually takes the place of thymine in RNA).

2. **Deoxyribose sugar moiety:** It is a pentose sugar with five carbon atoms.
3. **Phosphate molecule.**

Bonds between nucleotides: The **two nucleotide chains** of DNA are **held together** by two types of molecular forces.

1. **Hydrogen bonds:** These are formed between the nitrogenous bases on opposite nucleotide strands. They are always between a purine and pyrimidine nitrogenous base only.
   - Adenine base on one strand always pairs with thymine on the other strand (**A-T or T-A**).
   - Guanine base on one strand pairs with cytosine on the other (**G-C or C-G**).
2. **Phosphate diester bonds:** These bonds are between sugar molecules.

CELL DIVISION

Genetic information is passed from parent to all the descendant cells through cell division. There are **two types of cell division** namely **mitosis (somatic cell division** in the cells of the body) and **meiosis (germ cell division)**.

Cell Cycle

Definition: The cell cycle is defined as the **series of events that take place in a cell leading to its division** and duplication (replication).

Major Phases of Cell Cycle (Fig. 2.3)

Cell cycle consists of **two major phases** namely **interphase and mitotic phase**.

Interphase

It is the period between successive mitoses of the cell cycle. The interphase is subdivided into three phases: G_1, S and G_2 phase.
- G_1 **(gap 1/resting) phase**
- **S (synthetic) phase during which DNA is synthesized**
- G_2 **(gap 2/premitotic) phase.**

Mitotic phase: Described below.

Mitosis (Mitotic phase)

It is the final phase of cell cycle in which two identical (daughter) cells are produced. Mitosis is defined as the **process of somatic cell division to form two identical daughter cells**, each with the same chromosome complement as the parent cell.

Characteristic Features
- It produces **two genetically identical** "daughter cells" having complete set of genetic information.

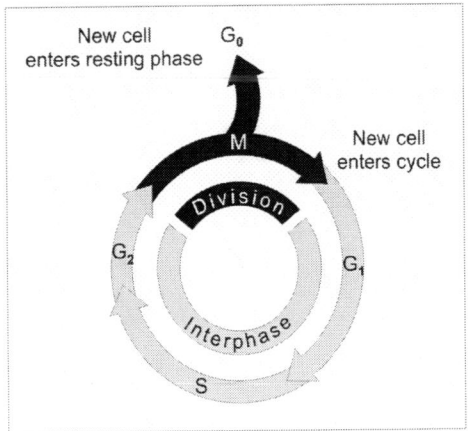

Fig. 2.3: Major phases of cell cycle.

- These daughter cells have exactly the **same normal number of chromosomes** (i.e. 46) as the original parent cell. The daughter cells are diploid because they contain 46 chromosomes (i.e. 2N = 2 × 23).

Sites of mitosis: It occurs **in all cells except the germ cells** or gametes.

Phases of mitosis (Fig. 2.4): There are **four different phases** of mitosis. They are: (1) prophase, (2) metaphase, (3) anaphase and (4) telophase.

1. **Prophase** *(Greek pro meaning "before"):* The changes occurring in this phase are:
   - Condensation of chromatin
   - Replication of centrosome
2. **Metaphase** (Greek μετα meaning "after"): The changes in this phase are:
   - Gradual breaking of nuclear membrane which later disappears.
   - Movement of the centrosomes and alignment of chromosomes.

   A mitotic karyotype can be constructed from cells arrested at metaphase.
3. **Anaphase** (Greek ανα meaning "up," "against," "back," or "re-"): The changes in this phase are:
   - Division and movement of chromosomes
   - Division of cytoplasm
4. **Telophase** (Greek *telo* meaning "end"): During this final phase, two identical, individual daughter cells are formed.

Meiosis

Meiosis the second form of cell division. Like mitosis, interphase of the cell cycle includes G_1, S, and G_2 phases. Interphase is followed by meiosis.

Definition: It is defined as **special form of germ cell division** that **produces reproductive cells** in which **each daughter cell receives half the number of chromosomes** (23) in the genome.

Sites of meiosis: Meiosis occurs **only in germ cells of the gonads** (sperms in males and ova in females).

- **In females:** Meiosis occurs in fetal and adult ovary. **Meiosis begins in fetal life but does not complete until after ovulation** (usually at about 12 years of age). A single meiotic cell division can thus take more than 40 years to complete. The second

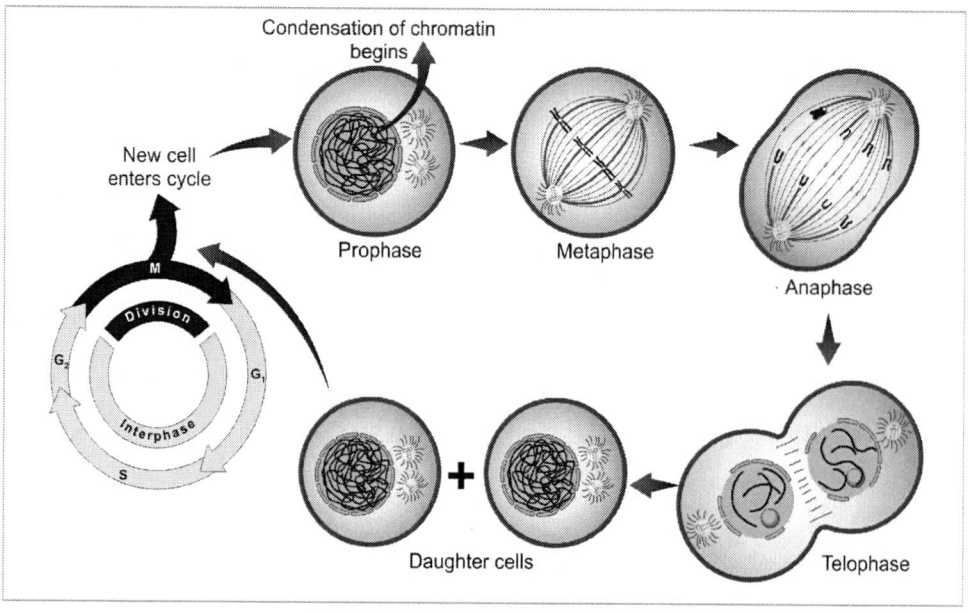

Fig. 2.4: Various phases of mitosis.

meiotic division normally is not completed until the oocyte is penetrated by sperm.
- **In males: Meiosis begins at puberty** and takes place in the seminiferous tubules of testis. **Both meiotic divisions are completed in a matter of days** in the testis. It continues throughout life.

Stages of Meiosis

Meiosis consists of two successive stages, namely, meiosis I and meiosis II.

Meiosis I: During this stage, **the number of chromosomes per cell is reduced by half** and is termed the **reduction division**. It is characterized by:
- **Pairing of homologous chromosomes:** In this stage, the replicated homologous chromosomes come together.
- **Recombination:** The **process of exchange of DNA** (swapping of genetic material/crossing over of chromosome segments) **between homologous chromosomes** (chromosomes with identical genetic material) is a unique event known as **recombination (synapsis)**. Recombination results in each chromosome having mixed segments of both maternal and paternal origin. This is responsible for significant **genetic diversity**/variability in humans.

After recombination, the homologous chromosomes separate to opposite poles and the chromatids consist of part of their original DNA and part of DNA from other homologous chromosome. There is no DNA synthesis (no S phase) between the two divisions (meiosis I and II).

Meiosis II: The second division in the meiotic process is termed the **equational division** because the events in this phase are **similar to those of mitosis**. However, meiosis II differs from mitosis in that the number of chromosomes has already been halved in meiosis I and the cell does not begin with the same number of chromosomes as it does in mitosis.

Result: The end result of meiosis is different in males and females. **Both sperm and ova are haploid cells (23 chromosomes-N)**.

- **Males:** Meiosis in males **produces four spermatozoa** from each original germ cell.
- **Females:** Meiosis I (the first meiotic division) in females gives rise to secondary oocyte and a small cell (polar body) that is discarded. During meiosis II, the secondary oocyte gives rise to one large mature ovum (egg) and a second polar body, which again is discarded. In females, the end result after the second meiotic division is **three polar bodies and one ovum**.

Main stages of meiosis in males and females are shown in Figure 2.5.

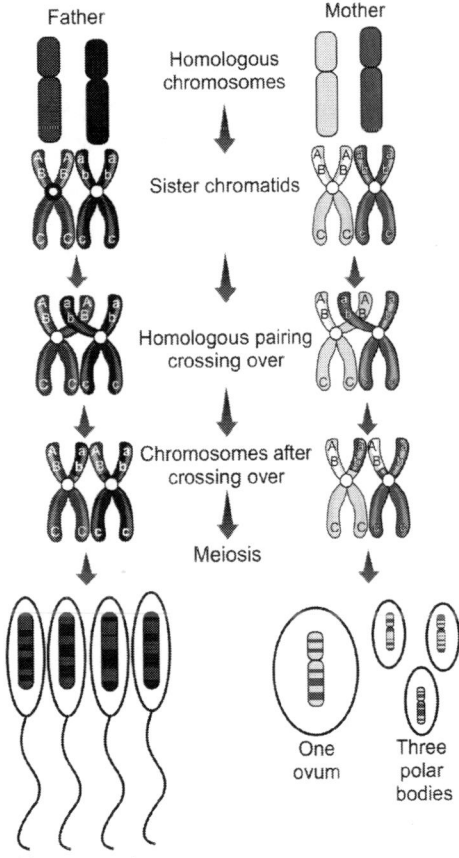

Fig. 2.5: Main stages of meiosis in males and females. A single homologous pair of chromosomes is shown in male, meiosis results in four spermatozoa. In the female, meiosis produces only one ovum (egg) and three polar bodies.

GENETIC PRINCIPLES IN BLOOD BANKING

Genes

Definition: Gene is defined as a **segment of DNA** which carries the genetic information. Gene is the basic **physical and functional unit of heredity**.

Genes are the basic units of inheritance on a chromosome. It is a unit of inheritance that encodes a particular protein and is the basic unit for inheritance of a trait. DNA has also segments which do not contain genes. The human genome contains about **21,500 genes,** and each gene varies in size.

Structure of Gene (Fig. 2.6)

Each gene consists of a specific sequence of nucleotides. **Genes may be silent or active.** When active, the **genes direct the process of protein synthesis**. Genes do not code for proteins directly but **by means of a genetic code**. The **genetic code** consists of a sequence code word called **codons**. A codon for an amino acid consists of a sequence of three nucleotide base pairs called a **triplet codon**.

Regions of Gene

- **Initiator and stop codons:** The boundaries of a gene are known as **start and stop codons**. The start codons tell when to begin protein production and stop (termination) codons tell when to end the protein production.
- **Coding region:** The **nucleotide sequence between the start and stop codons is** the core region known as **coding region**. This region is divided into two main segments namely exons and introns.
  i. **Exons:** This region codes for producing a protein.
  ii. **Introns:** These are the regions between exons and do not code for a protein (**noncoding region**).
  Most of the genes contain both exons and introns, the number of which varies with different genes.
- **Regulatory regions:** These are also noncoding regions which control gene expression.
  – **Promoters** are regions which bind to transcription factors, either strongly or weakly.

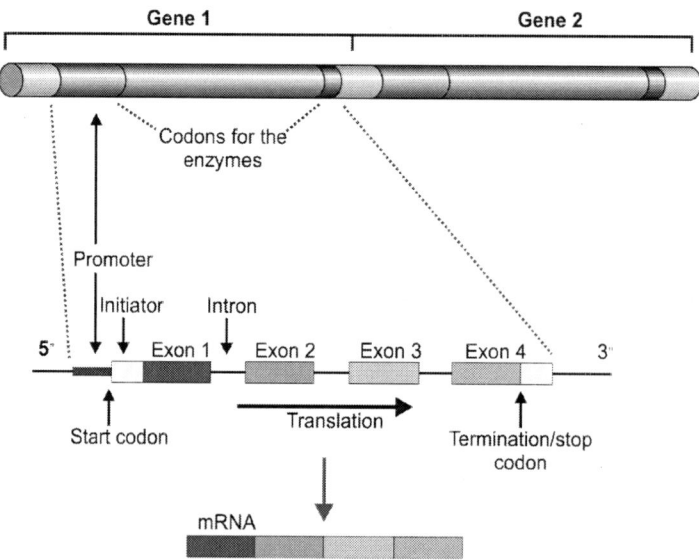

Fig. 2.6: Diagrammatic structure of a gene and its messenger ribonucleic acid (mRNA) product. Start and termination codons mark the limits of the gene. The coding portions of the gene are the exons (four in this example), and interspersed with introns which do not appear in the mRNA product.

- **Enhancers** are regions which can enhance the effect of a weak promoter.
- **Silencers** are regulatory regions that can inhibit transcription.

Allele

Chromosomes have many genes. Specific **genes** are **located at a specific place** (region) on every chromosome and this location is known as **genetic locus**. This genetic locus codes for particular characteristics. Every individual has two copies of each gene, one inherited from each parent. Each chromosome of a pair (homologous chromosomes) usually carries the same set of genes but not necessarily identical genes. These **different forms** of the **same gene** on **same position** (called locus) on a specific pair of homologous chromosomes are called **alleles**. Several different forms of alleles may exist for each locus. For example, *A*, *B*, and *O* are alleles on the *ABO* gene locus. Each allele determines a single inherited characteristic in an individual. For example, if a gene on a particular chromosome codes for a characteristic such as hair color, another gene (called an allele for hair color) at the same position on homologous chromosome also codes for hair color. However, these two alleles need not be identical: one might produce red hair and the other might produce blond hair. The terms, **"gene" and "allele" are often** used interchangeably. Therefore, **gene is the generic term and allele is specific term**.

Types of Allele (Figs. 2.7A to D)

- **Monoallelic:** About 70% of genes have one allele **(mono-allelic)**.
- **Diallelic:** They have only two alleles **(di-allelic)**.
- **Multiple alleles (poly-allelic/polymorphic):** They express two or more alleles at one locus. Multiple alleles of a given gene can occur, but any particular **individual can have only two of these alleles** for each gene, one from each parent and thus **allele occurs in pairs.** Examples for multiple alleles are the blood groups, hair color, hair texture, skin color, eye color, built, physical structures, etc.

Inheritance Patterns

ABO blood group system displays dominant, recessive, and codominant patterns of inheritance.

Dominant: In this, the gene product is expressed over another **unexpressed (recessive)** gene. A dominant expression would require only one form of the allele to express the trait. For example, group A phenotype inherits an A gene from one parent and an O gene from the other parent (A/O).

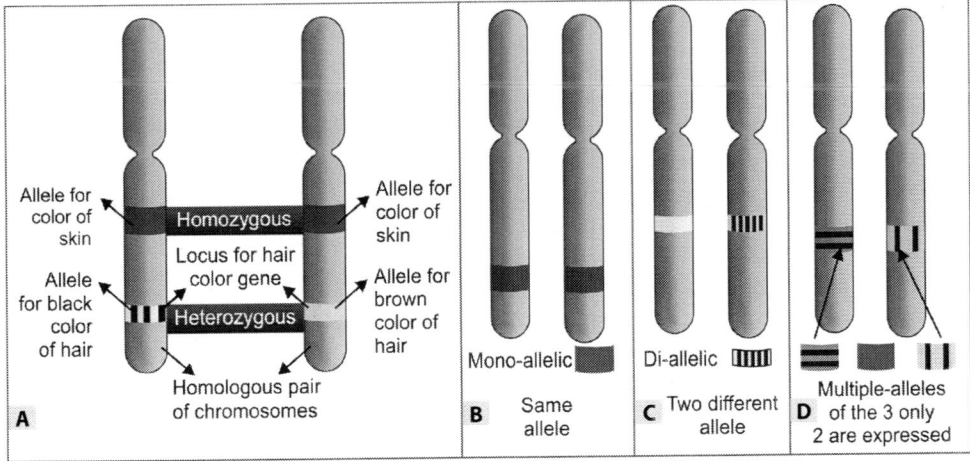

Figs. 2.7A to D: (A) Chromosome to show allele; (B to D) Different types of allele.

Recessive: It is a trait expressed only when inherited by both parents. Recessive inheritance needs the same allele from both parents to be inherited to show the trait. An example is inheritance of the group O phenotype that requires both parents to pass on an *O* gene (*O/O*).

If an individual inherits both the dominant and the recessive alleles, the dominant allele will be the one expressed. For example, the gene for right handedness being dominant over the recessive gene of left handedness.

Codominant: In this, there is equal expression of two different inherited alleles. The products of **both alleles of a gene pair exert** an observable **effect** and are thus equally dominant (e.g. the alleles A and B of the blood group system ABO; O is recessive to A and B).

Phenotype Versus Genotype

Phenotype

- **Trait** is **specific physical distinguishing appearance** of a characteristic condition (what you see) of a particular person. Trait is passed from parent to offspring. Physical expression of inherited traits is called phenotype.
- **Phenotype in ABO**: An individual's red blood cell (RBC) phenotype is determined by hemagglutination of red cell antigens using specific antisera. Serologic testing determines the presence or absence of antigens on the RBCs. The phenotype is determined by reacting red cells with known antisera and observing for the presence or absence of hemagglutination. For example, testing RBCs with anti-A or anti-B reagents can determine whether an individual has the A or B antigen on the RBC. If neither anti-A nor anti-B reagents shows agglutination, the RBCs are classified as group O. This determination is called the phenotype.

Genotype

The genotype (actual genetic makeup) refers to the actual complete set of genes/alleles present in an individual. For example:

- If an individual's **phenotype is A**, the **genotype may be** *A/A* **or** *A/O*.
- *A/A* **genotype** indicates that **both parents contributed the *A* gene**.
- *A/O* **genotype** indicates that **one parent contributed the *A* gene**, and the **other contributed the *O* gene.** Because the *O* gene has no detectable product, only the A antigen is expressed when the *A/O* genotype is inherited.
- If the *A/O* individual has a group O child, it indicates that the individual carried the *O* gene.
- Two individuals with group A red cells have the same phenotype but can have different genotypes.

Actual genotype is determined by family studies or molecular testing/typing (DNA-based assays). Hemagglutination cannot detect a genotype such as AO. These genes are inherited from each parent and may be inferred from the phenotype. Example of genotypes and phenotypes for the ABO blood group system.

Types of Genotypes

Classically, genotypes are described as:

Homozygous: If the **two gene copies of the allele** (for a given trait) are same/identical, the individual is called a homozygote and is homozygous for that gene. Examples: *AA, BB,* or *OO*.

Heterozygous: If **one gene copy or one allele differs from the other** (two alleles for a given trait are different), the individual is called heterozygous. In heterozygous individuals, one of the alleles is usually dominant, and the other is recessive. A dominant allele will override the traits of a recessive allele in a heterozygous pairing. An individual who has inherited different alleles from each parent, such as *AO, AB,* or *BO,* is called a heterozygote and is heterozygous for the genes.

Silent Genes

Null phenotypes: When certain recessive alleles are inherited, there is **no expression of the expected red cell antigens** and it is termed as null phenotype. In some blood

Blood Group Genetics

group systems, **genes do not produce any detectable antigen product.** These silent genes, known as **amorphs** (gene that does not express a detectable product) and they produce phenotypes called as null types. For example, in a Rh_{null} individual there is no Rh system antigens. The amorphic gene must be inherited from both parents (homozygous) to produce a null phenotype. Examples of null phenotypes include Rh_{null} and O.

Multiple Alleles and Blood Group

Presence of more than two alleles at a particular locus is called **multiple alleles.** The multiple alleles are responsible for a greater variety of genotypes and phenotypes.

ABO Blood Group

An excellent **example of multiple alleles** is the ABO blood group system. In ABO, there are at least **four alleles** namely A_1, A_2, B and O of a single ABO gene. These alleles **control the production of antigens on** the surface of the RBCs. An **individual can have any two of these four alleles**. These two alleles in an individual may be same or different and the blood group of individuals is determined by two of these alleles. For examples AA, A_1B, OO, A_2O. The "A" and "B" alleles are equally dominant to each other. Various combinations of these alleles can result in six ABO blood groups (Table 2.1). If an individual inherits A allele from one parent and B allele from the other parent, both alleles being dominant, the blood group will be AB. The "O" allele is recessive to both A and B alleles. An individual who inherits an A allele from one parent and an O allele from the other parent will have a genotype of AO and blood group will be A. If an individual inherits a B allele from one parent and an O allele from the other parent will have a genotype of BO and blood group B. An individual's blood group will be O if they have two O alleles from the both parents. "A" group has two subgroups namely A_1 and A_2.

■ POPULATION GENETICS

It is the study of distribution patterns of genes and the factors that maintain or change gene (or allele) frequencies.

- **Frequency:** It is used to describe prevalence at the genetic level. For example, occurrence of an allele (gene) in a population.
- **Prevalence:** It is used to describe the occurrence of a permanent inherited characteristic at the phenotype level (e.g. ABO blood group in any population).
- **Incidence:** It is used to describe the rate of occurrence in a population of a condition (e.g. disease) that changes overtime.

■ MOLECULAR GENETICS

Introduction

Molecule is the smallest physical unit of an element or compound. Molecular pathology/diagnostics is a term used for a family of techniques used to analyze biological markers in an individual's genetic code (genome) and to analyze how their cells express their genes as proteins (proteome). Molecular genetics is the procedures based on the detection or analysis of DNA and RNA, i.e. their molecules namely nucleic acids and proteins. Recent advances in molecular knowledge has revolutionized in the field of diagnostic medicine. DNA isolation is an essential technique in molecular biology. Molecular diagnostics is one of the fastest growing segments of laboratory medicine. Molecular immunohematology (MIH) is a rapidly emerging technology in transfusion medicine.

Table 2.1: Various genotypes and the corresponding phenotypes of ABO blood group system.

Genotype	Phenotype (blood group)	Genotype	Phenotype (blood group)
A^1A^1	A_1	A^2A^2	A_2
A^1O	A_1	A^2O	A_2
A^1A^2	A_1	BB	B
A^1B	A_1B	BO	B
A^2B	A_2B	OO	O

Application of Molecular Genetics to Blood Banking

Applications of molecular technology in blood banking and transplantation (refer chapter 23) are listed in Table 2.2. Nucleic acid testing (NAT) is a general term used for molecular-based methods of screening for infectious agents (discussed in chapter 17) One of the use of molecular technology in red cell typing is discussed below.

Molecular Testing Applications in Red Cell Typing

Classic hemagglutination testing is a simple and quick method used in blood bank testing to determine human RBC antigens However, there are several **limitations associated with hemagglutination testing.** These include:
1. In **recently transfused patients,** it is difficult to accurately determine the RBC antigen phenotype. When a patient presents with a positive direct antiglobulin test (DAT) due to anti-IgG, accurate phenotype results are challenging.
2. There is **short supply or nonavailability** of some **blood group antigen typing reagents**.
3. **Hemagglutination methods cannot determine the zygosity** (degree of similarity of the alleles for a trait) of the tested red cells.

Red blood cell antigen expression may be altered by variations in DNA sequences. Molecular techniques can identify the most important allelic variations attributable to the single nucleotide polymorphisms (SNPs) responsible for many of these variations. Thus, DNA-based/molecular methods for genotyping have supplemented traditional hemagglutination methods. With molecular techniques, it is possible to predict their presence or absence of antigens on the red cell membrane. For donor red cell antigen typing, molecular testing gives more accurate results and can be more cost-effective method

Table 2.2: Applications of molecular testing in the blood bank.

Application	Purpose
Transplantation	
HPC and organ transplantation	Human leukocyte antigen (HLA)-level and allele-level typing
Hematopoietic progenitor cell (HPC) transplantation	Engraftment studies to determine engraftment
Transfusion	
Red cell typing	In patients with multiple and recent transfusion
Determine blood types	When the direct antiglobulin test (DAT) is positive
Rh genotyping	Complex Rh genotypes, weak D expression
Screen for antigen-negative donor units	When antisera (antibody typing reagent) are not available (e.g. anti-Do^a, Do^b, Js^a, V, VS)
Donor antigen screening	To prevent alloimmunization
Antibody	To distinguish allo from autoantibody
RBC coated with immunoglobulins	DAT positive due to coating of RBC with immunoglobulins
Resolve group discrepancies	A, B and Rh discrepancies
HDFN (hemolytic disease of the fetus and newborn)	Determine parental RhD zygosity Type fetal blood
Donor testing by NAT	
Detect virus in donors (viral marker testing)	When they are below detectable levels by antibody detection methods (reduces the "window period")
Relationship testing	Establish paternity and legal relationships

in many situations. Molecular typing methods are useful when serologic typing cannot be performed due to limitations in the availability of sample or reagent. Applications of molecular tests for red cell typing in the blood bank are listed in Table 2.2.

Polymerase chain reaction–based red cell typing procedures

Bead-chip technology
Presently, the genes encoding the major blood group antigens have been sequenced and cloned. The increased knowledge about the correlation of the differences in DNA sequences with red cell antigen expression can be utilized for the development and standardization of laboratory tests. In many of the blood group systems, single-nucleotide substitutions, code for the unique blood group allele. The antigen-defining SNPs (single-nucleotide polymorphisms) are identified by PCR methods combined with bead-chip technology. This technology helps to provide compatible RBC units based on matching by DNA testing especially in patients requiring chronic multiple transfusion. Use of antigen-negative RBC units can prevent immunization to RBC antigens.

Principle: Bead-chip technology is one of the DNA arrays to predict human erythrocyte antigen (HEA) by DNA analysis. Human erythrocyte antigen bead-chip technology uses oligonucleotide primers. These primers are attached to silica beads of various colors. The beads in turn are attached to a substrate (e.g. a glass slide). A "map" identifying the color and the specific oligonucleotide (primer) is made.

HEA bead-chip molecular assay can detect 38 RBC antigens and phenotypic variants.

The advantages and limitations of RBC molecular testing are listed in Table 2.3.

Clinical applications of molecular testing (DNA analysis) for blood groups
- DNA-based assays are used to predict red cell phenotype of a fetus or of a patient who has been transfused or when red cells are coated with IgG.
- Others
  - Resolution of discrepancies in the ABO and Rh system
  - Identification of genetic basis of unusual serologic results
  - To distinguish alloantibodies from autoantibodies.

Prediction of red cell phenotype
- **In patients receiving large amounts of blood** (e.g. massive or chronic transfusions), the donor red cells can create problem when performing the phenotyping the patient's red cells. This especially problematic in recently transfused patients. Though cell separation techniques to obtain autologous red cells is available, they are time consuming and usually not successful. In such situations, PCR-based methods can help to derive red cell phenotype. An extended red cell phenotype can help in predicting the additional blood group antigens that may cause alloantibody formation in future transfusions.
- **Autoimmune hemolytic anemia (red cells coated with IgG)** is a condition characterized by formation of autoantibody against the patient's own red cells. In such situations, the bound immunoglobulin makes red cell typing difficult using serologic methods.

Table 2.3: Advantages and limitations of molecular tests for red cell antigens.

Advantages	Limitations
• No need for special reagents or rare antisera • No need for serologic confirmation • Can type red cell antigens in patients with positive DAT without extra efforts • Can be used in massive screening for rare antigen-negative donors	• Discrepancies between molecular and serologic confirmation can be found • All polymorphisms cannot be analyzed • Results can be challenging when patient or donor has altered alleles

- **Chemical removal**: IgG antibodies (autoantibodies) on the red cells must be removed chemically before proceeding with typing on the patient's red cells. The chemical that can be used include chloroquine diphosphate and EDTA-glycine acid. Disadvantage of this method is that these chemical treatments may denature an RBC antigen.
- **PCR-based methods**: It is alternative technique to derive red cell phenotype.
- **To distinguish alloantibody from autoantibody**: DNA-bases techniques will be helpful to know whether the antibody is allo- or autoantibody. This is mainly useful in patients with sickle cell disease and thalassemia who need long-term transfusion support and are at risk of alloimmunization.

Applications in prenatal practice
- **To know the risk of fetus for HDFN**: Molecular techniques can be used to identify a fetus which is not at risk for the development of hemolytic disease of the fetus and newborn (HDFN). When a mother has an alloantibody, fetal red cells can be tested for the antigen. If fetus is found to be antigen-negative, it is not at risk for HDFN, and there is no need for extensive monitoring of such mother.
- **Mother with an IgG alloantibody implicated in HDFN**: When a mother has an IgG alloantibody implicated in HDFN and the father is heterozygous or not available for testing, in such situations fetal DNA testing is useful.
- **Identify fetus at risk for anemia of the neonate**: DNA tests to detect anti-D in fetus by DNA testing.

Testing for antigen-negative blood donors
There are certain red cell antigens where typing is difficult because there are no commercially available antisera (suitable antibodies). Examples of these antigens include Hy, Jo^a, Js^a, Js^b, C^w, Do^a, Do^b, V, VS, S, and Fy$^{b.2}$. In such cases DNA assays can determine phenotype of such donor red cell antigens.

Confirm the D type of blood donors
Very weak expressions of D antigens can be found in some donors. This weak D antigen may not be detected by commercially available antisera and the unit may be labeled as D-negative. DNA assays can be used to confirm D negative phenotypes. This is especially useful in pregnant women and may guide RhIG prophylaxis.

Testing of paternal samples
When antibody is found in the maternal plasma, father's red cells should be tested for the corresponding antigen.
- **No antigen in father:** The fetus is not having any risk if father is negative for antigen.
- **Father positive for antigen:** In such case zygosity test should be performed to know whether father is homozygous or heterozygous for the gene coding the antigen. This is useful especially when there is availability of allelic antigen or antisera to detect allelic product.

Discrepancies between serologic (phenotype) and DNA (genotype) testing
Whenever there are discrepancies between serologic (phenotype) and DNA (genotype) testing, they should be investigated. Causes of this may be recent transfusions, stem cell transplantation and natural chimerism (chimerism is a mixture of donor and recipient cell populations after hematopoietic stem cell transplants. Chimerism can rarely occur naturally).

Silenced or nonexpressed genes: DNA test can detect either single or a few SNPs associated with antigen expression but cannot sample every nucleotide in the gene. The gene product may not be expressed on red cells due to mutation that either silences the gene or reduces its expression levels. In such situations routine hemagglutination tests cannot detect them. It can result in discrepancies in typing of patients and donors.

SUMMARY

- Blood group genetics deals with characteristic features by which blood groups are transmitted from parents to offspring.
- A gene is a segment of DNA and is the basic unit of inheritance. Specific **genes** are **located at a specific place** (region) on every chromosome and this location is known as **genetic locus**.
- When an individual has identical alleles at a given locus, the individual is called homozygous for the particular allele. If an individual has nonidentical alleles at a given locus, the individual is called heterozygous for the particular allele.
- The **different forms** of the **same gene** on **same position** (called locus) on a specific pair of homologous chromosomes are called **alleles**.
- **Deoxyribonucleic acid (DNA):** It consists of chain of nucleotides. Each nucleotide is composed of nitrogenous base, deoxyribose sugar and phosphate molecule.
- Each somatic cell of humans contains 23 pairs of chromosomes. Of this 22 pairs are called as autosomes and 1 pair is sex chromosomes of either XX (in females) or XY (in males).
- Genotype is the complement genes inherited from each parent.
- There are 36 blood group systems identified so far. Genetic bases of most antigens and phenotypes are known.
- Invention of DNA-based methods (genotyping) can be used to predict the phenotype of an individual. It has major applications in patient and donor testing.

SELF-ASSESSMENT EXERCISE

Write the essays on:
- Genetic principles in blood banking
- Molecular genetics
- Polymerase chain reaction

CHAPTER 3

ABO Blood Group System

CHAPTER OUTLINE

- Red blood cell groups
- ABO and H blood group system antigens
- Secretors and nonsecretors
- Subgroups of A, AB and B
- Null phenotypes
- Basic genetic features of ABO group system
- ABO/ABH antibodies

RED BLOOD CELL GROUPS

Introduction

Karl Landsteiner in 1901 **first described the existence of major human blood groups (ABO) based on the red cell antigens**. In immunohematology, after the initial discovery of ABO, many other blood group antigens which form part of the red cell membranes were detected. Many of these RBC antigens are more common (high-frequency antigens) and expressed by most donors (>90–99%), whereas other antigens are extremely rare (low-frequency antigens).

Blood Group Systems (Blood Group)

- Presently, **more than 700 red cell antigens** have been detected which have been organized (classified) into **36 blood group systems** (Table 3.1) by the International Society of Blood Transfusion (ISBT).
- Blood group systems **are groups of antigens** (defined system) **on the red cell membranes that share related serologic properties and genetic patterns of inheritance** (e.g. ABO system, Rh system).
- Blood group systems are **controlled by a genetic locus having a variable number of alleles** (e.g. A, B, and O in the ABO system).

In some systems, for example in Rh blood group system, the gene directly encodes a protein on the red cell, which is recognized by the immune system. With other blood group systems, several interacting genes encode a particular antigen on the red cell. For example, expression of the ABO antigens needs the interaction of the *ABO*, *Hh*, and *Se* genes.

- **Important blood group systems:** Only few blood group systems are clinically important and the two most important blood group systems are **ABO** and **Rh** systems. Accurate donor and recipient ABO phenotypes are fundamental to transfusion safety because the transfusion of ABO-incompatible blood to a recipient can result in intravascular hemolysis and other serious consequences of an acute hemolytic transfusion reaction (HTR).

Terminology of blood group systems: There is no consistency in the terminology used for blood group system.

- **Capital letters:** In some systems (e.g. ABO), antigens are given capital letters (e.g. B) or capital letters with subscripts (e.g. A_2). The corresponding alleles are denoted by italics, with superscripts when relevant (e.g. A^2).

Table 3.1: Blood group systems recognized by the ISBT working party.

ISBT number	Name (chromosome)	Abbreviation	Number of antigens
001	ABO (9q34.1)	ABO	4
002	MNSs (4q28.2)	MNS	46
003	P (22q13)	P	3
004	Rh (1p36.1)	RH	54
005	Lutheran (19q13.3)	LU	20
006	Kell (7q34)	KEL	35
007	Lewis (19p13.3)	LE	6
008	Duffy (1q23)	FY	5
009	Kidd (18q12)	JK	3
010	Diego (17q21.3)	DI	22
011	Yt or Cartwright (7q22)	YT	2
012	XG (Xp22.3)	XG	2
013	Scianna (1p34)	SC	7
014	Dombrock (2p13.2)	DO	8
015	Colton (7p14)	CO	4
016	Landsteiner-Wiener (19p13.3)	LW	3
017	Chido/Rodgers (6p21.3)	CH/RG	9
018	Hh/Bombay (19q13.3)	H	1
019	Kx (Xp21.1)	XK	1
020	Gerbich (2q14)	GE	11
021	Cromer (1q32)	CROM	18
022	Knops (1q32)	KN	9
023	Indian (11p13)	IN	4
024	Ok (19p13.3)	OK	3
025	Raph (11p15.5)	MER2	1
026	John Milton Hagen/JMH (15q24.3)	JMH	6
027	Ii (6p24.2)	I	1
028	Globoside (3q26)	GLOB	1
029	GIL (9p13)	GIL	1
030	Rh-associated glycoprotein (6p21-qter)	RHAG	4
031	Forssman (9q34.13)	Fors	1
032	Junior/Jr (4q22)	JR	1
033	Lan (2q36)	LAN	1
034	Vel (1p36.32)	VEL	1
035	CD59 (11p13)	CD59	1
036	Augustine (6)	AUG	2

- **Large and small letters:** In some systems (e.g. Kell), the main alleles are denoted by large and small letters. For example, *K* and *k*; in which the terminology indicates that the alleles are alternative forms.
- **Mixture:** In MNS system, a mixture of the above two systems are used. First antigens are called M and N, and the next pair S and s.
- **Standard numerical nomenclature:** It was devised by a Working Party of the ISBT. It consists of six numbers, the first three numbers represent the blood group system (ISBT No.—refer Table 3.1), for example 001, ABO; 002, MNSs; 003, P; 004, Rh, and the second three numbers represent a particular antigenic specificity within that system, for example 001001, A; 004001, D. In total, 36 (001–036) blood group systems have been given numbers so far. Blood group systems recognized by the ISBT working party are listed in Table 3.1.

Blood Type

- The term "**blood type**" refers to the antigenic phenotype. It is usually recognized by the using appropriate antibodies. Antigens present on an individual's red cells within a particular blood group system (e.g. ABO system, Rh [Rhesus] system) represent that person's blood type for that system. For example, ABO is the blood group and blood type may be A, B, AB or O. The number of possible blood types within one blood group system varies.
- Taking all blood group systems and type combinations into account, more than 500 billion different types of RBCs are possible.
- Only a few red cell antigens are specific to RBCs (Rh, LW, Kell and MNSs). Some blood group antigens are found (expressed) not only on RBCs but also in many other tissues and body fluids (e.g. saliva, plasma).

Red Cell Antigens

Biochemical Nature of Blood Group Antigens

Red blood cell (RBC) antigens are very diverse in structure and composition. There are two basic kinds of blood group antigens and these are either proteins (e.g. Rh, M and N blood group substances) or carbohydrates/glycolipids (e.g. ABH, Lewis, Ii, and P blood group substances). Because of these differences in structure, conformation, and molecular nature, not all blood group substances are equally immunogenic in vivo.

1. **Carbohydrate-defined antigens:** One group of antigens is determined by carbohydrates attached to either proteins (forming glycoproteins) or to lipids (**glycolipids**). The specificity of these blood group antigens is determined by sugars. The genes code for an intermediate product, usually an enzyme that creates the antigenic specificity by transferring sugar molecules onto a protein or lipid. The carbohydrate-defined antigens are ABO, Lewis, Hh, P, and I systems. These are indirect gene products.

2. **Protein-defined antigens:** These are second type of antigens (e.g. Rh, M and N blood group substances). They are direct gene products and their blood group specificity is determined primarily by inherited amino acid sequences of proteins that are directly determined by genes. Most of the blood group polymorphisms are due to single amino acid substitutions. Proteins carrying red cell antigens are inserted into the red cell membrane in one of three ways: single pass, multipass or linked to glycosylphosphatidylinositol (GPI-linked). Most blood group antigens are proteins or glycoproteins (protein-defined antigens).

Inheritance of Red Cell Antigens

Most of the antigens present on an individual's red cell (including white blood cell and platelet) membranes are inherited in a **Mendelian dominant fashion**. Most blood group genes are located at specific chromosomes (e.g. ABO system on chromosome 9, Rh system on chromosome 1). Each blood group system is a series of red cell antigens, determined either by a single genetic locus or by very closely linked loci.

- **Genotype:** The genotype refers to the **actual complete set of genes/alleles present in an individual**. Thus, the term genotype is used for the sum of the inherited alleles of a particular gene (e.g. AA, AO). Most red cell genes are expressed as codominant antigens (i.e. both alleles are expressed in the heterozygote).
- **Phenotype:** It refers to the recognizable product of the alleles (e.g. A, B, AB).
- **Alleles:** The different forms of the same gene on same position (called locus) on a specific pair of homologous chromosomes are called alleles (refer page 31 of chapter 2). In transfusion medicine, the various alleles for a particular blood group system are equally dominant, or codominant. If the gene is present (and there is a suitable testing solution available), it will be detected.

For detailed discussion refer chapter 2.

Immunogenicity of Blood Group Antigens

The ability to elicit an immune response by different blood group antigens varies greatly.
- The **A, B** and **RhD** antigens are the **most immunogenic**. Hence, all blood to be transfused must be matched for these antigens between the blood donor and the recipient. About 50–75% of D-negative individuals would produce anti-D if transfused with even one unit of D-positive blood.
- After the D antigen, **K** is the next most immunogenic, followed by **Fya**. The significance of antigens and antibodies is not limited to transfusion medicine.
- Apart from antigens of the ABO system, most of other antigens were detected by antibodies stimulated by transfusion or pregnancy.

Red Cell Antibodies

The ABO and Rh systems are of major clinical importance.
- **ABO system is the only blood group system in which individuals have antibodies in their serum to antigens that are absent from their RBCs.** These antibodies are found without any exposure to RBCs through transfusion or pregnancy. Because of these **naturally occurring antibodies**, transfusion of an incompatible ABO type may **result in immediate lysis of donor RBCs.** This results in very severe (if not fatal), transfusion reaction in the patient. Testing to detect ABO incompatibility between a donor and potential transfusion recipient is the fundamental test in transfusion. Anti-A and anti-B are naturally occurring antibodies and are capable of causing severe intravascular hemolysis after an incompatible transfusion.
- The RhD antigen is the most immunogenic red cell antigen after A and B. RhD antigen is capable of stimulating anti-D production after transfusion or pregnancy in the majority of RhD-negative individuals.
- Antibody production in most other blood group systems needs the introduction of foreign RBCs either by transfusion or pregnancy. If RBCs containing a foreign antigen are transfused into a recipient whose red cells do not contain that antigen, the recipient can form an antibody. **Antibodies from different members of the same species** are referred to as **alloantibodies**.

ABO AND H BLOOD GROUP SYSTEM ANTIGENS

The ABO system is the most important of all blood groups in transfusion medicine.

General Characteristics of ABO Antigens

Distribution of ABO Blood Group System Antigens

ABO is often referred to as a **histo-blood group system**. This is because, ABO antigens are not only **expressed on red cells** (cell membranes), they are also present on **most tissues** and in soluble form **in secretions**.

- **Association with cell membranes:** ABO antigens are distributed widely on cell membrane. They are found on red cells, on lymphocytes (adsorbed from plasma), platelets (adsorbed from plasma), most epithelial and endothelial cells, and organs such as the kidneys. ABO blood group system antigens, which are intrinsic to the red cell membrane, biochemically present are either **glycolipid or glycoprotein molecules.**
- **Soluble forms:** ABO blood group system antigens can also be found in soluble forms synthesized and secreted by tissue cells. Soluble antigens are found in secretions and all body fluids except cerebrospinal fluid (CSF). The soluble forms ABO blood group system antigens are **primarily glycoproteins.**

ABO antigens can be detected in utero at 5–6 weeks of gestation. ABO antigen development occurs slowly. The full expression of adult levels of ABO antigens is reached at about 2–4 years of age.

Number of copies of antigens per cell: A newborn has few copies antigen per red cell when compared with an adult (e.g. newborn red cells carry 200,000–320,000 B antigens whereas adult red cells carry 610,000–830,000 B antigens). In contrast to adult, antigen structure of the newborn's red cells is partially developed. This is responsible for weaker ABO phenotyping reactions in cord blood samples.

Formation of A, B and H Red Cell Antigens

In the formation of A and B antigen, H antigen plays a major role. Hence, H antigen is discussed along with A and B antigens.

Common Structure for A, B and H Antigens

Basic precursor substance: A, B, and H antigens are formed from the same basic precursor substance/material (i.e. common structure or antigen building block) called as ABH precursor substance. The basic precursor structure is (a **paragloboside** or **glycan**) an oligosaccharide (sugar) chain attached to either a protein/polypeptides (forming a glycoprotein) or a lipid (forming a glycolipid) carrier molecule. The precursor substance is a product of unidentified gene. The oligosaccharide chain of basic precursor substance consists of four sugar molecules (tetrasaccharides) linked either in simple linear forms or complex branched structures. Each sugar molecules are composed of hexoses (Fig. 3.1). Each hexose sugar molecules in turn consist of six carbon atoms and the attachment or linkage describes which carbon atoms are involved in binding the two sugar molecules together. Common carbohydrate precursor which forms antigens in several blood group systems namely ABO, H, Lewis, Ii, and P1 antigens (Fig. 3.2).

Type 1 and type 2 carbohydrate chains (refer Fig. 3.4): There are two major forms of the ABH precursor substance namely type 1 and type 2 carbohydrate (oligosaccharide) chains. The difference between these two types of precursor substances is the attachment or linkage of the last D-galactose sugar molecule and N-acetylglucosamine on the precursor substance.

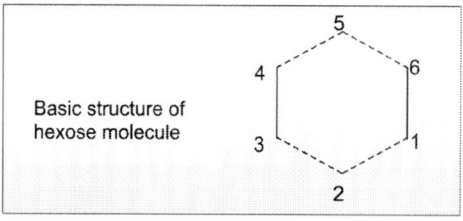

Fig. 3.1: Basic structure of hexose molecule with numbering from 1 to 6.

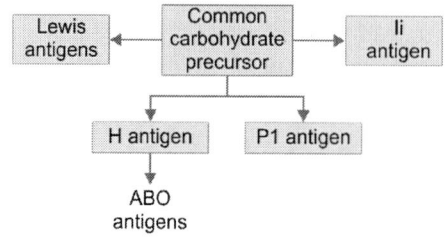

Fig. 3.2: Common carbohydrate precursor which forms antigens in several blood group systems namely ABO, H, Lewis, Ii, and P1 antigens.

ABO Blood Group System

- **Type 1 oligosaccharide chains:** These are formed when the number 1 carbon of D-galactose (Gal) is linked with the number 3 carbon of N-acetylglucosamine (GalNAc). This linkage is described as β1→3. Type 1 structures are associated mainly with body fluids. Thus, type 1 precursor substances are the major precursor substances found in the gut lining, plasma, and secretions such as urine, milk, and saliva. It is the substrate for the *FUT2* (*Se*) gene (discussed on page 47). Synthesis of type 1 chain ABO antigens is linked to the Lewis blood group system.
- **Type 2 oligosaccharide chains:** In this, the number 1 carbon of D-galactose Gal is linked with (connects) the number 4 carbon of N-acetylglucosamine (GalNAc). This linkage is described as β1→4. Type 2 structures are associated mainly with glycolipids and glycoproteins on the membrane of **blood cells**. Some type 2 glycoprotein structures are located in body fluids and secretions (e.g. saliva). They are the substrates for the *FUT1* (*H*) gene (discussed on page 47).

Inheritance and Development of A, B and H Antigens

Genetic loci controlling expression of ABO: The inheritance, formation and expression of ABO (A and B) antigens depend not only on *ABO* genes but also two other genes (i.e. *H* gene and *Se* gene) which are not part of the ABO system. Thus, expression of ABO antigen is controlled by the interaction of three separate genetic loci (i.e. *ABO*, *H* gene and *Se* [for secretor] gene). Both *H* and *Se* genes are inherited independently of the ABO blood group system antigens. H substance is a product of *H* gene which is needed for expression of ABO antigens. Hence, H gene is discussed first.

H Gene

Hh system is separate from the ABO system and the ABO and Hh genes are inherited independently of one another. The H antigen is the only antigen in the H blood group system. **H locus** has two alleles namely: (1) H and (2) h.

- The **H allele is a dominant allele**, whereas the **h allele** of the H locus is as an **amorphic gene** (like *O* gene) with no detectable/functional gene product or codes for an inactive fucosyltransferase. Most of the individuals are homozygous for the *H* gene (i.e. HH) and the *H* gene is present in more than 99.99% of the random population.
- If an individual has two copies of the *h* gene (hh), there is neither the production of an enzyme nor the H antigen. The phenotype hh (genotype hh) is extremely rare. The heterozygous Hh cannot be recognized.

The *H* **gene is also called** *FUT1*. It produces glycosyltransferase enzyme and the biochemical name for this enzyme is **α-2-L-fucosyltransferase**. Only one copy of the *H* gene is needed to make the H antigen. The *H* gene genetically influences the formation of the **ABO antigens on the RBCs.**

Formation of H antigen

- **Fucosylation of basic precursor substance:** The **L-fucosyltransferase enzyme** (product of *H* gene) transfers the sugar **L-fucose** (fucose) to the terminal D-galactose in the basic precursor substance of either type 1 chain or type 2 chain (Fis. 3.4). *FUT1* gene adds galactose to both oligosaccharide chains on red cells (type 2) and in secretions (type 1). Therefore, L-fucose is the sugar responsible for H specificity (blood group O). This enzymatic reaction produces H antigen and its formation is crucial for the expression of A and B antigens. This is because the gene products of the ABO alleles need the H antigen to be the acceptor molecule. Without this fucosylation, neither A nor B antigens can be made or formed. Two genes active in different tissues, produce L-fucosyltransferases: namely *FUT1* responsible for H on red cells; *FUT2* (discussed on page 47) for H in many other tissues and in secretions.
- **Immunodominant sugars:** The sugars that occupy the terminal positions (refer Fig 3.6) of the chain of the basic precursor substance are responsible for the blood

group specificity and are called the **immunodominant sugars**.

- The **H antigen** generates H substance which is the precursor substance or building block necessary for making both A and B antigens. Without any H antigen, there is no A or B antigen on the RBCs regardless of which *ABO* genes are present. Individuals of the *hh* genotype cannot covert the basic precursor substance into H substance which is the precursor required for the formation of the A and B antigens. Thus, the red cells from an h homozygote (genotype *hh*) are classified as the Bombay phenotype and para-Bombay phenotypes (Oh). These phenotypes are very rare and individuals with Bombay phenotype lack both H antigen and ABO antigen expression on their red cells (The Bombay phenotype is discussed in detail on page 51). There is a slightly higher prevalence of Bombay group in people of Japanese or Indian heritage.
- **H substance, the biochemical precursor of A and B:** The basic precursor substance is converted by L-fucosyltransferase enzyme (product of *H* gene) to H substance by the addition of sugar L-fucose (fucose) to the terminal D-galactose in the basic precursor substance. H substance is the biochemical precursor of A and B.
- Genes for three different blood group systems (ABO, Hh, and Sese) control the expression of ABH antigens. ABH antigen activity is not directly determined by ABH genes. *A*, *B*, and *H* genes do not synthesize antigen directly but they code for a different enzyme (glycosyltransferase). These enzymes catalyze the transfer of a biochemical group from one molecule to another and biochemically known as a glycosyltransferases. A glycosyltransferase enzyme catalyzes/facilitates the transfer of glycosyl groups (simple carbohydrate/sugar units, e.g. fucose) from its donor substrate to the acceptor substrate. Hence, the gene products of *A*, *B* and *H* genes are transferase enzyme which transfers different sugar on the polypeptide or lipid to produce the unique antigen.

Concentration of H antigen
- Some of the H substance remains unconverted. All A and/or B blood cells normally contain some H substance along with A and/or B antigen (refer Fig. 3.6).
- The amount of H substance on red cells depends on the ABO group (refer Fig 3.3). The H antigen content of red cells can be assessed by agglutination reactions with anti-H.
  - The *O* gene is an amorph and does not encode a functional enzyme. It produces an inactive transferase. The O cells have only H substance (H substance remains unchanged on group O cells). Adult group O red cells have highest concentration of H antigens (about 1.7 million H antigen copies/red cell).
  - Other ABO phenotypes have fewer copies of H antigens because the H antigen is the acceptor molecule for the A and B enzymes.
  - Group A_1B phenotype possesses the least number of unconverted H sites. The amount of H substance on red cells in order of decreased quantity is $O > A_2 > B > A_2B > A_1 > A_1B$ (Fig. 3.3).

ABO Genes and its Products

The *ABO* genes follow simple Mendelian genetic laws. In ABO, there are **three major alleles**, within the ABO locus: A, B and O. Two

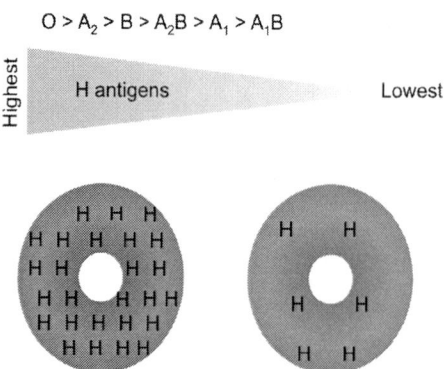

Fig. 3.3: Variation of H antigen concentrations in various ABO phenotypes. Group O red cells have highest H antigens and group A_1B red cells have lowest H antigens.

of these namely *A* and *B* alleles are codominant and the third O allele is recessive. A and B are termed codominant because both *A* and *B* alleles are expressed when present. These ultimately determine the four phenotypic products: A, B, AB, and O substances. The ABO locus is located on chromosome 9. Genes code only for proteins. ABO antigens are not proteins but are carbohydrates. The antigenic activity of ABO blood group antigens is determined by carbohydrate (sugars) structure and these antigens are not direct products of the genes (i.e. not produced directly by the genes).

The **inherited genes** (*A* and/or *B*) do not actually code for the production of antigens but **code for intermediate product**. This product of A or B gene (or both) is usually a specific enzyme namely **glycosyltransferase enzymes**. The enzyme product of *A* gene is N-acetylgalactosaminyltransferase (adds *N*-acetyl-D-galactosamine) and that of *B* gene is D-galactosyltransferase (adds D-galactose). The expression of A and B antigens depends on the presence of *H* gene. ABO antigens are the most important antigens in transfusion medicine. Figure 3.4 shows the site of action of *ABH* genes.

Flowchart 3.1 shows the flow of genetic information in the ABO blood group system.

A, B and H antigens and relationship with age: A, B, and H antigens are detectable early in fetal life. However, they are not fully developed on the red cells at birth. The number of antigen sites on red cells reaches "adult" level at the age of about 1 year. It remains constant until old age, when a slight reduction may be observed.

ABO Phenotypes
Blood Group A (A Phenotype)

- Individuals of blood group A may be homozygous **(AA)** or heterozygous **(AO)**. The *A* gene (*AA* or *AO*) does not code for the A antigen itself but rather codes for an enzyme that makes the A antigen. This enzyme is *N*-**acetylgalactosaminyltransferase** (GalNAc). In the formation of blood group A (Fig. 3.4), the N-acetylgalactosaminyltransferase enzyme converts H substance into A antigen by transferring (attaching) *N*-**acetyl-D-galactosamine (GalNAc) sugar** to the fucosylated galactose (Gal) of H (type 2 precursor substance) substance (i.e. the chain was previously converted to H antigen).
- *N-acetylgalactosamine* **(GalNAc)** is the immunodominant sugar and is responsible for A specificity (blood group A).
- The *A* gene tends to elicit higher concentrations of transferase than the *B* gene. This results in the conversion of almost all of the H antigen on the RBC to A antigen sites. Group A individuals have **A antigens on their RBCs and anti-B antibodies in their serum or plasma.**

Blood Group B (B Phenotype)

- Individuals of blood group B may be homozygous **(BB)** or heterozygous **(BO)**.
- B gene codes for the production of an enzyme that makes the B antigen. This enzyme is ***D-galactosyltransferase***. In the formation of blood group B (Fig. 3.4), D-galactosyltransferase (product of B gene) enzyme **converts H substance to B antigen by transferring** (attaching) **D-galactose** (Gal) sugar to the H substance. This D-galactose (Gal) sugar is the immunodominant sugar and is responsible for B specificity (blood group B).
- Group B individuals have **B antigens on their RBCs and have anti-A antibodies in their serum or plasma.** There are few weak

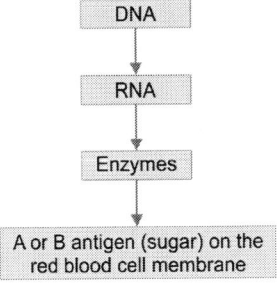

Flowchart 3.1: Illustration of flow of genetic information in the ABO blood group system.

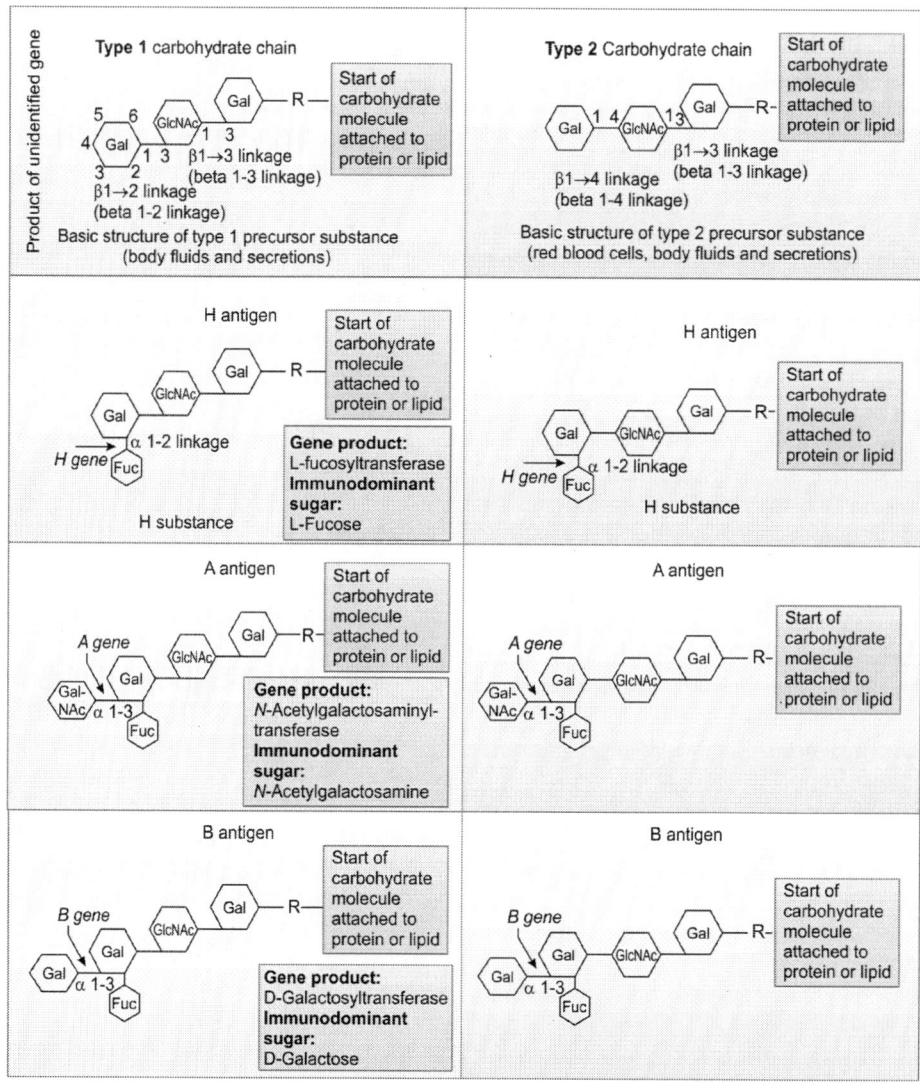

Fig. 3.4: Schematic diagram of the site of action of ABH genes.
(Gal: galactose; Fuc: fucose; GlcNAc: N-acetylglucosamine; GalNAc: N-acetylgalactosamine)

subgroups of B, but are less common than the rare A subgroups.

Blood Group O (O Phenotype)
- Group O individuals are homozygous with two *O* genes **(OO)** and inherit at least one *H* gene (genotype *HH* or *Hh*). Individuals with blood group O have neither A nor B antigens on their RBCs.
- The ***O* gene** at the ABO locus is sometimes called as an **amorph** (nonfunctional or silent gene), because it does not elicit the production of a catalytically active polypeptide transferase or produces an inactive transferase. Therefore, the **H substance remains unmodified/unchanged on group O cells** in the individuals with blood group O. They **have the highest concentration of unconverted H antigen**. The group O phenotype reflects the complete absence of ABO enzyme activity due to ABO-null alleles. They **have**

both anti-A and anti-B antibodies in their serum or plasma. Anti-AB antibodies are also found in the serum or plasma of group O individual. Probably the *O* and *B* genes arose by mutation of the *A* gene.

Blood Group AB (AB Phenotype)

- When both *A* and *B* genes are inherited, the B enzyme (D-galactosyltransferase) competes more efficiently for the H substance than the A enzyme (*N*-acetylgalactosaminyltransferase).
- It reflects **coinheritance of A and B**. Individuals of type **AB** possess both enzymes (*N*-acetylgalactosaminyltransferase, D-galactosyltransferase), and both the above processes occur resulting in production of blood group AB. Group AB individuals **lack both anti-A and anti-B antibodies in their serum or plasma**.

SECRETORS AND NONSECRETORS

Secretors (Genotype SeSe or Sese)

Some individuals secrete A, B and/or H antigens in a water-soluble form in secretions. A, B and H antigens may be found in the secretions of the goblet cells and mucous glands of the gastrointestinal tract (saliva, gastric juice, bile, meconium), genitourinary tract (seminal fluid, vaginal secretions, cervical secretions, ovarian cyst fluid, urine), and respiratory tract, as well as milk, sweat, tears, amniotic fluid and exudates. These **individuals who secrete H substance in the saliva and other body fluids** together with **A substance, B substance or both**, depending on their blood group are **called as secretors**. Secretors constitute about 80% of the general population. Secretor status of an individual can be determined by testing for ABH substance in saliva. Blood group secretors and antigen present in their secretions are listed in Table 3.2.

The secretion of A, B, and/or H antigens is controlled by *Se* gene/*FUT2* (dominant allele

Table 3.2: Blood group secretors and antigen present in their secretions.

Group of secretors	Antigen present in the secretions
Group O secretors	H antigen
Group A secretors	A and H antigens
Group B secretors	B and H antigens
Group AB secretors	A, B and H antigens

Se). The *Se* (for secretor) gene is also called *FUT2*. *Se* codes for a specific **fucosyl (Fuc) transferase** in secretory organs (e.g. exocrine glands), but is not active in RBCs. Secretors have inherited at least one secretor (*Se*) gene. The *Se* gene genetically influences the formation of the **ABO antigens in secretions**. The *Se* gene is on chromosome 19, close to the *H* gene. Individuals of *SeSe* or *Sese* genotypes secrete either or both A and B antigens whereas individuals of the *sese* genotype do not secrete. However, their RBCs can express the A and B antigens.

Nonsecretors (Genotype sese)

The *se* gene, like the *h* gene, is an **amorph**. Individuals with *sese* **do not produce any A, B or H antigen in their secretions** and are called **nonsecretors**. They do not or have only traces of H substance, A substance, B substance or both in saliva and other body fluids. The antigens are expressed normally on their red cells and other tissues. Nonsecretors constitute about 20% of the population. They do not produce a functional fucosyltransferase. Hence, the type 1 precursor substance secreted into their fluids is not converted to H substance and therefore cannot be converted into A or B antigens, irrespective of their ABO genotype.

Various glycosyltransferase enzymes produced by genes encoding antigens involved in ABO and H blood group systems are summarized in Table 3.3.

SUBGROUPS OF A, AB AND B

The most common subtypes of ABO are subgroups of the A antigen.

Table 3.3: Various glycosyltransferase enzymes produced by genes encoding antigens involved in ABO and H blood group systems.

Gene	Allele	Transferase	Antigen-determining sugar
FUT1	H	α-2-L-fucosyltransferase	L-fucose
	h	None	
ABO	A	α-3-N-acetyl-D-galactosaminyltransferase	N-acetylgalactosamine
	B	α-3-D-galactosyltransferase	D-galactose
	A and B	All the above	All the above
	O	None	
FUT2	Se	α-2-L-fucosyltransferase	
	se	None	

(FUT: fucosyltransferase)

Subgroups of A

Subgroups A1 and A2

There are two main subgroups of A antigen: (1) A_1 and (2) A_2.

The differentiation of A_1 and A_2 subgroups: During routine ABO phenotyping, both A_1 and A_2 red cells agglutinate with commercially available anti-A reagents. **A_1 red cells are distinguished from A_2** (and other weak A subtypes) **by using a lectin anti-A_1** (protein of nonimmune origin) reagent extracted from the seeds of the plant *Dolichos biflorus* (DBA) or human anti-A_1. This lectin reagent serves as a source of anti-A_1 (known as anti-A_1 lectin) and has some degree of specificity. These subgroups develop due to the inheritance of either the A_1 or A_2 alleles/genes. They differ slightly in their ability to convert H antigen to A antigen. The A_2 transferase is less efficient in transferring N-acetyl-D-galactosamine to available H antigen sites. Thus, **A_2 red cells have fewer A antigen sites than A_1 cells** and the plasma of group. The **anti-A_1 lectin is not used in routine ABO phenotyping/testing of blood from donors and recipients**. This is because for transfusion purposes, it is unnecessary to distinguish between the A_1 and A_2 phenotypes. However, this reagent is useful in resolving ABO typing problems and identifying infrequent subgroups of A.

Blood group AB has two subgroups namely A_1B and A_2B. Sometimes individuals with A_2 or A_2B may have anti-A_1 in their serum. However, this is usually weak and has no significance in selection of blood for transfusion.

- The anti-A_1 reagent agglutinates RBCs with the A_1 (or A_1B) antigen, but not red cells with the A_2 (or A_2B) antigen.
- About 80% of group A individuals and group AB individuals belong to group A_1 and group A_1B. The remaining 20% belong to group A_2 and group A_2B. Anti-A_1 can be found in 1–8% of group A_2 individuals.

Differences between A_1 and A_2 subgroups are listed in Table 3.4 and shown in Figure 3.5.

Other Weak Subgroups of A

- **Very rare:** There are several other subgroups of A, but are **extremely rare** (frequency of <1%) and are mainly of academic interest. The A subgroups have been classified as A_{int}, A_3, A_x, A_m, A_{end}, A_{el}, and A_{bantu} based on the reactivity of red

Table 3.4: Differences between A_1 and A_2 subgroups.

Feature	A_1 phenotype	A_2 phenotype
Nature of A antigen	Branched	Linear
Number of A antigens per adult red cells	2 million	500,000
Reaction with anti-A	Positive	Positive
Reaction with anti-A_1 lectin	Positive	Negative

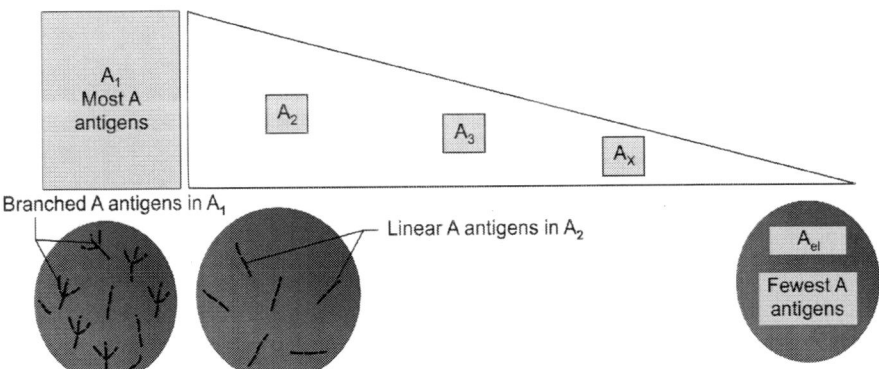

Fig. 3.5: Gradient of A antigens sites per red cell in various subgroups of A. A_1 phenotype has highest A antigens followed by A_2 phenotype and least in A_{el} phenotype. Comparison of A_1 and A_2 red cells with regard to nature and concentration of A antigens is depicted in the lower part of figure.

cells with human anti-A and anti-A,B. They result from mutant forms of the glycosyltransferases produced by the *A* gene. These mutant forms are less efficient at transferring *N*-acetyl-D-galactosamine onto H substance. The most common of these is A_3.

- **Weak or no agglutination with commercial anti-A reagents:** The decreased number of A antigen sites per red cell in these weak subgroups results in weak or no agglutination when tested with commercial anti-A monoclonal antibody reagents. This is a key factor in recognizing a subgroup in this category. Current anti-A, B monoclonal antibody reagents blend anti-A and anti-B clones and can detect the weaker subgroups.
- **Murine monoclonal blends:** Murine monoclonal blends of commercial anti-A can enhance the detection of some weaker subgroups in ABO phenotyping. Some subgroups (e.g. A_3 subgroup) may characteristically **demonstrate mixed-field agglutination patterns** with anti-A or anti-A,B reagents or possess anti-A_1 in the serum (e.g. A_3, A_x, and A_{el} subgroups). Mixed-field agglutination is a pattern of agglutination in which a population of the red cells has agglutinated and the remaining red cells remain unagglutinated.
- **Increased reactivity with *Ulex europaeus* (UEA):** Some subgroups of A may react weakly or not react even with murine monoclonal blends of anti-A. In such circumstances, saliva studies for the detection of soluble forms of A and H antigens and testing with anti-H lectin (*Ulex europaeus* plant lectin with specificity for the H antigen, i.e. anti-H) may provide additional information. The weak subgroups of A usually have amount of H antigen usually equivalent to group O red cells.
- **Special techniques of adsorption and elution:** They may also be required to demonstrate the presence of the A antigen (e.g. A_{el} subgroup). However, these techniques are not routinely done.
  - **Adsorption:** It is a **procedure which uses red cells (known antigens) to remove red cell antibodies** from a solution (plasma or antisera). Group A red cells can remove anti-A from solution.
  - **Elution:** It is a **procedure that dissociates antigen-antibody complexes on red cells.** The IgG antibody freed from the antigen-antibody complexes is tested for specificity.

Various techniques used to serologically differentiate weak A phenotypes are summarized in Box 3.1.

Various lectins used in blood banking are listed in Table 3.5.

> **Box. 3.1:** Various techniques used to serologically differentiate weak A phenotypes.
>
> - **Forward grouping** of A and H antigens with anti-A, anti-A, B, and anti-H
> - **Reverse grouping** of ABO isoagglutinins and the presence of anti-A_1
> - **Adsorption-elution tests** with anti-A
> - **Study of saliva** to detect the presence of A and H substances
> - **Additional special procedures:** (1) Molecular testing for mutations or (2) serum glycosyl-transferase studies for detecting the A enzyme.

Table 3.5: Lectins used in blood banking.

Lectins	Types of cells agglutinated
Dolichos biflorus	A_1 or A_1B cells
Bandeiraea simplicifolia	B cells
Ulex europaeus	O cells (H specificity) and other ABO blood groups depending on the amount of H antigen available
Vicia graminea	N
Iberis amara	M

Subgroups of B

Subgroups of B are very rare and much less frequent than A subgroups. They include B_3, B_m, B_x, B_{el}, and B_w. The criteria for the recognition and differentiation of these subgroups are similar to that of the A subgroups. They are usually recognized by variations in the strength of the reaction using anti-B and anti-A,B reagents.

Weak Phenotypes

In the ABO system, there are also several phenotypes associated with weakened, anomalous or complete absence of expression of ABO antigen. These include weak A and weak B phenotypes. They can cause ABO discrepancies during routine testing.

Weak ABO Phenotypes (Subtypes)

The ABO system contains several weak subtypes. Weak ABO subtypes are due to mutations at the *ABO* gene locus. All are characterized by reduced expression of A/B and a parallel increase in H-antigen expression. A_2, the most common weak A subtype. A_2 red cells possess 75% less A antigen than A_1 cells and can have an anti-A_1.

Anomalous ABO Expression

The ABO system also contains hybrid *ABO* alleles that can synthesize both A and B antigens.

It may be inherited (*cis*-AB, B[A]) or acquired (acquired B). The inherited (*cis*-AB, B[A]), and acquired B phenotypes are usually detected because of discrepancies during routine ABO typing.

- **Inherited:** The *cis*-AB and B(A) phenotypes are due to hybrid alleles and show characteristics of both A_1 and B gene. The cis-AB and B(A) individuals can synthesize both A and B antigens.
  - ***cis*-AB phenotype:** This is inherited as a single, autosomal dominant allele. In this, same enzymes are synthesized by both A and B antigens. In this, person carries both the *A* and *B* genes on the same chromosome. This rare occurrence is termed a ***cis-AB***. It results in the ability to genetically transmit both *A* and *B* genes to progeny. These individuals are typically A_2B with unusually weak expression of B and usually accompanied by alloanti-B.
  - **Inherited B(A) phenotype:** It is an autosomal dominant phenotype. In this, there is synthesis of A antigen by the *B* gene enzyme. This B(A) phenotype is a rare group B who has small/trace amount of A antigen expression on group B RBCs. This is detected when tested with certain anti-A monoclonal antibodies.
- **Acquired:**
  - **Acquired B phenotype:** It is an acquired enzymatic modification of group A_1 red cells in vivo. It usually occurs in the setting of bacterial infection or cancer, and due to enzymatic deacetylation of group A antigen to form a B-like antigen on RBCs.
  - **Acquisition of B antigen from bacterial infection:** Rarely individuals with group A may acquire B antigen from a

bacterial infection. Bacterial infection releases a deacetylase enzyme which converts N-acetyl-D-galactosamine into α-galactosamine, which is similar to galactose, the immunodominant sugar of group B. This may sometimes lead to interpretation of blood group as AB instead of A. If this group reported as AB (after the acquisition of B antigen) and is transfused with AB red cells, there is production of hyperimmune anti-B. It will result in a fatal hemolytic transfusion reaction. This was originally detected in patients with carcinoma of the gastrointestinal tract.

Importance of Subgroup Identification in Donor Testing

The subgroups of A and B are usually only of academic interest. However, failure to detect a weak subgroup can lead to serious consequences. Weak subtypes can cause **ABO typing discrepancies during serum grouping** because of the presence of unexpected anti-A or anti-B activity. On occasions, A/B expression is so weak that red cells may be misinterpreted as group O.

- **Missing a weak subgroup in a recipient:** If a recipient (the individual receiving the transfusion) has a weak subgroup and missed during ABO phenotyping, the recipient blood group will be reported as group O. Reporting weak subgroup as a group O probably **may not harm the recipient**. This is because for O group, only O red cells would be selected for transfusion and O red cells can be transfused to any ABO phenotype without any reactions.
- **Missing a weak subgroup in a donor:** If a donor with weak subgroup is reported as group O (rather than group A) during donor phenotyping, subsequently the donor unit will be erroneously labeled as group O (rather than group A). This may result in the **decreased survival of the transfused cells in a group O recipient's circulation**.

■ NULL PHENOTYPES

Two rare null phenotypes include (1) Bombay and (2) para-Bombay phenotypes/groups. They are characterized by an absence of all ABH antigens on RBCs and also loss of FUT1 activity. In the classic Bombay phenotype (Oh), neither AB nor H antigens are present on RBCs or in secretions. In para-Bombay, few or no ABH antigens are present on RBCs, but sometimes may show normal expression of ABH antigens in secretions and body fluids.

Bombay (Oh) Blood Group

- In 1952, Bhende, Bhatia and Deshpande from Bombay/Mubai, India discovered a new extremely rare blood group known as Bombay blood group (phenotype Oh).
- The classic Bombay phenotype is most frequently found in the children resulting from consanguineous marriages. Consanguineous marriages are marriages between people of close blood relationship, usually closer than third cousins.
- The (Oh) Bombay phenotype is inherited as an **autosomal recessive trait**. In the Oh Bombay phenotype, the individual is **homozygous for the inactive *h* allele** of *FUT1*. The molecular defect is most commonly due to **mutation in the gene *FUT1* (*H* gene)**. There is no normal expression of the ABH antigens because of the inheritance of the *hh* genotype. The ***hh* genotype does not produce of α-1,2-fucosyltransferase (H transferase) necessary to convert the ABO precursor substance to the H substance** (H antigen). This enzyme catalyzes the transfer of fucose in an α-1,2 linkage to the terminal galactose of the precursor molecule on RBCs forming the H antigen (Fig 3.6). Like the *O* gene, the *h* gene appears to be amorph and has no effect on precursor substance. These individuals lack the *H* gene and therefore L-fucose is not added to the basic precursor substance (type 2 chain). The basic precursor substance

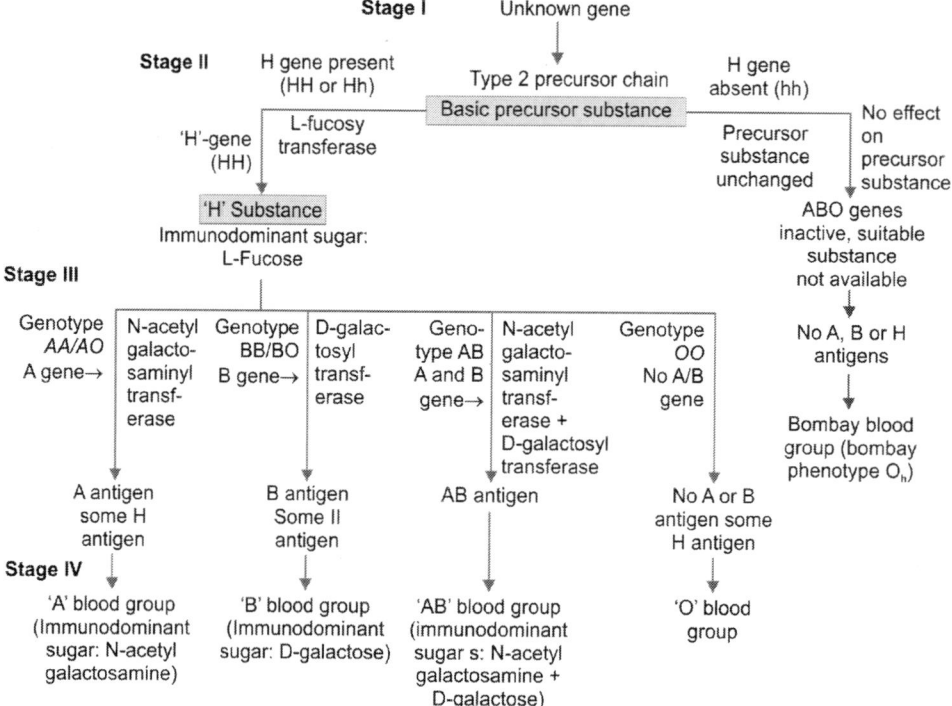

Fig. 3.6: Stages and interaction of the *Hh* and *ABO* genes in the production of ABO blood group and the role of *H* gene in the formation of A and B antigens.

cannot be converted into H substance. Hence, H substance is not expressed on the RBC. Even though Bombay (*hh*) individuals may inherit *ABO* genes, A, B, or H antigens do not form due to absence of H substance. This, in turn, results in failure to form A, B and H antigens and red cells lack these antigens.

- **Grouping:** When their blood sample is tested for routine ABO grouping, they will be **labeled as blood group O**. However, their serum/plasma contains anti-H in addition to anti-A, anti-B, and anti-A,B antibodies. When serum from the Oh is tested against group O red cells, after immediate-spin strong agglutination and/or hemolysis occurs. All these antibodies are active at 37°C. Therefore, these individuals with an Oh Bombay phenotype can only be safely transfused with only Bombay blood group (i.e. Oh red cells).
- The **mutation of *FUT1* (*H* gene)** in the Bombay phenotype is also associated with a silenced *FUT2* gene (*Se* gene), which codes a very similar α-1,2-fucosyltransferase and normally transfers a fucose to form H antigens in secretions. The classic Bombay phenotype is an **H-deficient nonsecretor (*hh, se/se*)**.
- **Confirmatory testing** is done using an **anti-H (lectin) reagent made from the *Ulex europaeus* plant**. RBCs of the **Bombay phenotype (Oh) do not react with the anti-H lectin** (*Ulex europaeus*), whereas **normal group O individual reacts strongly with anti-H lectin**.

Stages and interaction of the *Hh* and *ABO* genes in the production of ABO blood group and the role of *H* gene in the formation of A and B antigens are depicted in Figure 3.6. Salient features of the Bombay phenotype (Oh) are listed in Box 3.2.

Para-Bombay Blood Group

- The para-Bombay phenotypes are **rare phenotypes**. Their **red cells completely**

ABO Blood Group System

Box. 3.2: Salient features of the Bombay phenotype (Oh).

- *hh* genotype
- No formation of H, A and B antigens
- Absence of agglutination with anti-A, anti-B, or anti-H lectin
- Phenotypes as blood group O
- Serum contains anti-A, anti-B, anti-AB, and anti-H
- A, B, and H nonsecretors (no A, B, or H substances present in saliva)
- RBCs will not react with the anti-H lectin (*Ulex europaeus*)
- Absence of α-2-L-fucosyltransferase (H enzyme) in serum and H antigen on red cells
- Recessive mode of inheritance (identical phenotypes in children but not in parents)
- RBCs are compatible only with the serum from another Bombay individual. Hence, they can be transfused only with blood from another Bombay (Oh).

lack serologically detectable H antigen or have small amounts of H antigen.
- RBCs of these individuals **express weak forms** (small amounts) of **A and/or B antigen**. The expression of A and/or B antigen depends on the individual's genes at the ABO locus. If an individual is genetically A or B, the respective enzymes (products of respective gene) can be detected, but no H enzyme is detectable, even though there is small amount of production of H antigen on the RBC. The **terminology Ah and Bh** are used to describe these individuals. ABh individuals have also been reported.
- Probably in para-Bombay blood group, the homozygous inheritance of a mutant *H (FUT1)* gene produces low levels of H transferase. It produces small amount of H substance on the RBC and is completely used by the A or B transferase present. This results in production of small quantities of A or B antigen on the RBC with no detectable H antigen. The anti-H present in the serum is weaker in reactivity than the anti-H found in the Bombay phenotype.
- **Genetic basis for the para-Bombay:** The para-Bombay phenotype reflects the presence of **nonfunctional variant *H* gene but a normal *Se* gene**. They produce only small amount of H antigen. These products undergo conversion to A or B by the products of the *A* and *B* genes, respectively. **The serum of Ah and Bh individuals contains anti-H in addition to expected anti-A or anti-B.** The para-Bombay group may be due to a mutated *FUT1 (H gene)* with or without an active *FUT2* gene (*Se* gene) or a silenced *FUT1* gene with an active *FUT2* gene.
  - **Mutated *FUT1* gene para-Bombay:** The activity of encoded α-1,2-fucosyltransferase enzyme product of mutated *FUT1* gene is greatly reduced. This will produce very low amounts of H, A and B antigens. These antigens are serologically undetectable, but can be detected by using only adsorption and elution techniques with the appropriate reagents.
  - **Silenced *FUT1* gene with the active *FUT2* gene para-Bombay:** The α-1,2-fucosyltransferase enzyme associated with the active *FUT2* gene (α2FucT2) produces H, A, B, type 1 antigens in secretions (including plasma). The type 1 antigens present in plasma may adsorb onto the RBC membrane, yielding very weakly expressed H, A, and B antigens.
- **Test findings:** RBCs have little or no A, B, and H antigens. Tests with anti-A or anti-B will give weak reactions.
  - **Ah individuals:** Their serum contains anti-B and no anti-A, although anti-A_1 is usually present.
  - **Bh individuals:** Their serum always contains anti-A, and anti-B may be detected.
  - **Oh secretors:** Their RBCs are not agglutinated by most examples of anti-H but may be agglutinated by strong anti-H reagents.

BASIC GENETIC FEATURES OF ABO GROUP SYSTEM

Inheritance of genes from the *ABO locus* on chromosome 9 is inherited as per the Mendelian laws.

- The **three major alleles of the ABO** blood group system are **A, B, and O**. The A gene can be divided into the A_1 and A_2 alleles. Each individual inherits two ABO genes, one from each parent and these genes determine the ABO antigens on their RBCs.
- The **A and B genes** express a **codominant (equally dominant) mode of inheritance.** The O gene/allele is considered an amorph, as it does not produce any detectable antigen. Therefore, the group O phenotype is an autosomal recessive trait with the inheritance of two O genes that are nonfunctional. The A_1 allele is dominant over the A_2 allele, and both alleles are dominant over the O allele. O allele produces neither A nor B and therefore there is absence of both antigens, A and B on the red cells.
- **Correct terminology regarding the ABO blood group system:**
  - *Punnett square:* A Punnett square is a square diagram. Figure 3.9 depicts possible ABO blood group system gene combinations with Punnett squares.
  - **Phenotype and genotype:** The designations group A and B refer to phenotypes, whereas *AA, BO,* and *OO* denote genotypes. In the case of an individual with O group, both phenotype and genotype are the same, because that individual is homozygous for the *O* gene. An individual who has the phenotype A (or B) can have the genotype *AA or AO* (or *BB or BO*). The phenotype and genotype are the same in an AB individual because of the inheritance of both the *A* and *B* gene.
  - **In alleles—numbers should be superscript:** When reference is made to the alleles A^1 and A^2, the numbers should be always indicated as superscripts.
  - **In phenotypes—numbers should be subscript:** In references to the A_1 and A_2 phenotypes, the numbers should be always indicated in a subscript format.
- **Determination of genotype:** It is not possible to determine the genotype from the phenotype of an A or B individual by serological studies. Family studies or molecular assays are necessary to determine the exact genotype.

The major ABO phenotypes, antigens on their red cells, antibodies in plasma and possible corresponding genotypes for the phenotypes along with frequency in Indians are presented in Table 3.6.

A pedigree chart is a diagram that shows the occurrence and appearance of phenotypes of a particular gene. A pedigree chart with regard to ABO group is shown in Figure 3.7. Difference between phenotype and genotype of ABO system inheritance patterns is depicted in Figure 3.8.

Punnett Square

The Punnett square is a square diagram used to display the possible genotypes and phenotypes of the offspring from known genotypes of the parents. It is used to predict the genotypes and

Table 3.6: ABO blood group system.

Phenotype (blood group and subgroups)	Antigens on red cells	Antibodies in serum/plasma	Genotypes	Frequency in Indians
A				
A_1	$A+A_1$	Anti-B	$A^1/A^1, A^1/O, A^1/A^2$	3.16%
A_2	A	Sometimes (1–2%) anti-A_1	$A^2/A^2, A^2/O$	3%
B	B	Anti-A, anti-A_1	B/B or B/O	30%
AB				
A_1B	A, A_1 and B	None	A^1/B	9%
A_2B	A and B	Sometimes (25–30%) anti-A_1	A^2/B	1%
O	(H)+	Anti-A, anti-A_1, anti-B, and anti-A_1B	O/O	31%

possible combinations of maternal alleles with paternal alleles. Examination of family history is an important component in the investigation of inheritance patterns. Possible ABO blood group system gene combinations with Punnett squares are shown in Figure 3.9. For example, two group A parents can have a group O child and the parents of a group AB child can be group A, B, or AB but not group O.

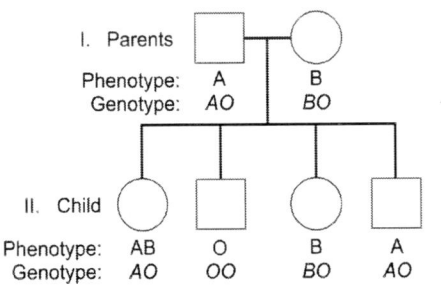

Fig. 3.7: Pedigree chart. In this illustration, parents are group A and group B phenotypes and their corresponding genotypes are *AO* and *BO*. They may produce children with group AB, O, B, and A phenotypes.

ABO/ABH ANTIBODIES

Natural ABO/ABH Antibodies

The ABH (ABO) system is unique in that it is the only blood group system in which there are naturally occurring antibodies in serum against missing ABH antigens

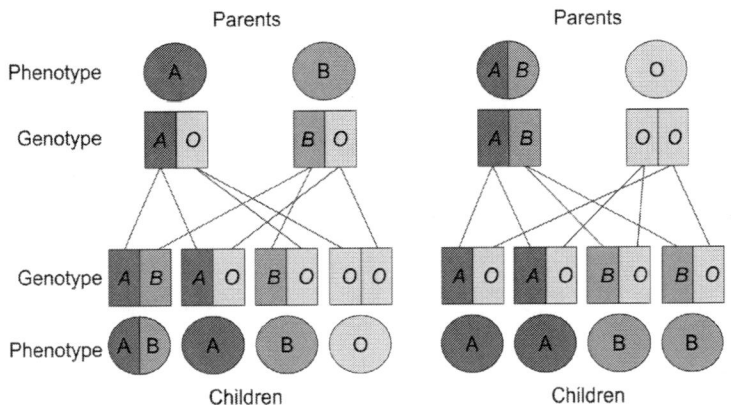

Fig. 3.8: Difference between phenotype and genotype of ABO system inheritance patterns.

	A	B
O	AO	BO
O	AO	BO

	A	B
A	AA	AB
B	AB	BB

	A	B
A	AA	AB
O	AO	BO

	A	B
B	AB	BB
O	AO	AA

	A	O
O	AO	OO
O	AO	OO

	A	O
A	AA	AO
O	AO	OO

	A	O
B	AB	BO
O	AO	OO

	A	A
B	AB	AB
B	AB	AB

	B	O
O	BO	OO
O	BO	OO

	A	O
B	AB	BO
O	AO	OO

	B	O
B	AB	AO
O	BO	OO

	B	B
O	BO	BO
O	BO	BO

Fig. 3.9: Punnett square showing ABO inheritance. First row of each square represents allele (separate column for each allele) of one parent and first column of each square represents allele (separate row for each allele) of another parent.

(Table 3.6). These natural antibodies are present in individuals who have not been previously transfused.

Naturally occurring antibodies: ABO antibodies were initially called naturally occurring because they were thought **to arise without antigenic stimulation**. However, presently they are believed to be stimulated by exposure to ABH antigen-like (ABO like) substances in the diet or the environment. There are bacteria, pollen particles, and other substances present in nature are chemically similar to A and B antigens. Bacteria are widespread in the environment and many bacterial species express ABH-like structures (i.e. A-like and B-like antigens) on lipopolysaccharide. These can cross-react with ABH antibodies and lectins. This exposure may be a source of stimulation of anti-A and anti-B. Thus, assumption that these so called "naturally occurring", antibodies develop without antigenic stimulation is incorrect. Consequently, the term naturally occurring is a misnomer because an immunologic stimulus is present for antibody development. The **term non-RBC stimulated is more appropriate for these ABO antibodies.**

Antibody development: Newborns do not produce their own ABO antibodies until they are 3–6 months of age. Hence, if ABO antibodies are detected before this time, they are maternal in origin. ABO antibodies appear in the blood at about 3 months after birth and gradually develop after 4–6 months of age. Their titer gradually increases and adult titers are reached by 5–10 years of life. Then they gradually become weaker as the age advances and may cause problems in ABO phenotyping. Various causes of reduction in ABO antibody titers are listed in Box 3.3. Their recognition can help in resolving ABO phenotyping problems in certain circumstances.

Types of Antibody

Anti-A, Anti-B and Anti-A,B

The types of antibody depend on the ABO group and its type is that antibody in which corresponding antigen/s is/are absent in

> **Box. 3.3:** Various causes of reduction in ABO antibody titers.
>
> **Physiological (age-related):**
> - Newborn
> - Elderly
>
> **Pathological:**
> - Congenital
>   - Congenital hypogammaglobulinemia
>   - Congenital agammaglobulinemia
> - Acquired
>   - Chronic lymphocytic leukemia
>   - Immunosuppressive therapy
>   - Bone marrow transplant
>   - Multiple myeloma
>   - Acquired hypogammaglobulinemia
>   - Acquired agammaglobulinemia

their red cells. These antibodies are against red cell A (anti-A)/B (anti-B)/A,B (anti-A,B) antigens (Table 3.6). Individuals of group A have anti-B, whereas anti-A will be found in group B individuals. If A is absent from an individual's red cells, anti-A agglutinins will be found in the serum, and if B is absent from and individual's red cells, the serum contains anti-B agglutinins.

Immunoglobulin class: The most important immunoglobulins in transfusion medicine are IgG and IgM. The titers of anti-A and anti-B can vary widely.

- **Anti-A and anti-B in A and B group:** The anti-A produced in group B individuals and the anti-B produced by group A individuals are mainly antibodies of the IgM class along with small amounts of IgG. The ABO antibodies are of **IgM type** and do not cross the placental barrier. Neonates may present the IgG type of ABO antibodies that have maternal origin, because IgG antibodies can cross the placenta. In adults, these antibodies are mostly IgM type although some may be IgG or IgA.
- **Anti-A and anti-B in O group:** The anti-A and anti-B antibodies of the serum of group O individuals are mainly of the **IgG class**. The IgG antibodies react at body temperature (37°C).

Temperatures and their reaction:
- **In vitro serologic reactions:** ABO antibodies directly agglutinate a suspension

of red cells in a physiologic saline environment and there is no need to add any additional potentiators. They are reactive at room temperature (15–25°C) and react immediately on centrifugation. The agglutination reactions do not require an incubation period.

- **Anti-A and anti-B** are usually immunoglobulin (Ig) M type. Usually IgM antibodies (except ***antibodies to ABO antigens***) react best at room temperature (20–22°C) or lower (to 4°C) and are usually not involved in the destruction of transfused red cells. The antibodies to ABO antigens are an important exception to this rule. IgM class antibodies to ABO antigens react in vitro at room temperature and in vivo at body temperature. Although they react best at low temperatures, IgM class antibodies to ABO antigens can cause lysis of red cells at 37°C.

Hemolytic properties: IgG and IgM forms of anti-A and anti-B are capable of the activation and binding of complement. This can result in hemolysis of red cells both in vivo or in vitro.

Relationship between ABO antigens located on RBCs and antibodies in plasma is depicted in Figure 3.10.

Less Common ABO Antibodies

Anti-A$_1$

Anti-A$_1$ is a naturally occurring antibody found occasionally (1–8%) in the serum of individuals with group A$_2$, not uncommonly (25–50%) in the serum of individuals with group A$_2$B and other weak A subtypes. **Anti-A$_1$ reacts only with A$_1$ and A$_1$B red cells, but not A$_2$ and other weak A phenotypes.** However, **normally anti-A1 acts as a cold agglutinin** and its reactive at 37°C is very rare. Although uncommon, anti-A$_1$ can cause transfusion reactions and solid organ rejection.

Anti-H

Anti-H antibodies are usually a **benign, naturally occurring antibody.** It can occur in **persons with little or no H antigen** on their red cells, i.e. **in the sera of A$_1$ and A$_1$B nonsecretors.** It **reacts most strongly with group O followed by A$_2$, B, A$_2$B, A$_1$, and A$_1$B red cells.** Because some degree of H antigen is present on all RBCs, anti-H is an autoantibody in most individuals. Normally, it also acts as a cold agglutinin (autoantibody). Only exception being occurrence of a very active anti-H alo-

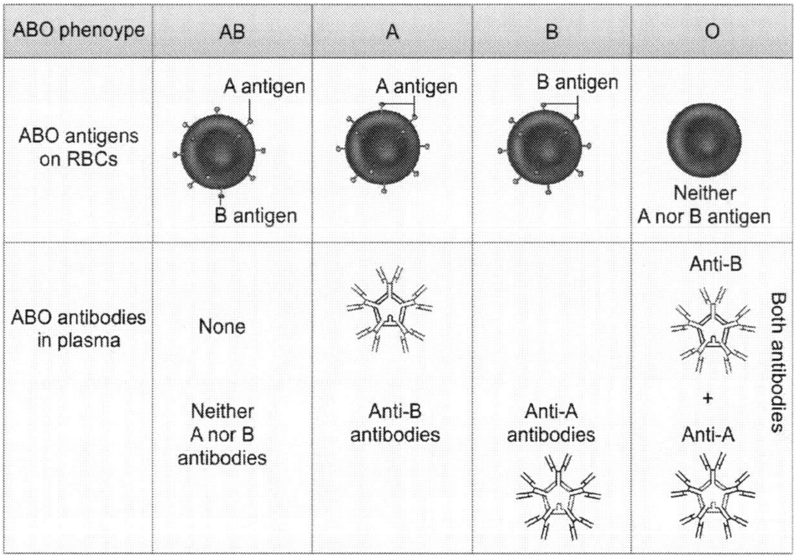

ABO phenoype	AB	A	B	O
ABO antigens on RBCs	A antigen / B antigen	A antigen	B antigen	Neither A nor B antigen
ABO antibodies in plasma	None / Neither A nor B antibodies	Anti-B antibodies	Anti-A antibodies	Anti-B + Anti-A / Both antibodies

Fig. 3.10: Relationship between ABO antigens located on RBCs and antibodies in plasma. Group AB RBCs have both A and B antigens but lack ABO antibodies in the plasma; group A RBCs have A antigens and have anti-B antibodies in plasma; group B RBCs have B antigens and have anti-A antibodies in plasma; group O RBCs lack both A and B antigens and have anti-A and anti-B antibodies in plasma.

antibody in the Oh Bombay phenotype (who lack the H gene and do not make H antigens), in which it is an IgM antibody. The **alloanti-H is a clinically significant alloantibody in Bombay (Oh) and para-Bombay individuals**. It binds complement and causes lysis of red cells (hemolysis) at 37°C. Thus, Oh Bombay phenotype needs Bombay blood for transfusion. A few individuals of group A or AB have anti-H, probably because almost all their H antigen has been converted to A or B. These anti-H antibodies usually do not react at body temperatures and do not cause hemolysis.

Acquired ABO Antibodies

The acquired antibodies are significant.

Hyperimmune Anti-A and Anti-B

An individual lacking a particular antigen may develop an antibody after (acquired) exposure to RBCs carrying the corresponding antigen. This is less frequent and causes immunization to A or B antigens producing **hyperimmune (high-titer antibodies) anti-A and anti-B**. Hyperimmune anti-A and anti-B occur **usually in response to exposure due to parenteral introduction of red cell antigens**. This may develop **during transfusion or pregnancy**.

- **Transfusion of incompatible red cells:** These acquired antibodies cause hemolytic transfusion reaction. It can occur in response to transfusion of incompatible red cells, transfusion of plasma containing soluble A or B antigens.
- **Pregnancy with an ABO-incompatible fetus:** Passage of fetal red cells (having paternal antigens foreign to the mother) into the maternal circulation during pregnancy may result in mainly IgG type of antibodies. These hyperimmune IgG anti-A and/or anti-B from group O or group A_2 mothers can cross the placenta barrier and cause hemolytic disease of the newborn (HDN). These antibodies react over a wide range of temperature and can produce more effective hemolysis than the naturally occurring antibodies. Group O donors should always be screened for high-titer anti-A and anti-B antibodies, which may cause hemolysis when group O platelets or plasma are transfused to recipients with A and B phenotypes. **The most important acquired *antibody* is anti-D**, which is a major cause of HDN.
- **Following injection/inoculation:** Very rarely, hyperimmune anti-A and anti-B may be formed following the injection/inoculation of some toxoids and vaccines containing A or B antigens. These are predominantly of IgG type/class. They are usually produced in individuals with O group and sometimes A_2 group.

Plasma-containing blood components prepared from such **high-titer universal donors** should be reserved for transfusion to recipients with O group.

Clinical Significance of ABO Antigens and Antibodies

Transfusion Medicine

The ABO blood group system (and its **ABO antigen**) is the **single most important** of all blood group system involved **in transfusion** of blood. In ABO blood group system, the only blood group system in which individuals have antibodies in their serum to antigens of ABO system that are absent (not present) from their own RBCs. These antibodies may be antibody anti-A and anti-B depending on the ABO blood group. These antibodies are found without any exposure to RBCs through transfusion or pregnancy. Hence, they are called as naturally occurring antibodies (refer page 55).

Hemolytic transfusion reactions

ABO antibodies are usually naturally occurring IgM type (though they may also have an IgG component). They have thermal activity at 37°C. The ability of ABO antibodies to activate the complement cascade with resultant hemolysis, they are of clinical significance in transfusion medicine. If blood is transfused without regard to ABO compatibility (i.e. incompatible ABO type), an antigen-antibody reaction can develop between a recipient's ABO antibody and the ABO phenotype of the transfused red cells. It can cause activation of complement and cause immediate, intravascular immune destruction of the transfused donor red cells *(hemolysis)* in the recipient possessing the corresponding antigen. The destruction of the red cells can cause very severe, transfusion reactions (dangerous/fatal immediate/acute HTR [hemolytic transfusion reaction]), anemia, and hemolytic disease of the fetus and newborn (HDFN). For example, a recipient of group A has circulating anti-B antibodies in serum. If this recipient is transfused with group B or AB donor red cells, the circulating anti-B would recognize the B antigen on the donor red cells and combine with the antigens. This antigen-antibody reaction will activate complement system causing a decreased survival of transfused red cells by causing hemolysis. Thus, testing to detect ABO incompatibility between a donor and potential transfusion recipient is the fundamental basis of all pretransfusion tests.

Hemolytic disease of the fetus and newborn (HDFN)

It is commonly also called as hemolytic disease of the newborn (HDN). **ABO antibodies seldom cause** HDFN but it is **usually mild**. The main reasons being:
- They are IgM type antibodies and **do not cross the placenta**.
- IgG ABO antibodies are often IgG2, which **do not activate complement or facilitate phagocytosis**.
- **ABO antigens are present on many fetal tissues and in body fluids**, so the hemolytic potential of the antibody is greatly reduced.

Transplantation

ABO antigens (epitopes) are also **expressed on many tissues and body fluids**. ABO antigens are important histocompatibility antigens expressed in **RBCs, platelets, most endothelial cells** and **epithelial membranes**. Because of their wide expressed, ABO antigens should be considered as a **major importance in solid organ and hematopoietic progenitor cell** (bone marrow) **transplantation**. The transplantation of ABO-incompatible solid organs increases the risk of hyperacute graft rejection. However, ABO-incompatible renal transplantation can be successfully carried out with plasmapheresis in addition to immunosuppression of the recipient. Major ABO-incompatible hematopoietic progenitor cell transplants (e.g. group A hematopoietic progenitor cells into a group O recipient) will cause hemolysis, unless the donation is depleted of RBCs.

For confirming the red cell phenotype

ABO antigens are useful for forward grouping and ABO antibodies are useful for reverse (serum/plasma) grouping (refer chapter 4 on pages 75, 76). Thus, they help in confirming the red cell phenotype.

Biological Role (ABO System and Disease)

The biological role of ABH antigens is not clear. Many studies have observed a higher incidence of many diseases according to ABO types. These include autoimmune, neoplastic, and infectious disorders.

ABO, Cancer and Possible Biological Role

- **Group A:** They have increased risk (1.2 times) of developing carcinoma of the stomach and pancreas than group O or B. The risk of the pancreatic cancer is found higher among A_1 than in A_2 subgroups of A type.
- **Group O:** Lung cancer in blood group O has higher mortality.
- **Weak expression of ABH antigens**—was found on the red cells of patients with leukemia.
- **Loss of A and B expression**—in lung, esophageal, and bladder cancers is associated with a poorer prognosis. Depression of A and B antigen expression can occur in malignancy and may be associated with increased risk of metastasis.

Predisposition to certain diseases

The inheritance of ABH antigens is also weakly associated with predisposition to certain diseases.
- **Group O:** They have increased risk (1.4 times) of developing peptic ulcer than non-group O (i.e. group A, B and AB) individuals.

- **Nonsecretors of ABH:** They have 1.5 times the risk of developing peptic ulcer than secretors.
- **ABO and coagulation:** There are a two-fold increased risk of venous thrombosis and pulmonary embolism in non-group O than O group individuals. There is also increased risk of coronary heart disease, increased low-density lipoprotein (LDL), and total cholesterol in nongroup O. It may be due to differences in circulating von Willebrand's factor (VWF), LDL, cholesterol, and P- and E-selectin.
- **Plasma levels of vWF and factor VIII:** ABO group also affects plasma vWF and factor VIII levels. Group O individuals have levels around 25% lower than those of other ABO groups. ABO blood group may accelerate the clearance of vWF.

ABO and malaria
ABO is considered a major host susceptibility factor in malaria. Blood group O provides a survival and reproductive advantage against malaria than non-group O. Group O may provide an advantage in parasite clearance. *Plasmodium falciparum* may bind A and B antigens with rosette formation which is a risk factor in cerebral malaria.

ABO and pathogens
- Group O is a receptor for many gastrointestinal pathogens. These include norovirus, rotavirus, *Helicobacter pylori*, *Campylobacter jejuni*, and *Vibrio cholerae* El Tor.
- Group O may be protective against some infections due to anti-A and anti-B. These infections include some enveloped viruses (HIV, SARS-CoV), schistosomiasis, *E. coli*, and other gram-negative organisms.

SUMMARY

- ABO and H group antigens are widely distributed in blood cells, tissues, body fluids and secretion. Biochemically, they may be glycolipids or glycoproteins. They have a common structure of type 1 or type 2 oligosaccharide chain.
- ABO blood group system has naturally occurring antibodies that are mainly belong to IgM class.
- ABO blood group system genes are located in the chromosome 9 and H system gene is located in the chromosome 19.
- ABO genes are inherited in a codominant manner. Major alleles of ABO group are A_1, A_2, B and O.
- ABH-soluble antigens are secreted by tissue cells and are found in all body secretions. The antigens secreted depend on the person's ABO group.
- ABO RBC antigens can be glycolipids, glycoproteins, or glycosphingolipids; ABO-secreted substances are glycoproteins.
- Glycoproteins in secretions are formed from type 1 precursor chains. The ABH antigens on RBCs are formed on type 2 precursor chains.
- N-acetylgalactosamine is the immunodominant sugar responsible for specificity of A antigen, D-galactose is the immunodominant sugar responsible for specificity of B antigen, and L-fucose is the immunodominant sugar responsible for specificity of H antigen.
- Major allele of H is H/H and H/h. The hh genotype is known as the Bombay phenotype or Oh. It has no expression of the ABO and H antigens.
- Individuals with O group have the greatest amount of H substance whereas group A_1B individuals contain the least amount of H substance.
- Serum of group A individuals has anti-B, group B individuals has anti-A, group AB individuals has neither anti-A nor anti-B and group O individuals contains both anti-A and anti-B.
- Majority of the individuals inherit the Se gene and are called as secretors. Their secretions and body fluids contain soluble H or ABO antigens, and the minority of individuals inherit the se gene and are called as nonsecretors. The Se gene codes for the production of L-fucosyltransferase.

SELF-ASSESSMENT EXERCISE

Write short notes on:
- Bombay blood group
- Bombay blood group and its significance in blood transfusion
- Para-Bombay blood group
- Secretors and nonsecretors
- Clinical significance of ABO antigens and antibodies
- Subgroups of A, AB and B

CHAPTER 4

ABO Blood Grouping: Methods and Discrepancies

CHAPTER OUTLINE

- Blood banking reagents
- ABO grouping/typing
- Methods of ABO grouping
- Alternative methods to the tube test
- Factors causing discrepancies during ABO testing
- ABO discrepancies, problem encountered and their solutions

BLOOD BANKING REAGENTS

Commercial antibodies and reagent red cells are used in the blood bank to detect antigen-antibody (Ag-Ab) reactions. These reagents help to provide safe and viable blood products. It is necessary for the blood bank technologists to know the correct usage of these reagents and also the limitations of each reagent. Technologists also should be competent enough to rapidly and accurately interpret the results from patient and donor testing. The reagents used in blood banking tests are discussed here. First the blood bank reagents used in testing to detect agglutination in test tubes are discussed followed by alternative methods in which the tubes are not used in the test.

Categories of reagents used in blood bank have been shown in Table 4.1.

Table 4.1: Categories of reagents used in blood bank.

Category	Content
Antisera	Known red cell antibodies
Antiglobulin reagents	Anti-IgG or anti-C3d or a combination of anti-IgG and anti-C3d
Potentiators	To enhance antibodies
Reagent red cells	Known red cell antigen phenotypes

There are many manufacturers of blood bank reagents. The routine blood bank reagents available commercially are shown in Figure 4.1.

The licensing of blood bank reagents: Commercial antisera and reagent red cell products are under regulations control. Before licensing the commercial reagent, the regulatory necessitates the minimum standards relating to product specificity and potency for use in blood banks and transfusion services.

- **Specificity** reflects the unique recognition of the antigenic determinant and its corresponding antibody molecule. For example, the specificity of the commercial anti-D should be such that it should react with red cells having D antigens and should not react with red cells without D antigens.
- **Potency** means the strength of an Ag-Ab reaction. For example, potent commercial anti-A reagents should produce strong agglutination (3+ to 4+) with red cells having the A antigen.

Reagent product insert: The manufacturer of reagent provides a package or product insert to the consumer along with the reagent. Thorough understanding of the product inserts is needed for proper use of blood bank reagents. The product insert (Box 4.1)

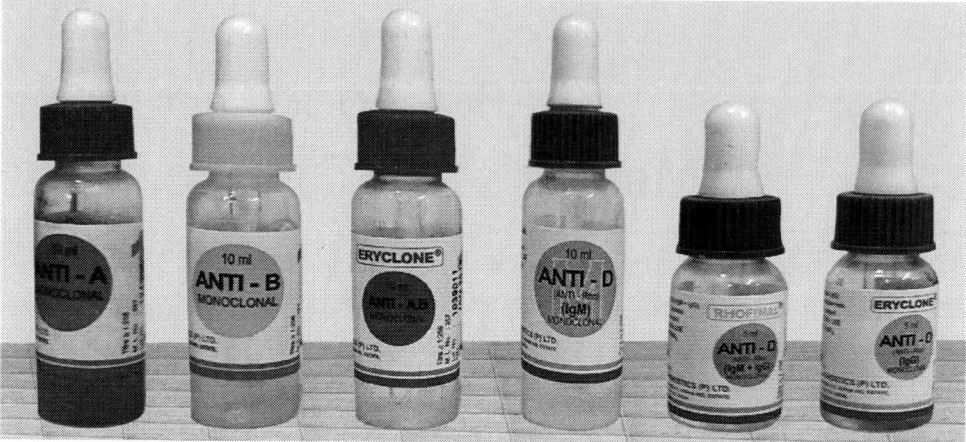

Fig. 4.1: Routine blood bank testing reagents (from left to right anti-A, anti-B, anti-A, B and anti-D [IgM, IgM+IgG and IgG]) *(For color version, see Plate 1).*

Box 4.1: Usual contents of reagent product insert.

- Description
- Intended use
- Principle
- Procedure for proper use
- Interpretations
- Performance characteristics
- Limitations of the reagent
- Quality control

describes in detail the intended use, summary, principle, procedure for proper use, the specific performance characteristics, and the limitations of the reagent. Standard operating procedures (SOPs) are written in the blood bank to reflect the procedures outlined in these product inserts. Whenever new reagent lots are received in the blood bank, the product inserts must be reviewed for any procedural changes. If there are any revisions, that must be incorporated into the SOPs before using the reagent in routine testing.

Quality control (refer Chapter 22): Reagents should be tested daily for performance. The results of quality control testing are recorded and reviewed. It is mandatory to maintain records of quality control testing that includes results, interpretations, date of testing, and the personnel who performed the test. If reagents do not meet performance criteria, appropriate corrective actions should be implemented.

- **Antisera:** They **should be clear** and should be inspected daily for any evidence of bacterial contamination. Any turbidity or cloudiness in the reagent bottles indicates contamination of the product.
- **Reagent red cells:** Inspect them for any evidence of hemolysis.

Commercial Antibody Reagents

Polyclonal versus Monoclonal Antibody Products (Fig. 4.2)

Ideally, an antibody reagent product should contain a concentrated suspension of highly specific, well characterized, uniformly reactive immunoglobulin/antibody molecules. Commercially available antibody reagents can be either polyclonal antibody-based or monoclonal antibody-based products.

- **Polyclonal antibody:** If multiple clones of B cells secrete antibodies in an immunologic response to a foreign antigen, the antiserum/antibody reagent produced is called polyclonal.
- **Monoclonal antibody:** If single clones of B cells secrete antibodies in an immunologic response to a foreign antigen, the antiserum/antibody reagent produced is called monoclonal.

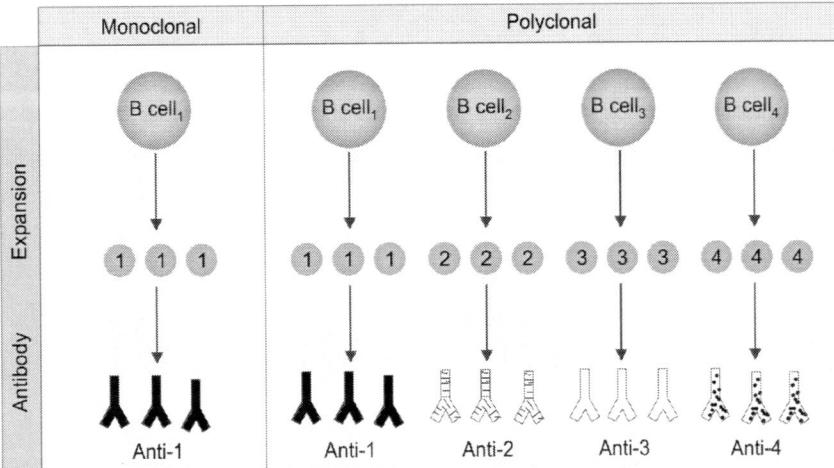

Fig. 4.2: Comparison of monoclonal versus polyclonal immune responses. In monoclonal immune responses, there is activation of single clone of B cells by the immune response and it secretes an antibody with one specificity (anti-1 in left part). In polyclonal immune responses, after exposure to the antigen, there is activation of multiple clones of B cells by the immune response and they secrete antibodies of different specificities. In the right part, these response to the antigen are named as anti-1, anti-2, anti-3, and anti-4. These were secreted by different clones of B-cell.

Polyclonal antibody reagents

In the early 1990s, the of monoclonal antibody-based blood banking reagents were introduced into transfusion medicine. Before this, commercial antisera used in blood bank were derived from polyclonal sources. These polygonal reagents were obtained from the immunization of animals and humans with purified antigens. The separation techniques used to produce the polyclonal antisera were time-consuming.

Polyclonal immune response: B cells produce antibodies that are specific for the multiple epitopes of the injected antigen. This produces a heterogeneous population of antibodies which can recognize different epitopes (epitopes are single antigenic determinants; functionally, parts of the antigen that combine with the antibody) on a single antigen. Polyclonal antiserum is prepared from several different clones of B cells that secrete antibodies of different specificities. Examples for polyclonal antiserum used in blood bank are antihuman globulin (AHG) reagents. Polyclonal antihuman immunoglobulin G (IgG) serum is produced by immunizing rabbits with purified human IgG molecules. This activates multiple clones of B cell in rabbits. Each clone of B cell produces an antibody directed at a specific epitope of the IgG molecule. The combination of the multiple clones of B cell secreting many antibodies in the rabbit serum makes a polyclonal antibody reagent (Fig. 4.2). (For details refer Chapter 9 page 175)

Monoclonal antibody reagents

Monoclonal antibodies are the products of a single clone of B cells that secrete antibodies of the same specificity. The monoclonal antibody technique is useful in producing high-titer antibodies with well-defined specificities. Monoclonal antibodies are produced by an immortal clone that manufactures antibodies of a defined specificity (Fig. 4.2). In vitro, the monoclonal antibodies are produced using hybridoma technology.

Hybridoma technology (Fig. 4.3): Hybridomas are hybrid cells formed by the fusion of myeloma cells and antibody-producing B lymphocytes and are used in the production of monoclonal antibodies. Monoclonal antibody is produced by immunizing the laboratory

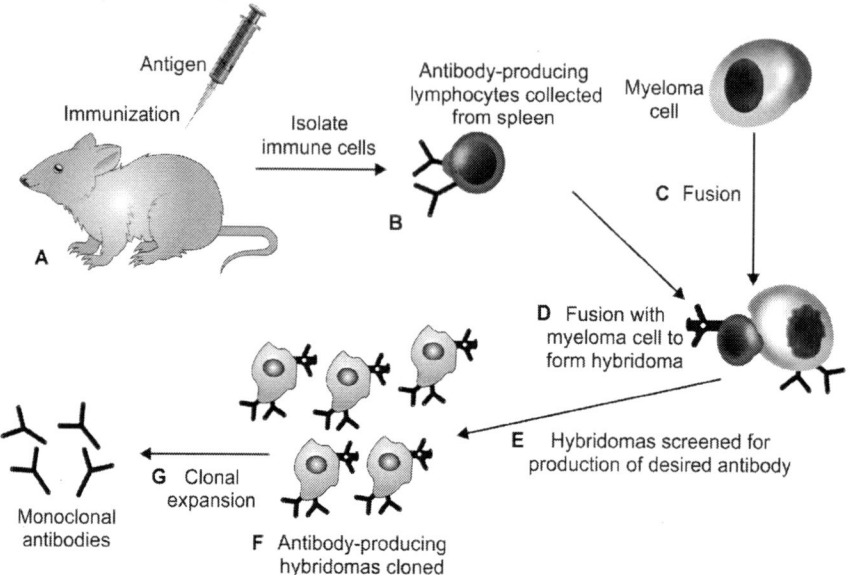

Fig. 4.3: Method of production of monoclonal murine antibody. Monoclonal antibodies are the products of a single clone of B lymphocytes. (A) **Immunization:** First mice are immunized with antigen. (B) **Harvesting:** The spleen B lymphocytes of mice are harvested. (C) **Fusion:** The antibody-forming B lymphocytes are fused with a myeloma cell from a mouse. (D) **Hybrid cells (hybridomas):** The resulting hybrid cells are cultured. (E) **Screening:** The hybridomas are screened for the production of desired antibody. (F) **Cloning:** Each hybridoma is descended from a single B cell clone. (G) **Monoclonal antibodies:** The hybridoma cell line is expanded and they produce the same antibody molecule.

animals, usually mice, with antigen. After a suitable immune response, antibody-secreting lymphocytes are obtained from spleen of the mice immunized with antigen. These antibody-secreting lymphocytes (B lymphocytes) from spleen are harvested and are fused with myeloma cells (i.e. abnormal cell from a mouse that has malignant tumor of plasma cells called myeloma). This results in fused hybrid cells called as "hybridomas". Each hybridoma is descended from a single clone of B cell. The hybridoma cells are propagated in tissue culture and they grow rapidly. They are screened for the production of antibody of required specificity and affinity. All cells of the hybridoma cell line produce the same antibody molecule, called a monoclonal antibody. These antibodies are identical in terms of antibody structure and antigen specificity. In contrast to polyclonal antibodies, monoclonal antibodies recognize one specific epitope of the antigen. In routine blood typing, murine (mouse) monoclonal antibodies have replaced polyclonal reagents for A and B antigens and complement proteins.

Human B lymphocytes transformed with Epstein-Barr virus (EBV): Human monoclonal antibodies also can be produced with blood group specificity. For this, human B lymphocytes are transformed with EBV. These transformed cells are grown in tissue culture and they secrete monoclonal antibodies. It was first derived by using B lymphocytes from D-immunized donors. Both IgG and IgM anti-D were obtained from the EBV-transformed cells.

Heterohybridomas: These are hybrid cells formed by the fusion of B lymphocyte of one species with the myeloma cell of a different species. Heterohybridoma is another method for the production of stable lines of human monoclonal antibodies. In this method, human B lymphocytes are fused with murine myeloma cells which form heterohybridomas. A number of human monoclonal antibodies are now available in the market for use in blood typing.

Use of monoclonal antibody-based reagents in blood bank in place of polyclonal antibody-based reagents has increased the accuracy and there is no need to depend on reagents prepared from human blood donated by volunteers. The approved monoclonal antibodies available for use in blood bank include anti-A, anti-B, anti-A,B, anti-D, anti-C, anti-E, anti-c, anti-e, anti-IgG, anti-C3b, anti-C3d. Desired monoclonal antibody reagents can be produced in large quantities with lot-to-lot consistency of a single specificity.

Disadvantage of monoclonal antibody reagents: In routine testing, discrepant reactions may be observed between human- or animal-source reagents and the monoclonal antibody reagents.

Differences between monoclonal and polyclonal antibody are presented in Table 4.2.

Monoclonal and polyclonal antibody reagents
Blending of monoclonal and polyclonal antibodies produces reagents with specific advantages in blood bank testing. Examples of monoclonal and polyclonal blend antibodies are antiglobulin reagents (discussed in Chapter 9 page 174) in which there is a combination of rabbit polyclonal antibodies and a murine (mouse) monoclonal antibody.

Reagents for ABO antigen typing are discussed on pages 70, 71. Reagents for D antigen typing are discussed in Chapter 5 on pages 105-6.

Low-Protein Reagent Control

To ensure that the ABO and Rh typing results were interpreted correctly, a reagent control is used. The reagent control should not show any agglutination (a negative result). The ABO and D typing reagents are produced with protein concentrations similar to human serum (approximately 6% bovine albumin).

- **Spontaneous agglutination** of red cells occurs less frequently at this low-protein concentration than with **reagents containing higher concentrations of protein**.
- **False-positive result during typing:** It can be due to (1) spontaneous agglutination of red cells during typing and (2) if blood specimen contains strong cold autoantibodies (antibodies to self-antigens) or has protein abnormalities.
- **Reagent control:**
  - **No need of reagent control:** A negative result using ABO low-protein reagents can act as a reagent control. An additional reagent control in ABO and D typing is **not needed when the patient or donor red cells show no agglutination with anti-A, anti-B, or anti-D in red cell testing.**
  - **Need for reagent control:** A reagent control is needed to interpret the results, **if red cells are agglutinated with anti-A, anti-B, and anti-D**. The reagent control should be performed according to the reagent manufacturer, example of which is presented in Table 4.3.

Reagent red cells: A_1 and B red cells for ABO serum testing (discussed on page 71)

Screening cells (discussed in Chapter 10 on page 191)

Antibody identification panel cells (discussed in Chapter 10 on page 198)

Antiglobulin reagents (discussed in Chapter 9 on page 174)

Table 4.2: Differences between monoclonal and polyclonal antibody.

	Monoclonal antibody	Polyclonal antibody
Production/secretion by clone of B lymphocytes	Production by a single clone of antibody-producing B lymphocytes	Production by several different clones of antibody-producing B lymphocytes
Immunoglobulins secreted	Single immunoglobulin class (IgG or IgM)	Mixture of IgM and IgG antibodies
Features of immunoglobulin	Unique specificity for a particular epitope	Mixture of antibodies that may be directed at different epitopes of the same antigen

Table 4.3: Example of situation where low-protein reagent control is necessary.

Reaction with			Red cell antigens present	Interpretation	Reagent control
Anti-A	Anti-B	Anti-D			
+	0	+	A and D	No agglutination with anti-B	Not needed
0	+	0	B	No agglutination with anti-A	Not needed
0	+	+	B and D	No agglutination with anti-A	Not needed
+	+	0	A and B	No agglutination with anti-D	Not needed
+	+	+	Typing cannot be interpreted	Agglutination with anti-A, anti-B and anti-D	Reagent control needed to determine the ABO and D typing

(+: agglutination, 0: no agglutination)

Antibody Potentiators or Enhancement Media/Reagents

Red blood cells (RBCs) have a negative charge at this surface which makes RBCs to repel each other. This natural repulsive force which holds the RBC apart is called zeta potential (refer page 14 of Chapter 1). This is protective and keeps RBCs from adhering to each other in the peripheral blood. In a physiologic saline solution, the zeta potential or the force of repulsion between red cells influences the agglutination reaction.

- **IgM antibody molecules** are larger in size, pentameric in shape (refer Fig. 1.3), and have multivalent properties. The **agglutination is facilitated** when the red blood cells have attached **IgM antibodies** and IgM antibodies can easily react in a saline medium.
- **IgG antibody molecules** are smaller in size (refer Fig. 1.4) and less able to span the distance between adjacent red cells generated by the zeta potential. IgG molecules may attach to red cells, but **visible agglutination may not be produced.**

The test methods in transfusion medicine use serum or plasma and red cells (either red cells provided by the manufacturer or saline-suspended red cells). To increase the sensitivity of the test methods/system, various enhancement reagents, or potentiators may be used. These enhancement reagents are commercially available which enhance or speed up the antibody-antigen reaction (Ag-Ab complex formation) in routine tests. They **help in the detection of IgG antibodies by increasing their reactivity**. Enhancement media can reduce the zeta potential of the red cell membrane (Fig. 4.4) in vitro test and promote agglutination. They may enhance antibody uptake (first stage of agglutination) or promote direct agglutination (second stage of agglutination), or serve both functions. They are added to the cell/serum mixture before the 37°C incubation phase. These reagents shorten the incubation time.

Types of potentiators: The major types of potentiators used in the blood bank laboratory are low ionic strength saline (LISS), polyethylene glycol (PEG), and proteolytic enzymes (ficin and papain).

Uses of potentiators: They are commonly used in both antibody screening and identification procedures. They increase the speed and sensitivity of the antibody attachment to the red cell antigen.

Low Ionic Strength Solution (LISS)

The incubation of serum and red cells in a reduced/lower ionic environment **increases the rate of binding of antibody to specific antigen receptor sites on red cells**. In physiologic saline, sodium and chloride ions cluster around the antigen and antibody molecules. Formation of Ag-Ab complex is influenced by the attraction of opposite charges. The clustering of sodium and chloride

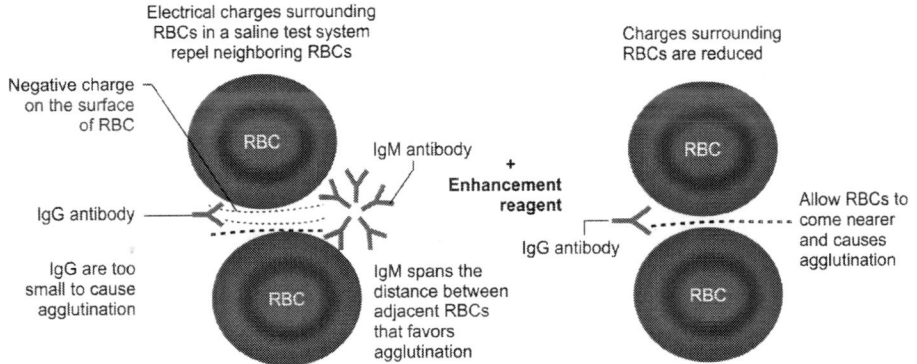

Fig. 4.4: Addition of enhancement reagents can lower the zeta potential and allows better interaction between RBCs and increasing the possibility of agglutination.

ions around Ag and Ab hinders the Ag-Ab complex formation. If the ionic strength is reduced/lowered, the antigen and antibody molecules can combine at a faster rate. The advantage of LISS is that it **increases the antibody uptake and reduces the incubation time and time needed for the result**. LISS reagent **contains sodium chloride, glycine and salt-poor albumin** (approximately 0.03 M) ionic strength compared with saline (approximately 0.17 M). It is formulated to prevent hemolysis of red cells, which is a concern when using LISS. It not only lowers the zeta potential, but also increases the uptake of antibody onto the RBC during the sensitization phase. This increases the possibility of agglutination.

Uses of LISS: It may be used to suspend test red cells for use in tube or column agglutination tests or as an additive medium for tube or solid phase tests. The LISS is **used mainly to enhance antibody uptake and improve detection at antiglobulin phases of testing**, with the antibody screen (speeds the agglutination, economical, and provides good sensitivity).

Disadvantages of LISS: These include (1) increasing serum in the test alters the ionic strength of a LISS procedure, decreasing the sensitivity of the test system and (2) enhances the cold autoantibodies (especially if the tubes are centrifuged at immediate-spin and microscopic evaluations).

Polyethylene Glycol

PEG is **water-soluble polymer** and **used as an additive in a low ionic saline medium**. In LISS solution, the **PEG removes water molecules** from the test system/environment and **allows a greater probability of collision between antigen and antibody molecules**. Thus, it effectively concentrates antibody in the test mixture, while creating a low ionic environment that enhances the rate of antibody uptake. This will concentrate any antibodies present, thereby increases the degree of RBC sensitization. Usually, PEG test systems are more sensitive than LISS, albumin, or saline systems. However, in patients with raised levels of plasma protein (e.g. multiple myeloma), PEG is **not used due to increased precipitation of proteins**. LISS and PEG enhance autoantibodies. Hence, their use in the blood samples containing both autoantibodies and alloantibodies makes their identification difficult.

Uses

- Polyethylene glycol can directly affect the aggregation of red cells. Hence, it can be **used only in indirect antiglobulin testing** (IAT) where it increases the sensitivity. Since, PEG can cause nonspecific aggregation of cells, the tubes used in the test should not be centrifuged after the 37°C incubation and they should be read before washing. Only monospecific anti-

IgG AHG reagent is suitable for use with PEG because polyspecific AHG reagents can cause nonspecific agglutination.
- Polyethylene glycol **increases the sensitivity of antibody detection and identification.** It often detects the antibodies which are not detected using bovine serum albumin (BSA) or LISS.

Antibodies usually considered as of little clinical significance (IgM type) and do not react well or at all with PEG. PEG can enhance warm autoantibodies.

Enzymes

Proteolytic enzymes are enzymes that **breakdown/denature certain protein molecules. Commonly used** proteolytic enzymes in the immunohematology laboratory that are commercially available are **papain, ficin, and bromelain.** Proteolytic enzymes originate from plants—ficin comes from figs, bromelain used in solid-phase red cell adherence assay (refer page 82) from pineapple, and papain from papaya. These enzymes can **remove the negatively charged molecules from the red cell membrane** and denature certain antigenic determinants. The loss of these negatively charged molecules from the red cell membrane reduces the zeta potential and **enhances the agglutination** of some antigens to their corresponding antibodies. Depending on the red cell antibody, the enzymes used in testing may enhance, depress, or inhibit entirely the Ag-Ab complex formation. Hence, it is necessary to have a good knowledge of the blood group systems in the interpretation of these enzyme tests.
- In Rh, Kidd, and Lewis blood group systems, the enzymes enhance the reaction.
- In red cell antigens such as M, N, S, Xga, Fya, and Fy, the proteolytic enzymes denature the red cell antigens.

Uses: Proteolytic enzymes (ficin or papain) are usually not used as potentiators in the antibody screen because they remove/eliminate some antigens from the red cells. They should not be used as the sole method in antibody screening. However, these enzymes **can be used as additional tools for investigating complex antibody problems.** In a mixture of antibodies, enzymes may enhance the reactions of one antibody or abolish the reactions of another antibody. Thus, it may provide important information in the solution of the problem. **Enzymes enhance cold and warm autoantibodies.**

Bovine Serum Albumin (BSA)

BSA is prepared from bovine serum or plasma. It is available commercially either in 22% or 30% concentration. It is **less commonly used** as a potentiator than other enhancement media. LISS influences both the stages of agglutination (refer page 11 of Chapter 1). In contrast, BSA influences the second stage of agglutination by allowing antibody-sensitized RBCs to come nearer to each other than in a saline medium without additives. BSA's enhancement action is by reducing the zeta potential and disperses the charges.
- **Enhances the sensitivity of the IAT:** The addition of BSA to reaction tubes causes the direct agglutination of Rh antibodies and increases the sensitivity of the IAT (indirect antiglobulin test) for a wide range of antibody specificities. For better results, incubation time may be increased.
- **No enhancement of warm autoantibodies:** BSA does not enhance warm autoantibodies. Thus, it is useful when dealing samples from patients with autoantibodies in their serum.
- **Reduces the repulsion between red cells:** BSA reduces the repulsion between red cells. However, it does not reduce the required incubation time.

Various mechanisms of antibody potentiators are mentioned in Table 4.4.

Lectins

Lectins were first discovered as plant seed extracts but were also found in bacteria to mammals. They are **useful as blood banking reagents because of their specificity toward certain red cell antigens.** Lectins are **used as alternatives to antisera for**

Table 4.4: Mechanism of antibody potentiators.

Type of antibody potentiator	Mechanism of action
Low ionic strength saline (LISS)	Rate of antibody uptake is increased
Polyethylene glycol (PEG)	Concentrates the antibody in the test environment in LISS
Proteolytic enzymes (papain and ficin)	Removes negative charges from the red cell membrane thereby reduces the zeta potential. Denatures some red cell antigens
Bovine serum albumin (BSA)	Reduces the repulsion between cells but the incubation time is not shortened

blood typing. Lectins are sugar-binding proteins of nonimmune origin. They behave **similar to that of antibodies but they are not immunoglobulin** (antibodies) in nature. For example, a lectin from the eel (a snake-like, catadromous fish) *Anguilla anguilla is* a useful anti-H reagent. Lectins bind specifically to the carbohydrate portions/determinants of certain red cell antigens and cause red cells agglutination. Although it does not produce antibodies, they can be used for identifying antigens present on patient or donor red cells. Refer Table 3.5 for the major lectins used in blood group serology.

ABO GROUPING/TYPING

It is advisable to use fully automated systems (where possible) for blood grouping to reduce the risks of interpretation and transcription errors. Blood grouping must be done by a validated technique using appropriate controls. All new batches of grouping reagents must be checked for reliability by the techniques used in the laboratory. Grouping reagents must be stored as per the manufacturer's instructions.

ABO grouping is the single most important serological test done in blood bank during compatibility testing. Hence, it is necessary that there should not be any compromise in the sensitivity and security of the test system. When the **ABO group** of an individual is to be determined, **it is necessary to do both cell grouping and serum grouping**. The naturally occurring antibodies namely anti-A and anti-B in the plasma should be tested against known A and B cells. This process is called "reverse" grouping (refer pages 75, 76). This acts as an excellent built-in check.

Landsteiner's Rule (Law)

It exists **only in the ABO system**.
- **Corresponding antigens and antibodies cannot normally coexist in the same individual's RBCs**.
  - Individuals with group A have A antigen on their RBCs will not normally have anti-A antibodies in their serum.
  - Individuals with group B have B antigen on their RBCs will not normally have anti-B antibodies in their serum.
  - Individuals with group AB with AB antigens on their RBCs will not normally have anti-A and anti-B antibodies in their serum.
- In the ABO system (unlike other blood group systems), **if an individual lacks A or B antigen on the red cell, the corresponding antibody will be found in the serum**. These are the so-called isoantibodies (naturally occurring) usually of IgM type. These antibodies are capable of causing intravascular hemolysis if incompatible blood is transfused.
  - Adults lacking group A antigen will have anti-A antibody in their sera.
  - Adults lacking group B antigen will have anti-B antibody in their sera.
  - Adults lacking group both A and B antigen (O group) will have anti-A or anti-B antibody.

Grouping Procedures

ABO typing procedures consist of two parts:
1. **Forward typing/grouping** (red cell grouping or front type) is defined as **using known sources of commercial antisera** (anti-A, anti-B) **to detect antigens on**

an individual's RBCs. In this technique, undetermined (unknown) test RBCs (antigen) is typed against known potent and specific antibody or antisera (namely specific anti-A and anti-B).
2. **Reverse typing/grouping** (serum grouping or back type) is defined as **detecting ABO antibodies in the patient's serum by using known reagent RBCs**, namely A_1 and B cells. In this technique, the undetermined/unknown (patient or donor) serum is tested against known group RBC antigens (namely A_1 and group B red cells). It is used to test for the expected ABO antibodies in the patient's serum.

The manufacturer's instructions must be followed for all commercial reagents. Both forward and reverse typing results must match to confirm the true ABO type of an individual. This is an excellent way to guard against errors in ABO grouping. Any discrepancy between the forward and reverse groups should be investigated further.

Interpretation of results of ABO blood grouping is presented in Table 4.5.

Reagents for ABO Antigen Typing/Blood Grouping

Monoclonal ABO Antibody Reagents

- ABO antibody reagents needed for ABO typing include monoclonal anti-A, anti-B and anti-A,B (ABO antibody). These commercial antisera reagents contain monoclonal antibodies obtained from cultures of cells secreting antibodies called hybridomas (refer pages 63, 64).
- Before this technology, polygonal ABO grouping reagents were used that are obtained from human donors with or without deliberate immunization.
- The advantages of monoclonal ABO reagents over polyclonal reagents include: (1) more specific, (2) more potent, (3) more batch to batch consistency, (4) absence of nonspecific antibodies, and (5) free from viruses (e.g. HIV and hepatitis virus).
- Anti-A and anti-B reagents are used to determine whether an individual's red cells have the A and B antigens of the ABO blood group system. These reagent ABO antibodies are suspended in a diluent with a concentration not exceed a 6% bovine albumin concentration and is considered a low-protein medium.
- ABO monoclonal antibody reagents are prepared in such a manner that they produce strong reactions with antigen-positive red cells and can detect weak expressions of the A and B antigens. The anti-A and anti-B red cell typing reagents produce strong agglutination (refer Table 1.4) reactions (3+ to 4+) for most antigen-positive red cells.
- Test is performed in immediate-spin phases (refer page 74) and it is recommended that test should be confirmed by checking for expected ABO antibodies using reagent red cells. In immediate-spin phases, the source antigen and source antibody used in immunohematologic testing are combined. It is immediately centrifuged, and observed for agglutination.
- **Coloring dyes for reagents:** Dyes were added to these ABO antibody reagents in order to reduce potential errors in testing.
  – Anti-A always contains a blue dye
  – Anti-B contains a yellow dye

Table 4.5: Interpretation of results of ABO blood grouping.				
Forward typing (red cell grouping)		Interpretation of ABO group	Reverse typing (red cell grouping)	
Anti-A	Anti-B		A_1 cells	B cells
++++	–ve	A	–ve	++++
–ve	++++	B	++++	–ve
++++	++++	AB	–ve	–ve
–ve	–ve	O	++++	++++

- Anti-A,B is a blending of clones for A and B antigen recognition and the reagent is clear.
- **Reagent labels:** ABO typing reagents are labeled with the antibody specificity and specify how it can be used. For example, a reagent bottle of anti-A may contain the phrase "**for slide, tube, and microplate testing**".
- **Product insert:** The detailed methods are provided in the product insert.

Known ABO Blood Group Red Cells

A_1 and B cells are used for reverse grouping; group O cells or an "autocontrol" may be included to ensure that reactions with A and B cells are not due to the presence of cold autoantibodies. Known red cells used in ABO grouping are obtained from pooled A cells, B cells, and O cells. The red cells are washed in saline to remove serum, plasma, hemolyzed cells and small clots which may give rise to false-positive reactions. The supernatant of final wash in saline should be clear. A 2–4% red cell suspension for tube, microplate typing techniques and 30–40% for slide technique is used. A diluent control should be included where recommended by the manufacturer.

Supplementary Reagents

With routine use of monoclonal reagents for blood grouping, the necessity of some of supplementary reagents has been reduced. The supplementary reagents are mainly used for testing the suspected subgroups. The main supplementary reagents used in ABO grouping include: anti-A_1 lectin, anti-H, monoclonal anti-A, and anti-B. Anti-A,B may be used to distinguish O group from A subgroups.
- **Anti-A_1 lectin (Fig. 4.5):** It is obtained from seeds of *Dolichos biflorus*. It reacts strongly only with A_1 (even if found in small quantities) individuals and is **used to differentiate between A_1 and A_2 subgroups**.
- **Anti-H (Fig. 4.5):** It reacts selectively with ABO group individuals with H substance. **Group O individuals** which contain only H **react strongly with anti-H**, whereas a

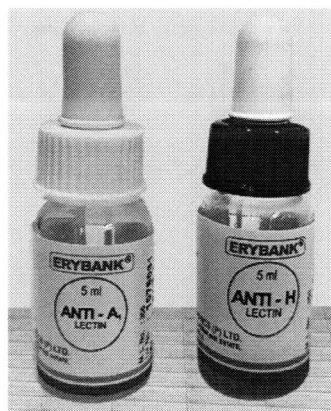

Fig. 4.5: Anti-A_1 lectin and anti-H reagents.

group A_1B individual contains very little H and thus reacts very weakly or negatively with anti-H.
- **Group "O" reagent screen cells:** They consist of two or three group O red cells with various antigen specificities. They are used in some donors **to detect antibodies other than anti-A or anti-B**. These antibodies do not occur naturally and are termed as **irregular antibodies**. They occur due to immunization either by prior transfusion or pregnancy. They help on ruling out ABO typing discrepancy caused by cold antibodies.
- **Group A_2 and group A_2B red cells:** These may be used to resolve discrepancies of ABO groping. A_2 red cells are used when suspected A subgroup has develops anti-A_1. Agglutination of reagent A_1 cells by patient serum, but without agglutination of A_2 cells suggests presence of anti-A_1.

METHODS OF ABO GROUPING

In ABO grouping technique (method or procedures), donor or patient red blood cells (unknown antigen) are combined with commercial antisera (known antibodies) and observed for the presence or absence of agglutination. Presence of agglutination indicates the presence of corresponding antigen and absence of agglutination indicates the absence of corresponding antigen on the red cells tested (Tables 4.5 and 4.6).

Table 4.6: Interpretation of ABO grouping.

Reaction with antisera added			Interpretation
Anti-A	Anti-B	Anti-A,B	ABO blood group antigen and phenotype
0	0	0	O
+	0	+	A
0	+	+	B
+	+	+	AB

(+: agglutination; 0: no agglutination)

Box 4.2: Various methods for ABO blood grouping.

- Manual methods
  - Traditional methods: Slide or tile technique
  - Tube technique
  - Microplate method
  - Column agglutination technique
    - Gel technology (ID Micro Typing System)
    - Glass microbead technology
  - Solid phase red cell adherence assay
  - Erythrocytes magnetized technology
- Automated or semiautomated method
- Molecular blood grouping and genotyping

The **procedure to determine ABO blood group system is called as ABO grouping**, ABO forward grouping, front typing, and ABO red cell testing. The Technical Manual of the AABB refers the procedure to the determination of an individual's ABO blood group as ABO typing (phenotype) and not an ABO grouping. However, many other references retain the terminology of ABO grouping and the FDA name for these reagents remains ABO grouping reagents.

Methods: Different methods available for routine ABO blood grouping are listed in Box 4.2. It is necessary to use the appropriate reagent, because not all reagents have been validated by the manufacturer for all techniques. Molecular techniques for ABO blood grouping are not used routinely since serology is superior, quicker, cheaper and accurate.

Forward Typing/Grouping

The basic principles of all the methods are same (except molecular blood grouping and genotyping). They are always performed at room temperature and agglutination is observed against well-lighted background. ABO grouping is carried out by making a 2% saline suspension of red cells and adding anti-A, anti-B, and anti-A,B sera. The slide and tube techniques are described here.

Slide or Tile Technique

Slide or tile grouping is **not very sensitive method**. It is performed only for emergency ABO grouping especially in outdoor blood camps and **used in under-resourced or developing countries**. The technique is satisfactory if potent grouping reagents are used.

Disadvantages: (1) Insensitive, (2) cannot detect weak antigens in forward typing and low-titer antibodies in reverse typing, (3) it dries up due to evaporation (hence must be read within about 5 minutes) and (4) needs confirmation either by tube or microplate technique.

Materials required:
- Clean glass slide or white tile
- Reagent antibody namely anti-A, anti-B, and anti-A,B sera
- Test red cells (30–40% suspension)
- Applicator sticks.

Method (Fig. 4.6)
- Take a slide/white tile and label to identify the cells used.
- Put one drop each of anti-A, anti-B, and anti-A,B sera on the marked slide/tile.
- Add one drop of 30–40% red cell suspension to each of anti-A, anti-B, and anti-A,B sera (not shown in Figures 4.6 and 4.7) on the marked slide/plate.
- Mix the cells and reagent antisera with clean applicator stick and spread the mixture over an area of 2 cm.
- Rock the slide or tile gently and look for "agglutination".
- Record the results within 2 to 5 minutes.

Interpretation: ABO blood is interpreted depending on the agglutination in the antisera

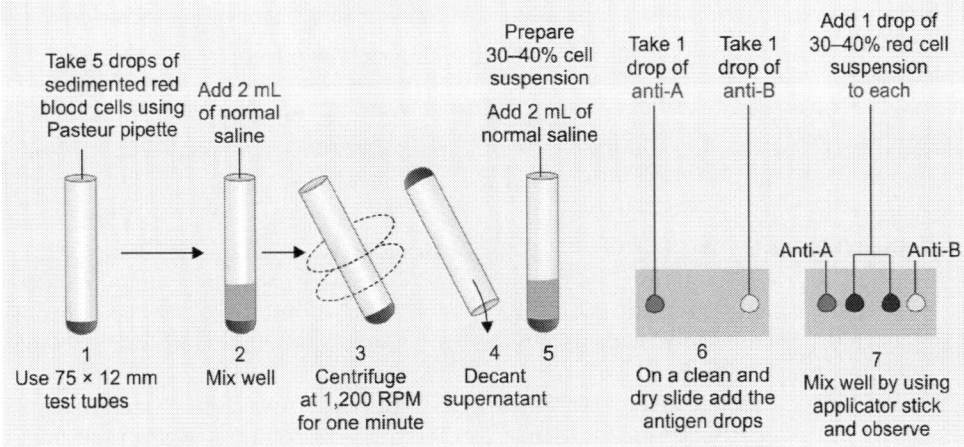

Fig. 4.6: Steps in ABO blood grouping by slide method.

(Table 4.6 and Fig. 4.7). Based on the interpretation of testing results, an ABO blood group type is assigned to the patient or donor. Four major blood phenotypes in the ABO blood group system are: (1) A, (2) B, (3) AB, and (4) O.
1. Group A individuals possess the A antigen and lack the B antigen.
2. Group B individuals possess the B antigen and lack the A antigen.
3. Group AB individuals possess both the A and B antigens.
4. Group O individuals lack both the A and B antigens.

Controls:
- Each blood group test should preferably have controls, both positive and negative.
- **Positive control:** This is run by performing the above techniques by using cells of known groups A, B, AB, and O. This is especially useful for testing the potency of antisera.
- **Negative control:** Run the above tests by adding saline instead of antisera. If agglutination develops, it indicates autoagglutination or pseudoagglutination.

Tube Method

Advantages: (1) It allows for long incubation without any drying. (2) The Ag-Ab reaction can be enhanced by centrifuging the tubes.

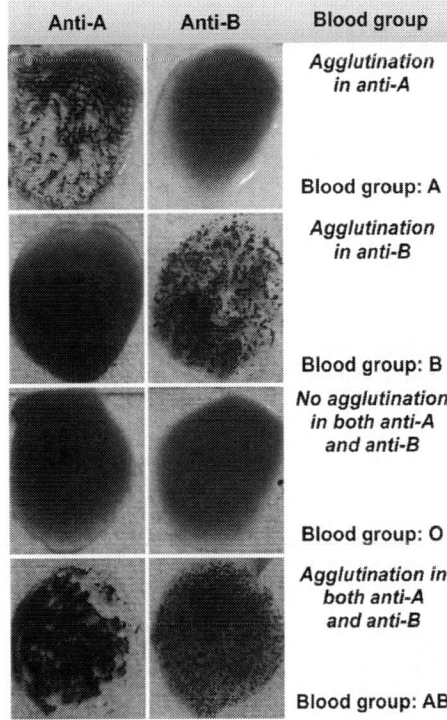

Fig. 4.7: Interpretation of blood group by slide method interpretation of blood group by slide method *(For color version, see Plate 1).*

Techniques: It can be performed either by (1) immediate spin technique or (2) saline room temperature technique.

1. **Immediate spin technique:** It is good method for rapid ABO grouping than slide technique.

   Materials required:
   - Clean test tubes (75 × 12 mm)
   - Antiserum: anti-A, anti-B, and anti-A,B
   - Test red cells (2–5% suspension)

   Method (Fig. 4.8):
   - Take three clean test tubes (75 × 12 mm size) and label them as anti-A, anti-B, and anti-A,B (not shown in Figure 4.8), respectively.
   - Add two drops of antisera, i.e. anti-A, anti-B, and anti-A,B (not shown in Figure 4.8) in prelabeled tubes.
   - Add one drop of 2–5% red cell suspension to each test tube.
   - Centrifuge (Fig. 4.9) all the three test tubes for 15–30 seconds.
   - Look for hemolysis or agglutination (Fig. 4.10) against well-lighted background and record the results.

2. **Saline room temperature technique**

   Materials required:
   - Clean precipitin tubes 50 × 7 mm or 75 × 12 mm tubes
   - Antiserum, i.e. anti-A, anti-B, and anti-A,B
   - Test red cells (2–5% suspension).

   Method:
   - Take three clean precipitin tubes (50 × 7 mm) or test tubes (75 × 12 mm size) and label them as anti-A, anti-B, and anti-A,B, respectively.
   - Add two drops of antisera, i.e. anti-A, anti-B, and anti-A,B in prelabeled tubes.
   - Add one drop of 2–5% red cell suspension to each test tube.
   - Gently mix the contents of each tube.
   - Incubate all the tubes at room temperature for 60 minutes.
   - Look for hemolysis or agglutination macroscopically under strong light, usually by tipping the tube over a mirror.

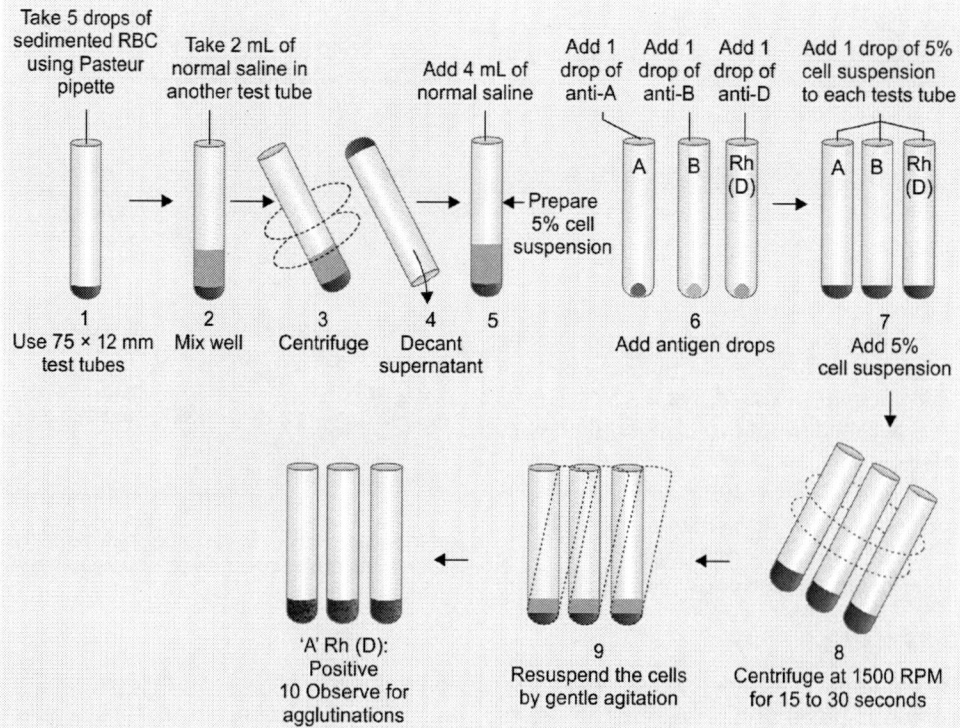

Fig. 4.8: Steps in ABO and Rh typing by tube method.

ABO Blood Grouping: Methods and Discrepancies

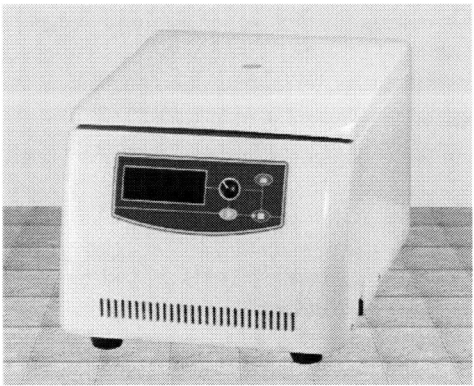

Figs. 4.9: Table top centrifuge.

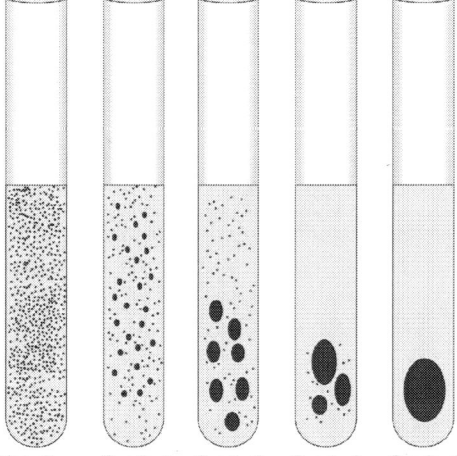

Fig. 4.10: Grading of results of ABO typing by tube test.

If agglutination is not observed using this macroscopic method, transfer one drop of mixture from each tube onto a glass slide, using a thin bore Pasteur pipette. Spread the cells over an area of 2 × 1 cm, using the pipette. Examine the slide under microscope for "agglutination" or to find very weak reactions.
- Record the results.

Serum Grouping or Reverse Typing

A_1 and B Red Cells for ABO Serum Testing

Testing a patient's serum or plasma with commercial group A_1 and group B red cells confirms the ABO typing performed on the patient's red cells. It is known as ABO reverse grouping or ABO serum testing. This procedure detects ABO antibodies in the serum of patient (Table 4.7). The results obtained by reverse grouping provide an additional confirmation or check of the assigned ABO typing (obtained by red cell testing using commercial anti-A and anti-B reagents, i.e. forward grouping). The serum of patients contains the antibody directed against the antigen of the ABO system that is lacking on their red cells.
- Patients with group A have A antigen on their red cells and lack the B antigen. Their plasma contains anti-B antibodies. Serum or plasma of group A individuals agglutinates with reagent B red cells but not with reagent A_1 red cells.
- Patients with group B have B antigen on their red cells and lack the A antigen. Their plasma contains anti-A antibodies. Serum or plasma of group B individuals agglutinates with reagent A_1 red cells but not with reagent B red cells.

Source and package: The reagent RBCs for reverse typing are obtained from selected human either a single donor or a pool of several donors. They are supplied in several optional packages and the most commonly

Table 4.7: ABO serum testing (reverse grouping).

ABO blood group antigen and phenotype	ABO antibody (in the serum)	Reaction with reagent A_1 red cells	Reaction with reagent B red cells
A	Anti-B	0	+
B	Anti-A	+	0
AB	No anti-A or anti-B	0	0
O	Anti-A and anti-B	+	+

(+: agglutination; 0: no agglutination)

available package consists of a two-vial set of A_1 and B red cells.

Preparation: During its preparation, all reagent red cells are washed to remove blood group antibodies. Then they are resuspended to a 2–5% concentration in a buffered preservative solution to minimize hemolysis and loss of antigenicity during the storage. These red cell preparations are usually negative for the Rh antigens D, C, and E.

Quality control: Each reagent lot is tested for specificity. Reagent red cells should not be used if the red cells darken, spontaneously agglutinate in the reagent vial, or show evidence of significant hemolysis.

Method: The test is conducted similar to tube method. However, in this typing, use donors/patient's serum and 3–4% pooled cell suspension of group A_1 cells, B cells, and O cells.

Interpretation of ABO serum testing (reverse grouping) is presented in Table 4.7.

ALTERNATIVE METHODS TO THE TUBE TEST

Blood bank reagents for grouping were designed to detect agglutination in the classic tube test. At present other techniques/methods are available for detecting Ag-Ab reactions. These are briefly discussed as alternative methods to tube test.

Microplate Method for ABO Grouping

In this method, microplates are used for testing. Microplate method is **ideal method for testing large number of blood samples** and it saves time. This method has replaced test tube method in many laboratories.

Microplates: These are polystyrene plates containing 96 small wells (Fig. 4.11A). Each well is considered a short test tube. Each well can hold 200–300 µL of reagent. The bottom of the microplate wells may be flat bottom type, conical (V-shaped) type, or U-shaped type (Fig. 4.11B). The results can be easily read in U type well plates. Hence, they are most commonly used for blood grouping. The microplates are usually disposable, but they can be reused after proper cleaning so that all foreign proteins are removed. It is advisable to use microplates for one type of test reagents each day and avoid using them for different tests.

Uses: The microplate technique can be adapted to red cell antigen testing (**ABO and Rh typing**) or serum testing for **antibody detection or identification**.

Principle: Microplate techniques apply the same principle of hemagglutination in tube test.

Materials Required

- Microplates (Fig. 4.11)
- Reagent antisera (anti-A, anti-B, and anti-A,B)
- Test red cells (2–5% saline suspension).

Method

- Place one drop of antisera (anti-A, anti-B, and anti-A,B) into the appropriate (separate) wells of the microplate (Fig. 4.12).
- Add one drop of 2–5% saline suspension of donor or patient's red cell (depending on

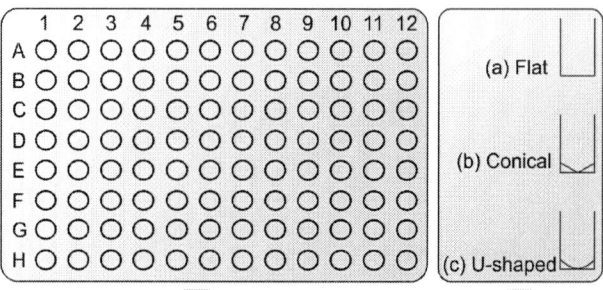

Figs. 4.11A and B: Diagrammatic appearance. (A) Microplates with 96 well plate; (B) Different shape of wells.

ABO Blood Grouping: Methods and Discrepancies

	Patient's cell									Control		
										A cells	B cells	O cells
Cell group	1	2	3	4	5	6	7	8	9	10	11	12
Anti-A	O	O	O	O	O	O	O	O	O	O	O	O
Anti-B	O	O	O	O	O	O	O	O	O	O	O	O
Anti-A, B	O	O	O	O	O	O	O	O	O	O	O	O
	Patient's serum											
Serum group	1	2	3	4	5	6	7	8	9	10	11	12
A_1 cells	O	O	O	O	O	O	O	O	O	O	O	O
B cells	O	O	O	O	O	O	O	O	O	O	O	O
O cells	O	O	O	O	O	O	O	O	O	O	O	O

Fig. 4.12: Various reagents and red cells used in microplate method.

whether forward or reverse grouping) to each of the antisera in the wells.
- Mix the contents of the well by gently shaking/tapping the plate.
- Incubate the microplate at room temperature for 20–30 minutes. The microtiter plates can also be centrifuged if needed at an appropriate time and speed.
- Look for any hemolysis and record.
- Gently shake the microplate to resuspend the cell button either by manually tapping the side of plate with the palm of hand or with the help of a mechanical microplate shaker. Alternatively, in tilt and stream method, the microtiter plates may be observed for a streaming pattern of red cells when the plate is placed on an angle.

Interpretation

Read the agglutination reactions either directly or with the aid of microplate reading mirror.
- **Positive reactions:** Agglutination or hemolysis in any well forms a concentrated button of red blood cells. A concentrated button of red cells is indicative of Ag-Ab reactions. The red cells remain in the center or fall in discrete button to the entire bottom of the well of the antibody-coated well.
- **Negative reactions:** In this, there is no agglutination and the red cells are dispersed throughout the well. There will be smooth suspension of red blood cells or a streaming pattern of blood cells when the plate is placed on an angle.

Interpretation of grading of reactions in microplate method has been shown in Table 4.8.

Alternatively, the results can also be obtained by automatic microplate reader

Table 4.8: Interpretation of grading of reactions in microplate method.

Grade	Description
++++	Complete agglutination all cells
+++	Majority of cells are agglutinated with few cells lying free
++	Many fairly large clumps of cells and many free cells
–ve	No agglutination

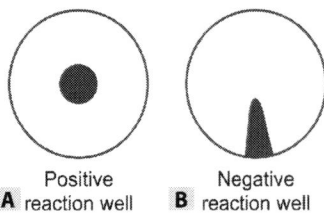

Figs. 4.13A and B: Positive and negative reactions in microplate method. (A) Positive reaction and (B) Negative reaction.

(photometric devices) at 570 nm wavelength. Automated devices can read and interpret the reactions on the microplates (Figs. 4.13A and B).

Column Agglutination Technology (Gel Card Technology/Microtyping System)

- In the traditional tube techniques/tests described above, the shaking of tube to resuspend the red cell button varies among technologists. This technical variation affects the grading and interpretation of the test results. To standardize, to improve sensitivity and specificity in blood bank serology, traditional tube testing methods, two alternative tubeless methods were developed. These are: (1) column agglutination/gel card/microtyping systems and (2) solid phase red cell adherence (SPRCA) assay.
- The gel technology by Micro Typing Systems, Inc. (Pompano Beach, Florida) as the ID-MTS Gel Card was introduced into the blood bank in 1994. It is an innovative technique, invented by Dr Yves Lapierre et al. (France) in 1985. It minimizes the problems associated with conventional techniques. In the gel test, the gel particles combined with diluent or reagents are predispensed into specially designed microtubes manufactured in plastic cards.

Features of Gel Card or a Glass Microbead Matrix (Fig. 4.14)

- The column-agglutination test (CAT) system consists of **either a gel card or a**

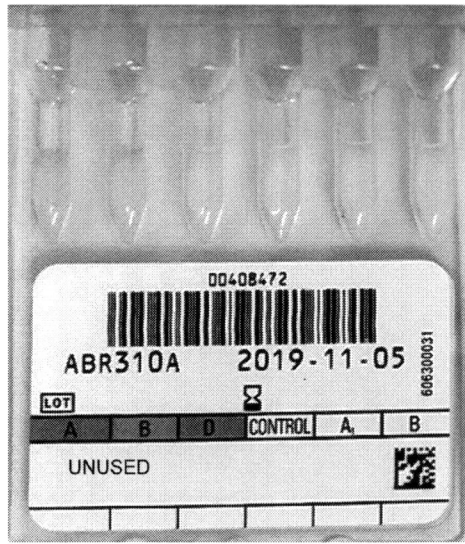

Fig. 4.14: A column-agglutination technology-appearance of glass microbead matrix (blank).

glass microbead matrix (Fig. 4.14). This card is a small plastic card about the size of a credit card and contains six to eight microtubes (vertical columns) per card.
- Each microtube of gel card consists of a **broad upper reaction chamber that narrows as a lower part** (refer Fig. 4.17).
- The **lower part is a column contains either a prefilled clear gel mixture** (buffered dextran-acrylamide gel particles) **or a glass microbead matrix and reagents**. The gel or microbead matrix contains sodium azide (preservative) and reagents as per requirements for a particular test. These constituents are incorporated into gel at the time of manufacture. Depending on the configuration of the card, the **gel or a glass microbead matrix is premixed with antisera/AHG/other reagents**. Two major categories of gel cards are used in blood bank. Specific reagent antibody is incorporated into the gel. These cards are:
  - **Group-specific antisera for blood grouping:** Cards for ABO (anti-A, anti-B, anti-AB) and D (anti-D) phenotype and other Rh antigens (C, c, E, e).
  - **Antihuman globulin cards** (anti-IgG and anti-IgG, -C3d) (for Coombs/

antiglobulin test). IAT (antibody screen, antibody identification, and compatibility testing) and direct antiglobulin test (DAT).
- On the **top of the gel card**, there is **a foil strip which prevents spillage or drying of microtube contents**.
- The six-microtube configuration of the gel card allows testing of more than one patient sample in one gel card. This technology is suitable for automation in blood bank.

Principle

This technology **uses hemagglutination reaction** and the dextran-acrylamide gel particles (or a glass microbead matrix depending on the type of column content) trap agglutinated red cells. This technology **utilizes the differential migration of RBC agglutinates through vertical columns of gel-filled microtube/glass microbead matrix.** When the red cells migrate through the gel matrix or glass microbead matrix, it separates agglutinated red cells from unagglutinated red cells. The movement of red cells in the gel column/glass beads depends on the principle of size exclusion. Thus, agglutinated red cells being too large to pass through the gel/glass bead are trapped at or near the top. The unagglutinated RBCs being smaller pass easily through the gel column/glass bead and form a pellet/button at the base/bottom of the microtube.

Technique

1. A weak suspension (0.8–1%) of red cells is prepared in a LISS.
2. Measured volumes of reagent red cell (RBC) suspension and/or plasma/serum (depending on the nature of test to be performed) are added to the reaction. For example, if the test is for ABO grouping, red cells are poured over the chamber of the microtube (top of the microtube/column).
3. The reaction mixture is incubated at 37°C. The reaction chamber allows red cell sensitization to occur during the incubation period.
4. Next step is centrifugation that drives the red cells into the gel/bead matrix to contact antisera (antibody) incorporated into the gel particles resulting in hemagglutination. The serum and cell reaction take place in a microtube. Centrifugation also separates positive and negative agglutination results.
5. The hemagglutinate gets trapped while other unsensitized red cells form a button at the bottom of the microtube.

Manual and automated methods for performing and interpreting these tests are now available.

Uses of Column Agglutination System (Box 4.3)

The column agglutination system is an open system and can be used for a variety of red cell serology testing requirements and other tests.

Interpretation (Figs 4.15, 4.16 and 4.17)

- **Positive reactions (antibody/antigen interactions):** If antibody is present, large red cell agglutinates form. The gel matrix acts as a sieve and agglutinated red cells

---

Box 4.3: Uses of column agglutination system.

- Blood grouping (ABO and Rh typing)
- Red cell antibody detection (identification) or screening
- Pretransfusion compatibility testing including cross-matching
- Typing for other blood group systems
- DAT/IAT and other Coombs phase tests
- Antibody classification: IgG, IgM, IgA, complement, etc.
- Specialized hematological tests, e.g. for paroxysmal nocturnal hemoglobinuria (PNH), sickle cell, heparin-induced thrombocytopenia (HIT)
- For diagnosis of syphilis, measles, diphtheria, parvovirus infection, leishmaniasis

(DAT: direct antiglobulin test; IAT: indirect antiglobulin test)

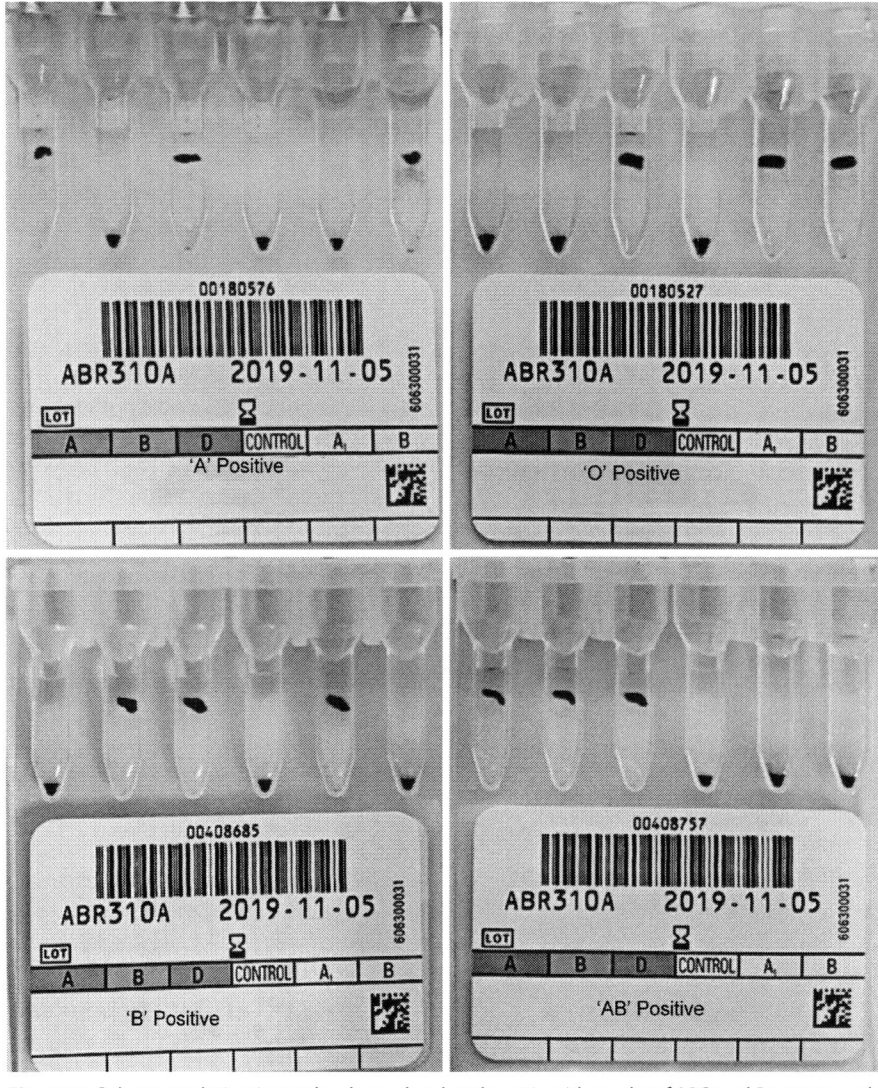

Fig. 4.15: Column-agglutination technology-glass bead matrix with results of ABO and D tests namely A, O, B and AB and all are D (Rh) positive.

are too large to pass through the gel are trapped at or near the top of the gel column (trapped at various levels, depending on the agglutination strength and size of the agglutinates). Reaction strength and size determine the migration of the agglutinates. The reactions may be graded from 1+ to 4+ and a card reader if used provides objectivity to the grading. The largest (4+) agglutinates (Fig. 4.17) at or near the top of the gel column and smaller agglutinates farther into the gel column.

- **Negative test:** If the specific antigen is not present on the red cells, hemagglutination does not occur. The unagglutinated RBCs pass easily through the gel column and form a pellet/button at the base/bottom of the microtube.
- **Dual populations of cells (mixed cells):** If there are dual populations of cells, it produces two distinct striking populations namely (1) unagglutinated cells at the bottom of the tube and (2) agglutinated cells at the top of the well (Fig. 4.17).

ABO Blood Grouping: Methods and Discrepancies

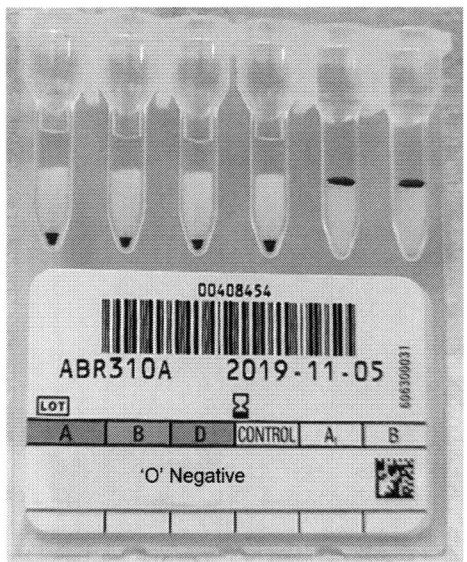

Fig. 4.16: Column-agglutination technology-glass bead matrix with result showing O(Rh) negative group.

Advantages Over Conventional Tube Procedures

- **Simple, rapid** to use, safe, easily readable, reproducible and cost-effective technique.
- **More standardized** than conventional tube testing.
- **Greater uniformity** between repeat tests.
- **Greater sensitivity** and more standardized when compared to conventional tube techniques. It uses small volumes of plasma and reagents.
- **Reliable, stable and defined hemagglutination** end point makes it an attractive method. Technical errors are eliminated and results are clear-cut. Objective and consistent interpretations of agglutination are possible.
- **Keeps the work place clean.** Special racks or sample tubes and typing cards are provided.
- For antiglobulin/Coombs test, red cells do not need saline washing.
- **Less sensitive to clinically insignificant cold antibodies.** Thus, eliminating unnecessary antibody workups.
- They have a **shelf life of 1 year** and easy storage at room temperature (18–25°C).
- It is **useful for performing blood group serology.** The card can also be used for antibody screening. It is available for pretransfusion cross-match (refer Box 4.3).
- Additional time savings because it eliminates the need of repetitive washing steps and manual macroscopic and/or microscopic readings in conventional techniques.

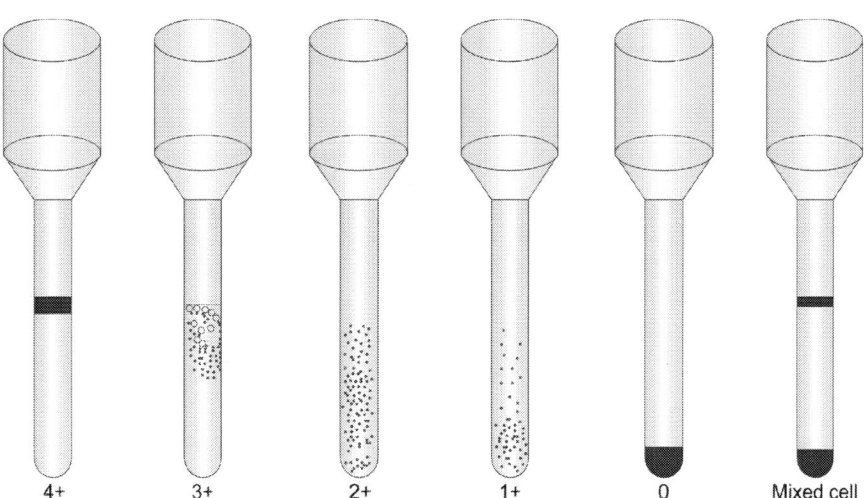

Fig. 4.17: Interpretation of Gel card technology.

- The **reactions are stable for hours or days** if the cards are closed with a tape and kept in a refrigerator. This is useful for a second or repeated reading if needed.
- **This testing can be automated**, permitting high-throughput testing, electronic interpretation and validation, and easy digital documentation of results by making photocopies.

Disadvantages

- **Needs special centrifugation for microtube cards**
- Needs special incubator top to incubate the microtube cards
- Expensive.

Factors affecting the test: (1) Size of particles, (2) RPM (revolution per minute) of the centrifuge, (3) weight and size of card and (4) constituents of the card.

Particle Gel Immunoassay (PaGIA)

In this gel technology, inert polymer particles are used for the detection of syphilis, leishmaniasis, detection of paroxysmal nocturnal hemoglobinuria (PNH) and fetomaternal hemorrhage.

Solid Phase Red Cell Adherence Assay

Solid phase red cell adherence assay is another alternative method to tube tests used in blood bank testing for detection of red cell alloantibody (also platelet antibody) and for ABO grouping. Commercial solid phase test procedures came to the market in late 1980s. Solid-phase assays use microplate test wells. In this technique, one of the components of an Ag-Ab reaction (i.e. either the antigen [reagent red cells] or antibody) is immobilized onto the solid medium present in bottom and sides of the microplate wells.

After reaction with a free antigen/antibody, the end point of the reaction is indicated by use of red cells, which may be a part of the Ag-Ab reaction or may be added as indicator cells.

Uses: Depending on the reagent (e.g. red cells or antibodies) used to coat the plates, solid phase technology can be used for various purposes in blood bank (Box 4.4).

> **Box 4.4:** Uses of solid phase red cell adherence (SPRCA) technology.
>
> - ABO and Rh typing
> - Antibody identification
> - Antibody detection/screening
> - Direct antiglobulin test
> - Weak D test
> - Compatibility testing (cross-matching) IgG cross-match
> - May also be adapted to platelet serology (platelet antibody screening and platelets cross-match)

Advantages of solid phase technology:

- Standardization and stable, defined end points. This leads to more objective and consistent interpretations of agglutination reactions.
- Sensitivity and specificity are higher (especially IgG antibodies) than other techniques including gel technology. Detects clinically significant antibodies, hence more specific.
- No need for predilution of reagents or samples.
- Automated washing of hemolyzed, icteric (i.e. sample from patient with jaundice) and lipemic (sample with hyperlipidemia) samples assures validity.
- Reagents (cell panels for antibody screening) are precoated on the test wells.
- Same method and procedure for all assays making handling easier.
- Turnaround time is less.
- Longer shelf life of antibody screening and identification plates (3 months) which avoids wastage of red cell-based reagents.
- Solid phase technology is **available as both automated and semiautomated testing** and is usually a part of a fully automated system.
- Wide range of uses (Box 4.4).

Types of Solid Phase Test Systems

It may be direct or indirect type. In a direct test, the antibody is fixed to the wells. In indirect method, reagent RBCs (target antigen) are fixed to the bottom of microplate wells.

Direct solid phase test systems

It is used for forward grouping. It is used for ABO and Rh typing of red cells.

Technique:

1. In forward grouping, U-shaped microplate wells are coated (fixed) with appropriate antibodies (e.g. antiserum—anti-A, anti-B, anti-A,B, and anti-D) and are dried.
2. A drop of 0.5% bromelain-treated test red cells from donor or patient are added to the well and incubated. Bromelain is proteolytic enzyme (refer page 68) that induces a marked decrease in the electronegative charge on the surface of RBCs enabling their agglutination by normally nonagglutination antibodies in saline medium.
3. Then the plates are centrifuged.

Interpretation:

- **Positive reactions:** Antigen-positive RBCs from donor or patient sources spread out. They adhere to the sides and entire bottom of the antibody-coated well.
- **Negative reactions:** Antigen-negative RBCs from donor or patient sources settle to the bottom of the well. After centrifugation, it produces a tightly packed cell button in the bottom of the well.

Indirect solid phase test systems (Fig. 4.18)

It is used for reverse grouping. For a reverse group, uncoated empty wells are used with standard reagent red cells (target antigen). The monolayer of RBC membrane is fixed/attached to the bottom of the microplate well.

Technique:

1. Unknown (test) patient or donor serum or plasma and enhancement reagent (often LISS-that enhances the antibody-antigen reaction) are added to the well. They are allowed to react with red cell membranes fixed to the bottom of microplate wells.
2. They are incubated at 37°C for 5 minutes and the alloantibody is allowed to bind to the solid phase. This step allows for the capture of IgG antibodies from the patient or donor serum to the red cell membranes.
3. After incubation, the plates are washed to remove unbound, excess serum globulins (IgG antibodies) washing step removes unbound IgG antibodies.
4. Then add indicator RBCs coated with antihuman IgG (AHG) (i.e. anti-IgG-coated indicator red cells) and the plates are centrifuged.

Interpretation: Wells may be read manually by a technologist or with an automated plate reader (reading device).

- **Positive indirect test:** It is characterized by the presence of alloantibody/antibody in the test serum or plasma. In this situation, a reaction will occur between the reagent RBCs and the alloantibody in the test serum. The alloantibodies bind to the reagent (indicator) RBCs present in the solid phase in the microplate wells and adhere to the sides and bottom of the well. Hence, the antiglobulin (AHG)-coated indicator red cells will bind and cover the bottom surface of the well. Similar to column agglutination, positive reactions are very stable. So, the plate may be covered, stored at 2–8°C, and can be read even up to 2 days after the test.
- **Negative indirect test:** It is characterized by the absence of antibody in the test serum. Hence, the antiglobulin (AHG)-coated indicator red cells settle to the bottom of the wells and form a discrete button after centrifugation in the bottom of the well (Fig. 4.18).

Capture-R Ready-Screen and Capture-R Ready-ID are configured as indirect solid-phase red cell adherence assays (SPRCA) tests. Red cell membranes are bound to the microtiter wells. For antibody screen and identification procedures, pretreated wells having red cell membranes bound to the surface of polystyrene microtiter plate are used.

Glass bead technology and erythrocyte-magnetized technology are discussed under Chapter 20 on page 427.

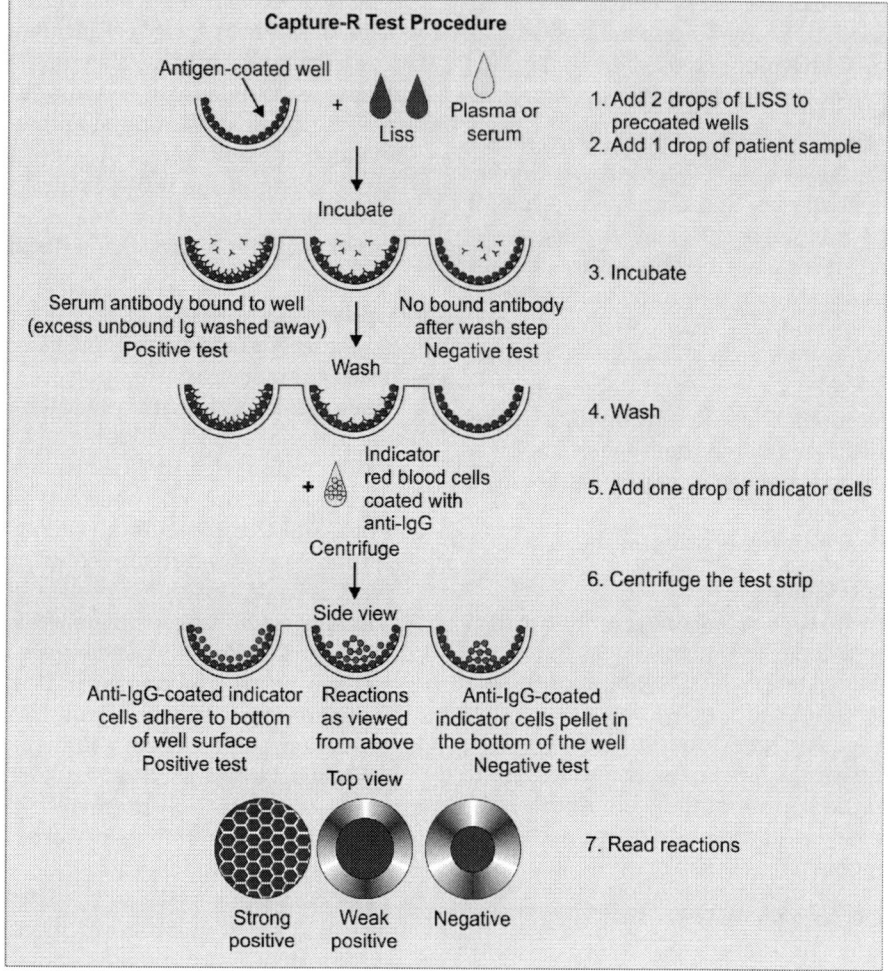

Fig. 4.18: Various steps in solid-phase red cell adherence assays (SPRCA) technology (indirect) and its interpretation.

Molecular Blood Grouping and Genotyping

With the advent of molecular technology, it is now possible to type the DNA of blood group antigens. Suitable techniques for genotyping of ABO, Kell, Duffy, Kidd, MN and SS have been used. However, the molecular genetic technology for blood grouping is now performed in only reference laboratories.

Advantages of Blood Genotyping

- Highly sensitive and specific.
- Helps in solving controversial issues in blood group genetics.

Applications of Molecular Blood Grouping

- In patients who received multiple transfusions.
- RBCs-coated with IgG (e.g. autoimmune hemolytic anemia)
- To resolve ABO and Rh typing discrepancies for patients and donors.
- To identify a fetus at risk of hemolytic disease of newborn (HDN).

- After ABO-incompatible hemopoietic stem cell transplantation.

Techniques for Molecular Blood Grouping

- Polymerase chain reaction-based methods
- DNA microarrays
- Mass spectrometry
- TaqMan allelic discrimination.

FACTORS CAUSING DISCREPANCIES DURING ABO TESTING

1. **Improper identification of blood specimen.**
2. **High ambient temperature** in the laboratory.
3. **Defect in the equipment:** Improper calibration of centrifuge can lead to either over or under centrifugation.
4. **Reagents:** Poorly standardized or stored reagents and incorrect use of reagents.
5. **Improper techniques**
   - **Procedure:**
     - Improper RBCs to serum ratio or improper concentration of cell suspensions
     - Failure to add proper reagent
     - Improper duration of incubation.
   - **Reading:**
     - Failure to identify hemolysis
     - Inaccurate/incorrect reading, recording or interpretation of test results (agglutination reactions).
6. **Factors related to recipient (patient)**
   a. **Due to antigen:**
      - **Failure to express ABO antigen on RBC**
        * Age: Newborn and old age
        * Disease: For example, leukemia, lymphoma
        * During pregnancy and women on oral contraceptives.
      - **Presence of acquired B antigen**
        * Infection (gram-negative septicemia)
        * Carcinoma of colon.
   b. **Due to acquired antibodies:** These include anti-A_1 in A_2 individuals, anti-H in Bombay phenotype, cold autoantibodies and unexpected alloantibodies.
   c. **Absence or presence of weak antibodies:** For example, immunodeficiency states, agammaglobulinemia. Acriflavine used as a dye in anti-B antisera reacts with anti-acriflavine antibody present in the sera of some individuals.
   d. **Occurrence of blood group chimera** (characterized by the presence of two populations of red cells). The various causes are mentioned here.
      - **Artificial chimera** may occur (1) during bone marrow transplantation or (2) due to transfusion of O group blood to patient of A or B blood group.
      - **Permanent chimera** which can occur due to (1) exchange of blood in twins in utero due to vascular anastomosis or (2) due to dispermy (two sperms fertilize one egg).
   e. **Rouleaux formation:** It may be found in patients when albumin/globulin ratio is abnormal. It can also occur in cord blood samples contaminated by Wharton's jelly.
   f. **Acquired antibodies:**
      - Anti-A_1 in A_2 individuals
      - Anti-H in Bombay phenotype
      - Cold autoantibodies
      - Unexpected alloantibodies.
   g. **Absence or weakening of antibodies:**
      - Immunodeficiency states
      - Agammaglobulinemia.
   h. **Excessive A or B substances.**

Controls for ABO and D Grouping

It is necessary to run positive and negative controls with every test or batch of manual tests. In fully automated systems, the controls should be run at least twice in a 24-hour period. If controls do not give the expected reactions, it should be investigated to determine the cause of the problem.

ABO DISCREPANCIES, PROBLEMS ENCOUNTERED AND THEIR SOLUTIONS

An ABO discrepancy occurs when there is discrepancy between the result of ABO phenotyping of red cell testing (forward typing) does not agree with the expected serum testing (reverse typing). The unexpected reaction may be due to an extra positive reaction or a weak or missing reaction in the forward and reverse grouping. Any discrepancy in ABO testing should be resolved before reporting a patient or donor ABO group. It must be resolved before transfusion of recipients or labeling of donor units.

Causes: These can be due to problems with:
1. The patient's serum (reverse grouping)
2. The patient's red cells (forward grouping)
3. Both the serum and cells.

Recognition and Resolution of ABO Discrepancies

The recognition and resolution of ABO discrepancies are challenges faced in the blood bank.

Indications of Discrepancies

The following observations during ABO phenotyping indicate ABO discrepancies.
- **Weaker agglutination than expected:** Agglutination strengths of the typing reactions are weaker than expected. Usually, RBC and serum grouping reactions are very strong (3+ to 4+). In ABO red cell testing, the agglutination reactions with anti-A and anti-B reagents are 3+ to 4+ and the results of ABO serum testing with reagent A_1 and B cells are 2+ to 4+. The ABO discrepancies are usually due to weaker reactions.
- **Missing expected reactions** in ABO red cell testing and serum testing. For example, in an individual with group O, there is missing one or both reactions in serum testing with reagent A_1 and B cells.
- **Presence of extra reactions** in either the ABO red cell or serum tests.

Whenever there are discrepancies in ABO typing, preliminary procedures should be performed to analyze the cause of ABO discrepancy (Box 4.5).

> **Box 4.5:** Preliminary procedures in case of ABO discrepancy.
>
> - Identification of documentation errors: Check
>   - Labels of all samples, reagents and records
>   - Results are properly recorded
>   - Interpretations are accurate and properly recorded
> - Reagent or equipment errors
>   - Check whether daily quality control on ABO typing reagents is satisfactory
>   - Inspect reagents for contamination and hemolysis
>   - Centrifugation time and calibration are confirmed
>   - Check the equipment used
> - Standard operating procedure (SOP) errors: Check whether
>   - Procedure follows as per manufacturer's directions
>   - Correct reagents were used and added to testing
>   - Red blood cell suspensions are at the correct concentration
>   - Cell buttons are completely suspended before grading the reaction
> - Obtain fresh sample of blood from the patient
> - Check patient's record especially for any previous history of transfusion, consumption of drugs or any illness or disease (if so the diagnosis)
> - Repeat the test procedure with new sample

ABO Discrepancies due to Technical Errors

The source of discrepancies in ABO typing can be **either technical or sample-related problems**. The first step in the resolution of an ABO discrepancy is to identify the source of the problem. Is it due to a technical error in testing (Box 4.6), or related to the sample itself?

Several types of technical errors can cause ABO discrepancies and lead to erroneous results. It is necessary to be aware and recognize these technical errors. Their recognition can assist in the resolution of an ABO discrepancy. These technical errors leading to ABO discrepancies in the forward and reverse groupings can be classified into several categories (Box 4.6).

ABO Blood Grouping: Methods and Discrepancies

Box 4.6: Technical errors for ABO discrepancies.

Errors before the procedure
- Incorrect labeling of the blood sample at the patient's bedside or in the laboratory
- Incorrect or inadequate identification of blood samples, test tubes or slides
- Clerical errors or incorrect recording of results
- A mix-up in samples

Errors in reagents and instruments
- Use of uncalibrated centrifuge
- Use of contaminated reagents

Errors during the procedure
- Cell suspension may be too heavy or too light
- Failure to add reagents or the addition of incorrect reagents
- Failure to add sample or the addition of incorrect sample
- Failure to follow manufacturer's instructions
- Over centrifugation or under centrifugation or warming during centrifugation

Errors during observation of result
- Missed observation of hemolysis
- Failure to record the result immediately after the test to avoid transcription errors

Resolution

- **Serum versus saline for RBC suspension:** If the initial test was done using RBCs suspended in serum or plasma, repeat testing the same sample using a saline suspension of RBCs. It can usually resolve the ABO discrepancy. The red cell suspensions prepared from patient samples can be washed three times before repeated testing.
- **Review all the technical factors** that might have given rise to the ABO discrepancy and correct if are identified.
- **Error in specimen collection or identification:** Obtain all information regarding the patient's age, diagnosis, transfusion history, medications, and history of pregnancy. If the discrepancy persists and appears to be due to an error in specimen collection or identification, obtain fresh sample from the patient and repeat the RBC and serum testing.
- **Withhold the interpretation:** If a discrepancy is found, the results must be recorded. However, the interpretation of the ABO type must not be done until the discrepancy is resolved.

When a technical error is detected and corrected, the ABO discrepancy can be quickly resolved with repeated testing. A fresh blood sample can be obtained from the patient to rule out the possible contamination or identification error. If the results of repeat tests on new sample are same as the previous test, then the problem is probably related to the sample itself (e.g. related to the patient or donor). Then use supplementary reagents and repeat the tests.

A stepwise approach to resolve when there is any ABO discrepancy is presented in Flowchart 4.1.

Sample-Related ABO Discrepancies

Sample-related ABO discrepancies can be divided into two groups: (1) ABO discrepancies that affect the ABO red cell testing and (2) discrepancies that affect the ABO serum or plasma testing.

- First step to solve the sample-related ABO discrepancies is **to detect whether the discrepancies** are **due to the patient or donor red cells** (red cell testing), or due to **patient or donor antibodies** (serum or plasma testing).
- Next observe the **strengths of agglutination reactions** in the testing of both the red cells and the serum or plasma. For this approach, it is necessary to know the potential problems relating to ABO red cell and serum testing (Table 4.9). The most commonly ABO discrepancies are due to weak or missing ABO antibodies in serum/plasma testing.

ABO Discrepancies Associated with Red Cell Testing

ABO discrepancies involving the testing of red cells (forward grouping) can be classified into three categories: (1) due to presence of extra antigens, (2) due to missing or weak antigens, and (3) mixed-field reactions.

Flowchart 4.1: Steps in resolving ABO discrepancies.

```
┌─────────────────────────┐          ┌─────────────────────────────┐
│   ABO discrepancy       │          │ If an error in specimen     │
│ forward and reverse     │──────────│ collection and              │
│ testing do not match    │          │ identification is suspected │
│ as expected             │          └──────────────┬──────────────┘
└───────────┬─────────────┘                         │
            │                                       ▼
            │                          ┌─────────────────────────┐
            │                          │ Request a new sample to │
            │                          │ be drawn from the patient│
            │                          └──────────────┬──────────┘
            │                                         ▼
            │                               ┌──────────────────┐
            │                               │  Repeat testing  │
            │                               └────────┬─────────┘
            │                                        ▼
  First rule out technical errors          ┌──────────────────┐
       (most common cause)                 │ No ABO discrepancy│
            │                               └────────┬─────────┘
            │                                        ▼
            │                               ┌──────────────────┐
            ▼                               │ Report out ABO   │
          Step 1                            │ group            │
                                            └──────────────────┘
```

Step 1

| Repeat ABO typing on the same sample. This will help to exclude technical error during initial testing | If during the initial test red cells were suspended in serum or plasma, then repeat the test after washing the red cells several time with saline |

→ No ABO discrepancy → Report out ABO group

ABO discrepancy shows disagreement between original test result and the repeat test on the initial sample

Step 2

Obtain a fresh blood sample and perform the tests. Possible contamination of initial sample to be excluded

ABO discrepancy still persists

Step 3

Obtain patient's medical history
- History of previous transfusions or transplant
- Current medications
- Diagnosis
- Pregnancy etc.

Consider the possibility of antigens or antibodies of following nature
- Weak
- Missing
- Extra

Step 4

Decide whether the problem with red cell testing or serum/plasma testing
- Investigate accordingly

Extra Antigens Present

These may demonstrate unexpected positive agglutination reactions with commercial anti-A or anti-B reagents during ABO red cell typing (forward grouping).

Causes of discrepancies: Examples include **group A with acquired B antigen** and the **B(A) phenotype**.

Group A with acquired B antigen: This is characterized by weak reactions with anti-B

ABO Blood Grouping: Methods and Discrepancies

Table 4.9: Overview of sample-related ABO discrepancies.

Problems with red cell testing	Problems with serum/plasma testing
Due to the presence of extra antigens	Extra antibodies
Group A with acquired B antigen B(A) phenotype Rouleaux Hematopoietic progenitor cell transplant	A subgroup with anti-A_1 Cold alloantibodies/autoantibodies Rouleaux Intravenous immunoglobulin (IVIg)
Due to the missing or weak antigens	Missing or weak antibodies
ABO subgroup Weakened A and B antigen expression in patients with leukemia or Hodgkin's lymphoma Transplantation	Newborn Elderly Immunotherapy for transplantation
Due to the mixed-filed reactions Transfusion of group O to group A, B or AB Hematopoietic progenitor stem cell transplants A_3 phenotype	

antisera due to acquired B phenomenon (refer page 50). It may be found in group A_1 individual with disease of the lower gastrointestinal tract, colorectal carcinoma, intestinal obstruction or gram-negative septicemia. These individuals give reactivity with anti-B reagents in ABO red cell testing and appear as group AB. This phenotype is usually associated with a bacterial deacetylating enzyme that alters the A immunodominant sugar, N-acetylgalactosamine, by removing the acetyl group. The resulting sugar, galactosamine, resembles the B immunodominant sugar, D-galactose, and cross-reacts with many anti-B reagents. These individuals should receive units of group A red cells for transfusion purposes.

Table 4.10 shows the ABO testing results of an acquired B phenomenon.

B(A) phenotype group B individual: They acquire reactivity with anti-A reagents in ABO red cell testing. Their B gene transfers trace amounts of the immunodominant sugar for the A antigen and the immunodominant sugar for the B antigen. The B(A) phenotype is due to the increased sensitivity of potent monoclonal antibody reagents for ABO phenotyping. These reagents can detect trace amounts of either A or B antigens. Table 4.11 shows the ABO testing results in B(A) phenotype group B individual.

Missing or Weakly Expressed Antigens

In this category of ABO discrepancies, patient or donor red cells show weaker-than-usual reactions with reagent anti-A and anti-B or may fail to demonstrate any reactivity. This is observed under the following:
- ABO subgroups
- Weakened A and B antigen expression in patients with leukemia or Hodgkin's lymphoma.

Table 4.10: ABO discrepancy due to acquired B antigen and its resolution.

	Forward grouping (reaction of patient's cells with)		Reverse grouping (reaction of patient's serum with)	
	Anti-A	Anti-B	A_1 cells	B cells
Patient	++++ (strong)	+ (weaker than usually expected)	Negative	++++
Group	Cell group AB (phenotype AB)		Serum group A	
Interpretation	Patient's probable group is A. Group A individual possesses an extra/acquired a B-like antigen which reacts with reagent anti-B (weaker agglutination). It can be seen in association with cancer of the colon or other diseases of the digestive tract			
Resolution	1. Acidify anti-B reagent to a pH of 6 2. Run DAT (direct antiglobulin test) 3. Run autocontrol			

Table 4.11: ABO discrepancy due to B(A) phenotype group B individual.

	Forward grouping (reaction of patient's cells with)		Reverse grouping (reaction of patient's serum with)	
	Anti-A	Anti-B	A_1 cells	B cells
Patient	+ (weak)	++++ (strong)	++++ (strong)	0
Group	Cell group B(A) phenotype		Serum group B	
Resolution	1. Know the patient's diagnosis and transfusion history 2. Test red cells with additional monoclonal antibody anti-A reagents from other manufacturers or a source of human polyclonal anti-A			

Table 4.12: ABO discrepancy in subgroup A individual.

	Forward grouping (reaction of patient's cells with)		Reverse grouping (reaction of patient's serum with)	
	Anti-A	Anti-B	A_1 cells	B cells
Patient	0	0	0	+++
Group	Cell group O phenotype		Serum group A	
Inference	These reactions are characteristics of a missing antigen in the red cell testing. The serum testing results are those expected in a group A individual. Anti-A, found in group O individuals, is absent in the serum testing			
Resolution	1. Know the patient's diagnosis and transfusion history 2. Repeat the red cell testing with extended incubation times and use human polyclonal anti-A,B or monoclonal blend anti-A,B. The extended incubation time may enhance the antigen-antibody reaction 3. Molecular genotyping of this patient can identify the subgroup of A and resolve the ABO discrepancy			

ABO subgroups: Missing or weakly expressed antigens can present as an ABO discrepancy and typically observed with a subgroup of A. Weak or missing reactions with anti-A and anti-B reagents correlate with subgroups of A and B. Table 4.12 shows the ABO discrepancy in subgroup A individual.

Additional test results may help in resolving ABO discrepancy (Table 4.13).

ABO discrepancy in leukemia has been shown in Table 4.14.

Mixed-Field Reactions

Mixed-field reactions are due to the presence of two distinct cell populations. It can be observed in red cell testing with anti-A or anti-B reagent. Mixed-field reaction contains mass of agglutinated and unagglutinated red cells.

Causes of mixed-field reactions
- **Recent transfusion of non-ABO-identical RBCs:** Testing red cells from a patient who was recently transfused with non-ABO-identical RBCs (group O donor RBCs to a group AB recipient) can show mixed-field reaction.
- It may occur with the transfusion of group O RBCs to group A, B, or AB individuals, recipients of **hematopoietic progenitor transplants**. They are called artificially induced chimerisms. Chimerism is defined as the presence of two cell populations in a single individual. It may also occur with exchange transfusions and fetal-maternal bleeding.

Table 4.13: Additional test results in subgroup A individual.

	Anti-A,B
Patient's red cells	+
Inference	Probably subgroup of A
	Anti-A,B
Patient's red cells	0
Next perform the adsorption and elution with anti-A	

ABO Blood Grouping: Methods and Discrepancies

Table 4.14: ABO discrepancy seen in leukemia.

Patient's phenotype	Forward grouping (reaction of patient's cells with)		Reverse grouping (reaction of patient's serum with)	
	Anti-A	Anti-B	A_1 cells	B cells
A	+	O	O	+++
B	O	±/+	++++	O
Interpretation	Weak reactivity in forward grouping with anti-A and anti-B is due to disease (e.g. leukemia) associated with weakened expression of the corresponding antigen			

- **Individuals with the A_3 phenotype.**

Recent transfusion of non-ABO-identical RBCs: For example, group B patients transfused with group O RBCs (Table 4.15).

ABO Discrepancies Associated with Serum or Plasma Testing

ABO discrepancies associated with serum or plasma testing (reverse grouping) may be due to the presence of additional antibodies other than anti-A and anti-B or the absence of expected ABO antibody reactions. The most commonly it is due to the absence of expected ABO antibody reactions.

Additional Antibodies in Serum or Plasma Testing

These additional antibodies include a **subgroup with anti-A_1, cold alloantibodies, cold autoantibodies, rouleaux** and administration of intravenous immunoglobulin (IVIg). Cold alloantibodies are red cell antibodies specific for other human red cell antigens that typically react at or below room temperature. Cold autoantibodies are red cell antibodies specific for autologous antigens that typically react at or below room temperature.

Group A_2 with anti-A_1

ABO discrepancy in group A_2 individuals with anti-A_1 has been shown in Tables 4.16 and 4.17.

Cold alloantibodies or cold autoantibodies in serum or plasma testing (Tables 4.18 and 4.19)

In addition to antibodies of ABO blood group system, donors and patients may have antibodies to other blood group system red cell antigens.

- **Alloantibodies:** These are additional serum antibodies which include anti-P1, anti-M, anti-N, anti-Le_a, and anti-Le_b. These antibodies react at or below room temperature; hence, they are called as cold antibodies. Reagent A_1 and B red cells used in ABO serum testing may contain these antigens in addition to the A and B

Table 4.15: ABO discrepancy in group B patients transfused with group O RBCs.

	Forward grouping (reaction of patient's cells with)		Reverse grouping (reaction of patient's serum with)	
	Anti-A	Anti-B	A_1 cells	B cells
Patient	O	++ mixed field	++++	O
Interpretation	The agglutination reaction strength with anti-B is weaker than expected for group B individuals. Anti-B mixed-filed reactivity ++ indicates unagglutinated red cells. The results of serum testing are typical of group B. These findings indicate that the group B patient is probably transfused with O group RBCs.			
Resolution	1. Check the patient's diagnosis 2. Enquire about recent transfusion or hematopoietic progenitor cell transplant 3. If possible, investigate pretransfusion ABO phenotype history			

Table 4.16: ABO discrepancy in group A_2 individuals with anti-A_1.

	Forward grouping (reaction of patient's cells with)		Reverse grouping (reaction of patient's serum with)	
	Anti-A	Anti-B	A_1 cells	B cells
Patient	++++	0	++	++++
Interpretation	The agglutination reaction with anti-A and absence of agglutination with anti-B indicates group A. The result of serum testing with A_1 and B cells suggests group O. The demonstration of extra reaction in the serum testing with reagent A_1 red cells (++). This may be due to the anti-A_1, cold alloantibody, cold autoantibody or rouleaux			
Resolution of ABO discrepancy	1. Ask for the patient's diagnosis and history of transfusion 2. Test the patient's red cells with anti-A_1 lectin to know whether a subgroup of A is present (Table 4.17) 3. Test the patient's serum with three examples of A_1 and A_2 reagent red cells to confirm the presence of anti-A_1 antibody. If agglutination is found with A_1 red cells without the agglutinate with A_2 red cells indicates the presence of anti-A_1			

Table 4.17: Additional test results in individual with group A_2 with anti-A_1.

Test the patient's red cells anti-A_1 lectin	
0	Probably subgroup of A. Suspect anti-A_1 antibody
Next perform the adsorption and elution with anti-A	

Table 4.18: ABO discrepancy due to cold alloantibodies or cold autoantibodies.

	Forward grouping (reaction of patient's cells with)		Reverse grouping (reaction of patient's serum with)	
	Anti-A	Anti-B	A_1 cells	B cells
Patient	++++	++++	0	+
Interpretation	Strong agglutination reaction with anti-A and anti-B indicates group AB. The result of serum testing with B red cells is weaker (+) and suggests group A. The demonstration of extra reaction in the serum testing with reagent B red cells (+). This may be due to the presence of cold alloantibody or cold autoantibody			
Resolution of ABO discrepancy	1. Inquire the patient's diagnosis and transfusion history 2. Test the patient's serum with screening O reagent cells and an autocontrol at room temperature. This helps differentiate cold alloantibody from cold autoantibody (Table 4.19) 3. If an alloantibody is detected, antibody identification techniques should be performed (see Chapter 10)			

antigens. Screening group O reagent red cells are used to detect these alloantibodies because O cells do not contain A and B antigens. Thus, these screening O reagent cells help in distinguishing between ABO antibodies and alloantibodies.

- **Autoantibodies:** Patients and donors may also have serum antibodies directed against their own red cell antigens. These antibodies are called as autoantibodies. If autoantibodies are reactive at or below room temperature, they are also called cold. Cold autoantibodies usually have the specificity of anti-I or anti-IH and react against all adult red cells, including screening cells, A_1 and B cells, and autologous cells.
- **Autocontrol:** Autocontrol is testing an individual's serum with their own red cells to determine whether an autoantibody is present. An autocontrol (autologous control) is tested to differentiate between a cold autoantibody from a cold alloantibody. If the autocontrol is positive, the reactions observed with the A_1 and B cells and

ABO Blood Grouping: Methods and Discrepancies

Table 4.19: Differentiation of cold alloantibodies from cold autoantibodies.

	Screening cells	Autologous red cells	Inference
Patient's serum	Positive reaction	Negative reaction	Cold alloantibody
Patient's serum	Positive reaction	Positive reaction	Cold autoantibody

screening cells are probably indicate that they are autoantibodies.

Rouleaux

It is a stacking of RBCs on top of one another in columns and they adhere in a coin-like (stacked coins) fashion under microscopic examination. It appears like and misinterpreted as weak or false-positive agglutination by inexperienced laboratory technologist. Rouleaux may occur in conditions associated with altered ratio of normal albumin to globulin (increased concentrations of serum proteins) in plasma (e.g. in multiple myeloma and Waldenström macroglobulinemia) and in the presence of plasma substitutes such as dextrans. Multiple myeloma is a malignant neoplasm of the bone marrow characterized by abnormal proteins in the plasma and urine. Table 4.20 shows an example of ABO discrepancy caused by rouleaux formation.

Resolution of ABO discrepancy due to rouleaux:

1. Know the patient's diagnosis and transfusion history.
2. Rouleaux can be **rectified by washing the patient's RBCs several times with saline and repeat the phenotyping.**
3. **Saline replacement technique:** Perform the saline replacement technique to distinguish true agglutination from rouleaux (Flowchart 4.2). In reverse grouping or typing, saline replacement

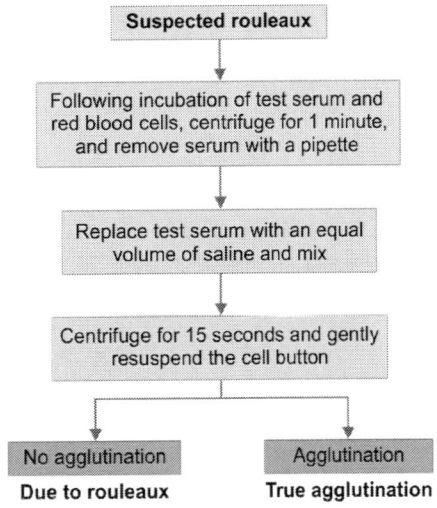

Flowchart 4.2: Saline replacement technique helps to distinguish rouleaux causing false-positive reactions from agglutination.

technique can be useful. In this technique, test is repeated by **removing the serum or plasma by an equal volume of saline** which will free the red cells in case of rouleaux. It can be seen on microscopic examination/rouleaux will usually disperse on a slide if a drop of saline is added. If it is true agglutination, RBC clumping will still remain after the addition of saline. Rouleaux is an in vitro problem not an in vivo problem that is observed during laboratory testing.

Table 4.20: Example of ABO discrepancy caused by rouleaux formation.

	Forward grouping (reaction of patient's cells with)		Reverse grouping (reaction of patient's serum with)	
	Anti-A	Anti-B	A_1 cells	B cells
Patient	++++	++++	++	++
Interpretation	Patient's probable group is AB. Agglutination with A_1 and B cells in reverse grouping is due to rouleaux formation caused either due to increased serum protein or plasma abnormalities in the patient			

4. **Microscopic examination.**
5. **Run antibody screen.**

Missing or Weak ABO Antibodies in Serum or Plasma Testing

In some patient-related situations, ABO antibodies may be missing or weakened and can result in an ABO discrepancy. Missing or weak ABO antibodies in serum/plasma testing are the most common cause of ABO discrepancies. Table 4.21 shows ABO discrepancy due to missing or weak ABO antibodies.

Bombay group

ABO discrepancy due to Bombay group and its resolution has been shown in Table 4.22.

Special test using anti-H and autocontrol to detect the cause of incompatibility in patients with Bombay group are presented in Table 4.23.

Summary of ABO Discrepancies

Summary of ABO discrepancies are presented in Flowchart 4.3.

False-Positive Reactions and False-Negative Reactions

False-Positive Reactions

T-activation/polyagglutination

Polyagglutination is the agglutination of red cells by all or most normal adult sera but not by the patient's own serum. This is due to IgM antibodies reacting with a hidden antigen on the red cells which usually becomes exposed by enzyme activity. The

Table 4.21: ABO discrepancy due to missing or weak ABO antibodies.

	Forward grouping (reaction of patient's cells with)		Reverse grouping (reaction of patient's serum with)	
	Anti-A	Anti-B	A_1 cells	B cells
Patient	0	0	0	0
Interpretation	The agglutination pattern with anti-A and anti-B reagents indicates patient's probable group O		The results of serum testing with reagent A_1 and B red cells indicate a group AB	
Resolution of ABO discrepancy	1. Enquire the patient's history, including age, diagnosis, and reduced immunoglobulin levels which may provide clues to explaining the missing reactions in the serum testing. The concentrations of ABO antibodies are reduced in newborns and elderly 2. Incubate serum testing with reagent A_1 and B cells for 15 minutes at room temperature, then centrifuge and examine for agglutination. This step often solves the problem 3. If the results are still negative, place the serum testing at 4°C for 5 minutes with an autologous control. The autologous control helps in ensuring that positive reactions are not due to cold autoantibody 4. By adding one or two drops more plasma or serum to the test			

Table 4.22: ABO discrepancy due to Bombay group and its resolution.

	Forward grouping (reaction of patient's cells with)		Reverse grouping (reaction of patient's serum with)	
	Anti-A	Anti-B	A_1 cells	B cells
Patient	Negative	Negative	++++	++++
	Cell group is O		Serum group is O	
Further tests	Patient's serum mixed with screen O cell gives reaction and cross-match with group O blood shows strong incompatible reaction. Special test necessary			

ABO Blood Grouping: Methods and Discrepancies

Table 4.23: Special test using anti-H and autocontrol to detect the cause of incompatibility in patients with Bombay group.

Antisera	Anti-H	Autocontrol (serum of patient)
Reaction with patient cells	Negative	Negative
Inference	Negative reaction with anti-H indicates that patient's group is not O	Negative reaction with autocontrol indicates that there is no autoantibody in the patient
Possible cause	Because of strong incompatible reaction with group O, the patient cannot be of O group. Negative reaction with anti-H antisera suggests the absence of H substance. Hence, patient is probable having a rare Bombay O phenotype. If such patients need blood, they should be given only Oh cells	

most common form is T-activation is brought out by bacterial enzyme neuraminidase. This cleaves N-acetylneuraminic acid from the red cell membrane and exposes the T antigen. This was observed when polyclonal reagents which contain anti-T were used for grouping. Present usage of monoclonal reagents does not produce this phenomenon.

Acquired B

It develops in patients with A_1 group where there is **reaction with anti-A** but an **additional weak reaction** also occurs **with anti-B**. The blood group appears to be "AB" in forward grouping with anti-B in the reverse grouping. This discrepancy may be overlooked if the patient's own anti-B is weak or if the reverse group is not performed. Usually, this acquired B antigen (B-like substance) is produced by the action of bacterial deacetylase enzyme on A_1 red cells. This is different from acquired B phenomenon described on pages 50 and 89.

Potentiators

Red cells may be coated with IgG due to in vivo sensitization. The use of potentiated

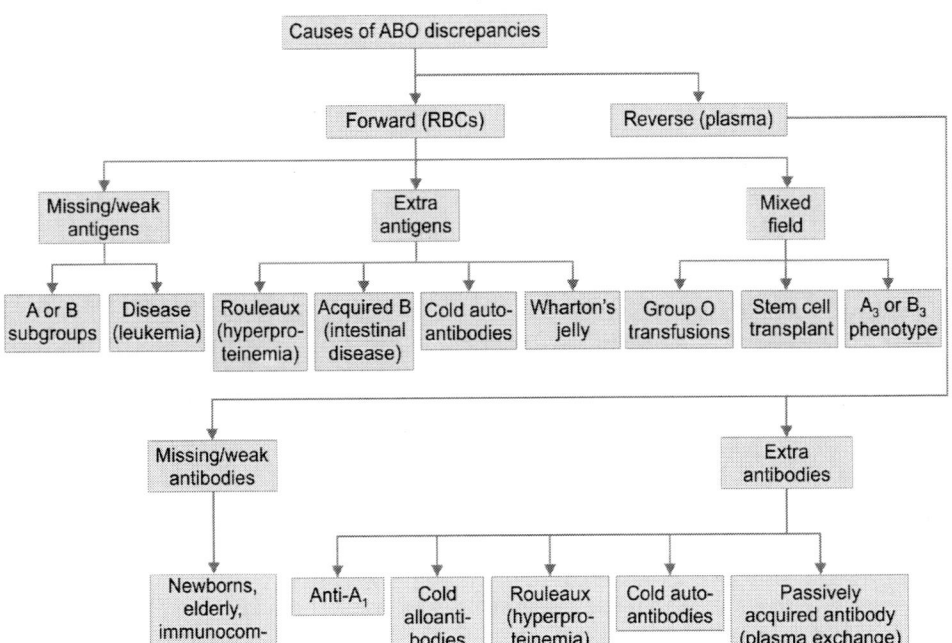

Flowchart 4.3: Summary of ABO discrepancies.

reagents (refer page 66) for ABO or D typing or potentiated techniques, such as the antiglobulin test for D typing may cause a false-positive reaction. Hence, it is not advisable to use potentiated techniques or reagents for blood grouping.

In vitro bacterial contamination of reagents, patients' red cells or reverse grouping cells may cause false-positive agglutination.

False-Negative Reactions

Failure to add reagents or test plasma
It is the most probable cause of a false-negative grouping result.

Loss of potency of blood grouping reagents
Inappropriate storage or freezing and thawing of blood grouping reagents may lead to loss of their potency. Hence, it is necessary to run regular controls.

Failure to identify lysis
In vitro, the presence of complement, anti-A and anti-B may cause lysis of reagent red cells. Failure to recognize this lysis as a positive reaction, falsely negative results may be recorded in reverse grouping tests. This can be avoided, by resuspended cells EDTA saline (using serum rather than plasma) in reverse grouping.

Mixed-field appearance
This is characterized by the appearance of dual population of agglutinated and non-agglutinated red cells. Its recognition is necessary and it should not be confused with weak agglutination. It may be seen in both ABO and D (Rh) grouping.

- It is most likely caused due to the **transfusion (either deliberate or accidental) of nonidentical ABO or D red cells**. Investigation is necessary to determine the actual blood group of the patient. The transfusion might have been given as an emergency or at a different establishment or might be an intrauterine transfusion. A mixed-field ABO group may be the first clue of a previous ABO-incompatible transfusion.
- **An ABO-or D (Rh)-incompatible hematopoietic stem cell transplant** can cause a temporary mixed-field picture till total engraftment occurs. It may subsequently reappear if the graft is failing. Rarely, a dual population of cells may be permanent and results from a weak subgroup of A (A_3) or a blood group chimerism.

Interpretation of a dual population of red cells depends on the technique used.
- In a tube, microscopic reading will show strong agglutinates in a background sea of free cells.
- In Column Agglutination Technology (CAT) cards/cassettes, it shows a line of agglutinated cells at the top of the column, with the nonagglutinated cells passing through to the bottom of the column.
- In liquid-phase techniques, if the reaction grade is not a strong positive or an obvious negative then the reaction needs further investigation (e.g. microscopic examination).
- In a solid-phase technique, a mixed field is seen as a dual population of cells, with the agglutination surrounded by free cells.
- Automated systems should be set up to identify mixed-field picture.

SUMMARY

- The reagents in the immunohematology laboratory are used to detect Ag-Ab reactions.
- These reagents should have specificity and potency. Specificity in blood banking reagents refers to recognition of antigen and antibody to make the Ag-Ab reaction. Potency in blood banking reagents refers to the strength of an Ag-Ab reaction.
- A package or product insert is supplied with the reagent and describes the use of reagent, summary, principle, procedure and the limitations of the reagent.
- The quality control of reagent red cells and antisera reagents is performed daily.
- Polyclonal antibodies are prepared from several different clones of B cells that secrete antibodies of different specificities.
- Monoclonal antibodies are derived from a single clone of B cells that secretes antibodies of the same specificity.
- Reagents for ABO typing are monoclonal origin and may be blended to create reagents that recognize the corresponding A or B antigen. These

(Contd...)

(Contd...)

- reagents contain IgM antibodies in a low-protein environment.
- The low-protein control reagent prevents the formation of spontaneous agglutination of patient or donor red cells in testing. The control should always show no agglutination.
- Reagent red cells are used as sources of antigen in antibody screens, ABO reverse grouping, and antibody identification tests.
- Antibody potentiators, or enhancement media, are reagents that enhance the detection of IgG antibodies by increasing their reactivity. These enhancement media used in blood bank include LISS, PEG, BSA, and enzymes. Enhancement media reduce the zeta potential of the red cell membrane and promote agglutination.
- Lectins are plant or other extracts that bind to carbohydrate portions of certain red cell antigens and agglutinate the red cells.
- ABO blood grouping can be done by test tube method or microplate techniques. The principles are agglutination in both techniques. Microplate techniques use a microtiter plate with 96 wells to serve as the substituted test tubes. They are presently replaced by gel technology.
- In gel technology, gel particles are combined with diluent or reagents to trap agglutination reactions within the gel matrix.
- Another recent technique is solid phase red cell adherence testing. In this, the antigen or antibody is immobilized to the bottom and sides of the microplate wells.
- Causes of ABO discrepancies can be due to problems with the patient's serum (reverse grouping), the patient's red cells (forward grouping) or both the serum and cells.
- False-positive reactions may occur due to T-activation/polyagglutination, acquired B, in vitro bacterial contamination or due to potentiators (if used).
- False-negative reactions may occur due to failure to add reagents or test plasma, loss of potency of blood grouping reagents, failure to identify lysis or mixed-field appearance.

SELF-ASSESSMENT EXERCISE

Write essay on:
- Describe Gel card technique and its application in hematological disorders and transfusion medicine. Comment on its advantages and disadvantages.

Write short essay/notes on:
- Various techniques of ABO grouping
- Precautions to be taken in ABO blood group detection and discrepancies in blood grouping
- Medicolegal aspect of ABO blood group
- Bombay blood group
- Gel card technology
- Application of Gel card techniques in transfusion medicine
- Solid phase red cell adherence testing
- Solving various ABO discrepancies encountered in blood bank

CHAPTER 5

Rh Blood Group System

CHAPTER OUTLINE

- Introduction of Rh (D) system
- Nomenclature
- Rh antigens
- Rh antibodies
- Rh (D) grouping/typing
- Problems encountered in Rh grouping and their solutions

INTRODUCTION OF RH (D) SYSTEM

Rh blood group system is the second system (after the ABO blood group system) of clinical significance in transfusion medicine. Though the original antibody (now called anti-LW) was subsequently found to be different from anti-D, the Rh terminology has been retained for the human blood group system.

Discovery of Rh System

The first human antibody against the antigen later called D was reported in 1939 by Levine and Stetson. The discovery of the Rh blood group system, as with many other blood group systems, occurred during the investigation of an adverse transfusion reaction or hemolytic disease of the fetus and newborn (HDFN). They found Rh blood group system in the serum of a woman whose fetus had hemolytic disease of the newborn (HDN) and who experienced a hemolytic reaction after transfusion of her husband's blood. It was formerly called the Rhesus system, because in 1940 Landsteiner and Wiener described the **original antibody that was obtained by injecting red blood cells** (RBCs) **of rhesus monkeys into rabbits** and guinea pigs. These antibodies reacted with most (approximately 85%) human RBCs and they called the corresponding determinant the Rh factor. The **antigen detected by animal anti-Rhesus was D antigen**. Later Levine and Stetson discovered an identical anti-Rh antibody in a mother.

Clinical Importance

Rh blood group is important because:
- It **can cause HDN in Rh-negative woman with Rh-positive fetus**.
- If **Rh-negative patients are given Rh-positive blood,** the patient will develop Rh antibodies and **leading to hemolytic transfusion reaction**.

Basic Genetics of Rh System

Types: The locus of Rh genes is on chromosome 1. The Rh blood group system is highly (most) complex and polymorphic. The Rh blood group system has grown to include more than 50 related antigens. There are **three pairs of genes involved in Rh system namely Cc, Dd and Ee**. However, they code only five principal antigens (C, c, D, E, and e) because there is **no antigen production by d gene**. These five Rh antigens (D, C, c, E, and e) are **found in blood only on red cells** and exist as transmembrane proteins. They are **fully developed in early fetal life** and remain so throughout life.

Transmission: Rh genes are transmitted in set of three, i.e. CDe, CDE, CdE, etc. One set is received from each parent, and this combination of genes on parent chromosomes determines the genes of their children. Transmission of D antigen follows an autosomal dominant pattern. Out of the various gene combination, the **presence or absence of D gene is important to determine whether an individual is Rh-positive ("D-positive") or Rh-negative ("D-negative")** (Table 5.1). Thus, the terms "Rh-positive" and "Rh-negative" refer to the presence or absence of the D red cell antigen. **In contrast to the ABO blood group system, the absence of the D antigen or other Rh blood group system antigens on the red cell does not typically correspond with the presence of the antibody in the plasma.** For example, individuals who phenotype as "group A, D-negative (Rh-negative)" would have anti-B in their serum but not anti-D. The **production of anti-D** and other Rh blood group system **antibodies needs immune red cell stimulation from red cells positive for the antigen.** This exposure may **occur during transfusion or pregnancy**. Normal pattern of Rh inheritance is presented in Figure 5.1.

In clinical practice five blood typing Rh system reagents are readily available namely: anti-D, anti-C, anti-E, anti-c, and anti-e. Of these, **D antigen is the only antigen in the Rh system which is immunogenic and clinically significant**. Hence, routine pretransfusion testing is done only for D antigen with anti-D. The immunogenicity of Rh antigens in decreasing order is expressed as: D>c>E>C>e.

NOMENCLATURE

The Rh system was discovered in the 1940s, and several terminologies for the Rh blood group system developed over the years. These are mainly due to differences in thinking regarding the inheritance of the Rh antigens.

Fisher and Race: DCE Terminology

In the 1940s, Fisher and Race proposed a nomenclature system based on genetic evidence of the allelic nature of the C/c and E/e antigens. They proposed that the Rh system consisted of three closely linked loci or subloci on each chromosome, which were inherited as a block of genes (haplotype). These include *D* at one locus, *C or c* at the second, and *E or e* at the third locus. Each gene was responsible for producing a product (or antigen) on the RBC surface. Fisher-Race developed a DCE nomenclature (Rh D, Cc, Ee terminology) and named the antigens of the system D, d, C, c, and E, e. Though "d" does not represent an antigen but simply represents the absence of D antigen, but the term was utilized with Fisher-Race terminology. Each antigen and corresponding gene were given the same letter designation (when referring to the gene, the letter is italicized). The terminology represents a "short-hand" notation for the eight possible (triplet) Rh gene combinations (Table 5.2). The **phenotype** (antigens expressed on the RBC detected by typing) of a given RBC is defined by the presence of D, C, c, E, and e expression. According to Fisher-Race theory, each individual inherits a set of *Rh* genes from each parent (i.e. one *D* or *d*, one *C* or *c*, and one *E* or *e*). The *Rh* genes were thought to be **codominant** and each inherited gene expresses its corresponding antigen on the RBC. The combination of maternal and paternal haplotypes determines the **genotype** (the *Rh* genes inherited from each parent) and

Table 5.1: Examples of gene combination and Rh status.

Examples of gene combination	Rh status
Dce/dce	Rh positive
DCe/DCe	
DcE/dce	
dce/dce	Rh negative
dcE/dce	
dCe/dce	

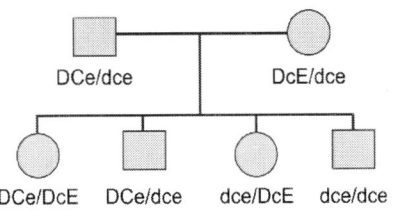

Fig. 5.1: Normal pattern of Rh inheritance.

Table 5.2: The haplotype of Fisher and Race and modified Wiener system for Rh.

Fisher-Race haplotype	Modified Wiener haplotype
Rh positive	
DCe	R^1
DcE	R^2
Dce	R^0
CDE	R^z
Rh negative	
dce	r
dCe	r'
dcE	r"
dCE	r^y

phenotype. The Rh phenotype of an individual is reported as DCE rather than CDE because Fisher postulated that the *C/c* locus lies between the *D/d* and *E/e* loci. It is necessary that C, c, E, and e represent actual antigens recognized by specific antibodies. There is no antibody that recognizes antigen which indicates the fact that d antigen does not exist. The **Fisher-Race notations/terminology** with five major Rh system antigens is the **most commonly used** because they fit most easily with the serologic reactions obtained in practice.

Drawbacks

The number of Rh antigens continues to grow and the original Fisher-Race terminology is becoming too limiting. Rarely, an individual may not express any allelic antigen at one or both Rh loci (i.e. an individual may lack E and e, or all CcEe antigens). The genotype for such Rh (D)-positive individual with a deletion phenotype can be written *DC-* or *Dc-*, or *D-*. A deletion of Cc with Ee has not been observed. An individual without any expression of Rh antigens on the RBC is said to be **Rh$_{null}$**, and the phenotype is written as _/_. An individual may have weakened expression of all Rh antigens and these individuals are said to have the **Rh$_{mod}$ phenotype. Placing parenthesis around (D), (C), and (e) indicates weakened expression of particular antigen.**

Wiener (Rh-HR) Terminology

This terminology was based on the belief that the Rh antigens were the products of a single (one) gene coding for an "agglutinogen" composed of multiple/several (series of) "blood factors." However, it is found that there are two Rh genes and not one gene. The agglutinogen may be considered the phenotypic expression of the haplotype.

Wiener's terminology is complex and unwieldy.

Modified Wiener terminology: Many uses modified Wiener terminology interchangeably with other nomenclatures. A modified version (Table 5.2) of Wiener's nomenclature is useful in spoken language to convey the **Rh haplotype**. In this, uppercase "R" indicates that D antigen is present and lowercase r (or little r) indicates that D is absent and a number or letter indicates the presence of C/c or E/e antigens. Thus, C or c and E or e Rh antigens carried with D are represented by 1 for Ce (R_1), 2 for cE (R_2), 0 for ce (R_0), and z for CE (Rz) (Table 5.2). The lower-case letter "r" indicates haplotypes lacking D with C/e and E/e antigens indicated using symbols: r' for Ce, r" for cE and r^y for CE. The symbols prime (') and double prime (") are used with r to designate the Cc and Ee antigens; for example, "prime" is used for Ce (r'), "double prime" for cE (r"), and "y" or "z" for CE (r^y). Dashes are used to denote the missing antigens of the rare deletion (or CE-depleted) phenotypes; for example, D__ (referred to as D dash, dash) lacks C/c and E/e antigens.

Rosenfield and Coworkers: Alpha Numeric Terminology

As the Rh blood group system expanded, it became difficult or impractical to assign names to new antigens using the existing terminologies. Rosenfield and associates proposed a numeric system of naming the antigens of the Rh system in 1962. The advantage of this nomenclature is that it depends on simple demonstration of the presence or absence of the antigen on the RBC. It neither had genetic basis nor based on a theory of Rh inheritance. A minus sign preceding number is used to indicate the absence of the antigen. If typing of an antigen is not done, its number will not appear in the sequence. An advantage of this nomenclature is that the RBC phenotype is provided in brief and clearly expressed manner. For the five major antigens are assigned numbers as: D is Rh1, C is Rh2, E is Rh3, c is Rh4, and e is Rh5. For example, RBCs with type D + C+ E + c negative, e negative, the Rosenfield nomenclature is Rh: 1, 2, 3, -4, -5. If the sample was not tested for, it would be Rh: 1, 2, 3, -4. All Rh system antigens have been assigned a number and this system is suitable to electronic data processing (including data entry and retrieval). Its limitation is that a similar nomenclature is also used for other blood groups such as Kell, Duffy, Kidd, Lutheran, Scianna, etc. In Kell blood group system, K: 1, 2 refer to the K and k antigens. Hence, it is necessary to use both the alpha (Rh:, K:) and the numeric (1, 2, -3, etc.) to indicate a phenotype.

International Society of Blood Transfusion: Updated Numeric Terminology

It is necessary to have a universal/uniform/ standardized nomenclature that is readable to both eye and machine and also to retain the genetic basis of blood groups language for terminology. Hence, the International Society of Blood Transfusion (ISBT) formed the Committee on Terminology for Red Cell Surface Antigens. The ISBT adopted a six-digit number for each authenticated antigen belonging to a blood group system. The first three numbers denote the system and the remaining three the antigenic specificity. Number 004 was given to the Rh blood group system, and then each antigen was given a unique number to complete the six-digit computer number. For example, for Fisher-Race D or Wiener Rh_0, it is 004001.

For each antigen, an alphanumeric designation similar to the Rosenfield nomenclature is used. The alphabetic names formerly used were not changed but were converted to all uppercase letters (e.g. Rh, Kell is converted to RH, KELL). Hence, D is RH1, C is RH2, and so forth. There is no space between the RH and the designate number.

Overview of Rh Terminologies

Phenotype: The *phenotype* is what is seen by tests made directly on the RBCs, even though other antigens may be present. The phenotype includes the alphabetical symbol (denotes the blood group), followed by a colon and then the specificity numbers of the antigens defined. A minus sign preceding the number is used to indicate that the antigen was tested for but was not present. For example, the phenotype D + C+ E- c + e + or DCe/ce or R1r would be written as RH:1, 2, -3, 4, 5.

Haplotype: It is the genetic constitution of an individual with respect to one member of a pair of allelic gene. It is short for haploid genotype. The *genotype* refers to the actual total genetic makeup of an individual. In haplotype, the symbols are italicized. A haplotype is followed by a space or an asterisk, and then the numbers of the specificities are separated by commas. Examples, *R1* haplotype or *Dce* would be *RH 1,2,5 or RH*1,2,5 and R2* haplotype or *DcE* would be *RH 1,3,4 or RH*1,3,4*.

■ Rh ANTIGENS

Rh blood group system is a very complete red cell antigen system that contains at least 55 different antigens. The most important of these is D. The **D antigen is the most immunogenic of all red cell antigens** and **most important in routine blood banking**. Rh antigens are **restricted to red cells**. Rh antigens **do not exist in soluble form** and thus are not secreted in body fluids. More than 80% of D-negative individuals who receive a D-positive transfusion will develop anti-D antibody. **Rh is the second most important blood group system in terms of transfusion**. It is necessary to routinely test blood of all recipients and donors for D to ensure that D-negative (Rh-negative) recipients are identified and given D-negative blood.

- The **first Rh antigen detected is the D antigen**. Other antigens namely C, c, E, and e were later identified and became part of the Rh system. Rh system as a gene complex which is inherited in various combinations of the antigens namely C or c, D or d and E or e. The D antigen is most/highly immunogenic of all the Rh antigens, resides on the RhD protein followed by c, E, C, and e. Cc and *Ee antigens* are weak antigens and therefore risk of sensitization to these antigens is less than the risk of sensitization to D. D antigen of the Rh system is the most immunogenic red cell antigen after A and B. D antigen is the basis for determining Rh positivity or negativity and is routinely used to designate blood type (for example, A-positive or A-negative). Hence, individuals can be classified as D-positive (Rh-positive) or D-negative (Rh-negative), depending on the presence of the red cell D antigen (Fig. 5.2).
- **Rh positive (+ve):** Individuals who have D antigen on the red cell surface are Rh positive (+ve).
- **Rh negative (–ve):** Individuals who lack the D antigens on the red blood cells are called as Rh negative (–ve).
- D antigen is capable of stimulating anti-D production after transfusion or pregnancy in the majority of RhD-negative individuals. Detection of D antigen is largely a preventive step to avoid transfusing a D-negative recipient with the cells expressing the D antigen.

Weak D Antigen

Most D-positive red cells show clear-cut macroscopic agglutination after centrifugation with reagent anti-D and can be readily classified as D-positive. In about 1% of D-positive individuals, demonstration of the D antigen requires additional steps like prolonged incubation with anti-D reagent or enhancement by addition of antiglobulin serum (antihuman globulin [AHG]) after incubation with anti-D owing to a quantitative decrease in RhD protein. **Red cells which are positive for D only by the indirect antiglobulin test (IAT) are referred to as weak D**. These were typed as weak D (historically these cells were known as D^u which is no longer used now). It is characterized by weakened expression of the normal D antigen (few normal antigens per red cell). They produce weak or absent RBC agglutination by anti-D during routine serologic testing. Some of these cells may even appear to be D-negative, depending on methodology. In **weak D individuals, cells have the D antigen** but have **fewer D antigens per cell than normal Rh-positive cells**. Recently the serologic weak D definition has been modified to reactivity of RBCs with anti-D reagent giving no or weak (≤2+) reactivity in initial testing with moderate or strong reactivity with AHG. The **weak D test needs a control** because the test uses an antiglobulin phase. Red cells with a positive direct antiglobulin test (DAT) will agglutinate in the IAT. A control for the routine D phenotype is present if negative reactions with anti-A and anti-B are observed. These reagents all have similar diluents.

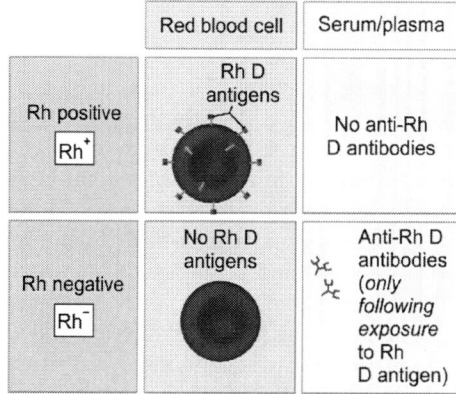

Fig. 5.2: Rh blood groups, Antibodies to Rh D antigen develop only in Rh-negative individuals who have been exposed to Rh positive blood during transfusion or Rh-negative mother delivering a Rh-positive infant.

Significance of Weak D

- **In donors:** Weak D is considered as D-positive.

- **In recipients:** Weak D recipients should receive only Rh-negative blood. Rh-negative mothers with "weak D" positive infants should be given Rh immunoprophylaxis.

Partial D Antigen

The D antigen is a multivalent structure. **Partial D antigens are RhD proteins with missing D epitopes** (i.e. there is lack part of the D antigen complex). Such red cells deficient in components of D are described as partial D. They **will be typed as D-positive**. The individuals with partial D antigens can produce alloanti-D antibodies to that missing part. This alloanti-D is nonreactive to their own cells (i.e. autologous RBCs) but can react with allogeneic red cells. The alloanti-D produced by these individuals recognizes D-specific epitopes missing on their own RBCs. The **partial D red cells react strongly when tested with anti-D**. Normally, it is not possible to detect this during routine testing. But once they produce anti-D, they can be recognized. This should be kept in mind while investigating a case of atypical antibodies.

Rh_{null} Type (Rh-Negative Phenotype)

Rarely, individual may **lack all the Rh antigens** (D–) and this is called Rh_{null} type. This has a genetic origin and may be due to the absence of the gene that regulates the expression of Rh antigens or to the presence of an amorphic gene. Rh_{null} cells have abnormalities in RBC morphology (spherocytes, stomatocytes), water content, cell volume and carbon dioxide (CO_2) permeability. Rh_{null} cells show increased osmotic fragility and a reduced survival/life span and may produce mild hemolytic anemia (Rh deficiency syndrome). These individuals are also prone to develop Rh antibodies.

Rh_{mod} Phenotype

The Rh_{mod} phenotype is similar to the Rh_{null}. In this phenotype, red cells **lack most of their Rh antigen** expression because of the inheritance of a modified RHAG gene. Hemolytic anemia is also a characteristic of this phenotype.

Enhanced D Antigen

In this, there is **altered expression of D antigen**. It may be due to inheritance of D--/D--genotype with no Cc/Ee.

Rh System Biochemistry

There are two closely linked genes encode Rh antigens namely, **RHD and RHCE**. They are located closely together on chromosome 1.
- The *RHD* gene encodes the D antigen.
- *RHCE* gene encodes CE antigens in various combinations (ce, cE, Ce, or CE).
- Rh-positive individuals possess at least one *RHD* gene and produce the RhD protein and the D antigen on their red cells. Rh-negative individuals, lack the RhD protein and the D antigen.
- A third gene, *RHAG*, located on chromosome 6, encodes for another protein RhAG (Rh-associated glycoprotein) and is associated with the production of the Rh_{null} phenotype.

RH ANTIBODIES

Characteristics of Rh Antibodies

ABO antibodies are found in individuals who lack the corresponding antigen. In contrast to ABO system, there are **no naturally occurring corresponding antibodies against Rh antigens** in Rh-negative individuals.
- **Acquired (immune) antibodies:** Rh antibodies develop only after exposure to Rh antigens on foreign red blood cells.
- **Causes of Rh antibody production:** The most common and clinically the most important Rh antibody is anti-D. Most Rh antibodies result from exposure to human red cells through **pregnancy or transfusion**.
  – During pregnancy in Rh-negative woman carrying Rh-positive fetus:
    - Transplacental hemorrhage
    - Abortion, amniocentesis, trauma or delivery.
  – Following transfusion of Rh incompatible blood or blood components: Rh+ve blood given to Rh−ve patients.

- **Amount of RhD-positive cells needed for sensitization:** Even exposure of 0.1 mL RhD-positive cells is enough to elicit antibody response in Rh-negative individuals. **Once produced, it is irreversible** and circulating Rh antibodies can persist for years at nondetectable levels. Subsequent exposure to Rh antigen produces a rapid secondary antibody response.
- **Nature of antibodies:** Most antibodies against Rh antigens are of **immunoglobulin G (IgG) isotype (IgG1 and IgG3)**, although rare examples of immunoglobulin M (IgM) and immunoglobulin A (IgA) are known. Anti-Rh antibodies are **reactive at 37°C,** and **do not bind complement effectively** (Rh antibodies do not fix complement). The incompatible RBCs are almost always cleared through extravascular destruction. The hemolysis develops due to Rh incompatibility is extravascular type and occurs predominantly in the spleen.
- **Enhancement of the reactivity of anti-Rh antibodies:** The reactivity of Rh antibodies can be enhanced **by high protein, low-ionic strength saline (LISS), polyethylene glycol (PEG), AHG or with enzyme-treated RBCs**. They **can be detected by antiglobulin test** (Coombs test). The gel method is very sensitive for the detection of Rh antibodies.
- Rh antibodies are directed against all Rh antigens, except d and include: anti-D, anti-C, anti-c, anti-E and anti-e. Rh antibodies may develop due to previous alloimmunization by previous pregnancy or transfusion, except for some naturally occurring forms of anti-E and anti-CW.

Clinical significance/importance: Rh blood group is important in individuals who are D-negative.
- **Hemolytic disease of the fetus and newborn (HDFN/HDN):** Rh incompatibility between mother and fetus results in hemolytic disease of the newborn. It can develop when the **pregnant woman is Rh-negative and have an Rh-positive fetus**. HDN develops when the D-positive fetal RBCs cross the placenta and reach mother's circulation. Once present, these anti-D can produce **HDFN** that used to cause of fetal death before the introduction of anti-D prophylaxis. To prevent sensitization to the D antigen, Rh-negative patients should be transfused with Rh-negative RBCs. This is especially true for young girls and women of childbearing age.
  - **Prophylaxis of Rh immune globulin (IgG anti-D):** All Rh-negative women should be prophylactically given Rh immune globulin (IgG anti-D) in mid pregnancy, following an invasive procedure (i.e. amniocentesis) and immediately after delivery **to prevent alloimmunization**. Rh immune globulin should be **administered within 72 hours of exposure** to prevent active immunization. Rh immune globulin should not give to Rh-negative women who are already immunized to D antigen (i.e. have anti-D).
- **Hemolytic transfusion reactions:** Rh incompatibility between donor and recipient results in hemolytic transfusion reactions. If Rh-negative patient is given Rh-positive (D-positive) blood, it stimulates the production of Rh (anti-D/anti-Rh) antibodies and can also cause serious hemolytic transfusion reaction.
- **Auto-Rh antibody may be found in individuals with warm autoimmune hemolytic anemia** (e.g. anti-e).

■ Rh (D) GROUPING/TYPING

Indications: Rh antibodies are fairly straightforward to detect and identify. Routine Rh grouping of RBCs are done using D antigens in patients and in weak D antigens in donors. **Tests for other than D antigens** are performed **only when there is specific indication**. These indications include:
- To identify unexpected antibodies
- To obtain a compatible blood for patients having unexpected antibody
- Selection of panel of donors having desired antigens (red cell panel)

- Investigation of disputed paternity
- In Rh-negative donors to prevent immunization due to other antigens
- Family studies.

Types of Rh Typing Reagents (Antisera)

Many types of reagent antisera derived from a variety of sources are available for routine Rh testing. The reagents may be high-protein, low-protein, chemically modified, saline-reactive, monoclonal, or blends of monoclonals. The most commonly monoclonal-polyclonal blends and monoclonal blends reagents are used. The goal is to obtain Rh typing of individuals' RBCs as quickly and accurately as typing for ABO.

Reagents for Rh (D) Grouping

In the D typing, anti-D is combined with patient or donor red cells. Development of agglutination indicates the presence of the D antigen on the red cells (e.g. D-positive), and if no agglutination indicates there is absence of the D antigen (e.g. D-negative). Running of a negative reagent control ensures that a false-positive result is not present (Table 5.3).

Historically, the reagents used in Rh grouping were divided into two categories: high-protein and low-protein reagents.

1. **High-protein reagents of human polyclonal origin** were first used for routine D typing. To polyclonal human anti-D sera, potentiating substances such as albumin, enzymes and AHG reagent are added with human IgG anti-D to enhance the agglutination.
2. **Low-protein reagents** are **monoclonal anti-D antibodies** or **monoclonal and polyclonal antibody blends**. They have replaced the high-protein reagents.

Monoclonal Antisera (Anti-D Reagents)

Conventional anti-D reagents are mainly of the IgG type and cause agglutination only if they are potentiated. They need control as the antisera are suspended in high-protein medium. As monoclonal antibody production

Table 5.3: Typing for D antigen with patient or donor red cells.

Reaction of red cells with anti-D	Reaction of red cells with reagent control	Inference (D antigen)
+	0	D-positive
0	0	D-negative
+	+	Cannot interpret typing

(+: Agglutination; 0: no agglutination)

became available, Rh monoclonal antibodies (monoclonal antisera) have become the reagents of choice.
- Monoclonal meaning protein or molecules from a single clone of cells. These monoclonal reagents are **derived from single clones of antibody-producing cells**. The antibody-producing cells are hybridized with myeloma cells (malignant tumor cells obtained from myeloma which has capacity to multiply) to increase their reproduction rate. This increases their capability to produce single type of antibodies (refer pages 62, 63).
- Monoclonal anti-D reagents have a low-protein diluent formulation similar in protein concentration to the diluent of the ABO reagents (approximately 6% bovine albumin). The low-protein diluent does not produce the false-positive agglutination associated with high-protein D typing reagents. There is no need for a separate Rh control test.
- Since they are prepared from hybridoma cell cultures rather than human sources, monoclonal reagents have no risk of transmitting infectious disease.

Various anti-D monoclonal reagents are mentioned in Box 5.1 and refer Figure 4.1.

IgM anti-D monoclonal reagent: It is highly specific and **saline reacting** reagent. It **works equally well at room temperature and at 37°C**. It is good for emergency slide test or immediate spin tube tests as well as for routine RhD typing. IgM anti-D is **unreliable for detection of weak Du by antiglobulin test**.

> **Box 5.1:** Various anti-D monoclonal (D phenotyping) reagents.
>
> - Monoclonal from single clone
>   - IgM anti-D monoclonal reagents
>   - IgG anti-D monoclonal reagents
> - Monoclonal blend: IgM and IgG (blend) anti-D monoclonal reagents of human-marine heterohybridomas
> - Monoclonal-polyclonal blend: Blend of IgM anti-D from human-marine heterohybridoma monoclonal and IgG polyclonal anti-D reagent

> **Box 5.2:** Different methods of Rh (D) grouping.
>
> - Slide or tile technique
> - Tube technique
>   - Immediate spin (IS) technique
>   - Tube sedimentation technique (using saline, albumin, enzyme or AHG test)
> - Microplate method
> - Column agglutination technique
>   - Gel Technology (I.D Micro-typing system)
>   - Glass microbeads technology
> - Automated or semiautomated method

Monoclonal blends: As already mentioned earlier, the D antigen is a complex antigen composed of many epitopes. The monoclonal Rh antibodies obtained from a single clone have a narrow specificity. Hence, most commercial anti-D reagents are usually obtained or prepared by a blending/combination of monoclonal anti-D reagents from several different clones. This ensures reactivity with a broad spectrum of Rh-positive RBCs. Some companies blend both IgM and IgG anti-D to **maximize visualization of reactions at immediate spin testing** and to allow indirect antiglobulin testing **for weak D antigen** with the same reagent. The production of stable IgM anti-D provided a major breakthrough in blood group serology. Monoclonal blends can be used for slide, tube, microplate/microwell, and most automated Rh testing methods.

Similar to reagents for ABO typing, D typing reagents are labeled with the antibody specificity and specify how to use it. The detailed methods and the characteristics are provided in the product insert. Apart from D typing reagents, products are available for the phenotyping of other antigens within the Rh blood group system, such as C, E, c, and e.

Controls for Rh (D) Grouping

For monoclonal anti-D reagents: Known O Rh (D) positive and O Rh (D) negative cells may be used as controls.

For polygonal anti-D reagents: AB serum or diluent control with the anti-D reagents or 22% bovine serum albumin may be used as negative control.

Rh (D) Grouping Techniques (Procedure)

Usually Rh (D) grouping is done along with ABO grouping using the same techniques used for ABO grouping. The different methods of Rh (D) grouping are listed in Box 5.2.

Slide or Tile Techniques

Slide or tile technique is not recommended for routine use and is only used for emergency Rh typing especially in outdoor camps. Because it may not detect weak Rh antigens and may give false-negative results. Slide tests give optimal results only when a high concentration of red cells and antibodies are combined at 37°C. IgM monoclonal anti-D reagent have become widely available and work equally well for slide test.

- Place one drop of anti-Rh (D) reagent (should be monoclonal IgM type) on a slide/white tile.
- Add one drop of 30-40%) red cell suspension.
- Mix them using a clean applicator stick.
- Observe for agglutination after 2 minutes.

Interpretation: Presence of agglutination indicates that the blood sample is Rh+ve.

Tube Techniques

The procedure depends upon the type of the anti-D reagent used. It is as important to carefully read the instructions supplied with the reagents by manufacturer and proceed accordingly. Monoclonal anti-D will work in saline can be done at room temperature, but others need to be incubated at 37°C.

Tube test using IgM monoclonal anti-D/saline agglutination test for Rh (D) typing.

Materials required:
- 75 × 10 mm tubes
- Test serum-IgM monoclonal anti-D/saline anti-D
- Test red blood cells
- Pasteur pipettes (Fig. 5.3)
- Rh-positive and Rh-negative control cells (for monoclonal anti-D)

Method (refer Fig. 4.8):
- Prepare 2–5% washed red cell (to be tested) suspension in isotonic saline warmed at 37°C. Warm saline removes cold antibodies and nonspecifically bound proteins. Wash three times with normal saline to remove all the traces of serum. Decant completely after the last washing.
- With clean Pasteur pipette, add one drop of anti-D to a small clean test tube (75 × 10 mm size).
- Add one drop of 2–5% saline red cell suspension to the above tube.
- Mix them gently and incubate at 37°C for 30 minutes (sedimentation technique) or centrifuge for 1 minute at 1,500 rpm (immediate spin technique) for 15–20 seconds.
- Resuspend the cells by gentle agitation. Look for agglutination and hemolysis against well-lit background.
- Transfer one drop of the mixture onto a glass slide, using a thin bore Pasteur pipette. Spread the cells over an area of 2 × 1 cm using the pipette.
- Examine the slide under microscope for "agglutination".
- If reaction is negative, incubate further at room temperature, centrifuge and read again. This additional incubation promotes positive reaction with the presence of complement.
- Initial testing is done with polyspecific AHG and can later be confirmed with monospecific AHG.
- Grade the reaction and record the results.

Other techniques such as albumin addition technique and enzyme technique for Rh(D) typing are not discussed here. These techniques are similar to tube test using IgM monoclonal anti D (saline agglutination test) descried above except the addition of albumin/enzymes after centrifugation step.

Weak D (D^u) Testing

An anti-D reagent, used for indirect antiglobulin test, is used for testing weak D antigens (Box 5.3).

Materials required:
- 75 × 10 mm tubes
- Suitable anti-D reagent (refer Box 5.3)
- Test red cells
- Antiglobulin (AHG) reagent
- Control IgG-coated red cells.

Method (Fig. 5.4):
- Take one drop of 2–5% suspension of test red cells in a tube and add one drop of suitable anti-D.
- Mix them gently and incubate at 37°C for 15 to 30 minutes.
- Wash three times with saline.
- Observe the tube for agglutination.

Box 5.3: Reagents used for testing weak D antigens.
- IgG monoclonal anti-D
- Polyclonal IgG anti-D
- Blend IgG monoclonal and IgM monoclonal anti-D
- Blend monoclonal IgM and polygonal IgG anti-D

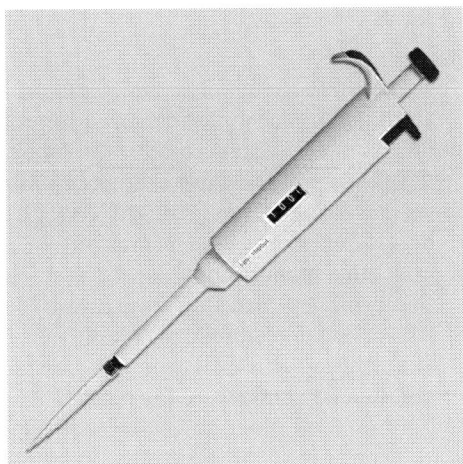

Fig. 5.3: Micropipette.

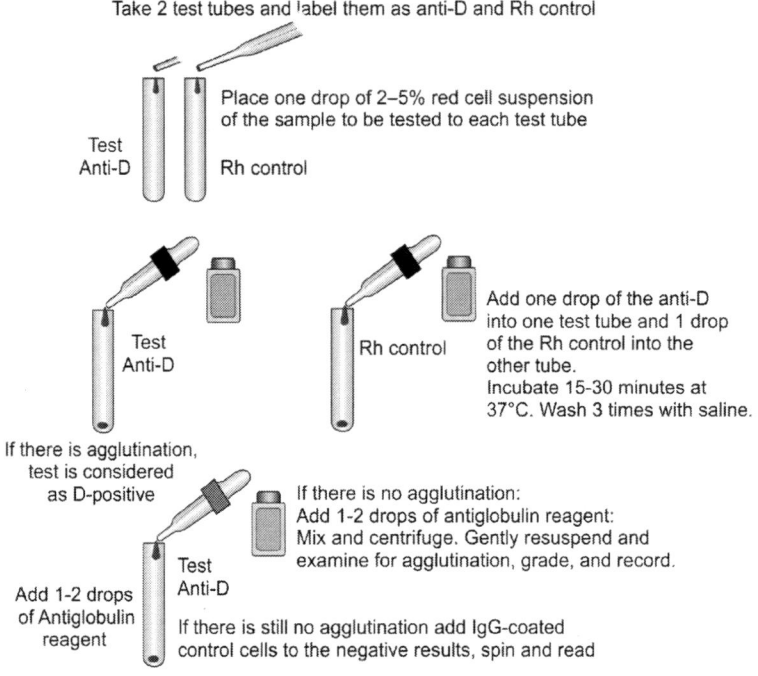

Fig. 5.4: Different steps in the procedure for detecting weaker D (D^u).

Interpretation
- **Positive test:** If there is agglutination, it indicates positive test and record the sample as D-positive.
  - If there is no agglutination then wash the cells three to four times with saline and decant the last wash completely.
  - Add two drops of antiglobulin (AHG) reagent and mix gently.
  - Centrifuge at 1,000 rpm for 1 minute.
  - Resuspend the cell button gently, look for agglutination and record the results.
- **Negative test:** All negative reactions should be confirmed by adding known IgG, sensitized control cells, recentrifuge and look for agglutination. The presence of agglutination confirms the test results and if there is no agglutination the test is considered as invalid.

The weak D test should not be performed on red cells with a positive direct antiglobulin test because of the false-positive results likely to occur.

Microplate Technique for Rh (D) Grouping (Fig. 5.5)

By using IgM monoclonal anti-D, Rh typing can be done simultaneously with ABO grouping on the same microplate.

Method:
- To the row G of microplate, add one drop of anti-D (1) to each well and then add one of the donor's/patient's red cells. The known Rh-positive, Rh-negative cells as controls are placed in column 11 and 12 (Fig. 5.5).
- Row H can be used for a second anti-D (2) from other manufacture.
- Gently mix the plate and cover it with the lid. Leave it undisturbed for 1 hour.
- Examine all the wells for hemolysis/agglutination and record the results.

Column Agglutination Technology (Gel Card Technology/Microtyping System)

Rh Blood Group System

		Donor/patient's cell									Controls		
											A cells	B cells	O cells
Cell group		1	2	3	4	5	6	7	8	9	10	11	12
A	Anti-A	O	O	O	O	O	O	O	O	O	O	O	O
B	Anti-B	O	O	O	O	O	O	O	O	O	O	O	O
C	Anti-AB	O	O	O	O	O	O	O	O	O	O	O	O
		Donor's/patient's serum											
Serum group		1	2	3	4	5	6	7	8	9	10	11	12
D	A cells	O	O	O	O	O	O	O	O	O	O	O	O
E	B cells	O	O	O	O	O	O	O	O	O	O	O	O
F	O cells	O	O	O	O	O	O	O	O	O	O	O	O
D typing		Donor's/patient's cells									Controls		
												Rh (−)	Rh (+)
G	Anti-D (1)	O	O	O	O	O	O	O	O	O	O	O	O
H	Anti-D (2)	O	O	O	O	O	O	O	O	O	O	O	O

Fig. 5.5: Diagrammatic microplate for ABO and Rh blood typing.

method is described under ABO grouping on pages 78-82 (refer Figs 4.14-4.17). Matrix gel system for D^u testing is also available.

Problems Encountered in Rh Grouping and their Solutions

Several common causes of false Rh typing results and corrective actions are presented in Table 5.4.

Problems in Rh Grouping

Various causes of problems encountered in Rh grouping have been shown in Box 5.4.

Resolving Rh Grouping Problems

Various steps in resolving problems encountered in Rh grouping have been shown in Box 5.5.

Table 5.4: False reactions with Rh typing reagents.

False-positives		False-negatives	
Probable cause	Corrective action	Probable cause	Corrective action
Defect in sample preparation		*Defect in sample preparation*	
Cell suspension too heavy	Use correct suspension and repeat the test	Failure to follow manufacturer's directions precisely	Follow the directions and repeat the test
Test incubated too long or drying (slide)	Strictly follow manufacturer's instructions	Saline-suspended cells (slide)	Use unwashed cells
		Resuspension too vigorous	Resuspend all tube tests gently

Contd...

Contd...

Reagent		Reagent	
Bacterial contamination of reagent vial	Use a new reagent vial and repeat the test		
Reagent contaminated by low-incidence antibody	Use reagent from another manufacturer or use a known serum antibody	Reagent deterioration	Open new reagent vial
Incorrect reagent selected	Repeat test using correct reagent	Incorrect reagent selected	Read vial label carefully and repeat the test
Centrifugation		**Centrifugation**	
Centrifugation too long	Repeat test by reducing the centrifugation time	Centrifugation too short	Repeat test using longer centrifugation time
RPM (revolution per minute) too high	Repeat test using lower RPM	RPM too low	Repeat testing using higher RPM
Problems in donor/patient		**Problems in donor/patient**	
Fibrin interference	Use saline-washed cells and repeat the test	Variant antigen	Submit sample for further investigation
Rouleaux			
Cold agglutinins	Wash with warm saline and repeat the test	Immunoglobulin-coated red cells (in vivo)	Use saline-active typing reagent

---

Box 5.4: Various causes of problems encountered in Rh grouping.

- Improper identification of specimen
- Poor quality of reagents
- Improper techniques
- Failure to add reagents
- Incorrect cells to serum ratio
- Fibrin clots
- Too much incubation
- Incorrect reading, recording or interpretation of test results
- Improper calibration of centrifuge: It can cause either over centrifugation or under centrifugation
- Problems in donor/patient
- Weak expression of D antigens
- Immunoglobulin coating of red cells
- Increased abnormal proteins in patients (e.g. multiple myeloma) can cause rouleaux and can give rise to false positive
- Polyagglutination

Box 5.5: Various steps in resolving problems encountered in Rh grouping.

- Check all labels, records and for any clerical errors
- Check patients record for history of pregnancy, diagnosis, medication and previous transfusion
- Check equipment and reagents for proper quality control
- Check Rh control sera
- Obtain a fresh blood sample of patient and repeat tests of new sample by alternative procedures such as:
  - Washing of cells with warm saline
  - Enzyme treatment of cells
  - Absorption/elution
  - Direct antiglobulin test
  - Microscopic analysis
- Carry out family studies

SUMMARY

- Rh system was first discovered as a cause of HDFN. It can also cause erythroblastosis fetalis and hemolytic transfusion reactions.
- According to Fisher-Race DCE terminology, the antigens of the system are produced by three closely linked sets of alleles and that each gene is responsible for producing a product (or antigen) on the RBC surface.
- Two closely linked genes control the expression of Rh. One gene (RHD) codes for the presence of RhD,

(Contd...)

(Contd...)

- and a second gene (RHCE) codes for the expression of CcEe antigens.
- Rh antigens are nonglycosylated proteins in the RBC membrane and they are inherited as codominant alleles.
- Blood donor units for transfusion are considered Rh-positive if either the D or weak D test is positive; if both the D and weak D tests are negative, blood for transfusion is considered Rh-negative.
- Most Rh antibodies are IgG type and react optimally at 37°C or following antiglobulin testing.
- Rh antibodies are IgG and can cross the placenta and coat fetal (Rh-positive) RBCs.

SELF-ASSESSMENT EXERCISE

Write short notes on:
- Various methods of Rh typing
- Weak D (D^u) testing
- Clinical significance of Rh blood group system

CHAPTER 6

Other Blood Group Systems

CHAPTER OUTLINE

- Lewis blood group system (ISBT No. 007)
- MNS blood group system (ISBT No. 002)
- Kell and Kx blood group systems (ISBT No. 006 and 019)
- Duffy blood group system (ISBT No. 008)
- Kidd (JK) blood group system (ISBT No. 009)
- Lutheran blood group system (ISBT No. 005)
- The P blood group: P1PK (ISBT No. 003), GLOB (028), and FORS blood group systems (031)
- I blood group system (ISBT No. 027)
- Diego blood group system (ISBT No. 010)
- Cartwright (Yt) blood group system (ISBT No. 011)
- XG blood group system (ISBT No. 012)
- Scianna blood group system (ISBT No. 013)
- Dombrock blood group system (ISBT No. 014)
- Colton blood group system (ISBT No. 015)
- Landsteiner-Wiener blood group system (ISBT No. 016)
- Chido/Rodgers blood group system (ISBT No. 017)
- Gerbich blood group system (ISBT No. 020)
- Cromer blood group system (ISBT No. 021)
- Knops blood group system (ISBT No. 022)
- Indian blood group system (ISBT No. 023)
- OK blood group system (ISBT No. 024)
- RAPH blood group system (ISBT No. 025)
- JMH blood group system (ISBT No. 026)
- GIL blood group system (ISBT No. 029)
- JR blood group system (ISBT No. 032)
- LAN blood group system (ISBT No. 033)
- VEL blood group system (ISBT No. 034)
- CD59 blood group system (ISBT No. 035)
- Application of other blood groups to routine blood banking

INTRODUCTION

In addition to the ABO and Rh antigens, there are over 300 unique other blood group antigens located on red cells. So far, the International Society of Blood Transfusion (ISBT) has defined 36 blood group systems. These blood group donors may also elicit antibodies if transfused to recipients/patients. Hence, it is necessary to test screen all patients' blood samples to detect any unexpected antibody. If the antibody screen is positive then the antibody should be identified and transfuse blood lacking the corresponding antigen. The other important blood group systems are listed in Box 6.1. Most of these are weak antigens and have no clinical significance.

Functional Roles of Blood Group Systems

The functional roles of blood group systems have been shown in Table 6.1.

Box 6.1: Important blood groups other than ABO and Rh.

- Lewis system
- MNS system
- Kell system
- Duffy system
- P system
- Kidd system
- Lutheran system
- Yt system
- Dombrock system
- Colton system
- Diego system

Other Blood Group Systems

Table 6.1: Functional roles of blood group systems.

Functional roles	Blood group systems
Glycosyltransferases (enzymatic activities)	ABO, P1PK, Lewis, and H
Structural relationship to red cell (structural proteins to maintain red cell shape and mechanical deformability)	MNS, Diego, and Gerbich
Transport proteins (transporting water-soluble molecules across the lipid bilayer for intake of nutrients and excretion of waste products)	Rh, Kidd, Diego, Colton, and Kx
Complement pathway molecules	Chido/Rodgers, Cromer, and Knops
Adhesion molecules (ability of cells to adhere to other cells)	Lutheran, XG, Landsteiner-Wiener, and Indian
Microbial receptors [for infection by microorganisms (bacteria, viruses, or protozoan parasites)]	MNS, Duffy, P, Lewis, and Cromer
Biologic receptors	Duffy, Knops, and Indian

LEWIS BLOOD GROUP SYSTEM (ISBT NO. 007)

The Lewis blood group system was assigned the ISBT system number 007 and the system symbol LE.

The Lewis blood group system is unique and unusual because the Lewis antigens are not intrinsic to RBCs and are not synthesized or manufactured by RBC. They are type 1 glycosphingolipids manufactured in the gastrointestinal tract and secreted into the fluids and the plasma. From the plasma they are passively adsorbed or incorporated onto the RBC membrane. They are the result of the interaction of two fucosyltransferases encoded by independent genes namely (1) *Le* and (2) *Se*. The *FUT3* or *Lewis* gene resides on chromosome 19p13.3. Phenotypes of Lewis system are presented in Box 6.2.

Lewis Antigens

- **Poorly developed at birth.**
- They are reversibly adsorbed or incorporated onto the RBC membrane from plasma.
- Not found on cord blood or newborn red cells.

Box 6.2: Phenotypes of Lewis system.

- Le(a+b−)
- Le(a−b+)
- Le(a−b−)

- It mainly consists of two antigens: (1) Lewis a (Le^a, LE1) and (2) Lewis b (Le^b, LE2) and three common Lewis phenotypes are observed in adults: (1) Le(a+b−), (2) Le(a−b+), and (3) Le(a−b−). The Le(a+b+) is rare and observed on RBCs of very young children.
- Four additional antigens reflect the influence of ABO on Lewis (Le^a and Le^b) synthesis and antigenicity. These include (1) Le^{ab} (L3), (2) Le^{bH} (LE4), (3) ALe^b (LE5), and (4) BLe^b (LE6). The amount of Lewis antigen on RBCs is also influenced by ABO type.
- **Antigen expression:** Tissues and fluids expressing Lewis include plasma, saliva, RBCs, platelets, lymphocytes, endothelium, uroepithelium, and bowel mucosa.

Le and Se gene interaction:
- Le without Se: Le^a on RBCs and in saliva
- Le and Se: Le^b on RBCs, Le^a and Le^b in saliva
- lele, secretor status irrelevant: Le(a−b−) on RBCs and in saliva
- sese: No H in secretions.

Lewis Antibodies

- Similar to ABO, Lewis antibodies are often **naturally occurring** and made by Le(a−b−) persons. Thus, they occur without any known RBC stimulus and antibodies occur against Le^a and Le^b antigens.
- They are generally **immunoglobulin M (IgM) antibodies** but unlike ABO

antibodies, anti-Lewis antibodies are seldom clinically significant. They **do not cross the placenta**. Since the Lewis antigens are not well developed on fetal RBCs and do not cross placenta, these antibodies **do not cause hemolytic disease of the fetus and newborn** (HDFN).

Detection of antibodies: Anti-Le^a is the most commonly encountered of the Lewis antibodies that agglutinate saline suspended RBCs at room temperature. These agglutinates are often fragile and can be easily dispersed if the cell button is not gently resuspended after centrifugation. Some are reactive at 37°C and in the indirect antiglobulin test (IAT).

- **Enhancement:** Le^a and Le^b are glycosphingolipids and their antibody reactivity can be enhanced by pretreatment of RBCs with enzymes.
- **Neutralization:** Antibody reactivity can be neutralized by the adding commercially available soluble Lewis substance or plasma containing the soluble Lewis antigen of interest.

Antibodies and Phenotype

- **Anti-Le^b** can be found in individuals of **Le(a+b–) or Le(a–b–) phenotype**. Anti-Le^a is not observed in the Le(a–b+) phenotype because these individuals synthesize a small amount of Le^a. Some Le(a–b+) women can transiently become phenotypically Le(b–) during pregnancy due to the development of anti-Le^b.
- **Anti-Le^a** can be found only individuals of **Le(a–b–)** phenotype.

Significance of Antibodies

- They are **not associated with HDFN** and only rarely may cause hemolytic transfusion reactions (HTRs).
- **May play a role in renal graft rejection** in Le(a–b–) individuals.
- **Transfusion:** Lewis antigens are not intrinsic component of the RBC membrane and they are readily shed from transfused RBCs within a few days of transfusion. Also, Lewis blood group substance present in transfused plasma neutralizes Lewis antibodies in the recipient. This is responsible for very rarity for anti-Le^a or anti-Le^b to cause hemolysis of transfused RBCs.
  - **Anti-Le^a:** When fresh serum is tested, anti-Le^a may cause in vitro hemolysis of incompatible RBCs. It is most often seen with enzyme-treated RBCs than with untreated RBCs. Rarely HTRs may occur in patients with anti-Le^a are transfused with Le(a+) RBCs. Hence, anti-Le^a that is reactive at 37°C and that causes in vitro hemolysis, should not be ignored.
  - **Anti-Le^b:** It is neither common nor as strong as anti-Le^a. It is usually an IgM agglutinin and can bind complement.

Biological Role of Lewis Blood Group

The Lewis blood group antigens play an important role in disease.

- Le(a–b–) is associated with **increased risk of atherosclerotic disease and coronary death**.
- **Tumor:** Aberrant expression of sialyl-Le^a seen in many **gastrointestinal** and **uroepithelial cell cancers** and may contribute to tumor metastasis. Sialyl-Le^a is a ligand for the endothelial adhesion molecule E-selectin and this may be responsible for interaction of tumor cell with endothelium.
- **Infections:**
  - *Helicobacter pylori* which causes gastritis and ulcers, binds H, Le^b, and Le^y antigens.
  - A Lewis null and/or nonsecretor phenotype has a higher incidence of **recurrent *Candida* vaginitis and urinary tract infection**.
  - Le^b and type 1 H antigen are also **receptors for most norovirus and rotavirus strains**. Nonsecretors have inherent resistance against infection whereas nonsecretor acts as risk factor for necrotizing enterocolitis and sepsis in premature infants.

MNS BLOOD GROUP SYSTEM (ISBT NO. 002)

Following the discovery of the ABO blood group system, in 1927, the MNS blood group was the second blood group system identified. MNS blood group system consists of more than 46 antigens. However, only four (M/N and S/s) are commonly encountered in the clinical setting. In 1953, an antibody to a high-prevalence antigen, U (for almost *universal* distribution), was named by Wiener. Following observation by Greenwalt and colleagues that all U– RBCs were also S–s–, it resulted in the inclusion of U into the MNS system. Thus, presently the system has five major antigens: (1) M, (2) N, (3) S, (4) s, and (5) U. Similar to Rh antigens, the MNS blood group antigens are **expressed only on RBCs**. The genes encoding the MNS antigens are located on chromosome 4.

Box 6.3: Common phenotypes of MNS system.

- M+N–
- M+N+
- M–N+
- S+s–U+
- S+s+U+
- S–s+U+

MNS Antigens

M and N Antigens

The **M and N antigens are found on** a well-characterized major RBC membrane glycoprotein called **glycophorin A** (GPA/GYPA), the major RBC **sialic acid-rich** glycoprotein (sialoglycoprotein, SGP). The M and N antigens differ in their amino acid residues. These antigens are **well-developed at birth**. Since M and N are located at the outer end of GPA; they **can be easily destroyed by the routine enzymes used in blood bank** such as ficin, papain, and bromelain as well by the less common enzymes trypsin and pronase. If RBCs are treated with neuraminidase, which cleaves sialic acid (also known as *neuraminic acid* or *NeuNAc*), it abolishes reactivity with only some examples of antibody.

S/s and U Antigens

S/s and U antigens reside on a smaller glycoprotein called **glycophorin B** (GPB/GYPB) that is very similar to GPA. S and s antigens are **less easily degraded by enzymes**. This is because these antigens are located farther down the glycoprotein, and enzyme-sensitive sites are less accessible. The **enzymes used in blood bank** such as ficin, papain, bromelain, pronase, and chymotrypsin **can destroy S and s activity**. However, the amount of degradation depends on the strength of the enzyme solution, the duration of treatment, and the ratio between the enzyme-to-cell. Common phenotypes of MNS system are presented in Box 6.3.

Null Phenotypes

The MNS system also consists of three major null phenotypes namely (1) U–, (2) En(a–), and (3) M^k.

- **U– phenotype:** It is most common. In S–s–U– individuals, there is either complete loss or a recombination of glycophorin B occurs. This leads to altered expression of S/s and U antigens. Recombinant glycophorin B (Henshaw phenotype) can react weakly with some human anti-U and are known as U variants (S–s–U var).
- **En(a–) phenotype:** It is the result of recombination between glycophorin A and B genes to form a Lepore-type A-B hybrid lacking most of glycophorin A (GYPA).
- **M^kM^k phenotype:** It lacks all MNS antigens, including En(a), as the result of recombination and deletion of glycophorins A and B (GYPA and GYPB).

MNS Antigens and Encoding Genes

The genes for GYPA (*GYPA*) and GYPB (*GYPB*) are closely linked genes found on chromosome 4 and encode glycophorin A (GPA) and glycophorin B (GPB), respectively.

M and *N* are alleles of *GYPA* (encoding the M and N antigens on GPA) and *S* and *s* are alleles of *GPYB* (encoding the S and s antigens on GPB). Many rare variants can occur due to gene deletions, mutations and segmental exchanges. The M and N antigens include both protein and carbohydrate as part of the immune epitope. S/s antigen is an amino acid and the U antigen is a high-incidence antigen (occur in greater than 99% of the population). Loss of S, s, and U antigens is found with M^k and some recombinant *GYPB* alleles such as Henshaw.

MNS Antibodies

Anti-M and Anti-N

Features: Antibodies against M and N antigens are **naturally occurring antibodies usually of IgM isotype** (may also be IgG or have an IgG component). They are **usually detected as room temperature (react below 37°C) saline agglutinins**.
- They **do not bind complement**, regardless of their immunoglobulin class.
- They **do not react with enzyme-treated RBCs**.
- Anti-M and anti-N **may show dosage**, and react better with M+N– or M–N+ RBCs (genotype *MM or N/N*) than with M+N+ heterozygous RBCs (genotype *MN*). Very weak anti-M may not react with M+N+ RBCs at all and makes it difficult to identify this antibody.
- **Enhancement of antibody:** Antibody reactivity can be enhanced **by increasing the serum-to-cell ratio or incubation time**, or both, **by acidification of serum to pH 6.5**, by **decreasing incubation temperature or by adding a potentiating medium** such as albumin diluent, low ionic strength saline solution (LISS), polyethylene glycol (PEG) or by adding glucose-containing solution.

Anti-M: It is more **common in children** than in adults and particularly in patients with bacterial infections. Anti-M very rarely causes HTRs, decreased red cell survival or HDFN.

Anti-N: It is distinctly **uncommon** and of **no clinical significance**. In the past, an autoanti-N was found in patients regardless of their MN type, who were dialyzed on equipment sterilized with formaldehyde.

Anti-S and anti-s: They are usually **IgG-type** reactive at 37°C, and both are rarely implicated in HTRs and HDFN. Enzymatic modification of RBCs with proteases can reduce the reactivity of some anti-S and anti-s.

Anti-U: It is a rare immune antibody and usually contains IgG_1 component reactive at 37°C. It can cause fatal HTRs and occasionally severe HDFN. The reactivity of anti-U is resistant to proteolytic digestion.

KELL AND Kx BLOOD GROUP SYSTEMS (ISBT NO. 006 AND 019)

The Kell (KEL) blood group system was first identified in 1946 and consists of **mix of 36 high- and low-frequency antigens**. In 1946, K antigen (KEL1) was identified followed by its antithetical (directly opposed) k (KEL2) was identified 3 years later. Kell antigens are **numbered from KEL1 to KEL39 of which three are obsolete**. Anti-K was identified in a patient Mrs Kelleher. It was the first blood group system discovered after the introduction of antiglobulin testing. The Kell system consists of seven pairs (K/k, Js^a/Js^b, K11/K17, K14/K24, VLAN/VONG, KYO/KYOR, and KHUL/KEAL) and one triplet ($Kp^a/Kp^b/Kp^c$) of Kell antithetical antigens. Of the different sets of alleles, three very closely linked sets of alleles are clinically important namely (1) *K* (KEL1) and *k* (KEL2); (2) Kp^a (KEL3), Kp^b (KEL4) and Kp^c (KEL21), and (3) Js^a (KEL6) and Js^b (KEL7). Kell phenotypes are presented in Box 6.4.

Kell Antigens

The Kell antigens are **found only on RBCs** and its expression occurs by about the 10th

---

Box 6.4: Kell phenotypes.

- K+k–
- K+k+
- K–k+
- Kp (a+b–)
- Kp (a+b+)
- Kp (a–b+)
- Js (a+b–)
- Js (a+b+)
- Js (a–b+)
- K_o
- K_{mod}
- McLeod

week of life and is **well developed at birth**. The glycoprotein that contains Kell system antigens (CD238) is encoded by a gene at the *KEL* locus on **chromosome 7**, but their production also depends on genes at the *KX* locus on the X chromosome. The Kell antigens are **not denatured by the routine blood bank enzymes** ficin and papain **but are destroyed by trypsin and chymotrypsin when used in combination**.

Kx Antigen (XK1)

Kx is the only antigen of the Kx blood system and its product is Xk protein. Its ISBT number is 019 and symbol XK. The Kell glycoprotein is linked through a single disulfide bond to the Xk protein. This Xk protein is an integral membrane protein and expresses the Kx blood group antigen. This Xk protein is encoded by the XK gene on chromosome Xp21.1. The Xk protein is found in erythroid and megakaryocyte progenitors, skeletal muscle, heart, brain, and testis.

K and k Antigens

- **K antigens: Excluding ABO, K is the second to D in immunogenicity**. Most anti-K are induced by pregnancy and transfusion. However, the prevalence of K antigen is low, and the chance of transfusing a K+ unit is small. Even if anti-K develops, it is easy to find compatible units.
- **k antigens:** Antibodies to k antigen are very rare.

Kp^a, Kp^b, and Kp^c Antigens

Alleles Kp^a and Kp^c are produced due to low-prevalence mutations of their high-prevalence partner Kp^b.

Null and Weak Phenotypes

Like most blood group systems, Kell has a null phenotype that was discovered in 1957. The null phenotype is designated as K_0. K_0K_0 is an autosomal recessive, null phenotype in which none of the Kell antigens are expressed. These individuals can produce an alloantibody to the Kell glycoprotein (anti-Ku).

- **McLeod RBCs: Kell antigens are markedly depressed/absent** on McLeod RBCs. McLeod syndrome is an X-linked recessive disorder characterized by the absence of XK protein on RBCs, an acanthocytic morphology, compensated hemolysis with slow progression of cardiomyopathy, skeletal muscle wasting and neurological defects. McLeod syndrome can also be associated with chronic granulomatous disease (CGD). Lack of XK and Kell proteins in these individuals results in **formation of alloantibodies** against both proteins. These patients are incompatible with both Kell-positive and K_0K_0 RBCs.
- **Transient depression** and masking **of Kell antigens** may occur in **septic patients** and in **autoimmune hemolytic anemia due to anti-Kell autoantibodies**.

K_{mod} is the result of missense mutations and may occur on either K1 or k background.

Kell Antibodies

Anti-K

- **Naturally occurring anti-K is rare.** Most naturally occurring anti-K are IgM type which usually react best at room temperature. They have been associated with bacterial infections.
- K is very immunogenic and **immune anti-K** (anti-KEL1 or K1) is the most common immune red cell antibody found outside the ABO and Rh systems. Most anti-K appear to be **induced by pregnancy and transfusion**. It accounts for about two-thirds of non-Rh immune red cell alloantibodies. Alloantibodies against antigens in the Kell blood group system are **clinically significant**. It is commonly IgG_1 and occasionally complement binding. They **can cause both immediate and delayed hemolytic transfusion reactions (DHTRs)**. Anti-Kell antibodies are also associated with **HDFN**. HDFN secondary to maternal anti-Kell antibodies usually shows reticulocytopenia, with little or no bilirubinemia.

Other Kell antibodies (e.g. anti-k, anti-Kp^a, anti-Kp^b, anti-Js^a, and anti-Js^b) are rare.

DUFFY BLOOD GROUP SYSTEM (ISBT NO. 008)

The Duffy (FY) blood group system was discovered in 1951. It was named for Mr Duffy, a multiply-transfused hemophiliac who was found to have the first described example of anti-Fy^a. One year later, the antibody defining its antithetical antigen, Fy^b, was detected in the serum of a woman who had three pregnancies. Phenotypes in the Duffy System are presented in Table 6.2.

Duffy antigens and encoding genes: It contains five antigens: (1) Fy^a, (2) Fy^b, (3) Fy^3, (4) Fy^5, and (5) Fy^6.

The Duffy (Fy) locus is on chromosome 1. Fy^a and Fy^b are autosomal codominant antigens, whereas Fy^3, Fy^5, and Fy^6 are high-incidence antigens present on all RBCs except the Duffy null phenotype. The Fy^4 antigen, originally described by Sanger and colleagues on Fy(a–b–) RBCs, is in fact a distinct, unrelated antigen and is no longer included in the FY system.

Antigen expression: Duffy antigens are expressed on RBCs, cerebellar Purkinje cells and postcapillary venule endothelial cells. It may also be expressed on endothelial cells of renal glomeruli, vasa recta, thyroid, and pulmonary capillaries, alveolar type 1 squamous cells and epithelial cells of renal collecting tubules.

Table 6.2: Phenotypes in the Duffy system.

Reactions with anti-			RBC phenotype
Fy^a	Fy^b	Fy^3	
+	–	+	Fy(a+b–)
+	+	+	Fy(a+b+)
–	+	+	Fy(a–b+)
–	–	–	Fy(a–b–)
±	Weak reactivity	Weak reactivity	Fy(a–b^w)

Fy^a (FY1) and Fy^b (FY2) Antigen and Antibodies

These are two Duffy antigens most important in routine blood bank serology. They can be identified on fetal RBCs as early as 6 weeks gestational age and are well-developed at birth. These two antigens give rise to three phenotypes namely (1) Fy(a+b–), (2) Fy(a+b+), and (3) Fy(a–b+). The Fy^a and Fy^b antigens are very sensitive proteolytic enzymes but are not destroyed by trypsin. An extremely weak form of Fy^b expression is called Fy^x.

- Anti-Fy^a and anti-Fy^b are the antibodies against Fy^a and Fy^b. They can cause HDFN and both immediate and delayed HTRs. They are usually of IgG isotype, reactive at 37°C. They are detected only in the IAT.
- Antibodies against Fy^a, Fy^b, and Fy^6 antigens can be inhibited by prior protease digestion of RBCs. Anti-Fy^a is the most common alloantibody and can be detected in Fy(a–) individuals. Anti-Fy^b is relatively rare.

Fy^3 Antigen and Antibody

Anti-Fy^3 is rare antibody found in the serum Fy(a–b–) individuals who lack the Duffy glycoprotein. It reacted with all RBCs tested except those of the Fy(a–b–) phenotype. Fy^3 antigens are relatively resistant to enzymes/protease digestion.

Fy^5 Antigen and Antibody

Initially it was thought to be a second example of anti-Fy^3, because it reacted with all Fy(a+) or Fy(b+) RBCs but not with Fy(a–b–) red cells. However, it was found that it did not react with Fy(a+) or Fy(b+) Rh$_{null}$ RBCs and reacted only weakly with Fy(a+) or Fy(b+) D– RBCs.

The molecular structure of Fy^5 is not known, but probably it results from the interaction between the Rh complex and the Duffy glycoprotein. Individuals who are Fy(a–b–) or Rh$_{null}$ do not make Fy^5 antigen and are at risk of producing the antibody. Alloantibodies against Fy^5 are relatively rare and occur in Fy$_{null}$

individuals. Similar to Fy³, Fy⁵ is not destroyed by enzymes.

No human example of anti-Fy⁶ has been reported so far.

Duffy Glycoprotein and Malaria

The **Duffy glycoprotein is a receptor for merozoites of *Plasmodium vivax*.** Red cells with Fy(a–b–) phenotype are resistant to invasion by merozoites of *P. vivax*.

KIDD (JK) BLOOD GROUP SYSTEM (ISBT NO. 009)

The Kidd system is designated by the symbol JK or 009 by the ISBT. In 1951, Allen and colleagues found an antibody in the serum of Mrs Kidd, whose infant had HDFN. The antibody was named anti-Jkᵃ. Phenotypes in the Kidd system are presented in Table 6.3.

Significance: It has a special significance because **its antibodies may be difficult to detect to routine blood banking** and are **strongly associated with DHTRs** and with **intravascular hemolysis** (in contrast hemolysis with non-ABO antibodies is extravascular). Kidd antibodies may cause **acute transplant rejection.**

Kidd Antigens

Kidd gene is located on chromosome 18. The Kidd blood group is a simple and straightforward system. It consists primarily of two allelic antigens namely (1) Jkᵃ (JK1) and (2) Jkᵇ (JK2). Inheritance is autosomal codominant with three predominant phenotypes (Table 6.3). A fourth phenotype, Jk_{null} or Jk(a–b–), is very rare.

Expression of Kidd antigen: Kidd antigens are expressed on **RBCs** and along descending vasa recta **endothelial cells of the renal medulla.** Low level of expression may be found on heart, skeletal muscle, colon, small intestine, thymus, brain, pancreas, spleen, prostate, bladder and liver.

Null Phenotypes

The null phenotype Jk(a–b–) was described in 1959.

1. **Jk(a–b–) phenotype and the recessive allele, Jk:** Jk_{null} is **autosomal recessive**, reflecting homozygosity for a JK_{null} or amorph allele. Jk_{null} has a Jk(a–b–) phenotype and lack Jkᵃ, Jkᵇ, and the common antigen Jk3. Family studies show that most Jk(a–b–) nulls are homozygous for the rare "silent" allele *Jk*. Jk_{null} RBCs are resistant to lysis by 2M urea. The 2M urea is a lytic agent commonly used to lyse RBCs in a sample before it is used by some automated platelet-counting hematology analyzers.

2. **Jk(a–b–) phenotype and the dominant In (Jk) allele:** Another genetic explanation for the Jk(a–b–) phenotype is its association with a dominant gene called ***In (Jk)***, for "inhibitor". This type shows a **dominant pattern of inheritance**. Dominant type Jk(a–b–) RBCs adsorb and elute anti-Jk3 and anti-Jkᵃ or anti-Jkᵇ (depending on which genes were inherited). This suggests that the antigens are expressed but only very weakly. Individuals with the dominant

Table 6.3: Phenotypes in the Kidd system.

	Reactions with anti-		
Jkᵃ	Jkᵇ	Jk³	RBC phenotype
+	0	+	Jk (a+b–)
+	+	+	Jk (a+b+)
0	+	+	Jk (a–b+)
Null phenotype (Jk_{null})			
0	0	0	Jk (a–b–)
0/Weak reactivity	0/Weak reactivity	Weak reactivity	Jk (a–b–)

type Jk(a–b–) phenotype do not produce anti-Jk3. The molecular basis is not known.

Kidd Antibodies

Anti-Jk

Anti-Jk^a is more common than anti-Jk^b. Clinically anti-Jk or Kidd antibodies are a common cause of HTRs. They are usually of IgG$_1$ or IgG$_3$ isotype and can activate complement. Anti-Jk antibodies may be difficult to detect or identify in the blood bank. Anti-Jk antibodies have weak avidity, usually present in low titer, they demonstrate dosage and are frequently transient, disappearing rapidly after immune stimulation. On transfusion, these antibodies may produce an anamnestic response and post-transfusion hemolytic reaction. Hence, a previous history of antibodies is important before transfusion. Antibody reactivity can be enhanced with enzyme-treated RBCs and by the presence of complement. Although uncommon, anti-Jk can produce mild HDFN.

Anti-Jk3

The antibody anti-Jk^{a}Jk^b (i.e. inseparable) is also known as anti-Jk3 and it reacts with all RBCs except Jk$_{null}$, is found in Jk$_{null}$ individuals. Anti-Jk3 is produced by individuals of the rare Jk (a–b–) phenotype. Alloanti-Jk3 is an IgG antiglobulin-reactive antibody. Like other Kidd antibodies, anti-Jk3 reacts optimally by an antiglobulin test, and the reactivity is enhanced with enzyme pretreatment of the RBCs. Anti-Jk3 can cause severe, immediate, and delayed HTRs and with mild HDFN.

LUTHERAN BLOOD GROUP SYSTEM (ISBT NO. 005)

In 1945, anti-Lu^a was first detected (and described in detail a year later) in the serum of a patient who was transfused by a unit of blood carrying the corresponding low-prevalence antigen. This recipient was suffering from systemic lupus erythematosus. This blood donor's last name was Lutheran and new antibody was named Lutheran; the but the donor blood sample was incorrectly labeled.

The Lutheran (Lu) blood group system contains 22 antigens, numbered through Lu24. Two numbers (Lu10 and Lu15) are obsolete. This includes four pairs of allelic antigens and 11 high-incidence antigens. The four antithetical pairs are (1) Lu^a/Lu^b, (2) Lu6/Lu9, (3) Lu8/Lu14, and (4) Au^a/Au^b of which Lu^a, Lu9, and Lu14 are of low prevalence.

Lutheran antigens are resistant to the enzymes ficin and papain and to glycine-acid EDTA treatment. The Lutheran antigens are destroyed by treatment of red cells with trypsin or α-chymotrypsin, 2-aminoethylisothiouronium bromide (AET), and dithiothreitol (DTT).

The enzymes papain and ficin do not have any effect. Phenotypes in Lutheran system are presented in Table 6.4.

Antigens in the Lutheran System

The antigens in the Lutheran system are not well developed at birth. Hence, Lutheran antibodies do not cause clinically significant hemolytic disease of the newborn.

Table 6.4: Phenotypes in Lutheran system.

	Reactions with anti-		
Lu^a	Lu^b	Lu^3	RBC phenotype
+	0	+	Lu(a+b–)
+	+	+	Lu(a+b+)
0	+	+	Lu(a–b+)
Null phenotype (Lu$_{null}$)			
0	0	0	Lu(a–b–)
0/Weak reactivity	0/Weak reactivity	Weak reactivity	Lu(a–b–)
0/Weak reactivity	0/Weak reactivity	Weak reactivity	Lu(a–b–)

Antigen expression: Lutheran is a minor constituent of RBC membranes and appears on red cells at the orthochromatic erythroblast stage. Though these antigens are detected on fetal RBCs as early as 10–12 weeks of gestation, they are poorly developed at birth. Hence, HDFN is rare and only mild.

Blood bankers rarely deal with the serology of the Lutheran blood group system. This is because most of these antigens are high prevalence, so only a few individuals lack the antigen and can make an alloantibody. Consequently, the antibodies are seen infrequently.

Apart from RBCs, Lutheran glycoprotein is widely distributed/expressed in human tissues. These tissues include colon, small intestine, ovary, testis, prostate, thymus, spleen, pancreas, kidney, skeletal muscle, liver, lung, placenta, brain, heart, and bone marrow.

Lu^a and Lu^b antigens: Lu^a and Lu^b are antigens produced by allelic codominant genes.

Null/Weak Phenotypes

Lu(a–b–) phenotype can occur in three settings with distinct patterns of inheritance.

These include (1) autosomal recessive, (2) autosomal dominant (*In[Lu]*), and (3) X-linked recessive.

- **Autosomal recessive phenotype:** It is a true null phenotype and is extremely rare. This phenotype arises from inheritance of two silent amorph *LU* alleles. There is complete absence of all Lutheran antigens on RBCs. These individuals can develop an alloantibody to Lutheran glycoprotein (anti-Lu3) which can react with all Lu-positive RBCs except those from Lu(a–b–) individuals. It is not associated with altered expression of other red cell antigens.
- **Autosomal dominant and X-linked recessive:** These forms are characterized by very weak Lutheran expression. They are usually detected only after adsorption and elution.
  - *In(Lu)* is an **autosomal dominant Lu_{mod} phenotype**. Apart from Lutheran antigens, *In(Lu)* RBCs can show weakened expression of P1, i, Indian/CD44, and Knops/CD35 antigens and enhanced expression of CDw75. *In(Lu)* RBCs can show minor abnormalities, such as increased poikilocytosis and increased hemolysis, during in vitro storage.
  - X-linked Lu_{mod} phenotype: It shows weakened Lutheran; enhanced i and CDw75; and normal P1, i, and CD44 expression.

Since both *In(Lu)* and X-linked recessive Lu_{mod} phenotypes express some Lutheran antigens on RBCs and other tissues, both of them are not associated with the development of anti-Lu3.

Lutheran Antibodies

Lutheran antibodies are not clinically significant. They are only rarely associated with HDFN and HTRs. Most Lutheran antibodies do not react with RBCs treated with the sulfhydryl reagents AET, and DTT.

- **Anti-Lu^a** is the most common Lutheran alloantibody and rarely of clinical significance. It is usually IgM, room temperature agglutinin.
- **Antibodies against Lu^b and other Lutheran antigens** are of IgG isotype and react best in the IAT. It may cause extravascular hemolysis.

Biological Role

Lutheran is a high-affinity receptor for laminin. The laminin is a basement membrane protein involved in cell differentiation, adhesion, migration, and proliferation.

- **Overexpression of LU glycoprotein in ovarian carcinoma** and other cancers that **facilitate tumor cell adhesion and metastasis**.
- **Sickle cell anemia: Increased Lutheran expression on reticulocytes and sickle cells** may **contribute to the pathophysiology of vaso-occlusive crises**.
- **Polycythemia vera:** LU glycoprotein may contribute to thrombosis.

- In normal erythropoiesis, LU **may play a role in migration of maturing erythroid cells from the marrow.**

THE P BLOOD GROUP: P1PK (ISBT NO. 003), GLOB (028) AND FORS BLOOD GROUP SYSTEMS (031)

The "P group" is classified into three separate blood group systems:
1. **P1PK** blood **group system** (ISBT 003) comprised of P^k, P_1, and NOR antigens. The gene for P^k, P_1 and NOR resides on chromosome 22q13.
2. **Globoside blood group system/GLOB** (ISBT No. 028) contains P and LKE/Luke antigen and PX2 are assigned to the Globoside collection (209, symbol GLOB). The LKE is still classified under GLOB collection. The gene for Globoside or P antigen resides on chromosome 3q25.
3. **FORS** (ISBT 031) contains a single antigen, Forssman, present on rare Apae. Forssman antigen is expressed on many animal species but is typically absent from humans. Forssman expression can be found in the rare weak Apae RBC phenotype. Forssman antigen can react with human polyclonal anti-A.

P Blood Group Antigen

P blood group antigens are glycosphingolipids (similar to the Lewis system).

P blood group antigen expression:
- **P^k and P antigens:** P^k and P antigens are high-frequency antigens on RBCs (>99.9%). They are also expressed on nonerythroid cells, including lymphocytes, platelets, plasma, kidney, lung, heart, endothelium, placenta, uroepithelium, fibroblasts, and synovium.
- **P_1 antigen** is uniquely expressed on RBCs.
- PX2 is expressed by rare p cells and can react with alloanti-P.

Various phenotypes of P blood group system are mentioned in Table 6.5. There are two common phenotypes namely (1) P_1 and

Table 6.5: RBC phenotype, RBC antigen and possible antibodies in P blood group system.

RBC phenotype	RBC antigens	Possible antibodies
P_1	P^k, P, P_1	None
P_2	P^k, P	Anti-P_1
Null phenotypes		
P_1^k	↑P^k, P_1	Anti-P
P_2^k	↑P^k	Anti-P, anti-P_1
p	None	Anti-$P^k PP_1$ (Tj^a)
Weak phenotypes		
Variant P^k	↑P^k, ↓P	Anti-P
Weak P	↑P^k, ↓P	None

(2) P_2 phenotypes constitute more than 99%. Both P_1 and P_2 phenotypes have P^k and P antigens but P_2 phenotype does not express P_1 antigen.

Null/Weak Phenotypes

Three rare autosomal recessive null phenotypes (p, P_1^k, and P_2^k) and two weak variants (variant P^k and weak P) have been identified (Table 6.5). An association between the P^k variant and Luke (LKE)-negative phenotype has been noted. Because they lack P antigen, p and P^k individuals are resistant to parvovirus B19.

P Blood Group Antibodies

Anti-P_1

- The **most common antibody** is anti-P_1 found in P_2 donors. **Anti-P_1 is a naturally occurring antibody of IgM isotype.**
- It is **usually detected as a weak, room temperature agglutinin.** Anti-P_1 can bind complement and may be detected in the IAT by using polyspecific antihuman globulin (AHG). Antibody reactivity can be eliminated either by prewarming sera or by adding soluble P1 substance obtained from hydatid cyst fluid, earthworms, and bird eggs.
- Anti-P_1 titers **may be raised in patients with hydatid cyst disease or fascioliasis** (liver fluke) and in bird fanciers.
- Anti-P_1 is **not clinically significant** and does not a cause of HDFN.

Alloanti-PP₁Pᵏ

- Anti-PP₁Pᵏ (originally called as anti-Tja) is a separable mixture of anti-P, anti-P₁, and anti-Pᵏ **found in the sera of p individuals**.
- These antibodies are **naturally occurring** and may be **IgM only or IgM plus IgG** (IgG₃).
- They are **potent hemolysins**. Hence, patients should be transfused only with p RBCs. In women, alloanti- PP₁Pᵏ and alloanti-P are associated with HDFN and spontaneous abortion. Early and frequent plasmapheresis will be helpful in alloimmunized pregnant women of the p and Pᵏ phenotypes.

Alloanti-P

- Anti-P is a **naturally occurring IgM** alloantibody found in the serum of Pᵏ (and p) individuals.
- It is a **potent hemolysin** and can produce hemolysis following transfusion of P-positive (P₁ and P₂) RBCs. Some alloanti-P can react with PX2 present on p red cells with hemolysis.
- Alloanti-P can cause of HDFN and is associated with spontaneous abortions.

Autoanti-P (Donath-Landsteiner)

Paroxysmal cold hemoglobinuria (PCH): Autoanti-P (Donath-Landsteiner) is an autoantibody with anti-P specificity. It was observed in patients with PCH. PCH is a clinical syndrome which may **develop in children following viral infection**. In PCH, **autoanti-P is an IgG, biphasic hemolysin**. It **binds to RBCs at colder temperatures** and **produces intravascular hemolysis at body temperature**. This characteristic can be demonstrated in vitro by the Donath-Landsteiner test (Fig. 6.1).

Biological Role

The physiologic role of the P blood group antigens is not known.
- **Pᵏ antigen-apoptotic marker:** The Pᵏ antigen is a marker of apoptosis in germinal center B cells, Burkitt lymphoma, and lymphoblastic leukemia.

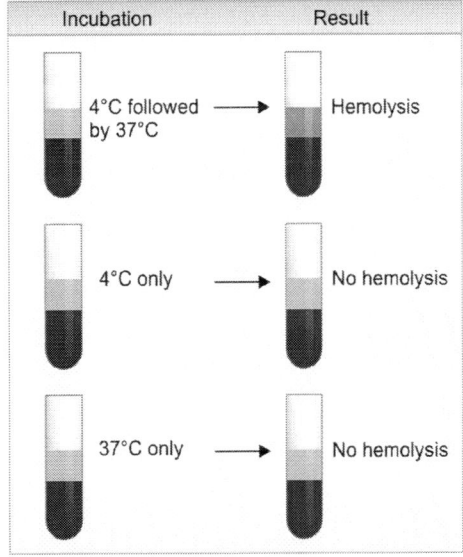

Fig. 6.1: Donath-Landsteiner test. After the patient's freshly drawn serum and red cells are incubated, complement binds only at lower temperatures and causes hemolysis when the tube is warmed to 37°C. No hemolysis occurs when incubated separately only at 4°C or 37°C.

- **LKE is a marker of embryonic and mesenchymal stem cells.** It is involved in adhesion, cell signaling, and metastasis in renal cell and breast carcinoma.
- **Receptors for microbial pathogens:** Several P blood group antigens are receptors for microbial pathogens.
  - The P blood group antigen is the **receptor for parvovirus B19**. It is a single-stranded DNA virus associated with multiple clinical sequelae such as aplastic crises.
  - **Pᵏ can bind human immunodeficiency virus** (HIV) and may cause resistance to HIV infection.
  - *Escherichia coli*: P, Pᵏ, and LKE blood group antigens on uroepithelium act as cell receptors for P fimbriae, a bacterial adhesin and colonization factor expressed on uropathogenic *E. coli* strains.
  - The P₁ and Pᵏ antigens are **receptors for shiga toxins**, produced by *Shigella*

dysenteriae and enterohemorrhagic *E. coli* (EHEC) strains. EHEC infection can cause gastroenteritis and community-acquired hemolytic-uremic syndrome. Probably its toxin binds to P^k antigen on glomerular vascular endothelium and platelets.
- The P^k antigen can also act as a **receptor for *Streptococcus suis*.**

I BLOOD GROUP SYSTEM (ISBT NO. 027)

It has long been recognized the existence of cold agglutinins in the serum of normal individuals and in patients with acquired hemolytic anemia. Wiener and coworkers (1956) named one of such agglutinins as antigen "*I*". It was termed "*I*" *for* "individuality" because after an extensive search of 22,000 individuals only five adult donors had I antigen.

I Blood Group Antigens

- The I blood group system contains two related antigens: (1) **I** and (2) **i**. The I and i are **not antithetical antigens**. The i antigen is biosynthetic precursor of I antigen and I is formed by the action of glycosyltransferases on i.
- The **i antigen is strongly expressed on cord cells** because of developmental delays in the enzyme responsible for I antigen synthesis from i. By 3 months of age, there is a significant decrease in i antigen, accompanied by increased I antigen. Some individuals do not to change their i status after birth. They become the rare adult i. Adult i RBCs generally express more i antigen than do cord RBCs.
- The adult I+i– phenotype develops by 18–24 months of age. Increases in I antigen are accompanied by parallel increases in A and B antigens.
- Both I and i antigens are high-prevalence antigens that widely expressed on glycolipids and glycoproteins on red cells and other tissues.
- Both i and I can be further modified to yield ABH, LeX, and related antigens.
- The gene for I antigen is on chromosome 6p24.
- Treatment of RBCs with enzymes ficin and papain enhances reactivity of the I and i antigens with their respective antibodies. The I and i antigens are resistant to treatment with DTT and glycine-acid EDTA.
- An early association of I and i to ABH was demonstrated. I and i antigens are precursors for the synthesis of ABO and Lewis antigens.

Null Phenotype

The i_{adult} phenotype is a rare, autosomal recessive phenotype.

Elevated i antigen: It is also observed:
- On cord RBCs and reticulocytes and in megaloblastic anemia, leukemia, and chronic hemolytic states associated with stressed erythropoiesis.
- In HEMPAS (hereditary erythroblastic multinuclearity with positive acidified serum lysis test). HEMPAS is a congenital dyserythropoietic anemia associated with chronic hemolysis, binucleated erythroblasts, and altered red cell glycosylation.

Anti-I and Anti-i Antibodies

Anti-I and anti-i are antibodies of **IgM isotype** and are **reactive at room temperature**.

Anti-I

- **Autoantibodies to I:** They are relatively common and are usually low-titered cold agglutinins. Generally benign, hemolysis secondary to high-titered anti-I can develop in cold autoimmune hemolytic anemia (CAIHA). CAIHA may occur in association with malignancy and occasionally infection (e.g. *Mycoplasma pneumoniae*). These antibodies often agglutinate RBCs at temperatures of 30–34°C.

- **Alloanti-I:** It is relatively rare and is occur as a naturally occurring antibody in i adult individuals.

Anti-i

Alloanti-i has never been described. **Autoanti-i** is rare antibody and can occur in **CAIHA**, **infectious mononucleosis** (Epstein-Barr virus infections), **choriocarcinoma**, and **alcoholic cirrhosis**.

Biological Role

- The **developmental delay in I antigen** synthesis may play a **protective role against HDFN**.
- I and i are **oncofetal antigens** and can show variable expression with malignancy.
- The **i antigen is a marker of human mesenchymal stem cells**.

DIEGO BLOOD GROUP SYSTEM (ISBT NO. 010)

Diego system is designated DI and number 010 by the ISBT.

Diego Antigens

The Diego blood group system (DI) is composed of **22 antigens**. These including **five sets of allelic antigens** namely (1) Di^a/Di^b (DI1/DI2), (2) Wr^a/Wr^b (DI3/DI4), (3) Hg(a+)/Mo(a+) (DI12/DI11), (4) Wu/DISK (DI9/DI22), and (5) Sw(a)/SW1 (DI14/DI22). Most antigens (20/22) are rare and low-incidence antigens.

Antigen expression: Apart from RBCs, Diego antigens are expressed in kidney along the collecting ducts.

Diego Antibodies

Antibodies against Diego blood group antigens can be immune stimulated or naturally occurring.
- **Immune stimulated:** These types of antibodies include those against Di^a, Di^b, Wr^b, and ELO. These antibodies are of IgG isotype and are detected in the AHG phase of testing. Anti-Di^a, Di^b, and Wr^b may be associated with reduced red cell survival, HTRs, and HDFN. Anti-Wr^b may also be associated with autoimmune hemolytic anemia.
- **Naturally occurring:** Antibodies against the majority of other Diego antigens are usually naturally occurring, room temperature, saline agglutinins. Anti-Wr^a is common.

CARTWRIGHT (YT) BLOOD GROUP SYSTEM (ISBT NO. 011)

It was discovered in 1956 and used the last letter "t" for this group derived from the patient's last name, which was Cartwright. Apparently why "T" became "Yt".

Cartwright Antigens

Cartwright (Yt) blood group system consists of two autosomal codominant antigens: Yt^a and Yt^b. Yt^a is the high-prevalence antigen and Yt^b is the low-prevalence antigen. The Yt antigens are antithetical. They are found on glycosylphosphatidylinositol (GPI)-linked RBC glycoprotein acetylcholinesterase (AChE). AChE is a critical enzyme required for the rapid degradation of neurotransmitter acetylcholine and involved in neurotransmission. However, the function of RBC-bound AChE is not known. The gene for AChE is located at chromosome 7q22.

Yt antigens show variable sensitivity to ficin and papain and are sensitive to DTT. They are resistant to glycine-acid EDTA treatment.

Antigen expression: The antigens are developed at birth but are weakly expressed on cord RBCs than on adult RBCs. They are not present on RBCs of patient with paroxysmal nocturnal hemoglobinuria (PNH)-III. In PNH, no GPI-linked glycoproteins are found. Apart from RBCs, Cartwright antigens are expressed on neural synapses and neuromuscular junctions.

Phenotypes

There are **three phenotypes**: the common **Yt(a+b−)** and **Yt(a+b+)**, and the rare **Yt(a−b+)**. No Yt(a−b−) phenotype has been reported.

Cartwright Antibodies

Anti-Yt^a and anti-Yt^b are usually clinically benign, though reduced red cell survival and DHTRs may rarely occur. Neither antibody is associated with HDFN. Anti-Yt^a and anti-Yt^b are of IgG isotype, developing due to immune stimulation by pregnancy or transfusion. They are usually detected in the IAT. Though Yt^a has a high incidence, anti-Yt^a is found more commonly than anti-Yt^b. This suggests that Yt^a is more immunogenic antigen than Yt^b and its antibody anti-Yt^b is rare. Yt antibodies may cause accelerated red cell destruction but usually do not cause HDFN.

XG BLOOD GROUP SYSTEM (ISBT NO. 012)

The XG system is designated by the symbol XG and number 012.

Xg Antigen

The XG blood group system contains a single antigen, Xg^a. This results in only two phenotypes namely: (1) Xg^a-positive and (2) Xg^a-negative. The antigen was named after the X chromosome and g for "Grand Rapids", where the patient was treated. The antigen is sensitive to ficin and papain but resistant to DTT treatment.

Location of gene: The gene for Xg^a antigen is located on the X chromosome Xp22.3. Hence, the incidence of the Xg^a-positive phenotype is higher among women.

Xg^a antigen association with CD99: The Xg^a antigen is located on an XG protein. In the RBC membrane, the XG protein is associated with CD99. CD99 is also known as 12E7 and MIC2. The gene responsible for CD99, *MIC2*, is located at Xp22.2. CD99 became part of the XG system because the *MIC2* and *XG* genes are adjacent and homologous.
- Xg^a has a phenotypic relationship to CD99.
- All Xg(a+) individuals show high expression of CD99 on their RBC.
- All Xg(a–) women have low CD99 expression and majority of Xg(a–) men have high expression of CD99.

Both Xg^a and CD99 escape X chromosome inactivation. Since males have only one X chromosome, Xg(a+) males are hemizygotes. Females, having two X chromosomes, can be homozygotes or heterozygotes.

Antibodies

- Anti-Xg^a may be **immune stimulated or naturally occurring**. Most of them are of **IgG** isotype and some may activate complement. Due to the differences in Xg(a+) phenotype between men and women, most of anti-Xg^a are found in men. Anti-Xg^a is not associated with HTRs or HDFN.
- Alloanti-CD99 is very rare.

SCIANNA BLOOD GROUP SYSTEM (ISBT NO. 013)

The Scianna (Sc) blood group system, designated by the ISBT with the symbol SC and number 013.

Scianna Antigens

Scianna is specific for RBCs and erythropoietic tissues. These antigens are expressed on cord RBCs. The Scianna blood group system contains seven antigens.
- Sc1 and Sc2 are antithetical antigens, with most individuals typing as Sc: 1, –2.
- Sc2 and Sc4/Rd are low-incidence antigens (Rd is Sc4).
- Sc3, Sc5 (STAR), Sc6 (SCER), and Sc7 (SCAN) are high-incidence antigens. Sc3 is a high-incidence antigen present on all RBCs except very rare Sc$_{null}$ (Sc: –1, –2, –3) phenotype.

The Scianna antigens are resistant to enzymes ficin and papain but can be weakened by DTT and AET treatment.

SC gene: It is located on chromosome 1 at 1p34. The product of the gene is a RBC adhesion protein called **er**ythroid **m**embrane **a**ssociated **p**rotein (ERMAP). Similar to Lutheran, Ok, and LW proteins, ERMAP is a member of the immunoglobulin superfamily. The biological role of ERMAP is unknown. Possibly it may play a role in RBC adhesion and signaling.

Null Phenotypes

Two Sc-null alleles are reported namely: (1) *SC01N.01* and (2) *SC01N.02*.

Antibodies

Anti-Scianna antibodies are rare.
- **Alloantibodies** to Scianna antigens are rare and are of no clinical significance. They are generally benign, usually of IgG isotype, some bind complements and reactive in the antiglobulin test. They are mostly immune stimulated and few are naturally occurring (e.g. anti-Sc2 antibodies). Anti-Scianna antibodies can be neutralized with soluble recombinant ERMAP protein.
- **Autoantibodies** to Sc1 and Sc3 have been rarely reported.

Significance: They do not cause of transfusion reactions but can lead to delays due to difficulty in finding crossmatch-compatible blood. Anti-Sc4 and anti-Sc2 may produce HDFN. Autoantibodies against Sc1 and Sc3 antigens may cause warm autoimmune hemolytic anemia.

DOMBROCK BLOOD GROUP SYSTEM (ISBT NO. 014)

The Dombrock blood group system, designated by the ISBT with the symbol DO and number 014. It was named for the first antibody maker, Mrs Dombrock in 1965.

Dombrock Antigens

The Dombrock blood group system contains seven antigens. Two autosomal codominant antigens are Do^a (DO1) and Do^b (DO2). It resulted in three phenotypes namely: (1) Do(a+b–), (2) Do(a+b+), and (3) Do(a–b+). The high-incidence/prevalence antigens Gy^a, Hy, Jo^a, DOYA, and DOMR are found on almost all donors. The phenotypes in Dombrock blood group system are presented in Table 6.6. The Do^a and Do^b antigens are poor immunogens and the antibodies are rarely found; however, Gy^a is highly immunogenic.

Antigen expression: Apart from RBCs, Dombrock mRNA has been identified in fetal

Table 6.6: Phenotypes in Dombrock blood group system.

	Reactions with anti-Dombrock antibodies						
Do^a	Do^b	Gy^a	Jo^a	Hy	DO^6	DO^7	RBC phenotype
+	0	+	+	+	+	+	Do(a+b–)
+	+	+	+	+	+	+	Do(a+b+)
0	+	+	+	+	+	+	Do(a–b+)
Null/Weak phenotype							
0	0	0	0	0	0	0	Gy(a–) or Do_{null}
0	w	w	0/w	0	w	+	Hy(–)
w	0/w	+	0	w	w	0/w	Jo(a–)
0	0	w	w	w	0	?	DOYA(–)
0	+	0	w	w	?	0	DOMR(–)
+	0	+	+	+	?	?	DOLG(–)
+	0	+	+	+	+	/	DOLC(–)

(W: weak reaction)

liver and spleen. The antigens are present on cord RBCs, but are absent from PNH-III RBCs. The gene for Dombrock is located on chromosome 12p12.3.

Null/Weak Phenotypes

The Do_{null} or Gy(a–) phenotype is a rare, autosomal recessive phenotype. An acquired Do_{null} phenotype may be found in patients with PNH-III. PNH-III is a hematopoietic stem cell disorder characterized by chronic hemolysis due to an absence of all GPI-linked glycoproteins, including Cromer, Dombrock, and Cartwright antigens. Loss of one high-incidence Dombrock antigen is usually associated with weakened expression of other Dombrock antigens.

Dombrock Antibodies

Anti-Dombrock antibodies may be clinically significant. Anti-Do^a and anti-Do^b can cause DHTRs but no clinical HDFN. The Dombrock antibodies are usually IgG isotype, arising from immune stimulation by transfusion or pregnancy.

Enhancement: Antibody reactivity can be enhanced by the use of papain or ficin enzyme-treated RBCs. Conversely, antibody reactivity is reduced or abolished by the treatment of red cells with sulfhydryl-reducing agents (DTT, AET), trypsin, chymotrypsin, and pronase.

These antibodies are usually found in mixtures of alloantibodies, weakly reactive and disappear. These factors make their identification difficult.

Significance: Dombrock antibodies can reduce the survival of RBC and produce acute and delayed HTRs. Transfusion reactions and accelerated clearance due to anti-Dombrock antibodies as well as their deterioration in vitro storage can false-negative results for these antibodies in the blood. This may cause false interpretation during routine pretransfusion testing. The units often may be labelled as crossmatch-compatible, even in a full IAT crossmatch.

COLTON BLOOD GROUP SYSTEM (ISBT NO. 015)

The Colton blood group system, ISBT symbol CO and number 015. It was initially identified in 1967.

Colton Antigen

It consists of two autosomal codominant antithetical antigens, Co^a (high-incidence/prevalence) and Co^b (low-prevalence), and a third high-incidence antigen ("TOR"). Another antigen called Co^3 is present on all RBCs except those of the very rare Co(a–b–) phenotype. The Colton antigens are resistant to treatment with ficin and papain, chloroquine, and DTT.

The Colton blood group antigens reside on aquaporin-1 (AQP-1) or channel-forming integral protein, a water-selective membrane channel. *AQP-1* gene is located on chromosome 7p14. AQP-1 is a major molecular water channel on RBCs that account for 80% of water reabsorption in the kidneys and thereby facilitate the concentration of urine in kidney.

Antigen expression: Apart from RBCs (including RBCs of newborns), Colton antigens are expressed in renal proximal tubules, thin descending limb of Henle, renal vasa recta endothelium, choroid plexus, ciliary body, microvessels, gallbladder, placenta and some epithelial cells.

Colton Antibodies

Anti-Colton antibodies can be clinically significant. They **can shorten RBC survival, HTRs, and HDFN**.
- Antibodies to Co^a and Co^b are usually of the IgG isotype that develop from immune stimulation by transfusion or pregnancy. Some of these antibodies can bind complement. Anti-Colton antibodies are detectable in the AHG phase of testing. These antibodies can be enhanced with protease enzyme-treated RBCs. Anti-Co^a

can cause HTRs and HDFN and anti-Co^b can cause HTRs and mild HDFN.
- Rare Co$_{null}$ and "TOR-negative" individuals can make an anti-Co^3 (anti-Co a+b), an alloantibody that reacts with both Co(a+b−) and Co(a−b+) RBCs.

LANDSTEINER-WIENER BLOOD GROUP SYSTEM (ISBT NO. 016)

The Landsteiner-Wiener (LW) blood group system, ISBT symbol LW and number 016. It was discovered along with the D antigen of the Rh blood group system. In 1940, it was named in honor of its discoverers, the LW or Landsteiner-Wiener.

LW Antigens

The LW blood group system consists of two allelic antigens: (1) LW^a and (2) LW^b. LW^a is a high-frequency and LW^b is of low-prevalence antigen. Expression of LW antigen depends on the expression of RhD protein. There is highest expression found on RhD-positive red cells and whereas RhD-negative cells had weaker expression. The null phenotype of LW is LW(a−b−) in which both LW^a and LW^b are absent. Rh$_{null}$ RBCs are also LW(a−b−). The LW antigen is expressed on RBCs and placenta. The LW antigens reside on intracellular adhesion molecule type 4 (ICAM4, CD242). ICAM is a member of the immunoglobulin superfamily. The *ICAM4* gene resides on chromosome 19p13. LW phenotypes are presented in Box 6.5.

LW Antibodies

- Antibodies include anti-LW^a and anti-LW^b and LW$_{null}$ individuals can make an anti-LW^{ab}, which reacts with both LW(a+b−) and LW(a−b+) RBCs.

Box 6.5: LW phenotypes.
- LW(a+b−)
- LW(a+b+)
- LW(a−b+)
- LW(a−b−) Big
- LW(a−b−) Rh$_{null}$

- Anti-LW antibodies usually rarely produce HTRs or HDFN.
- They are usually IgG isotype and are detected in the IAT. Anti-LW usually reacts strongly with D+ RBCs weakly (or without any reaction) with D− RBCs from adults. Antibody activity can be reduced by ethylenediaminetetraacetic acid (EDTA) and pretreatment of RBCs with sulfhydryl reducing agents (DTT, AET).

Biological Role

- LW expression is **elevated in sickle cell patients** and may be involved in microvascular occlusion.
- LW antigens may be **depressed during pregnancy** and in certain diseases, such as **lymphoma and leukemia**.
- Autoanti-LW can be found in serum of patients with warm autoimmune hemolytic anemia.
- Anti-LW **does not cause serious HDFN or transfusion reactions**.

CHIDO/RODGERS BLOOD GROUP SYSTEM (ISBT NO. 017)

The Chido/Rodgers (Ch/Rg) blood group system, designated by the ISBT with symbol CH/RG and number 017. It was named after the first two antibody producers namely: (1) Ch for Chido (in 1967) and (2) Rg for Rodgers (in 1976).

Chido/Rodgers Antigens

The Chido/Rodgers blood group system consists of 10 antigens and most are high-incidence antigens. This includes two pairs of antithetical antigens and three conformational antigens. The conformational antigens need coexpression of two spatially distinct Ch/Rg antigens and together produce a third, conformational antigen. Similar to Lewis blood group antigens, Ch/Rg antigens are not intrinsic to the RBC membrane. Rather, they are on the fourth component of complement (C4), and are passively adsorbed onto RBC membranes from plasma.

- Ch/Rg antigens are weakly expressed on cord RBCs and some GYPA-deficient RBCs. C4 is the product of two highly homologous genes *C4A* and *C4B*, on chromosome 6p21.3 near the HLA locus. In general, Chido antigens are on C4B, and Rodgers antigens are on C4A.
- The antigens can be destroyed by ficin and papain but are resistant to treatment with DTT and glycine-acid EDTA.

Chido/Rodgers Antibodies

- Antibodies against Ch/Rg antigens namely anti-Ch and anti-Rg are usually **IgG isotype** and react weakly. Both anti-Ch and anti-Rg can be neutralized by plasma.
- Anti-Ch and anti-Rg are **clinically insignificant** for transfusion and do not cause hemolytic transfusion reactions or HDFN.
- Anti-Ch/Rg antibodies are usually detected with AHG and antibody reactivity can be enhanced by incubating RBCs in a low-ionic sucrose solution. Antibody reactivity can be inhibited by plasma or by treatment of RBCs with proteases.

Biological Role

C4 deficiency is associated with autoimmune disorders (e.g. rheumatoid arthritis and Graves' disease) and **increased susceptibility to bacterial meningitis**.

GERBICH BLOOD GROUP SYSTEM (ISBT NO. 020)

The Gerbich blood group system was named in 1960 after Mrs Gerbich, the first antibody producer and became a system in 1990. It is designated by the ISBT as GE and number 020.

Gerbich Antigens

The Gerbich (Ge) blood group system contains 11 antigens: six high-frequency/prevalence (Ge2, Ge3, Ge4, GEPL, GEAT, and GETI) and five low-frequency/prevalence antigens (Wb, Ls^a, An^a, Dh^a, and GEIS). The gene is located on chromosome 2 at 2q14.3.

Antigen expression: Gerbich antigens are expressed on fetal and adult RBCs, platelets, and kidney and fetal liver. Gerbich antigens are resistant to treatment with DTT, chymotrypsin and glycine-acid EDTA. Ge2 and Ge4 are ficin and papain sensitive, but Ge3 is ficin-resistant. **Gerbich-negative RBCs show increased resistance to *Plasmodium falciparum* infection**.

Null/Weak Phenotypes

There are three autosomal recessive Gerbich-negative phenotypes. These are associated with the loss of one or more high-prevalence/incidence Gerbich antigens. These include Yus type (Ge: –2, 3, 4), Gerbich type (Ge: –2, –3, 4), and Leach type (Ge: –2, –3, –4). All three null phenotypes are **associated with ovalocytosis**. Gerbich antigens are also reduced in patients with hereditary elliptocytosis. The Leach type is the Gerbich null phenotype.

Gerbich Antibodies

Anti-Gerbich antibodies can be of IgM or IgG isotype. Most are immune stimulated. Anti-Ge2 is the most common of the Gerbich antibodies produced by the Ge: –2, 3, 4 phenotype individuals.

- Anti-Gerbich antibodies are **sometimes clinically significant**. It can shorten RBC survival and delayed hemolysis following transfusion of Gerbich-incompatible RBCs.
- Autoantibodies against Gerbich antigens **may be associated with severe autoimmune hemolytic anemia**.
- They can be detected at room temperature and are enhanced by AHG.

CROMER BLOOD GROUP SYSTEM (ISBT NO. 021)

Cromer Antigens

The Cromer system (Cr/CROM) has 16 antigens of which 5 are antithetical antigens. There are 13 high-incidence and 3 low-incidence antigens. It has 23 possible phenotypes. Cromer antigens are present on decay accelerating factor (DAF, CD55), which is widely expressed on tissues and in secretions.

Antigen expression: DAF is a complement regulatory protein identified on all hematopoietic cells, vascular endothelium, gastrointestinal and genitourinary epithelium, brain, and body fluids. Cromer is expressed on cord RBCs and placental trophoblasts. The *CD55* gene is located at chromosome 1q32. Cromer system antigens are resistant to treatment with ficin and papain as well as glycine-acid EDTA. They are destroyed by α-chymotrypsin and pronase. Cromer antigens are weakened, but not destroyed, by AET and DTT treatment.

Null/Weak Phenotypes

Inab or Cromer null phenotype is a very rare autosomal recessive phenotype. It is characterized by complete absence of all Cromer antigens but the expression of CD59 and other GPI-linked glycoproteins is normal. The Inab phenotype individual may suffer from chronic gastrointestinal disorders, particularly a chronic protein-losing gastroenteropathy. PNH-III RBCs are deficient in DAF and they also lack Cromer antigens.

Cromer Antibodies

Anti-Cromer antibodies are usually of IgG isotype formed due to immune stimulation. The clinical significance of anti-Cromer antibodies is variable. In some, they are associated with decreased RBC survival and HTRs. DAF is strongly expressed on trophoblast epithelium of placental tissue and will adsorb Cromer antibodies. Hence, Cromer antibodies do not cause HDFN. They are detected in the IAT. Anti-Cromer can be inhibited by plasma, urine, and platelet concentrates.

Biological Role

- **CD55/DAF protects cells from complement** by promoting the decay of two C3 convertases: (1) C4b2a and (2) C3bBb.

- **CD55 is an alternate ligand for *H. pylori*** and is upregulated in chronic infections.
- **CD55 is also a receptor for several viruses.**

KNOPS BLOOD GROUP SYSTEM (ISBT NO. 022)

Knops blood group system, designated by the ISBT as KN and number 022. It was named after Mrs Knops, the first antibody maker.

Knops Antigens

The Knops blood group contains nine allelic antigens, including six antithetical antigens.

The antithetical pairs of antigens are Kn^a and Kn^b, Mc^a and Mc^b, and Sl1 (Sla) and Sl2 (Vil).

Serologically, these antigens are grouped together because their corresponding antibodies demonstrate variable reactions, are not neutralized by pooled normal serum (unlike anti-Ch and anti-Rg), and are difficult to adsorb and elute.

Antigen expression: Knops antigens are expressed on adult and cord RBCs, neutrophils, B lymphocytes, and dendritic cells. The antigens are weakened by treatment with ficin and papain and are destroyed by sulfhydryl-reducing agents (AET, DTT). The antigens are resistant to glycine-acid EDTA.

Knops resides on a complement regulatory protein called complement receptor 1 (CR1, CD35). The *CR1* gene is located on chromosome 1q32.

Knops Antibodies

- Knops antibodies are **clinically insignificant**. Following Knops-incompatible transfusion, RBCs have normal survival.
- Knops antibodies are of IgG isotype formed due to immune stimulation, and are usually detected only with AHG. Antibody reactivity can be enhanced with longer incubation (e.g. 1 hour at 37°C).

Biological Role

- Knops/CR1 may be decreased in infection and autoimmune disorders due to presence

of high levels of circulating immune complexes
- Complement receptor 1 (CR1) can bind the complement component fragments C3b and C4b. They process immune complexes and promote their clearance from the circulation. CR1 can bind to C5a and accelerate the decay of C3 and C5 convertases.
- CR1 also enhances phagocytosis of C3b/C4b-coated particles.
- CR1 also acts as a receptor for several pathogenic organisms such as *P. falciparum*. The low expression of CR1 may be protective against malaria.

INDIAN BLOOD GROUP SYSTEM (ISBT NO. 023)

The Indian blood group system was designated IN and number 023 by the ISBT. It was named because the first In(a+) individuals were from India.

Indian Antigens

The Indian (IN) blood group contains two autosomal codominant antigens: (1) In^a (IN1) and (2) In^b (IN2).
- In^a was reported in 1973 and it is relatively rare except among Indian (4%) and Iranians (11%) and Arabs (12%).
- In^b is the antithetical high-prevalence/frequency allele.
- Three other high-incidence antigens include: (1) IN3, (2) IN4 and (3) AnWj.

These antigens are carried by the CD44 glycoprotein which is an adhesion molecule present on many cell membranes. The gene encoding CD44 is located at chromosome 11p13.

Antigen expression: Indian antigens are widely expressed on all hematopoietic cells, epithelial cells, and neural tissue. In^a and In^b are weakly expressed on cord RBCs and are destroyed (except AnWj) by treatment with ficin, papain, and DTT but are resistant to glycine-acid EDTA.

Null/Weak Phenotypes

Indian antigens (including AnWj) are depressed on *In(Lu)* RBCs. These antigens are transiently depressed on cord RBCs during pregnancy and autoimmune hemolytic anemia due to the presence of autoanti-AnWj.

Indian Antibodies

- Antibodies against both Indian and AnWj antigens **may be clinically significant**. Decreased RBC survival (with anti-In^a) and immediate HTRs (due to anti-In^b) have been reported. They are not associated with clinical HDFN.
- Autoimmune anemia due to autoanti-AnWj has been detected.

Anti-Indian antibodies are usually of IgG isotype formed due to immune stimulation. They can present as saline agglutinins and are reactive/enhanced in the antiglobulin test. Anti-Indian antibodies are inhibited by plasma, which contains soluble CD44. They do not bind complement.

Biological Role

- **CD44 is a major adhesion molecule** present on leukocytes. It can bind to a spectrum of extracellular matrix proteins, including collagen, fibronectin, laminin, and hyaluron.
- **Bone marrow:** CD44 may be responsible for the adhesion of erythroid progenitors to stromal fibroblasts in the bone marrow.
- **Leukocytes:** CD44 may facilitate white blood cell (WBC)-endothelial adhesion, thereby localize WBC to sites of inflammation.
- CD44 may play a role in tumor metastasis, wound remodeling, and embryonic differentiation.
- CD44 is a receptor for invasive *Streptococcus pyogenes* and CD44 plays a critical role in *Shigella* and *Listeria* invasion. The AnWj antigen may act as a receptor for *H. influenzae* type b.

OK BLOOD GROUP SYSTEM (ISBT NO. 024)

The OK system is designated by the ISBT with symbol OK and number 024.

OK Antigens

The OK system resides on CD147 or Basigin and contains three high-frequency antigens: (1) Oka, (2) OKGV, and (3) OKVM. CD147 is a member of the immunoglobulin superfamily that mainly functions as receptors and adhesion molecules. The gene for CD147 resides on chromosome 19p13.3.

Antigen expression: Oka is well developed on RBCs from newborns. CD147 is widely expressed on epithelium, blood cells, retina, and neural cells. The Oka antigen is resistant to treatment with enzymes (e.g. ficin and papain), sialidases, and sulfhydryl-reducing agents DTT, and glycine-acid EDTA.

CD147 Antibodies

Anti-Oka is rare and is of IgG isotype, arising from immune stimulation. It is associated with shortened RBC survival following transfusion of Oka-incompatible RBCs. Anti-Oka has not been reported to cause HDFN. It is reactive in the antiglobulin test.

Biological Role

- On WBCs, CD147 is a leukocyte activation-associated protein. It **may participate in cell adhesion, tumorigenesis, and wound healing**.
- CD147 may play a role in **red cell trafficking and splenic recirculation**. Loss of CD147 with aging is associated with splenic clearance of senescent red cells.
- CD147 is the **receptor for** PfRH5, **a malarial adhesion protein** absolutely needed for *P. falciparum* infection. It may be **responsible for *P. falciparum*'s tropism** for humans.
- CD147 is a **receptor for cyclophilin A and B**. Cyclophilins are incorporated into several viral proteins and facilitate infection by HIV, SARS coronavirus, and measles.

RAPH BLOOD GROUP SYSTEM (ISBT NO. 025)

Antigen

The RAPH blood group system contains only single antigen, RAPH or MER2, located on CD151 or tetraspanin (TM4). The system was named Raph for the first patient to make the alloanti-MER2. The antigen name MER2 is derived from **M**onoclonal, and Eleanor **R**oosevelt, the laboratory where the antibody was produced. CD151 or tetraspanin (TSPAN24) is located on chromosome 11p15.

Antigen expression: CD151 is widely expressed on epithelium, fibroblasts, endothelium, muscle, renal glomeruli and tubules, CD34 cells, early erythroid precursors, megakaryocytes, and platelets. CD151/MER2 is strongly expressed in early normoblasts but its expression is progressively lost over time with increasing maturation of erythroid cells. This is responsible for the variable MER2 expression among adult donors. MER2-negative donors strongly express CD151 on other cell lines such as platelets and lymphocytes.

The MER2 antigen is resistant to treatment with ficin and papain. It is sensitive to treatment with trypsin, α-chymotrypsin, pronase, and AET.

Null Phenotypes

A MER2-negative, autosomal recessive phenotype was detected in three individuals of Indian ancestry. All developed nephrotic syndrome with end-stage renal disease and neurosensory deafness.

MER2 Antibodies

Six examples of anti-MER2 were found in patients of Indian, Turkish, and Pakistani origin. All were of IgG isotype which developed following transfusion and pregnancy.

Reactivity is sensitive to disulfide-reducing agents and most proteases except papain. There is no documentation of HDFN due to anti-MER2. MER2 can cause HTRs in some patients.

Biological Role

MER2 is located on CD151, a tetraspanin that is essential/**critical** for the **function** and assembly of basement membranes in the **kidney**, **inner ear** and skin.

Raph is a receptor for HPV and HCV and **facilitates** *Neisseria meningitidis* adhesion.

JMH BLOOD GROUP SYSTEM (ISBT NO. 026)

The JMH (John Milton Hagen) system was designated by the ISBT with symbol JMH and number 026. It was established after the discovery of JMH protein as a GPI-linked glycoprotein CD108.

The antibody was named anti-JMH for the first antibody maker, John Milton Hagen.

JMH Antigens

JMH (John Milton Hagen) blood group system contains six high-incidence antigens and their strength can vary among individuals. The antigens include JMH1 through JMH6. JMH is a high-prevalence antigen. JMH1 antigen is recognized by antibodies made by individuals lacking the JMH protein. JMH is carried on CD108 (SEMA7A) glycoprotein. *SEMA7A* gene is located at chromosome 15q24.1.

Antigen expression: Apart from RBCs, JMH is expressed on lymphocytes, activated macrophages, thymus, brain, respiratory epithelium, placenta, testes, and spleen. JMH is weakly expressed on cord RBCs. It is destroyed by treating RBCs with proteases (e.g. ficin and papain), and DTT. The antigen is resistant to treatment with glycine-acid EDTA.

Variant and Null Phenotypes

JMH weak, JMH variant, and JMH negative have been identified. An acquired, JMH weak to negative phenotype can occur in the elderly individual, accompanied by the JMH autoantibodies.

JMH Antibodies

Anti-JMH antibodies are generally considered clinically insignificant. They **do not cause HTRs or HDFN**. However, in some JMH-variant individuals, it may shorten RBC survival due to true alloantibodies.

Anti-JMH antibodies are usually of IgG isotype (predominantly IgG_4 in acquired JMH-negative people) and can be naturally occurring. They are not neutralized with pooled plasma.

Biological Role

Semaphorin proteins are involved in cell signaling. SEMA7A has following roles:
- It can modulate cellular immunity in hematopoietic cells.
- It inhibits NK cell proliferation and acts as a negative regulator of T cell activation.
- It stimulates chemotaxis, secretion of inflammatory cytokines, and dendritic cell maturation in monocytes.
- It may a receptor for the *P. falciparum* invasive protein MTRAP, which is expressed by merozoites.

GIL BLOOD GROUP SYSTEM (ISBT NO. 029)

The ISBT Gill system symbol is GIL and number 029.

GIL Antigens

The GIL blood group system has only one high-incidence antigen: GIL.

Antigen expression: The GIL protein is expressed on RBCs, kidney, small intestine, stomach, colon, spleen, eye, and respiratory tract.

GIL antigen is found on the glycerol transporter aquaglyceroporin 3 (AQP3). AQP3 is a member of the major intrinsic protein family of water channels. AQP3/Gil is a membrane channel can transport urea and glycerol. The *AQP3* gene is located at chromosome 9p13.

GIL Antibodies

Anti-GIL is associated with HTRs. There are no reports of clinical HDFN due to anti-GIL even with positive DAT.

Anti-GIL is usually of IgG isotype and reactive at 37°C. Reactivity with anti-GIL is enhanced with AHG and also treatment of RBCs with ficin and papain. The antigen is resistant to proteases, sialidases, DTT, and glycine-acid EDTA treatment.

Biological Role

- **On red cells:** AQP3 may play a **role in malaria infection**. AQP3 may be internalized during *P. falciparum* infection. AQP3 protects against hydroxyl radicals and osmotic stress. Hence, internalization and loss of AQP3 from the red cell extracellular membrane can accelerate red cell damage.
- **On immature dendritic cells:** AQP is implicated in the **uptake of soluble antigen by micropinocytosis.**
- **Epidermis:** AQP3 is highly expressed in epidermis and cutaneous T cells. It plays a role in skin differentiation, hydration, and inflammation.

JR BLOOD GROUP SYSTEM (ISBT NO. 032)

Jr Antigen

Jr is a high-prevalence RBC antigen present on ABCG2 (ATP-binding cassette, subfamily G, member 2). ABCG2 is a membrane transporter glycoprotein involved in folate, porphyrin, urate transport, multidrug resistance, and removal of toxic metabolites. The *ABCG2* gene is located on chromosome 4q22. Jr contains a single high-incidence antigen Jr(a).

Antigen expression: Jr/ABCG2 is widely expressed. These include cord and mature RBC, stem cells, placenta, cerebral endothelium, lung, intestinal epithelium, renal proximal tubules, liver, and breast. The antigen is resistant to treatment with ficin and papain, DTT, and glycine-acid EDTA.

Jr Antibodies

Anti-Jra is a rare antibody and usually of IgG isotype. It develops due to immune stimulation by transfusion or pregnancy. Anti-Jra can shortened RBC survival and cause DHTRs. Anti-Jra can produce mild to severe HDFN, probably due to suppression of erythropoiesis. Antibody reactivity can be enhanced by enzyme treatment.

LAN BLOOD GROUP SYSTEM (ISBT NO. 033)

Lan Antigen

This system has a single antigen namely Lan. Lan is a high-incidence antigen expressed on ABCB6 (ATP-binding cassette, family B, member 6).

Antigen expression: ABCB6 is expressed on RBC (including its precursors), fetal liver, heart, and skeletal muscle. ABCB6 is a glycoprotein present on cell membranes as well as intracellular organelles (e.g. lysosomes and Golgi). The gene resides on chromosome 4q22.

Lan Antibodies

Anti-Lan is usually of IgG isotype and develops due to from immune stimulation.

Anti-Lan can be enhanced by enzyme-treated RBC. Anti-Lan can cause HTRs and HDFN.

VEL BLOOD GROUP SYSTEM (ISBT NO. 034)

The Vel blood group system contains a single high-incidence antigen namely Vel.

Vel Antigen

Vel resides on SMIM1 (small integral membrane protein 1). SMIM1 is a type I transmembrane protein. *SMIM1* gene is located on chromosome 1p36 near the *RHD* gene. The antigen is resistant to glycine-acid EDTA and DTT treatment.

Antigen expression: SMIM1 is highly expressed on normoblasts and red cells but not expressed on other hematopoietic cells. Thus, it may be an erythroid-specific protein.

Vel Antibodies

Anti-Vel was first described in 1952 and was named after the first antibody maker. Anti-Vel is most often IgG but can be IgM. These antibodies are highly significant and can activate complement. They can produce severe, acute, and delayed HTRs, as well as HDFN. Anti-Vel is a high-titer, low-avidity antibody and can be missed in routine testing. Reactivity with anti-Vel can be enhanced with enzyme-treated RBCs.

CD59 BLOOD GROUP SYSTEM (ISBT NO. 035)

CD59 Antigen

CD59 (membrane inhibitor of reactive lysis, membrane attack complex inhibitory factor) is a high-incidence antigen. Similar to CD55 (DAF, Cromer blood group), CD59 is a GPI-linked glycoprotein and is absent on PNH-red cells. The gene for CD59 is located on chromosome 11p13.

Antigen expression: It is expressed on RBCs, white cells, placenta, seminal fluid, and other tissues. It protects cells from complement-mediated lysis through inhibition of the terminal C5b-C9 membrane attack complex. CD59 is also involved in T cell activation, LPS binding, apoptosis, and reproduction.

CD59 Antibodies

The CD59 antibody is an IgG isotype, enhanced by enzymes and inhibited by soluble CD59. This antibody may be clinically significant.

APPLICATIONS OF OTHER BLOOD GROUPS TO ROUTINE BLOOD BANKING

The major blood group systems include ABO and Rh. Other blood group systems assume its importance only after patients develop unexpected antibodies. Hence, it is necessary to have a fundamental knowledge of antibody characteristics, clinical significance, and antigen frequency to help in confirmation of antibody specificity and to select appropriate units for transfusion.

Usually only a few antibody specificities are observed in practice. M, P1, and I antibodies react at room temperature and are not clinically significant. K, S, s, Fy^a, Fy^b, Jk^a, and Jk^b antibodies react in the antiglobulin phase and are clinically significant.

Resolving problems: Not all antibody problems can be easily solved and even panel reactions are sometimes inconclusive. It is to be borne in mind that the presence of silent, regulator, and inhibitor genes can affect antigen expression. This chapter will be a starting point for serologic problem-solving. Resolution of antibody problems may need the assistance of an immunohematology reference laboratory.

Clinical significance of blood group systems is presented in Table 6.7.

Table 6.7: Clinical significance of blood group systems.

Clinical significance	Blood group system alloantibodies
Clinically significant	ABO, Rh, Kell, Kidd; Duffy; S, s, and U, Lutheran (Lu^b)
Usually not clinically significant	I, Lewis, M, N, P1, Lutheran (Lu^a)

SUMMARY

- The ISBT terminology for RBC surface antigens is a standardized numeric system for naming authenticated antigens of various blood group systems.
- In the ISBT classification, RBC antigens are given a six-digit identification number: the first three digits represent the system, collection or series, and the second three digits identify the antigen.
- Blood group systems are also involved in several functions in the body.
- Lewis blood group antigens are not synthesized by the RBCs. They are found in plasma and red cells. They are adsorbed from plasma onto the RBC membrane. The Le gene codes for L-fucosyltransferase. It adds L-fucose to type 1 chains. Lewis antigens are poorly expressed at birth. Lewis antibodies are not considered significant for transfusion medicine.
- The P blood group consists of the biochemically related antigens P, P_1, Pk, and LKE. P_1 antigen is poorly developed at birth. Antibodies may demonstrate in vitro hemolysis, and can cause severe HTRs. Anti-PP_1P^k is associated with spontaneous abortions. Alloanti-P is found as a naturally occurring alloantibody. Autoanti-P is most often the specificity associated with the cold-reactive IgG autoantibody in patients with PCH. The autoanti-P of PCH usually does not react by routine tests and shows a biphasic hemolysin only in the Donath-Landsteiner test. Parvoviruses bind to P antigens on RBCs, causing pure RBC aplasia.
- I and i antigens are not antithetical; they have a reciprocal relationship. Most adult RBCs are rich in I and have only trace amounts of i antigen. Anti-I is a benign, weak, naturally occurring, saline-reactive IgM autoagglutinin, usually detected only at 4°C. Patients with *M. pneumoniae* infections may develop strong cold agglutinins with autoanti-I specificity.
- Anti-M and anti-N are cold-reactive saline agglutinins that do not bind complement or react with enzyme-treated cells. Anti-S and anti-s are IgG antibodies. They are reactive at 37°C and the antiglobulin phase. They may be associated with HDFN and HTRs.
- The Kell blood group antigens are wel-developed at birth. Excluding ABO, the K antigen is second only to D antigen in immunogenicity. Anti-K is an IgG antibody reactive in the antiglobulin phase. It has been implicated in severe HTRs and HDFN.
- The McLeod phenotype, affecting only males, is a rare phenotype with decreased Kell system antigen expression. The McLeod syndrome consists of abnormal RBC morphology, compensated hemolytic anemia, and neurological and muscular abnormalities. Some may have the X-linked chronic granulomatous disease.
- Duffy blood group system: Duffy (Fy) antigens namely Fya and Fyb antigens are well developed at birth. Fy(a−b−) RBCs resist infection by the malaria organism *P. vivax*. Anti-Fya and anti-Fyb are usually IgG antibodies and react optimally at the antiglobulin phase of testing; both antibodies may cause DHTRs and HDFN.
- Kidd blood group system: Kidd system antibodies are a common cause of DHTRs.
- Lutheran blood group system: Lu^a and Lu^b are antigens produced by codominant alleles. Anti-Lu^a may be a naturally occurring saline agglutinin that reacts optimally at room temperature. Anti-Lu^b is usually an IgG antibody reactive at the antiglobulin phase and can be produced in response to foreign RBC exposure during pregnancy or transfusion. Antibodies may show mixed-field reaction.
- The Diego system: Anti-Di^a, anti-Di^b, and anti-Wr^a are clinically significant and can cause severe HTRs and HDFN.

SELF-ASSESSMENT EXERCISE

Write short notes on:
- Minor blood groups and their significance
- MNS blood group system
- Lewis blood group system
- P blood group
- Kell blood group system
- Duffy antigen

CHAPTER 7

Donor Selection and Blood Collection

CHAPTER OUTLINE

- Types of donors and donation
- Donor selection
- Blood collection
- Hemoglobin estimation of donor
- Processing of the donor blood

INTRODUCTION

Transfusion medicine is a multidisciplinary consisting of all aspects of blood banking (i.e. blood donation, blood component preparation, blood cell serology, and blood transfusion therapy), immunohematology, transfusion therapy, clinical practice, transplantation science and regenerative medicine. The term **blood banking** has been replaced by *transfusion medicine* to stress the importance of patient care and clinical outcomes.

Branches of Transfusion Medicine

Operationally, transfusion medicine can be divided into blood centers and transfusion services. Blood centers and transfusion services are collectively called *blood establishments*.

1. **Blood centers** collect blood from donors and prepare and distribute blood components.
2. **Transfusion services** perform pretransfusion compatibility testing, select and issue blood components, and provide medical support for blood transfusion.

All blood establishments must be registered with the regulating authority and must have license. Blood cannot be synthesized artificially. So, the source of blood is from a healthy human donor.

Blood transfusion is the process of transferring blood/blood products from donor into the circulating system of recipient. It is important to properly collect the blood from donor, prepare its components (if required) and store blood/components in a proper way and transfuse in such a way to avoid any risks or hazards.

Basic Principles in Blood Transfusion

1. **Blood donation should be harmless to the donor.**
2. **Blood donation should be beneficial and not harmful to the recipient/the patient.** The transfusion service should aim at eliminating the risks and hazards of blood transfusion.

Benefits and Reasons for Transfusion

The indications for the transfusion of red blood cells (RBCs) and blood components can be divided into the following four major categories:

1. **Transfusion to restore or maintain oxygen-carrying capacity or hemoglobin.** This is done by the transfusion of RBCs with plasma removed, i.e. **packed RBCs**.

The most commonly used component is packed RBCs.
2. **Transfusion to restore or maintain blood volume.**
   a. **Transfusion of whole blood** is now limited to conditions involving massive resuscitation (severe bleeding during trauma/accidents). This is necessary **to prevent shock in cases of acute blood loss**, as in massive bleeding. It may be necessary in pregnancy with bleeding before, during or after delivery. It may be needed during major surgeries (e.g. heart surgery).
   b. In **actively bleeding patients** who have **lost more than 25-30%** of their blood volume, **RBCs and a volume expander** such as crystalloid (electrolyte) solutions such as 0.9% sodium chloride (isotonic saline) or **thawed plasma** are used.
3. **Transfusion to replace coagulation factors to maintain hemostasis.** This is done with a variety of blood components depending on the cause of bleeding. These components include platelet concentrates (platelet disorders) and cryoprecipitate (coagulation factor deficiencies, e.g. hemophilia).
4. **Transfusion to restore or maintain leukocyte functions.** It is rare indication and may be necessary for severely granulocytopenic patients with infections that do not respond to antibiotics.

TYPES OF DONORS AND DONATION

Types of Donors

No synthetic substitute is available for blood and we depend only on the human source. The types of donors include:
1. **Voluntary nonremunerated donors:** They donate blood own free will without any pressure and monetary benefit for recipients that are unknown to them. This type should be encouraged and practiced for safe donation because they belong to low-risk category and their blood is of better quality. They are usually willing to donate at regular intervals and mostly respond to request during emergencies. It is important to encourage voluntary nonremunerated donors for safe blood supply. Voluntary blood donation is the most important aspect of blood transfusion services. It is the source of blood needed to meet the demands of the patients in need. It is the one of the main responsibilities of the blood transfusion services to motivate donor and to constantly expand the voluntary blood donor base.
2. **Replacement or relative donors:** They are the either family members (relations) of the patients requiring blood or friends who replace the unit of blood used for the patient. Replacement donation is a common practice in our country. Sometimes, donors request that their blood should be given to the specific patients. Such donations are called directed donations (refer page 140).
3. **Professional or commercial paid donors:** These donors receive direct or indirect monetary benefits for the blood they donate. They do not reveal the truth about their illness, previous donations and personal life. Thus, they are not safe for blood donation. They frequently donate blood and their blood may give little or no benefit to the patient.

Types of Blood Donations

Allogeneic Donation

It is commonly referred to as **whole blood donation** is the process of voluntarily donating a unit of blood. Allogeneic donation is for use by the general patient population. In this, one unit (450 mL) of whole blood is collected in an anticoagulant.

Autologous Donation

In this type, blood is collected and reserved for an individual in advance for subsequent transfusion (e.g. elective or scheduled surgery for later use) to the same individual from whom the blood is collected. This blood is transfused to the same patient during or after the procedure to compensate for expected blood loss. This is discussed in detail in Chapter 19 on pages 411-3.

Apheresis Donation

In this type of donation, whole blood is removed from donor and a specific component (desired portion) of the blood or parts of the whole blood is collected/retained. The remaining components are returned to the donor. Blood components can also be collected by apheresis. The advantage of apheresis donation is that a more quantity of the desired components may be obtained from a single donation.

- The apheresis donation is **most commonly used for the collection of platelets** (commonly called **single donor platelets**).
- **Plasma may also be collected**, along with platelets.
- Apheresis donation is **useful for the collection of two units of RBCs from suitable donors**.
- **Leukocytes** may also be collected by apheresis; and apheresis donation is most commonly used for the collection of **hematopoietic progenitor cells for autologous or allogeneic transplantation**. Granulocytes or mononuclear cell apheresis may be collected for special applications.

Directed or Designated Donation

In this type, the **donation reserved for use by a specific patient**. Thus, patients like to select donors (usually relatives or friends) for themselves rather than receiving blood from the community donors, for their anticipated transfusion needs. Though patients feel greater safety, there is no evidence that it reduces the risk for transfusion-transmitted disease. Directed donors must meet all criteria for allogeneic blood donation and also the donor's blood must be compatible with the intended recipient. In some situations, directed donation is contraindicated. For example, donation of any plasma-containing blood component from a mother to her child is particularly risky. This is because the formation of human leukocyte antigen (HLA) antibodies in the mother's plasma to fetal antigens is common in pregnancy. Transfusion of such antibodies can result in transfusion-related acute lung injury. In recipients of hematopoietic progenitor cell transplants, transfusions from close relatives should be avoided. Because there is a risk for immunization to HLA and other histocompatibility antigens. This may reduce graft survival. The directed donation **may be desirable in rare occasions**. These include rare blood group compatibility requirements and long-term need of transfusion such as aplastic anemia. In neonatal alloimmune thrombocytopenia, collection of maternal platelets may be the best method for providing compatible antigen-negative platelets.

DONOR SELECTION

Donor selection is the **most important preliminary step** and primary responsibility of blood banking service. The blood must be collected from healthy, nonremunerated and safe donors so as to avoid any unwanted effects of the recipient. Every donor must be treated courteously and any doubts they may have must be clarified with genuine interest.

Donor Screening

Once the donor is found to be eligible and suitable, the screening has to be done before collection of the blood. Screening of donor can be divided into four phases (Fig. 7.1): (1) registration of the donor, (2) educational materials, (3) obtaining the donor's medical/

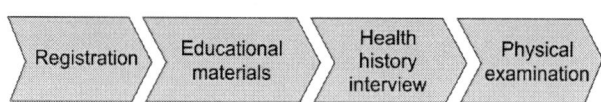

Fig. 7.1: Four steps in the screening of donors.

Donor Selection and Blood Collection

health history (health history interview) and (4) performing a "mini" physical examination.

Registration of Donor

First step before each donation (blood collection) is obtaining and recording donor identification and link the donor to existing donor records (if already present). To prevent an ineligible donor from donating again, every donor must be checked against a permanent record of previously deferred donors. The following information should be obtained and recorded (hard copy or electronically) during the registration process:

- **Full name of the donor** (first, last, middle)
- **Father's/husband's name**
- **Gender**
- **Age or date of birth:** The donor should be in the age group of 18–65 years. For **autologous** donation (donating blood to be used for oneself), there is no age restriction.
- **Date and time of donation**
- **Permanent address**
- Occupation
- **Telephone number:** This will help to recall the donor especially for group specific emergency need or to mail them their blood group card.
- **Date of last donation:** There must be:
  - Eight weeks gap between whole blood donations
  - Sixteen weeks after a two-unit RBC collection
  - Four weeks after infrequent plasmapheresis
  - Two days or more after plasmapheresis, plateletpheresis or leukapheresis.
- **Additional information:** Cytomegalovirus (CMV) status, because some patient groups (e.g. neonates) require CMV-negative blood in certain circumstances.
  - Intended use of the donation: allogeneic donation, directed donation, autologous donation, or apheresis donation.

Donor selection requires two most important aspects to know whether donor is suitable for donating blood. These include:

1. A detailed **medical history**
2. **Routine** limited **physical examinations** (preliminary health checkup) done on the day of the donation.

When selecting the donor, two points must be borne in mind: whether the donation of about 450 mL of whole blood and the procedure is harmful to the donor? and whether blood drawn from the donor is likely to be harmful to the recipient and transmit any disease to the recipient? If the answer is no for both of these questions, then blood can be collected.

Educational Materials and Donor Consent

Educational materials

Before donating, all donors must be provided with educational materials describing the donation process and donor eligibility. It must include risk factors for relevant transfusion-transmitted infections (RTTIs), human immunodeficiency virus (HIV) and acquired immunodeficiency syndrome (AIDS) and information regarding risks of other infectious diseases transmitted by blood transfusion. It should also describe the possible side effects and risks associated with the donation process. The educational materials must inform the signs and symptoms associated with HIV infection and AIDS. It is also necessary to stress the need of honest answers in view of window period. The donor is asked for high-risk activities and foreign travel.

Information and consent to donate

Information: Donors should be informed about the procedure for donating blood and its possible donation related adverse effects/risks, and tests done on their blood. Donors must be informed about health conditions and high-risk behaviors that make them unsuitable to donation of blood.

Consent to donate: Before donation, the donor must sign a statement documenting (a written informed consent for blood collection and its use) that they have given consent to the donation. Donor should be asked to read it carefully and give consent for phlebotomy and is done at the end of the donor history questionnaire (DHQ). It should be obtained from allogeneic, autologous, and apheresis donors before collecting the blood.

Medical History Questionnaire

Obtaining an accurate medical history of the donor is essential to ensure protection of the donor and benefit to the recipient. Donor is provided with a standardized medical history questionnaire (Fig. 7.2). The questions are designed so that a simple "yes" or "no" can be answered but elaborated if indicated. It should be filled by the donor itself or the donor clinic staff (interviewer). The questionnaire helps to collect information systematically from each donor and helps staff in transfusion medicine

---

BLOOD BANK
BLOOD DONOR RECORD, QUESTIONNAIRE AND CONSENT FORM

License No.: _____ Blood Unit No.: _____

CONFIDENTIAL
(O) Tick wherever applicable
Please answer the following questions correctly. This will help to protect you and the patient who receives your blood

Name:		Male:	Female:
Date of Birth:	Age:	Father's Name:	
Occupation		Organization:	

Address for communication:

Telephone No: Mobile No:
Would you like us to call on your mobile: ☐ Yes   ☐ No
Fax No: Email:

Have you donated previously: ☐ Yes   ☐ No
If yes, how many occasions: When last:

Your blood group: Time of last meal:
Did you have any discomfort/after donation?   ☐ Yes   ☐ No

(Ö) Tick appropriate answer:
1. Do you feel well today?   ☐ Yes ☐ No
2. Did you have something to eat in the last 4 hours?   ☐ Yes ☐ No
3. Did you sleep well last night?   ☐ Yes ☐ No
4. Have you any reason to believe that you may be infected   ☐ Yes ☐ No
   by either hepatitis, malaria, HIV/AIDS and venereal disease?

5. In the last 6 months have you had any history of the following?
   ☐ Unexplained weight loss   ☐ Repeated diarrhea
   ☐ Swollen glands   ☐ Continuous low-grade fever

6. In the last 6 months have you had any?
   ☐ Tattooing   ☐ Ear piercing   ☐ Dental extraction

7. Do you suffer from or have suffered from any of the following diseases:
   ☐ Heart disease   ☐ Lung disease   ☐ Kidney disease
   ☐ Cancer/Malignant diseases   ☐ Tuberculosis   ☐ Epilepsy
   ☐ Diabetes   ☐ Jaundice (last 1 year)   ☐ Hepatitis B/C
   ☐ Abnormal bleeding tendency   ☐ Malaria (6 months)   ☐ Allergic disease
   ☐ Fainting spells   ☐ Sexually trans disease   ☐ Typhoid (last 1 yr)

Fig. 7.2: Contd...

Are your taking or have taken any of these in the past 72 hours?
- ☐ Antibiotics
- ☐ Dog bite/rabies vaccine
- ☐ Vaccinations
- ☐ Steroids
- ☐ Aspirin
- ☐ Alcohol

8. Is there any history of surgery or blood transfusion in the past 6 months?
- ☐ Major
- ☐ Minor
- ☐ Blood transfusion

9. For Women donors
   - Are you pregnant? ☐ Yes ☐ No
   - Have you had an abortion in the last 3 months? ☐ Yes ☐ No
   - Do you have a child less than one year old? ☐ Yes ☐ No

10. Would you like to be informed about any abnormal test result at the address furnished by you?
    ☐ Yes ☐ No

Have you need and understood at the information presented and answered all the questions truthfully, as any incorrect statement or concealment may affect your health or may harm the recipient.
☐ Yes ☐ No

I understand that
a) Blood donation is a totally voluntary act and no inducement or remuneration has offered
b) Donation of blood/components is a medical procedure and that by donating voluntarily, I accept the risks associated with this procedure
c) My blood will be tested for hepatitis B, hepatitis C, malarial parasite, HIV/AIDS and venereal diseases in addition to any other screening tests required to ensure blood safety
d) I have been informed about the process of fractionation of fresh frozen plasma for therapeutic purposes. I give my consent for transport and use of my blood product for fractionation as might be deemed fit by Blood Bank

I prohibit any information provided by me or about my donation to be disclosed to any individual or government agency without my prior permission.

Date: —————— Time: —————— Donor's Signature: ——————

General physical examination:
Weight: —————— Pulse: —————— Hemoglobin: ——
Blood pressure: —————— Temperature: ——————

☐ Accept ☐ Defer Reason: ——————

Signature of medical officer: ——————

FOR OFFICE USE ONLY

BIOOD GROUP | A | B | AB | O   SUB GROUPS [   ]   Rh | POS | NEG

VOL. COLLECTED [   ] ML

PHLEBOTOMIST [   ]

Signature of the technician

Blood safety begins with a Healthy donor

Fig. 7.2: Donor history questionnaire (DHQ).

department to make quick assessment whether to accept, temporary defer or permanently reject the donor. Questions are usually divided into two categories: (1) questions intended to protect the donor and (2) questions intended to protect the recipient. The questionnaires must be reviewed by trained personnel before collecting blood. The medical history is conducted on the same day of the donation and should be inquired about: (1) history of any long-term illness, (2) if donor is taking any medication and (3) history of allergy to any substance/medication, etc.

Donor deferral

Deferrals: Blood centers should maintain a registry of deferred donors. Each donor must be checked against this registry before any donation is made and every donation must be tested for infectious disease markers. **Depending on the causative reason, deferrals may be temporary** for a defined interval of time **or permanent**.

Rejection: A **donor with history or certain risk factors should not be considered as suitable for donation**. An individual having multiple sex partners, homosexual males or a drug addict/chronic alcoholic should not be accepted as donors. The donor should be free from diseases of heart, lung, liver and kidney. Donor also should not suffer from cancer, diabetes, epilepsy, tuberculosis, bleeding disorder, allergy, malaria, sexually-transmitted disease. It is important to know whether the patient has history of diseases like hepatitis, AIDS, syphilis and if so, blood should not be obtained from them. In the blood center, blood is routinely screened for few common infections.

Types of deferral (Box 7.1): Donors may be deferred indefinitely, permanently, or temporarily depending on medical history or prior tests. The donor should be provided with a full proper explanation of the reason for the deferral in case a donor is rejected. It should be handled tactfully. They should be informed whether the deferral is temporary or permanent.

- A **permanent deferral** should not donate blood forever. Example for permanent deferrals for donors include a **confirmed positive test for hepatitis B surface antigen** (HBsAg), and **reactive nucleic acid tests for hepatitis C virus or HIV** during re-entry testing. These donors may be eligible to donate autologous blood. Some permanent deferrals may be determined from the testing performed on a previous donation. Box 7.2 lists conditions for current indefinite and permanent deferrals.
- A **temporary deferral** is recommended if the donor would be eligible at a specific time in the future. For example, a donor who has received a blood transfusion; defer for 12 months from date of transfusion. Major conditions for temporary donor deferral and period of deferral are listed in Table 7.1.

Conditions which can affect health of donor

There are certain conditions (Box 7.3) which adversely affect the health and may harm donor. Donor with these should not be accepted for blood donation. If the donor is deferred for any reason, the same must be recorded.

Criteria for the protection of the recipient

Donors should be thoroughly asked regarding the possible exposure to diseases that can be transmitted through the transfusion. These include relevant transfusion-transmitted infectious diseases (such as hepatitis, HIV, malaria, and others), risk for bacteremia, ingestion of certain medications, vaccinations and history of malignancy.

Physical Examination

Donor selection is the most important and preliminary steps of blood banking service. The blood must be collected from healthy, nonremunerated and safe donors to avoid any unwanted effects of the recipient. Perform a limited physical examination designed to protect both the donor and recipient. The following selection criteria/parameters should be checked each time the donor comes to donate blood.

- **General appearance:** The donor should be in good health. Healthy means that patient feels well and can perform normal

---

Box 7.1: Types of deferral.

- **Temporary deferral:** Prospective donor is not allowed to donate blood for a limited period of time
- **Permanent deferral:** Prospective donor will not be eligible to donate blood for someone else

Donor Selection and Blood Collection

Box 7.2: Conditions for donor rejection or permanent deferral.

- Infectious diseases—indefinite deferral:
  - Hepatitis B infection
  - Positive test for hepatitis B surface antigen or hepatitis B virus (HBV) nucleic acid testing (NAT)
  - Repeat reactive test for antibody to hepatitis B core antigen (anti-HBc) on more than one occasion
  - Clinical or laboratory evidence of HCV, HTLV, HIV or *Trypanosoma cruzi* infection
  - Previous donation associated with hepatitis, HIV or HTLV transmission
  - Signs and symptoms suggestive of HIV infection/AIDS, e.g. lymphadenopathy, persistent cough, unexplained weight loss, night sweats/fever, prolonged diarrhea
  - History of babesiosis or Chagas disease
  - Family history of Creutzfeldt-Jakob disease (CJD)
  - Recipient of dura mater or human pituitary growth hormone
- Abnormal bleeding tendency: Donors with a history of a coagulopathy
- Cardiovascular/heart disease: Prospective donors with active or past serious cardiovascular disease (e.g. myocardial infarction, coronary artery disease, angina pectoris, rheumatic heart disease with residual damage) except congenital abnormalities with complete cure. Open heart surgery including bypass surgery
- Chronic kidney disease
- Liver disease
- Malignant diseases except in situ cancer with complete recovery
- Unexplained weight loss
- Diabetes controlled on oral drugs and insulin
- Allergic subjects: Individuals with very severe allergy
- A history of serious central nervous system (CNS) disease
- Repeated episodes of syncope or a history of convulsions, seizure and epilepsy
- Stigma of parenteral drug use: Intravenous (IV) or intramuscular (IM) drug use, injection of nonprescribed drugs
- Donors taking drugs: Examples, antiarrhythmics, anticonvulsants, Dilantin, anticoagulants, antithyroid drugs, immunosuppressive/cytotoxic drugs, pituitary growth hormones of human origin, sedatives or tranquilizers in high dose, vasodilators, digitalis, etretinate (teratogenic) to treat psoriasis, drugs used for Parkinson's disease

Note: Ingestion of oral contraceptives or replacement hormones such as thyroxine is not a disqualification for blood donation.

Table 7.1: Major conditions for temporary donor deferral and period of deferral.

Conditions	Period of deferral
History of	
• Abortion	6 months
• Breastfeeding	6 months
• Acute glomerulonephritis	6 months after recovery
• Hepatitis in family members or close contact	6 months
• Alcoholism	Till intoxicated
• Jaundice	12 months
• Recipient of blood transfusion or tissue transplant	12 months from time of transfusion (blood, blood components)/transplant or grafts
• Aspirin ingestion	3 days for platelet donation
• Exposure to risk of acquiring a transfusion-transmissible infection	
○ Tattooing	6 months
○ Minor surgery	3 months
○ Major surgery	6 months
○ Tooth extraction or dental manipulation	3 days
○ Dental surgery under anesthesia	1 month

Contd...

Contd...

Conditions	Period of deferral
• Pregnancy	12 months after delivery and also during lactation
• Measles/mumps/chickenpox	8 weeks
• Typhoid fever	12 months after recovery
• Infectious disease: Nonsterile skin or needle penetration, sexual contact with an individual with a confirmed positive test for hepatitis B surface antigen, sexual contact with an individual with viral hepatitis, history of syphilis or gonorrhea	12 months
• Malaria—duly treated	3 months (endemic area) and 3 years (for nonendemic area)
Vaccination/immunization/inoculations	
• Vaccination protecting against viral infection: To avoid the possibility of transmitting live viruses (e.g. those of measles, mumps, rubella, Sabin oral polio vaccine, yellow fever, smallpox)	3 weeks following vaccination and donor is well following vaccination
• Vaccination/immunization with killed microbes or with antigens (cholera, typhoid, influenza, hepatitis A and B, Salk polio, plague, gamma globulins) or toxoids (tetanus, diphtheria, pertussis)	48 hours following vaccination and donor is well following vaccination
• Donors who have received immunoglobulins after exposure to infectious agents	For a period slightly longer than the incubation period of the disease in question
○ Hepatitis B immunoglobulin after exposure to the virus	9 months to 1 year
○ Tetanus immunoglobulin	4 weeks
○ Rabies vaccination for rabid animal bite	1 years after bite

Box 7.3: Conditions which can affect health of donor if blood is donated.

- Heart and lung disease
- Kidney disease
- Chronic peptic ulcer
- Epilepsy
- Circulatory disorders
- Cancer
- Anemia
- Diabetes
- Pregnancy
- Breastfeeding
- Excessive menstrual bleeding

activities. Donor should be healthy with normal vital signs. The donor should be mentally alert, and physically fit.

- **Age:** The donor should be in the age group of 18–65 years.
- **Weight:** The weight of the donor should not be less than 45 kg for donation of 350 mL of blood. Those weighing 55 kg and above can donate 450 mL of blood. A donor can donate blood 8–9 mL/kg body weight.
- **Blood pressure:** Systolic pressure in the range of 90–180 mm Hg and diastolic pressure 50–100 mm Hg.
- **Pulse:** Regular and between 50 and 100 beats/minute.
- **Body temperature:** Should not exceed 37.5°C/99.5°F. Raised temperature may indicate a possible infection in the donor, which can danger to the recipient.
- **Physical assessment of donor** for any skin rashes and swollen glands. Scars of needle pricks at venipuncture site on the arms and forearms of the donor might indicate drug addiction or frequent blood donation in professional donors. The donor should be free from any skin diseases at the site of phlebotomy. Vein selection is very important for blood component products; it should flow freely by a clean single vein puncture. On systemic examination, liver and spleen should not be palpable. There should not be any abnormality in heart or lungs.

- **Interval between blood donations:** The interval between blood donations should be at least 8 weeks after whole blood donation, 4 weeks after infrequent apheresis, and at least 2 days after plasma, platelet, or leukocyte apheresis. In India, the interval between blood donations should not be less than 3 months and for platelet apheresis donation, interval time is 7 days.
- **Hemoglobin or hematocrit level:** Blood for the hemoglobin or hematocrit test is obtained from venipuncture or finger stick. For males, minimum hemoglobin level required is 13.0 g/dL or minimum hematocrit is 39%. For females, minimum hemoglobin level should be 12.5 g/dL or minimum hematocrit is 38%. Methods for determining the donor's hemoglobin include the copper sulfate method and spectrophotometric methods.
- **Vaccinations and immunizations:** Recipient of live attenuated viral or bacterial vaccine should differ from donation for 2- or 4-week from the time of vaccination.
- **Malaria:** If there is confirmed diagnosis, defer for 3 years after becoming asymptomatic.
- The donor should be free from acute respiratory diseases.
- **Pregnancy and nursing:** Pregnant women are not eligible to donate. Only 6 weeks after giving birth, they can donate.

Summary of physical examination requirements is presented in Table 7.2.

Table 7.2: Summary of physical examination requirements.

Criteria checked	Acceptable limit
General appearance	Should be in good health
Age	>16 years
Weight	Minimum 45 kg
Blood pressure	Systolic: 90–180 mm Hg Diastolic: 50–100 mm Hg
Pulse	50–100 beats/minute
Temperature	≤37.5°C (99.5°F)
Hemoglobin	≥13.0 g/dL (130 g/L) for males ≥12.5 g/dL for females
Hematocrit	≥38% for females ≥39% for males

BLOOD COLLECTION

Blood collection is the most important and essential function of blood transfusion services. The phlebotomy should be performed carefully to minimize any potential donor reactions or potential contamination of the unit.

Two steps are involved in the donation process namely (1) donor eligibility and (2) suitability of the donation.

1. **Donor's eligibility:** It is to determine whether the donor is qualified to donate blood and blood components. Phlebotomy should be performed only in donor eligible for donation.
2. **Donation suitability:** To determine whether the donation is acceptable for transfusion.

Identification

Identification of donor: It is very essential to confirm the donor's identity at each step of the blood donation process from donor registration to final issue of each component. The phlebotomist is often different from the individual who takes the donor's health history. Hence, phlebotomist should confirm the identity of the donor before starting the venipuncture. Before beginning the collection, identify the donor record, at least by name, with the donor.

Inspection of site of phlebotomy: Next step is to inspect the antecubital area of both donor arms. This inspection gives the phlebotomist the idea about the arm with the best vein (Fig. 7.3) and to check for skin lesions and intravenous drug use.

Donor Preparation

The collection of blood should be done in a pleasant, convenient, well-ventilated area.

Materials required for collection of blood are listed in Box 7.4.

Labeling: This is the first and extremely important step in the collection process. **Properly label all bags** (primary and satellite bags/containers) and **sample tubes** and related materials used for blood collection. The donor registration form must be labeled

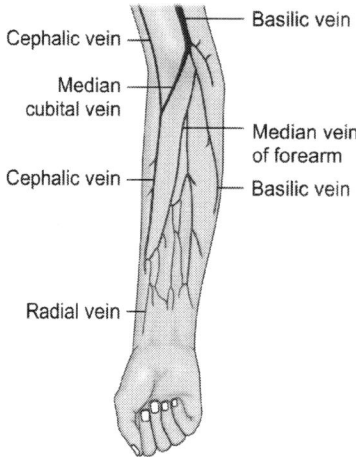

Fig. 7.3: Diagram of the arm showing the various antecubital (in front of the elbow) veins which is the site for the donor's venipuncture and subsequent donation.

Box 7.4: Materials required for collection of blood.

- Blood collection bags of 350 mL or 450 mL capacity [single, double, triple, triple ADSOL/ saline-adenine-glucose-mannitol (SAGM) or quadruple bags] containing citrate-phosphate-dextrose (CPD) or citrate-phosphate-dextrose-adenine (CPDA-1) as anticoagulant-preservative solution
- Sphygmomanometers
- Stethoscope
- Test tubes for sample collection (pilot tubes)
- Test tube racks
- Cotton wool swabs
- Scale for weighing the blood collected in bags
- Tube sealer, roller and cutter (dielectric sealer)
- Artery forceps and scissors
- Antiseptic solution
- Band aids
- Disposable needles and syringes
- Labels
- Emergency drugs
- Blood mixers (optional)

---

with a unique identification number (i.e. unique donation identification number [DIN]). The label consists of both numbers and letters readable by the phlebotomist and barcodes used for computer scanning, recheck all numbers. Almost all blood centers use barcoded labels, and much of the subsequent tracking of specimens, test results, and individual components is done by computers using these labels.

Selection of the vein and preparation of the venipuncture site (Box 7.5): Blood is drawn from a vein in the antecubital fossa.

- Before phlebotomy, inspect the donor's antecubital skin area of both arms to select the appropriate vein. The vein selected should be prominent, firm, and large enough to accommodate a 16-gauge needle and provide good blood flow.
- A blood pressure (sphygmomanometer) cuff is applied just above the cubital fossa is usually used to impede venous return and distend the vein. Inflate the cuff to 60–70 mm of Hg. Donor is asked to make fist to make the veins appear prominent. After palpating the vein, release the pressure of the cuff and prepare the venipuncture site.
- The skin over the venipuncture site should be (1) free of lesions, (2) adequate for donation and (3) without any evidence of injection of drug use (multiple needle punctures, i.e. small scars line forming tracks). Blood is collected by phlebotomy under aseptic conditions in a manner to minimize the risk for bacterial contamination. The skin at the venipuncture site must be cleaned with an antibacterial scrub (using disinfectants such as povidone-iodine or isopropyl alcohol plus iodine tincture). The **selection of the venipuncture site and its sterilization are very important steps**, since bacterial contamination of blood can be a serious and even fatal complication can occur.

Donation chair (donor couch) used for collecting blood from donors and process of blood collection is shown in Figures 7.4A and B.

Process of Blood Collection of Whole Blood

Closed system bag: Whole blood is collected into sterile, plasticized polyvinyl chloride

Donor Selection and Blood Collection

Box 7.5: Procedure for donor arm preparation for blood collection.

- Make the donor to lie down on the donor couch
- Apply tourniquet or blood pressure cuff over the upper arm
- Identify venipuncture site and then release tourniquet or cuff
- Scrub area of skin at least 4 cm (1.5 inches) in all directions (i.e. 8 cm or 3 inches in diameter) from intended venipuncture site for a minimum of 30 seconds using povidone-iodine 1% or isopropyl alcohol plus iodine tincture. Start at intended venipuncture site and move outward in a concentric spiral and let stand for 30 seconds. Then again scrub the area with 70% ethyl alcohol or methylated spirit in similar manner. Let stand for 30 seconds. After the skin is prepared, do not touch the area again. Do not repalpate the vein at the intended venipuncture site. Note: For donors sensitive to iodine, green soap is acceptable
- **Optional step:** A local anesthetic injection of 1% lignocaine (0.3 mL) may be given intradermally at the venipuncture site. Local anesthetic sprays can be used
- Cover the area with dry, sterile gauze until the time of venipuncture
- Position the bag below the level of donor arm on weighing balance. If automatic weighing is available (e.g. Biomixers), adjust it to the amount of blood to be drawn. Pass the donor tubing of the collection set through the automated clamp and start the mixer
- Clamp the tubing of the blood bag, just close the needle and remove the needle cap

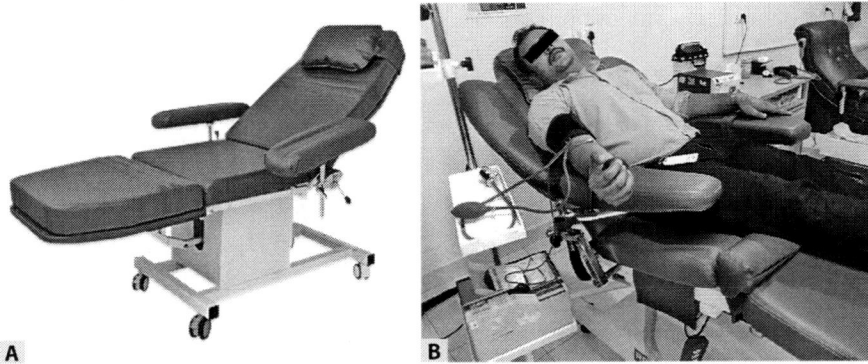

Figs. 7.4A and B: (A) Donor couche used for collecting blood from donors; (B) Process of blood collection.

(PVC) bag sets. These blood containers consist of combinations of multiple satellite bags connected by tubing. The advantage is that the components can be transferred between bags without being exposed to air and it minimizes the chance of bacterial contamination. This is known as a "closed system" (refer Fig. 8.1). Inspect bag for any defects and discoloration. Apply pressure and check for leaks. The anticoagulant and additive solutions should be inspected for appropriate volume, color and particulate contaminants.

Phlebotomy (venipuncture):

- Position bag below the level of the donor's arm. Adjust the blood monitoring balance system for the blood to be drawn (discussed below under volume of blood to be collected). Make a very loose overhand knot in the tubing. Place the bag on the monitor pan and route tubing through the pinch clamp. A hemostat should be applied to the tubing before the needle is uncapped to prevent air from entering the line.
- Reapply tourniquet or inflate blood pressure cuff. A tourniquet or blood pressure cuff inflated to 40–60 mm Hg makes the vein more prominent for venipuncture. Ask the donor to open and close the fist by squeezing rubber hand press (rubber ball) until previously selected vein is again prominent.
- Usually blood collection equipment uses a 16-gauge needles and the entire set is closed and connected so that the needle

is integral. Uncover sterile needle and perform the venipuncture immediately. A clean, skillful venipuncture is necessary for collection of a full clot-free unit of blood. Most phlebotomists follow a two-step process. In first step, the needle penetrates the skin, then after a brief pause and as second step the needle is inserted into the vein. The pause is so brief that it may not be noticeable to the donor. The phlebotomist must place the needle in such a way so as to minimize the likelihood of puncturing a nerve or artery. Introduce the needle into the vein. Remove the clamp of the tubing and also reduce the pressure of sphygmomanometer to 40-50 mm of Hg so that there is free flow of blood into the bag. Hold the needle in position by using two pieces of acceptable/adhesive tape on the bulb of the needle and cover site with a sterile gauze.

- Remove the hemostat. Open the temporary closure between the interior of the bag and the tubing. Ask the donor to open and close hand slowly every 10-12 seconds during collection.
- Observe the donor throughout the donation process. Never leave the donor unattended during or immediately after donation.

Note: If an attempt of venipuncture fails needle is withdrawn. New venipuncture is attempted but a fresh collection unit should be used (original to be discarded) and preparation of the site must be repeated as described earlier.

Collection of blood: During phlebotomy, the rate of blood flow must be sufficient to prevent formation of clot. There is possibility of bacteria entering into the blood bag from skin at the venipuncture. Hence, most blood collection sites now contain a small pouch for diverting the first few mL of blood which can reduce the bacterial contamination rate. The blood must flow freely and remains fairly brisk, so that coagulation activity is not triggered. Collection bag should be gently and periodically/frequently (every 45 seconds) mixed as it fills the container

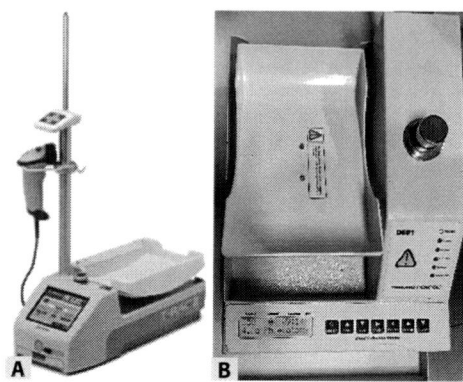

Figs. 7.5A and B: (A) Blood collection monitor; (B) Mechanical mixing device.

during the collection. This will ensure uniform distribution of anticoagulant and avoids the development of small clots. Mechanical mixing devices (Biomixers) that continuously mix the blood (Fig. 7.5) and anticoagulant during phlebotomy are also available and preferable than manual mixing.

Types of disposable blood collection bags (Table 7.3): PVC sterile bags with attached tubing and needle are easy to store. For blood component preparation, bag selection is very important.

Volume of blood to be collected:
- Blood has to be drawn in proportion with the amount of anticoagulant in the blood bag. The ratio of anticoagulant-preservation solution to blood collected should be 1.4 cc of anticoagulant to 10 mL of blood (1.4:10).
- Blood bags are designed in two types depending on the volume of blood (Box 7.6) to be drawn.
  - **450 mL blood bags:** In this, 450 mL of blood is collected into 63 mL of anticoagulant solution.
  - **350 mL blood bags:** In this, 350 mL of blood is collected into 49 mL of anticoagulant solution.
- Monitor the volume of drawn blood being drawn. Since it is difficult to directly measure the volume of blood drawn into the bag, indirect measurement is done

Donor Selection and Blood Collection

Table 7.3: Types of disposable blood collection bags.

Type of bag with amount of blood and anticoagulant	Use	Life of the blood
Single bag: 350 mL with 49 mL CPDA anticoagulant	For whole blood	35 days
Double bag: 450 mL with 63 mL CPDA anticoagulant	For component preparation packed red blood cells (PRBCs) and fresh frozen plasma (FFP)	35 days
Triple bag: 450 mL with 63 mL CPDA anticoagulant	Collect 350 mL/450 mL of blood in anticoagulant-containing primary bag. For preparation of FFP, packed red blood cell (PRBC), random donor's platelets. The satellite bags are used for the preparation of FFP and random donor's platelets	Half-life period of PRBC depends on the anticoagulant
Quadruple bag: 450 mL with 63 mL CPDA anticoagulant	Collect 350 mL/450 mL of blood in anticoagulant-containing primary bag. Used for all types of components preparation like PRBCs/leukodepleted PRBC/FFP/platelets concentrate and cryoprecipitate	Depends on the component

Note: Nowadays 78 mL SAGM-2 preservatives for 350 mL of triple bag and 100 mL SAGM-2 preservatives for 450 mL of quadruple bag are added. If SAGM-2 is used of preservative, the red cell life span is 42 days. In quadruple/triple bags, one satellite bag is specially made for platelet concentrate preparation.

Box 7.6: Formula for the amount of blood to be collected.

- Total weight of blood bag with capacity of 350 mL
  = (350 × 1.05) + weight of the empty blood bag
- Total weight of blood bag with capacity of 450 mL
  = (450 × 1.05) + weight of the empty blood bag

---

by weighing the blood bag using a blood collection scale or single pan weighing scale. This indirect measurement depends on the factor that weight of 1 mL of blood is equivalent to 1.053 g of blood (Box 7.6). Hence, a unit containing 400–500 mL should weigh 429–525 g plus the weight of the container and the anticoagulant. Use of blood monitor (Fig. 7.5A) will interrupt blood flow after proper amount has been collected.

- The volume of blood withdrawn should be not be more than 15% of the donor's estimated blood volume and should be less than 10.5 mL/kg body weight (including samples for testing). Usually, whole blood collection consists of 450 mL or 500 mL. If flow of blood stops and only 100 mL or less has been collected, phlebotomy can be tried with a fresh collection unit from the other arm (if the donor gives consent). If more than 100 mL has been collected and flow stops then the donor is given the credit of having donated (either on voluntary or replacement basis). The donor card should be preserved and reason for the insufficient quantity stated and the blood bag discarded. Units containing 300–404 mL can be used for transfusion but must be labeled as low volume units.
- The amount or volume of blood withdrawn must be within the manufacture's specified range to ensure correct ratio between whole blood and anticoagulant, otherwise the blood cells may be damaged or anticoagulation may not be satisfactory.

Time needed for collection: The average time needed for collecting 500 mL of blood is <10 minutes. Blood units requiring more than 15–20 minutes for collection time may not be suitable for preparation (collection) of platelets or plasma (FFP or cryoprecipitate) for transfusion. If the volume of blood available for test samples obtained from the diversion pouch is not sufficient, a second phlebotomy may be performed immediately after phlebotomy. Extremely rapid flow of blood or the appearance of bright red blood may indicate a puncture of artery puncture. This can be confirmed by feeling the pressure building in the blood container.

Post-Donation Care and Adverse Reactions to Blood Donation

Post-Donation Care (Donor Care after Phlebotomy)

- After the required amount of blood is obtained, clamp the tubing of the bag using artery forceps or plastic clip. Deflate the sphygmomanometer cuff (remove tourniquet). Immediately the needle used for phlebotomy is removed or withdrawn. Burn the needle tip in the electric needle burner and discard into a protective sleeve to prevent accidental injuries.
- Place cotton gauze over the venipuncture site and ask the donor to apply local pressure by fingers of the other hand to the gauze over the vein in the antecubital fossa for at least 1 or 2 minutes.
- Asking the donor to raise their arm (elbow straight) to minimize the venous pressure while pressure is applied over phlebotomy site with the other hand may be beneficial. The pressure is applied till hemostasis is achieved. After the bleeding stops, apply a bandage or band aid and apply a bandage or tape. The bandage can be removed after 10–12 hours. If there is no bleeding, discoloration, or evidence of a hematoma at the venipuncture site, the donor should be examined for other symptoms of a reaction to donation (mentioned below).
- Strip the donor tubing as completely as possible into the bag, starting at the seal. Prevent the blood from clotting in the tubing by inverting the bag several times to mix thoroughly. Then allow tubing to refill with anticoagulated blood from the bag. Repeat this procedure again.
- Seal the tubing attached to the collection bag into multiple segments using dielectric tube sealer (Fig. 7.6). It must be possible to separate segments from the unit for compatibility testing without breaking the sterility of the bag. Reinspect the container for defects.
- Collect pilot samples from the tubing in prelabeled pilot tubes. Seal the tubing or put the knot in the tubing and cut the distal to the seal to separate the needle. Recheck the numbers on the container, pilot tubes and donor card.
- Immediately after collection, the **whole blood should be placed at 1–6°C except in cases where platelets are to be separated**. If **platelets** are to be harvested, blood should not be chilled, but stored **at a temperature of 20–24°C until platelets are separated**. Platelets and FFP should be separated within 8 hours after collection of the whole blood.

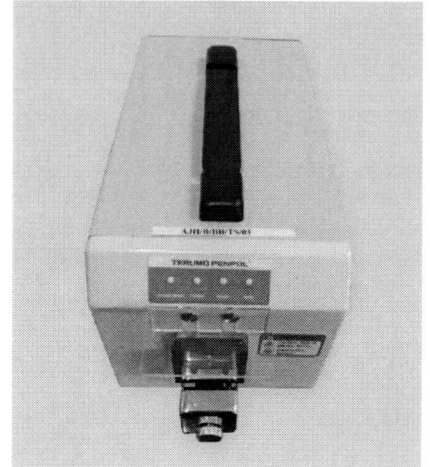

Fig 7.6: Tube sealer for sealing blood collection bag.

Post-Donation Management of Donors

- The donor should remain on the bleeding couch for 10 minutes under the observation of the staff. If the donors feel comfortable in sitting posture without problems, they are allowed to move from the donor bleeding couch to recovery or refreshment room. The donor should be observed during this time, as the movement from supine to an upright posture may bring on lightheadedness or even fainting.
- In the recovery/refreshment room, donor should be provided with drinking fluids and snacks. They should remain in the recovery room for about 15 minutes or till they feel comfortable to leave.

- Thank the donor for his blood donation and encourage the donor to be a regular voluntary donor.

Post-Donation Instructions to Donors

- Donors are advised to drink extra fluids usual in the next 4 hours to replace lost blood volume. They should not remain hungry.
- They should not smoke or consume alcohol for the next 24 hours.
- They should not indulge in strenuous physical activity in the next 24 hours.

Problems Encountering During Donation

- **Difficulty with flow of blood:** It may be due to spasm of vein, reduced sphygmomanometer cuff pressure or occlusion of lumen of the needle by wall or valve within the vein. In such situations, reassure the patient and check the cuff pressure. Lightly adjust the needle. Excessive move of needle leads to formation of hematoma at the site as well discomfort to the donor. If this does not help, remove the needle and discard the bag. If donor agrees, blood may be obtained from another arm.
- **Hematoma during or after phlebotomy:** If it occurs, stop the donation and reassure the donor.
  - Remove the tourniquet and the needle from the donor's arm.
  - Place 3 or 4 sterile gauzes or cotton over the venipuncture and apply firm digital pressure till stops bleeding (for 7–10 minutes). Raise the donor's arm above the heart level. Alternatively, a tight bandage may be applied, which should be removed after 7–10 minutes to allow inspection. Apply ice to the area for 5 minutes, if desired anti-inflammatory cream and oral anti-inflammatory drugs may be used if needed.
- **Signs of reaction or adverse effects** (discussed below) may occur during the phlebotomy.

Adverse Effects in Donors (Table 7.4)

Most donors do not develop side effects after or during donation. But adverse reactions can occasionally occur. It is important to recognize adverse reactions and to provide initial treatment. Special equipment and emergency medical kit should be available to handle any emergency situations (Box 7.7). Post-donation care consists of observing the donor for signs and symptoms of reaction. These reactions may occur with blood donations either at the time of donation or after donation. Repeat donors are less likely to have reactions than first-time donors. Majority occur within 1 hour of donation. Donors who develop reactions are more likely to be younger, unmarried, have a higher predonation heart rate and lower diastolic blood pressure.

Minor reactions

- **Needle-related injuries:** Mild **phlebitis and cellulitis** at the venipuncture site common, self-limited and usually of little consequence. Others include arm bruise or hematoma (management described above).
- **Systemic reactions:** Mostly vasovagal reactions (prefaint or **presyncope**) occur during 2.5% of whole blood donations. These include dizziness, sweating, nausea and vomiting (in about 1%), weakness, hypotension, bradycardia.

Box 7.7: Contents needed in emergency kit.

1. Emesis basin
2. Towels
3. Oropharyngeal airway
4. Tongue depressor
5. Oxygen and mask
6. Emergency drugs
   - IV fluids: 5% dextrose, 10% dextrose, dextrose normal saline, normal saline
   - Thrombophleb
   - Betadine solution and cream
   - Ampoules of adrenaline, dopamine, betamethasone, dexamethasone, hydrocortisone, metoclopramide, antihistamine
   - Aspirin/disprin tablets
7. Disposable syringe with needles of various sizes
8. IV stand
9. IV infusion set

Major reactions
- **Needle-related injuries:** Accidental injury to nerve or artery (refer below) is very rare complication. Needle injury to the nerve may cause pain, and motor and sensory loss, which can be prolonged.
- **Systemic reactions:** These include loss of consciousness, allergic reaction and citrate reaction. They occur during about 0.07% of whole blood and 0.05% of apheresis platelet collections. The vasovagal symptoms may progress to syncope (loss of consciousness) in about 5%, and nausea and vomiting. Smaller donors are more prone for risk of post-donation syncope. Mostly they occur shortly after donation. However, delayed reactions can occur, and if the donor is at work or is driving, these can be very serious.

Management of adverse effects

Laboratory personnel at a collection site should be trained well to treat donor reactions.

If possible, move donor who experiences an adverse reaction to an area where donor can be attended to in privacy. Depending on the adverse effects, follow the measures suggested below. If there is no rapid recovery, call the blood center physician or the physician designated for such purposes.

- **Accidental puncture of the artery:** It is seen as an extremely rapid flow of blood or the appearance of bright red blood may indicate a puncture of artery puncture. This can be confirmed by feeling the pressure building in the blood container. If it occurs, manage it as follows:
  - If an arterial puncture is suspected, stop the donation and immediately withdraw needle.
  - Apply hard pressure for 10 minutes to the venipuncture site and raise the limb above the level of head. The pressure should be applied for a minimum of 15–20 minutes. Check for the presence of a radial pulse. If pulse is not palpable or weak, call a blood center physician.
  - Wait till blood completely stops and donor is complete fine.

Puncture of artery may cause extensive bruising, fistula, aneurysm, distal ischemia, compartment syndrome.

- **Vasovagal syncope (fainting):**
  - In case of vasovagal syncope, immediately stop the phlebotomy. Donor should be managed by immediately placing the donor in the Trendelenburg position (supine/recumbent position with feet higher than head, i.e. raise the legs and lower the head). Apply a cold wet towel (or cold compress) to the forehead, shoulder and back of neck area. Place the donor on their back with legs raised above the level of the head. Loosen the donor's tight clothes.
  - Administer aromatic spirits of ammonia by inhalation if donor does not respond to initial measures. Test the ammonia on yourself before passing it under the donor's nose, as it may be too strong or too weak. Strong ammonia may injure the nasal membranes whereas weak ammonia is not effective. The donor should respond by coughing, which elevates the blood pressure.
  - Ensure adequate airway.
  - Monitor blood pressure, pulse and respiration periodically until the donor recovers.
  - Rarely, in cases of prolonged hypotension, intravenous infusion of normal saline may be required. The decision to initiate such therapy should be made by the blood center physician.
  - A physician should be available at the donation site for consultation, and emergency medical support, if necessary. It is preferable to shift these donors to another room to prevent other donors from apprehension. Vasovagal reactions can be minimized by prior hydration of the donor, or by the use of caffeine. The donors are advised not to return to work for the remainder of the day in an occupation where fainting would be hazardous to themselves or others. Donors should avoid strenuous exercise for the remainder of the day of donation.
- **Nausea and vomiting:**
  - Make donor as comfortable as possible and instruct to breathe slowly and deeply. Apply cold compress to the

donor's forehead and/or back of neck (similar to mentioned above under vasovagal syncope).
- Turn donor's head to the side to prevent aspiration of vomitus.
- Provide a suitable receptacle if the donor vomits and have cleansing tissues or a damp towel ready. After bout of vomiting has stopped, provide some water to rinse out donor's mouth.
- **Hyperventilation or deep breathing:** Some extremely nervous or apprehensive donors may hyperventilate and may lead to respiratory alkalosis and tetany. It may result in lowering of carbon dioxide. This may cause faint muscular twitching/spasms, tingling sensations or tetanic spasms of donor's hands or face. Donor room personnel should watch closely for these symptoms during and immediately after the phlebotomy. It may be managed by:
  - Diverting the donor's attention by engaging in conversation, to interrupt their hyperventilation pattern.
  - Ask the donor to breathe quickly and slowly. If this fails to relieve the spasm, ask the donor to breathe into paper/plastic bag which provides prompt relief. Do not give oxygen.
- **Convulsions:** It is very uncommon.
  - The donors should be prevented from injuring themselves due to convulsions. During severe seizures, some individuals exhibit great muscular power that is difficult to restrain.
  - Maintain adequate airway.
  - Keep the tongue depressor between teeth to prevent biting of own tongue, loosen the tight clothing and check the pulse frequently. Jaws should be separated by a padded device after convulsion has passed. If convulsion persists, it should be managed by medical specialist.
- **Serious cardiac difficulties:** Call for medical aid and/or an emergency care unit immediately. If the donor is in cardiac arrest, begin cardiopulmonary resuscitation (CPR) immediately and continue it until help arrives.

The nature and treatment of all reactions should be recorded on the donor record or a special incident report form. This should include a remark whether the donor should be accepted for future donations.

Reactions following blood donation in donor are summarized in Table 7.4.

Table 7.4: Adverse effects/reactions following blood donation in donor.

Reactions following blood donation in donor	Treatment
General	
Vasovagal attack or syncope or fainting	Cold compresses on back of neck
Weakness, sweating, dizziness, pallor, nausea and vomiting	Remove needle and tourniquet; elevate legs above head; apply cold compresses to forehead and back of neck
Hyperventilation	Diverting the donor's attention by engaging in conversation; ask the donor to breathe quickly and slowly
Convulsions	Prevent donor from falling from the donor chair (couch) or injuring himself or herself; ensure donor's airway is adequate. Use emergency measures by medical officer
At the site of venipuncture	
Hematoma	Remove the tourniquet and the needle from the donor's arm. Place sterile gauzes or cotton over the venipuncture and apply firm digital pressure
Infection of venipuncture site and thrombophlebitis	Self-limited and usually of little consequence
Rarely puncture of artery	Stop the donation and immediately withdraw needle. Apply hard pressure for 10 minutes to the venipuncture site and raise the limb above the level of head

HEMOGLOBIN ESTIMATION OF DONOR

Methods of Hemoglobin Estimation

Blood for the hemoglobin or hematocrit test is obtained from venipuncture or finger stick. For males, minimum hemoglobin level required is 13.0 g/dL or minimum hematocrit is 39%. For females, minimum hemoglobin level should be 12.5 g/dL or minimum hematocrit is 38%. Methods for determining the donor's hemoglobin include the copper sulfate method, hemo-cue blood hemoglobin system, cyanmethemoglobin method and by autoanalyzers.

Copper Sulfate Specific Gravity Method

It is an indirect reliable but not accurate method used mainly for determination of hemoglobin in blood donors.

Principle

Hemoglobin is the largest single component of the blood that affects the specific gravity of blood. Allow a drop of blood to fall into a series of solutions of copper sulphate of varying specific gravity and note the behavior of the drop and estimate the specific gravity of blood. If the blood drop sinks to the bottom, its specific gravity is more than that of the copper sulphate solution. If the blood drop rises after its initial fall, then its specific gravity is less than the specific gravity of copper sulphate solution.

Preparation of Copper Sulphate Solution

- **Preparation of stock solution:** Mix 350 g of copper sulphate in 500 mL of distilled water. Decant the crystals and filter the solution. This stock solution has a specific gravity (SG) of 1.000.
- **Preparation of working solution:** The working solution for 100 tests is prepared as follows:
  - For SG 1.053 take 5.2 mL of stock solution in a volumetric flask and make it up to 100 with distilled water.
  - For SG 1.055 take 5.4 mL of stock solution in a volumetric flask and make it up to 100 with distilled water.

Procedure

In this method, standard copper sulfate solutions of specific gravity ranging from 1.052 to 1.055 are prepared. A precalibrated chart gives the hemoglobin value corresponding to the specific gravity of copper sulphate solution closest to that of the blood. In blood banks, a solution of specific gravity of 1.053 is used for determining the hemoglobin level of 12.5 g/dL for selecting the donor.

1. Dispense 30 mL of copper sulphate solution (specific gravity 1.053) into appropriately labelled clean, dry tubes or bottles. Change the copper sulphate solution daily or after 25 tests and be sure that the solution is properly mixed before performing tests daily.
2. Clean the site of the skin puncture (i.e. finger tip) with antiseptic solution and allow it to dry.
3. Use a disposable lancet for puncture and puncture the skin to produce a free flow of blood.
4. One drop of blood is collected either in capillary tube or pipette and is allowed to fall from a height of 1 cm above the surface of copper sulfate solution. The drop of blood gets encased in a sac of copper proteinate, which prevents any change in specific gravity for about 12 seconds.
5. If the drop of blood remains on the surface or rises from the bottom of the solution, then the drop is lighter than the copper sulphate solution and hemoglobin content of the blood is below normal levels (i.e. less than 12.5 g/dL).
6. If the drop of blood has the specific gravity which is same or is higher than the copper sulphate solution, the drop of blood will sink within 15 secs. Thus its hemoglobin

will be equal to or higher than 12.5 (±0.1g) g/dL.

Sources of Errors in Hb Estimation
- Taking first drop of blood from finger prick
- Squeezing the finger because blood is not flowing freely
- Inside of blood pipette is not flushed out completely
- Dirty pipette
- Chip off of delivering end of blood pipette.

Hemo-cue blood hemoglobin system
It is a WHO approved method for Hb estimation in blood donors.

Principle
The reaction in the cuvette is a modified azide methemoglobin reaction. The microcuvette contains three reagents (Table 7.5) in dried form which convert Hb into azide methemoglobin (HiN3). The photometer uses a double wavelength measuring method, 570 nm and 880 nm (for compensation of turbidity) and determines the Hb.

Apparatus (Fig. 7.7)
The hemo-cue blood hemoglobin system consists of:
- Disposable microcuvette with reagent in dry form
- Microcuvette holder
- Single purpose derived photometer.

Technique
- Apply microcuvette to a drop of blood. The exact amount of blood is drawn into the

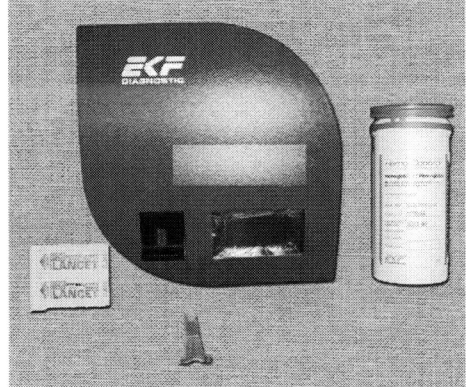

Fig. 7.7: Hemo-cue blood hemoglobin apparatus.

microcuvette by capillary action (capillary, venous or arterial blood can be used).
- Wipe off any excess blood from the sides of microcuvette.
- Place microcuvette in the cuvette holder and insert it into the photometer.
- The results are automatically displayed.

Advantages
- Quick and easy method.
- It is a single use device. Sterile and safe for blood donors.
- It can be used for outdoor blood donation camps.

Cyanmethemoglobin (Hemiglobin Cyanide; HiCN) Method

Cyanmethemoglobin is a photoelectric method which is the most accurate, convenient, readily available and preferred method for estimation of hemoglobin concentration. It is the standard method used in most of the centers.

Principle
Blood is diluted in a stable standard solution of potassium ferricyanide and potassium cyanide. RBCs are lysed and produces evenly distributed hemoglobin solution. **Hemoglobin is first oxidized to methemoglobin** (Hi) by the potassium ferricyanide. The cyanide ions (CN^-) of potassium cyanide convert **methemoglobin (Hi) to stable cyanmethemoglobin** (HiCN).

Table 7.5: Constituents and action of reagents in microcuvette.

Constituent	Action
Sodium deoxycholate	Hemolyses the RBC and releases the hemoglobin (Hb)
Sodium nitrite	Converts Hb (ferrous; Hb) to methemoglobin (ferric; Hi)
Sodium azide	Converts methemoglobin (Hi) to azide methemoglobin (HiN3)

The cyanmethemoglobin has a broad absorption, maximum being at a wavelength of 540 nm. Thus, the color of this solution is compared against a standard HiCN solution of known Hb value in a spectrophotometer or photoelectric colorimeter at 540 nm.

Apparatus

- Photoelectric colorimeter with a green filter or spectrophotometer at a wavelength of 540 nm is used.
- Sahli's pipette (mark of 20 mm)
- 5 mL pipette.

Reagents

- The diluent is **detergent-modified Drabkin solution**, the composition of which is shown in Table 7.6.
  Drabkin solution should be clear and pale yellow and when measured in the photoelectric colorimeter should give zero reading at 540 nm against water blank. The detergent enhances lysis of RBCs and decreases turbidity due to precipitation of proteins.
- Cyanmethemoglobin standard solution with known hemoglobin value.

Specimen

Blood sample required is either blood collected in EDTA or from skin puncture.

Technique

- Take 5 mL of Drabkin solution in a test tube.
- Take 20 μL/microliter (0.02 mL) of blood (1:251 dilution) in a hemoglobin pipette (similar to Sahli's method) and add it to the above test tube. Rinse the Hb pipette at least twice by drawing in Drabkin solution.
- Stopper the test tube and thoroughly mix the blood with Drabkin solution.
- Allow it to stand for 5 (at least 3) minutes at room temperature. This time is adequate for conversion of hemoglobin into cyanmethemoglobin.
- Pour test solution into the cuvette. Read the absorbance of the test sample in the spectrophotometer at 540 nm or photoelectric colorimeter using yellow-green filter.
- Take the absorbance of the HiCN standard solution at room temperature, in the same instrument in a similar fashion.
- Absorbance should be measured against the reagent blank (Drabkin's solution).

  Hb (g/dL) =

  $$\frac{\text{Absorbance of test sample} \times \text{concentration of standard}^* \times 251 \text{(diluent factor)}^{**}}{\text{Absorbance of standard (mg dL)} \times 100^{***}}$$

The standard must be kept in a dark place while not in use and should be discarded at the end of the day.

Preparation of Standard Graph and Standard Table

When many blood samples have to be tested, it is advisable to prepare a standard graph or table relating absorbance readings to hemoglobin in g/L for the individual instrument. It will help in obtaining the hemoglobin value quickly. This graph should be prepared for each photometer or when a bulb or other component is replaced. It can be prepared as follows:

- Prepare 5 dilutions of the HiCN reference standard with the cyanide-ferricyanide

* Concentration of standard is given for each standard, e.g. 50 mg/100 mL.
** Since 0.02 mL of blood has been added to 5 mL Drabkin, dilution is 1 in 251.
*** Divide by 100 to get the value in g%.

Table 7.6: Constituents of Drabkin solution (pH 7.0–7.4)

Constituent	Quantity
Potassium ferricyanide	400 mg
Potassium cyanide (KCN)	100 mg
Potassium dihydrogen phosphate (anhydrous)	280 mg
Non-ionic detergent (*Sterox SE*)	1 mL
Distilled water	2 L

Table 7.7: Dilutions of hemiglobincyanide (HiCN) reference solution for preparation of standard graph.

Tube	Hemoglobin (%)	HiCN volume (mL)	Reagent volume (mL)
1	100 (full strength)	4.0 (neat)	None
2	75	3.0	1.0
3	50	2.0	2.0
4	25	1.0	3.0
5	0	None	4.0 (neat)

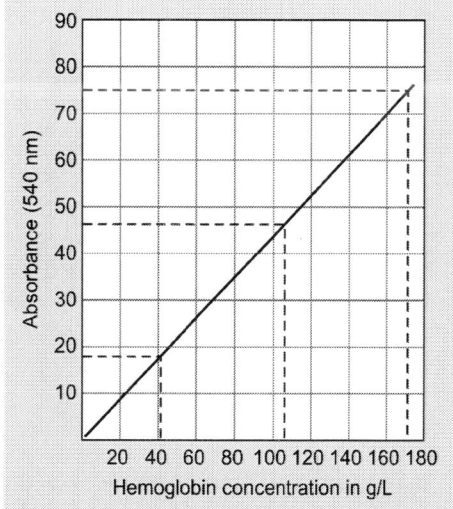

Fig. 7.8: Standard graph for determination of hemoglobin concentration by cyanmethemoglobin method.

reagent as mentioned in Table 7.7. It is necessary to perform the dilutions accurately. Because the graph will be used to determine the hemoglobin measurements.

- The hemoglobin concentration of the reference preparation in each tube is plotted against the absorbance measurement. For example, if the reference preparation contains 800 mg/L (i.e. 0.8 g/L) and the dilution used for hemoglobin estimations is 1:201, the respective hemoglobin concentrations of tubes 1–5 would be 160 g/L, 120 g/L, 80 g/L, 40 g/L and zero.
- On a linear graph paper, plot the absorbance values on the vertical axis and the hemoglobin values (absorbance; formerly called optical density) on the horizontal axis (Fig. 7.8). The points should fit a straight line that passes through the origin. From the graph, construct a table of readings and corresponding hemoglobin values.

Advantages of the Method

- Hb value obtained is **accurate** since almost all forms of hemoglobin (hemoglobin, oxyhemoglobin, methemoglobin, carboxyhemoglobin, but not sulphemoglobin) are converted into cyanmethemoglobin.
- Being a colorimetric method there is direct comparison with HiCN Standard. Thus, **visual error** during matching the color like in Sahli's method is **eliminated**.
- Cyanmethemoglobin is a stable compound and **color does not change with time**. So readings can be made at the operator's convenience delay in taking reading does not alter the value.
- **Easy** to perform the test.
- The **standard is stable** and certified cyanmethemoglobin standards are available.
- Reagents are readily available.

Disadvantages of the Method

- **Turbidity interferes with the reading:** Any turbidity due to abnormal plasma proteins (e.g. multiple myeloma, Waldenström's macroglobulinemia), hyperlipidemia, high WBC count (>25,000/mL) or fat droplets (hypertriglyceridemia) or in the Drabkin solution itself alters value and therefore inaccurate Hb values are obtained.
- **Poisonous diluents:** Potassium cyanide in the solutions is poisonous, though it is present only in a very low concentration. Hence the reagents should be handled carefully.
- **Explosive reagent:** Explosion can occur if undiluted reagents are poured in the sink. Hydrogen cyanide is released by

acidification and the gas, if it accumulates, can result in explosion. Reagents and samples should be disposed off along with the running water in the sink.

Precautions

- Do not pipette Drabkin solution by mouth. Use either suction bulb or auto-dispenser.
- Hemoglobin standard should be used that is supplied by International Committee for Standardization of Hematology.

PROCESSING OF THE DONOR BLOOD

- Before proceeding further, recheck the identification number of blood bag, pilot tube and donor registration number.
- Check all the donor samples for ABO and Rh grouping both for cell and serum grouping.
- All Rh (D) negative blood units must be tested for D^u phenotype by antihuman globulin (AHG) reagent.
  - Blood units which are Rh (D) negative but D^u positive should be labeled as Rh positive. They should be considered as D positive as donors but D negative as recipient.
  - Blood units which are Rh (D) negative but D^u negative should be labeled as Rh negative.
- All donor blood should be tested for unexpected antibodies, especially pregnant or have received blood transfusion.
- Test all the units must be tested by sensitive and specific tests for common blood transmissible disease such as hepatitis B and C (HBsAg, anti-HCV), HIV, syphilis and malaria.
- The blood bag should be properly labeled and results of tests should be mentioned on the label of the blood bag.

SUMMARY

- Careful donor selection is the most important ealement in ensuring a safe blood supply.
- An allogeneic blood donor should weigh at least 48 kg, pulse rate should be between 50 and 100 beats/minute and the hemoglobin/hematocrit level should be at least 12.5 g/dL/38% for females and 13 g/dL/39% for males.
- A donor deferral may be temporary or permanent.
- An individual with a history of hemophilia A or B, von Willebrand's disease, or severe thrombocytopenia must be permanently deferred from donating blood.
- Donors who have tested positive for the HIV antibody must be indefinitely deferred.
- Attenuated live viral vaccines such as smallpox, measles, mumps, yellow fever, and influenza (live virus) carry a 2-week deferral.
- Registration and donor identification: determine whether sufficient time has elapsed for donating and whether the donor was previously deferred.
- Donors are discouraged from donating if they have the potential of transmitting infection through the blood supply.
- Blood is not tested for certain diseases and therefore questions regarding exposure and travel are important for screening purposes.
- The safety of the donor and the recipient is an important element of the screening process. It includes medical history questions and a brief physical examination to determine eligibility.
- Arm preparation at the site of venipuncture is important to avoid contamination with bacteria.
- Signs of adverse donor reactions during phlebotomy are uncommon. But must be recognized and responded to quickly.
- Post-donation instructions to the donor include avoiding activities and the importance of increasing fluid intake after the donation process.
- Estimation of hemoglobin is one of the important investigations for the selection of blood donors. There are several methods of hemoglobin measurement. Hemo-cue blood hemoglobin system is a WHO approved method. Copper sulfate specific gravity method may also be used especially in blood camps. Standard method used is cyanmethemoglobin (HiCN) method and presently automated analyzers are used.

SELF-ASSESSMENT EXERCISE

Write short notes on:
- Types of donors
- Collection of blood from donors
- Adverse reactions in donors
- Donor selection and screening for allogenic blood transfusion
- Donor screening for blood transfusion
- Screening of blood donors

CHAPTER 8

Preservation, Storage and Transport of Blood

CHAPTER OUTLINE

- Preservation of blood
- Storage of blood
- Changes in stored blood (effects of storage of blood)
- Platelet preservation
- Pathogen reduction technology

PRESERVATION OF BLOOD

Blood is collected into a primary bag that contains an approved anticoagulant-preservative mixture solution. This solution prevents clotting and maintains cell viability and function during storage.

Aims of Preservation (Box 8.1)

Best preservation is obtained if following are observed:
- Use of proper container
- Collected appropriate volume of blood
- Use of suitable anticoagulant and preservative
- Store at optimum temperature
- Prepare components immediately after collection to get a better yield.

Box 8.1: Aims of preservation.
- Prevent or delay the physical and chemical changes (storage lesions) which occur when blood is stored
- Maintain viability and effective function of all constituents
- Prevent bacterial contamination
- Ensure prolonged shelf life

Blood Bags

Quality of blood bags: The blood collection bag should be sterile uncolored, transparent, pyrogen-free and hermetically (completely airtight) sealed. The bags should be flexible, pliable, and tough. They should be kink and scratch resistant. They should allow adequate gas exchange of O_2 and CO_2, but prevent evaporation of the liquid. Most bags are products of plasticized polyvinyl chloride (PVC). The addition of the plasticizer di-(2-ethylhexyl) phthalate (DEHP) allows many different PVC configurations to be produced ranging from very rigid to soft and highly flexible materials. These bags contain adequate amount of anticoagulant for the amount of blood to be collected. Before use, it should be properly inspected for any leakage, defect and clarity of anticoagulant solution. Previously glass bottles were used for collecting blood.

Blood Bag System

- **Closed system (refer Fig 8.1 and 8.2):** The entire blood collection bag set (including integrally attached satellite bags and tubing) is a sterile and considered a closed system. The primary blood bag with it may have one or more satellite bags/containers. A closed system collection set maintains the sterility of the blood. During the production of blood component, there will be no introduction of external air into the system. There is an internal access port or cannula which allows the transfer of components from one bag to the other bag. Collecting blood in a closed system and using the integral satellite bags allows the maximal allowable storage time for all blood components.

- **Open system:** If for any reason the sterile system becomes an open system in which the seal is broken or compromised and administration ports or other areas are exposed to air. This reduces the allowable storage time (reduces the expiration date) because of potential bacterial contamination.

Figure 8.1 shows triple bag blood collection sets with integral satellite bags. Diagram representation of unit of whole blood and integral plastic bag system used for preparing blood components is depicted in Figure 8.2.

Types of Blood Bags

The number of satellite bags on a collection set depends on the type of blood components to be prepared (Table 8.1).

1. **Single bag:** It consists of a single bag containing an anticoagulant-preservative solution into which blood is collected.
2. **Double bag and triple bag (Fig. 8.1):** It consist of a main bag to which one or two satellite bags are attached. The satellite bags are empty and can be used to make different components in closed circuit.
3. **Quadruple bag:** It consists of a main bag to which three satellite bags are attached.
4. **Penta bags (Pediatric bags):** For pediatric purposes, smaller volumes of whole blood are needed. Hence, blood is collected in main bag with attached satellite bags of small volumes in closed circuit.

Table 8.1: Examples of bag types and components that can be collected.

Bag type	Number of satellite bags	Components
Single	0	Whole blood
Double	1	Red blood cells/plasma
Triple	2	Red blood cells/platelets/plasma or red blood cells/cryoprecipitate/plasma
Quadruple	3	Red blood cells/platelets/cryoprecipitate/plasma

Anticoagulant-preservative Used

Whole blood is collected in a sterile, plasticized PVC bags containing an approved anticoagulant-preservative solution. These anticoagulant-preservative solutions work together to prevents clotting, maintains cell viability and function during storage and prolongs the shelf life (i.e. extend the storage of red cells). Mix the blood and anticoagulant gently and periodically during its collection. The different anticoagulant-preservative solutions available are:

- Acid-citrate-dextrose (ACD): Shelf life—21 days. It is not used nowadays.
- Citrate-phosphate-dextrose (CPD): Shelf life—21 days.
- Citrate-phosphate-dextrose-dextrose (CP2D): Shelf life—21 days.
- Citrate-phosphate-dextrose-adenine (CPDA-1): Shelf life—35 days

The chemical composition of these anticoagulant-preservative solutions is given in the Table 8.2.

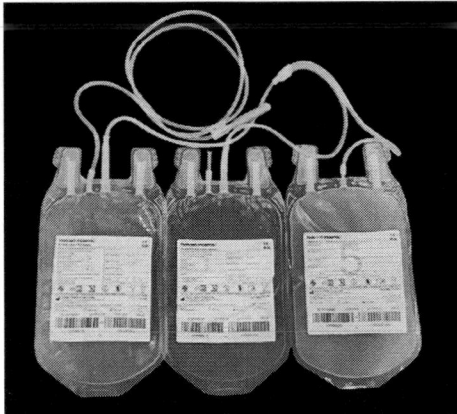

Fig. 8.1: Triple plastic bag for blood collection.

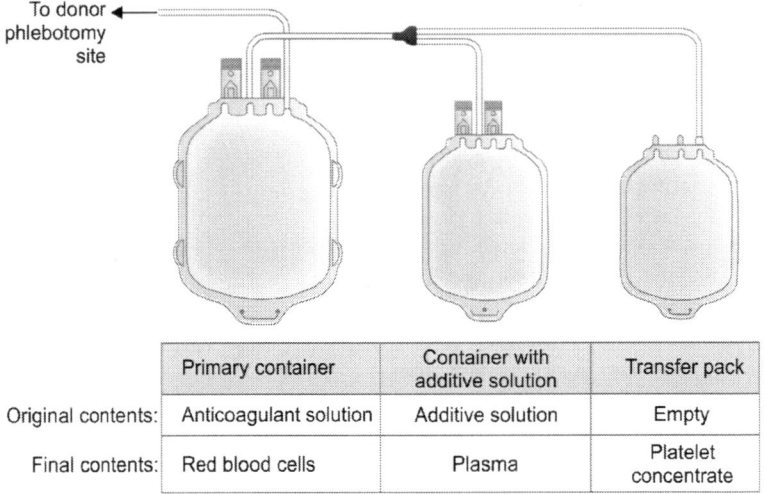

Fig. 8.2: Diagram representation unit of whole blood and integral plastic bag system used for preparing blood components.

Table 8.2: Various constituents in different anticoagulant-preservative solutions for collection of 450 mL whole blood.

Variable	Citrate-phosphate-dextrose (CPD)	Citrate-phosphate-dextrose-dextrose (CP2D)	Citrate-phosphate-dextrose-adenine (CPDA-1)*
	450 mL	450 mL	450 mL
pH	5.0–6.0	5.3–5.9	5.0–6.0
Ratio	1.4:10 (mL solution to blood)		
Shelf life	21 days		35 days
Content	mg in 63 mL	mg in 63 mL	mg in 63 mL
• Sodium citrate dehydrate	1,660	1,660	1,660
• Citric acid, anhydrous	188	206	188
• Dextrose, monohydrate	1,610	3,220	2,010
• Monobasic sodium phosphate, phosphate, monohydrate	140	140	140
• Adenine	0		17.3

*CPDA-1 is the anticoagulant preservative used in most blood banks.

Functions of Various Chemicals Used in Anticoagulant-preservative Solution (Table 8.3)

- **Citrate:** It prevents clotting by chelating calcium and is one of the main components of anticoagulant-preservative solution.
- **Dextrose:** It is needed for generation of adenosine triphosphate (ATP) via the glycolytic pathways. It is necessary for the viability of red blood cells (RBCs). Enhanced ATP levels in red cells indicate enhanced post-transfusion viability.
- **Citric acid:** Citric acid is a weak acid that prevents destruction of dextrose during autoclaving. Along with trisodium citrate which is alkaline it gives optimum pH.

Preservation, Storage and Transport of Blood

Table 8.3: Summary of functions of various chemicals used in anticoagulant-preservative solution.

Chemical used	Function
Dextrose	Needed for ATP (adenosine triphosphate) generation for viability of red cells
Adenine	Substrate for red cell synthesis of ATP
Citrate	Prevents clotting by chelating calcium, also protects red cell membrane
Sodium biphosphate	Buffers the end product of glycolysis (lactic acid) thereby prevents excessive decrease in pH
Mannitol (refer additive solution)	Osmotic diuretic acts as membrane stabilizer

- **Adenine:** It provides a substrate for red cell synthesis of ATP, thereby enhances ATP production. Thus, it increases the post-transfusion survival of RBCs.
- **Sodium biphosphate:** It acts as a buffer to control the decrease in pH expected from the buildup of lactic acid, an end product of glycolysis.

Volume of Blood to be Collected

The volume of anticoagulant-preservative solutions in the primary collection bag is either 63 mL (for 450 ML blood bags) or 49 mL (for 350 ML blood bags). The standard whole blood collection volume is: 450 ± 45 mL or ±10% for blood collected in a bag containing 63 mL of anticoagulant-preservative or

If collection is planned for less than 300 mL, the volume of anticoagulant-preservative solution should be reduced proportionately to maintain the correct anticoagulant-to-whole blood ratio, i.e. 1.4:10 (mL solution to blood).

If a donor is weighing less than 110 lb, it is necessary to reducing the amount of anticoagulant and the volume of blood to be collected.

Red blood cells low volume: If the whole blood collection does not meet the standard volume requirements of the collection bag and the anticoagulant has not been adjusted, the RBCs prepared from the unit are labeled as "red blood cells low volume."

Other components such as platelets, fresh frozen plasma (FFP), and cryoprecipitated antihemophilic factor (AHF) collected **from low-volume units should be discarded.**

Red Cell Additive Solutions (Additive Systems)

The storage environment of red cells can be altered by adding certain nutrients (nutritive solutions) after removal of plasma from whole blood. These nutrients constitute additive system. Additive system contains sodium chloride, dextrose, adenine and other substances that support red cell survival extend the red cell function and storage to 42 days. Additive solutions (AS-1, AS-3, AS-5, or AS-7) are provided as an integral part of the collection bag system. Additive systems consist of a primary collection bag containing an anticoagulant-preservative (e.g. CPD) with at least two satellite bags integrally attached, one is empty and one contains 100 mL of additive solution, adenine saline (AS).

- **Separation of plasma from blood in primary bag:** After withdrawal of whole blood (WB) into the primary pack of the blood bag containing CPD or CP2D, blood is centrifuged and plasma is separated from the RBCs. The plasma from primary bag is moved into the second bag.
- **Adding additive solution from satellite bag to packed red cells in primary bag:** The attached satellite bag contains a nutritive additive solution called adenine saline (AS). The **volume of AS in a 450 mL collection set is 100 mL.** After removing most of the plasma from primary bag, additive solution adenine saline from satellite bag is added to only the packed red cells (allowed to flow into the RBCs) in the primary bag, as it enhances survival and function of only red cells. More plasma can be removed from the RBC units because the added additive solution maintains the metabolism of red cell during storage.

- The additive solution must be **added to red cells within 72 hours** the whole blood collection (**after phlebotomy**).

Advantages of additive system:
- Extends the shelf/storage life of red cells (extended to 42 days).
- Lowers/reduces the viscosity of packed red cells that offers excellent (improves) flow rates and easy administration of transfusion because the hematocrit values of these units in the range of 55–65%.
- Maintains ATP levels.
- Helps in harvesting (to use or recover) maximum amount of fresh plasma (thus optimizes the production of platelets and cryoprecipitate).
- It minimizes hemolysis during storage to less than 1%.

Composition of the Additive Solutions (Table 8.4)

These solutions are composed of saline, adenine, glucose/dextrose and mannitol (in AS-1, AS-5, and AS-7). The various additive solutions available are:
- AS-1 (Adsol [adenine, dextrose, sorbitol, sodium chloride and mannitol]): AS-1, AS-5, and AS-7 solutions contain mannitol apart from saline, adenine, and dextrose.
- AS-3 (Optisol): It contains additional sodium citrate and does not contain mannitol.
- AS-5 (Nuricel/SAG-M): It contains dextrose, adenine, mannitol, saline.
- AS-7 (SLOX): It contains dextrose, adenine, mannitol, saline, citrate, sodium bicarbonate.

The absolute composition of the additive solution varies (Table 8.4) by blood collection set manufacturer.

Anticoagulant acid-citrate-dextrose A (ACD-A) is used in apheresis procedures. It has a shelf life of 21 days.

STORAGE OF BLOOD

Red blood cells and plasma: If RBCs and plasma are to be produced, the **blood is stored between 1°C and 6°C**. The aim is to keep cool without freezing. After collection, the whole blood is stored at 1–6°C in a special type of blood storage refrigerator or walk in cooler/cold room having temperature monitoring system with alarm facility. Reasons for storing within the range of 1–6°C are:
- Lowers the rate of glycolysis and metabolism so that there is slow down in the utilization of dextrose.
- Prevent or minimize the proliferation of any bacterial contamination which might have occurred during venepuncture.
- Minimizes the rate of diffusion of electrolytes across the RBC membrane.

Red blood cells are very sensitive to freezing and freezing will hemolyze RBC unless treated by glycerol. The lower limit of 2°C prevents freezing. Whole blood collected at

Table 8.4: Composition of the additive solutions (AS-1, AS-2 and AS-5).

Constituents	Additive solution AS-1 (volume of 100 mL)	Additive solution AS-3 (volume of 100 mL)	Additive solution AS-5 (volume of 100 mL)
Dextrose/glucose	2.20 g	1.10 g	900 mg
Adenine (0.25 mM)	27 mg	30 mg	30 mg
Mannitol	750 mg	-	525 mg
Sodium chloride (saline)	900 mg	410 mg	877 mg
Trisodium citrate	-	588 mg	-
Sodium dihydrogen monophosphate	-	276 mg	-
Citric acid (monohydrate)	-	42 mg	-
Storage limit	42 days	42 days	42 days

room temperature must be shifted to the cold room within 30 minutes.

Platelets: If platelets are to be prepared from the whole blood, the blood should be **maintained at room temperature (20–24°C)**. This is because alteration of the platelets after exposure to cold. Maintenance at room temperature is done by placing the units in containers specially designed to maintain that temperature.

Storing of Blood in Refrigerator/Cold Room

Following should be kept in mind:
- **Temperature maintenance:** The red cells should be stored in refrigerators with good air circulation and those designed for storage of blood. Household refrigerators are not suitable. Do not frequently open the door of refrigerator/cold room to avoid fluctuation of temperature during storage. Make sure that the temperature is uniform in all the areas of refrigerator. Check and record the inside temperature of refrigerator/cold room periodically (continuously is preferable) at least every 4 hours with the help of a precision thermometer. It **should have an alarm system** to warn staff if the temperature moves out of the acceptable range.
- If there are frequent power failure or power cuts, refrigerator **must have an alternate power supply**.
- **Other materials: Should not keep anything** (e.g. food or drinks) **other than blood**.
- **Areas:** There should be separate areas in the refrigerator or separate refrigerator for unprocessed/untested blood, processed/tested blood and cross-matched blood.
- **Arrangement of blood unit:** Blood unit **should be preferably kept in upright position** so that there is free circulation of cold air inside the refrigerator.

Storing of Blood during Transportation

Careful transportation of blood is also equally important as storage. The blood must be kept within the **temperature range of 2–8°C during transportation** in mobile camps. This can be achieved by:
- Using insulated cold boxes with compartments or insulated carrier boxes. The blood should be packed into the cold boxes surrounded by ice packs. However, the blood should not directly contact/touch the ice packs. It is very essential to measure/check the temperature of container/blood at the time of arrival and also check the units for any evidence of hemolysis.
- By using insulated carrier boxes, e.g. blood transport containers from Electrolux.

Transport of blood within hospital: Always record the time of issue of blood. Once a unit of blood is issued from the blood bank, it **must be transfused within 30 minutes**. Blood should not be left unmonitored. If any delay is anticipated, blood bag must be returned back to the blood bank or stored in a refrigerator having a temperature monitoring system. The bags should be transported in cold box or insulated carriers.

For improving the viability of other constituents of blood, they must be separated out immediately and stored at optimum temperature. Table 8.5 shows the temperature specifications during storage and transportation of various blood components, their expiration dates and quality control requirements for components.

Rejuvenation Solution

Extension of expiration date: Sometimes it may be necessary to restore 2,3-diphosphoglycerate (2,3-DPG) and ATP levels in RBC units collected in CPD or CPDA-1 during storage or up to 3 days after expiration. This may be achieved by using rejuvenation solution that contains pyruvate, inosine, phosphate, and adenine. The rejuvenation solution extends the expiration date for freezing or transfusing the RBC unit. This extension of expiration date may be needed when a rare or autologous unit is involved. Before transfusion, rejuvenated RBCs

Table 8.5: Storage, transportation and expiration of blood components.

Category	Storage	Transport	Expiration limits	Quality control requirement
Whole blood	1–6°C	1–10°C	ACD/CPD/CP2D = 21 days CPDA-1 = 35 days	
Red blood cell (RBC)				
RBC	1–6°C	1–10°C	ACD/CPD/CP2D = 21 days CPDA-1 = 35 days AS-1, AS-3, AS-5, and AS-7 = 42 days	Hematocrit = $\leq$80% in CPDA-1 units
Frozen RBCs	$\leq$–65°C	Maintain frozen state	CPD, CPDA-1 = 10 years	None
RBCs (washed, rejuvenated, or open system)	1–6°C	1–10°C	24 hours	Visual hemoglobin check; method known to provide a $\geq$80% RBC recovery
RBC, additive solution	1–6°C	1–10°C	42 days	
Irradiated RBC	1–6°C	1–10°C	Original expiration as mentioned above or 28 days from date of irradiation or whatever is shorter	Irradiator QC applied 2,500 cGy/rad in center of unit
RBCs leukocyte reduced	1–6°C	1–10°C	ACD/CPD/CP2D = 21 days CPDA-1 = 35 days Open system = 24 hours	$<5.0 \times 10^6$ residual leukocytes and 85% of original red cells retained
Platelets				
Platelets	20–24°C with continuous gentle agitation	20–24°C, maximum time without agitation is 24 hours	24 hours to 5 days depending on the collection system	$\geq 5.5 \times 10^{10}$ platelets in 90% units tested; pH $\geq$6.2
Platelets pheresis	20–24°C with continuous gentle agitation	20–24°C with agitation is 24 hours	5 days	
Platelets pooled or in open system	20–24°C with continuous gentle agitation	20–24°C	4 hours unless otherwise specified	None
Platelets leukocyte reduced	20–24°C	20–24°C	4 hours open system 5 days closed system	
Platelets pheresis, leukocyte reduced	20–24°C with continuous agitation	20–24°C	Open system = within 4 hours Closed system = 5 days	$<5.0 \times 10^6$ residual leukocytes in 95% of units; $\geq 3.0 \times 10^{11}$ platelets in 90% of units tested; pH $\geq$6.2
Platelets irradiated	20–24°C	20–24°C	4 hours open system 5 days closed system	
Apheresis granulocytes	20–24°C	20–24°C	24 hours	$\geq 1.0 \times 10^{10}$ granulocytes in 75% of units tested
Plasma				
Fresh frozen plasma (FFP)	$\leq$18°C or $\leq$65°C	Maintain in frozen state	12 months (–18°C) 7 years (–65°C)	None

Contd...

Contd...

Category	Storage	Transport	Expiration limits	Quality control requirement
FFP, PF24, thawed	1–6°C	1–10°C	24 hours	None
Plasma (frozen within 24 hours after phlebotomy-PF24)	≤–18°C	Maintain in frozen state	12 months (1 year)	None
Thawed plasma	1–6°C	1–10°C	>24 hours <5 days	
Liquid plasma	1–6°C	1–10°C	5 days after expiration of RBC	
Cryoprecipitated antihemophilic factor (AHF)	≤–18°C	Maintain in frozen state	12 months (1 year)	Factor VIII: ≥80 IU and ≥150 mg fibrinogen
Pooled cryoprecipitated AHF, thawed	20–24°C	20–24°C	As soon as possible or within 4 hours, if open system or pooled, 6 hours if single unit or pooled prior to freezing	Factor VIII: ≥80 IU and ≥150 mg fibrinogen

(ACD: acid-citrate-dextrose; CPD: citrate-phosphate-dextrose; CP2D: citrate-phosphate-double dextrose; CPDA-1: citrate-phosphate-dextrose-adenine; AS: additive solution; PF24: plasma frozen within 24 hours of phlebotomy; QC: quality control)

must be washed to remove the inosine which it may be toxic to the recipient.

CHANGES IN STORED BLOOD (EFFECTS OF STORAGE OF BLOOD)

Storage Lesion

The physical/morphologic (cell membrane shape) and biochemical changes occur when blood is stored at 1-6°C. These changes affect red cell viability and function. These changes together are called as storage lesions. These changes are **of little clinical significance** even in massively transfused recipients. This is because the recipient compensates or reverses them except in severely compromised patients and neonates. Hence, they should be given blood less than 7 days old.

Physical/Morphologic Changes

The storage limits and temperature criteria for each preservative solution should be such that at least 75% of the original red cells remain in the recipient's circulation 24 hours after transfusion with less than 1% hemolysis. The various physical changes in blood during storage at 1-6°C are due to aging of anticoagulant-preservative solution. These include:

Effect on cellular elements:
- **Changes in RBCs**
  - **Shape:** Change from disk shape to spherical shape.
  - **Loss of lipid in RBC membrane:** Causes decrease in deformability.
  - **Decrease in critical hemolytic volume (CHV):** CHV is the largest volume to which RBCs swell before hemolysis. CHV is decreased in parallel with lipid content of membrane.
  - **Osmotic fragility:** Increased.
- **Granulocytes:** If blood is stored for more than 24 hours at 1-6°C, only few granulocytes will be found. **WBCs lose their phagocytic and bactericidal property within 4–6 hours of collection** and become **nonfunctional after 24 hours of storage**. They do not lose their antigenic property and are capable of sensitizing the recipient to produce nonhemolytic febrile transfusion reactions.
- **Lymphocytes:** Viable lymphocytes **persist throughout the storage**. Few lymphocytes may remain viable even after 3 weeks of storage.

- **Platelets:** If **blood is stored for more than 24 hours at 1–6°C, only few platelets** will be found. Platelets lose their hemostatic function within 48 hours in whole blood stored at 4⁰C.
- **Effect of anticoagulant-preservative:** With trisodium citrate only 50% cells remain viable after 1 week.

Effect on heat labile coagulation factors (Factor V and Factor VIII):
- **First 48–72 hours: Decrease their activity** up to 50% within 48–72 hours of storage in whole blood stored at 4°C. Later the decrease is comparatively slow.
- **21-day storage:** Factor V activity is 30% and factor VIII activity is 15–20%.

Effect of temperature
For whole blood and red cells concentrate, optimum storage temperature should be between 1°C and 6°C. As red cells consume glucose for their continued metabolism, storing a blood unit at 1–6°C will also decrease the rate of glycolysis.
- **Fall of temperature:** A fall in temperature causes freezing injury to red cells and leads to **hemolysis**.
- **Rise of temperature:** If the temperature is more than 6°C, there will be **overgrowth of nonspecific bacteria**.
- **Room temperature: Platelets and granulocyte retain better function** when stored at room temperature. Platelets should be stored at 22°C in plasma under conditions in which the pH is maintained at values about 6.8.
- **Temperature of –30°C: Labile coagulation factors in plasma are best maintained** at temperature of –30°C or lower.

Table 8.6: Biochemical changes in CPDA-1 stored blood.

Constituents	CPDA-1	
	0 day	35 days
Plasma dextrose (mg/dL)	432	282
Plasma pH	7.6	6.98
ATP (% of initial value)	100	56
2,3-diphosphoglycerate (% of initial value)	100	<10.6
Plasma K⁺ (mEq/L)	3.3	17.2
Plasma Na⁺ (mEq/L)	169	153
% of viable cells 24 hours after transfusion	100	79

Biochemical Changes (Table 8.6 and Fig. 8.3)

One of the aims of the preservative solutions is to minimize the effects of the biochemical changes, thereby maximize the shelf life of the components.

Effect on pH: Gradual fall in pH on storage due to accumulation of lactic acid.
- A fall of pH of platelet concentration due to lactic acid production from platelet glycolysis leads to loss of viability of platelets.
- **Platelets concentrates must be gently and constantly agitated**. This is because without agitation there is rapid fall in pH due to lactic acid metabolites.

Effect of delay in refrigeration: There will be increased loss of 2,3-DPG over this period.

Effect on electrolytes: Important electrolyte change in stored blood is that of potassium (**plasma K⁺**). During blood storage, there is a

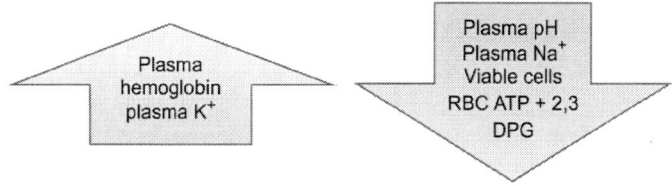

Fig. 8.3: Main biochemical changes in storage lesions.

slow but constant leakage of K⁺ from cells into the surrounding plasma.

- **Patient with severe kidney disease:** In these patients, even small amount of K⁺ fluctuations can be dangerous. Hence, they should be transfused with relatively fresh or washed red cells.
- **Neonates:** Due to a higher K⁺ content of stored blood, blood <5 days old is to be transfused for neonatal exchange and top-up transfusion.

Effect of anticoagulant-preservative: With ACD, storage viability is for 28 days and DPG levels better maintained at 1 week because of higher pH.

Heparin: It prevents coagulation of blood by inactivating thrombin and coagulation factors (i.e. Xa, IXa, XIIa) and plasmin. Nowadays, it is not in use in transfusion medicine.

PLATELET PRESERVATION

Factors which determine the viability and function of platelets depend on **temperature and pH**. Platelets should be **stored at 22–24°C** (controlled temperature) **with continuous agitation in platelet agitator and incubator**. The pH should be above 6.0.

Types of Plastic Bags and Shelf Life of Platelets

Types of plastic bags and shelf life of platelets have been shown in Table 8.7.

Note: Pooled platelets can be stored for 4 hours at 22–34°C before they are transfused.

Table 8.7: Types of plastic bags and shelf life of platelets.

Type of material used for bag	Shelf life of platelets
Polyvinyl chloride (PVC) bags with plasticizer di-(2-ethylhexyl) phthalate (DEHP)	3 days
Polyolefin bags with no plasticizer	7 days (recommended to store for 5 days only from the date of collection—considered as day 0)
Thin-walled PVC tri-(2-ethylhexyl) trimellitate (TOTM) plasticizer	

Platelet Additive Solutions

Traditionally, platelet components prepared from platelet-rich plasma derived from whole blood or those obtained by apheresis are stored in their own native plasma. Platelet components prepared from pooled buffy coats derived from whole blood are stored in plasma separated from one of the units of whole blood. Though this is clinically efficient, sometimes hazardous substances present in the donor's plasma may produce harm to the recipients. These hazardous substances include antibodies, allergens, foreign proteins or sometimes drugs. Transfusion-associated acute lung injury (TRALI) may occur due to cellular components and/or antibodies in donor's plasma.

The above disadvantages of plasma can be avoided or reduced by using certain synthetic mediums which replace about 65–80% of the plasma volume in a platelet component. These mediums are known as **Platelet Additive Solutions (PASs)**. PAS is a buffered salt solution used to store platelets. PASs **increase platelet viability during storage**, minimize the amount of plasma in platelet products, and plasma obtained can be used for other needs. PAS cannot be used alone and is used to replace a portion of the plasma. Plasma is necessary to provide a physiological environment for storage of platelets. Hence, it is recommended to combine 30% plasma and 70% PAS. The platelets can be stored up to 5 days at 20–24°C with continuous agitation.

Advantages of Platelet Additive Solutions

Advantages of platelet additive solutions have been shown in Box 8.2.

Various Platelet Additive Solutions

Various platelet additive solutions have been shown in Box 8.3.

Main primary constituents of PAS are citrate (to prevent coagulation), acetate (serves as a substrate for oxidative metabolism) and saline (provides osmotic strength). Glucose is needed throughout storage.

Box 8.2: Advantages of platelet additive solutions.

- *Replacement of plasma by additive solution:* Reduces allergic and transfusion reactions due to reduced levels of plasma proteins and antibodies
- *Reduced titer of ABO agglutinins:* No need for ABO compatibility between donor plasma and recipient cells
- Plasma not used for platelet storage can be utilized for other uses (e.g. fractionation)
- Improves the efficiency of platelet collections, increases the cost-effectiveness and facilitates pathogen inactivation
- *Immunological advantages:* Reduced levels of anti-human leukocyte antigen (HLA), human neutrophil antigen (HNA) antibodies which may be responsible for TRALI
- Increases storage life for 7 days
- Reduce allergic transfusion reactions and enhance plasma recovery

Box 8.3: Example of platelet additive solutions.

- T-Sol (PAS II)
- InterSol (PAS III)
- SSP+ (PAS III M)
- Composol
- M-Sol

PATHOGEN REDUCTION TECHNOLOGY

Pathogen reduction is a post-collection process in which pathogens in the blood are reduced for cellular blood components. The purpose is to reduce the risk of certain transfusion-transmitted infections (TTIs) in components.

Techniques: Pathogen reduction technology uses ultraviolet (UV) irradiation and photosensitizers. They produce damage to pathogen nucleic acids and prevent their replication and growth. Thereby it reduces the infectivity of any residual pathogens in the blood components. Psoralen treatment is a specific process for reduction of pathogen used in whole blood-derived pooled plasma; apheresis plasma; or apheresis platelets. Psoralen and UV light treatment inactivates a broad spectrum of viruses, gram-positive and gram-negative bacteria, spirochetes, and parasites.

SUMMARY

- Blood from donor is collected into a primary bag that contains an anticoagulant-preservative mixture solution. This solution prevents clotting and maintains cell viability and function during storage.
- There are different types of blood collection bags and the number of satellite bags on a collection set depends on the type of blood components to be prepared. These include single bag, double bag, triple bag, quadruple bag and penta bags (pediatric bags).
- Anticoagulants used include (1) CPD, (2) CP2D, and (3) CPDA-1.
- The storage environment of red cells can be altered by adding certain nutritive solution after removal of plasma from whole blood.
- Red blood cells and plasma are stored between 1°C and 6°C.
- Platelets are prepared from the whole blood maintained at room temperature (20–24°C).
- Careful transportation of blood is also equally important as storage.
- The physical and biochemical changes occur when blood is stored at 1–6°C. These changes together are called as storage lesions.
- The viability and function of platelets depend on temperature and pH.
- Platelet additive solution is used to store platelets that increase platelet viability during storage.
- Pathogen reduction is a process in which pathogens in the blood are reduced for cellular blood components.

SELF-ASSESSMENT EXERCISE

Write short notes on:
- Various preservatives used in blood collection
- Additive solutions in blood bank
- Storage of blood in blood bank
- Changes in the blood in stored blood (storage lesions)
- Various type of blood collection bags for blood banking especially enlisting their contents and use of these contents
- Pathogen inactivation of blood components

CHAPTER 9

Antihuman Globulin Test

CHAPTER OUTLINE

- Antihuman globulin reagents
- Principles of the antiglobulin test
- Direct antiglobulin test
- Indirect antiglobulin test
- Alternative methods to the tube test
- Sources of error in antiglobulin test
- Quality control for antiglobulin test

INTRODUCTION

Types of Blood Group Antibodies

Two major types of blood group antibodies are: (1) immunoglobulin M (IgM) and (2) immunoglobulin G (IgG).

1. **IgM antibodies:** They have a large pentamer structure (refer Fig. 1.3). In transfusion medicine, they bind to corresponding antigen on the red blood cells (RBCs) thereby **directly agglutinate RBCs** suspended in saline.
2. **IgG antibodies:** Some IgG antibodies are called as **nonagglutinating**, or **incomplete antibodies**. They have a too small monomer structure (refer Fig. 1.4) and cannot directly agglutinate sensitized RBCs. Hence, they may not be detected. Sensitized RBCs means that immunoglobulin or complement attached to the red blood cells from the immune system (in vivo) or from a test procedure (in vitro).
   - **Antihuman globulins (AHGs)** are obtained from immunized nonhuman species **bind to human globulins such as IgG** (anti-IgG) **or complement**, either free in serum or attached to antigens on RBCs. If AHG-containing anti-IgG is added to RBCs sensitized with IgG antibodies, this **allows hemagglutination of** these **sensitized cells**. Thus, an anti-antibody (anti-IgG) is used to detect the formation of an antigen-antibody (Ag/Ab) complex, which would otherwise go undetected.
   - **Addition of anticomplement component:** Some blood group antibodies are capable of binding complement to the RBC membrane. In such cases, an anticomplement component can be added to the AHG reagent.

History of Antiglobulin (Coombs) Test

In 1945, Coombs, Mourant, and Race observed that RBCs may combine with antibodies without producing agglutination (however, the principle was described much earlier in 1908 by Moreschi). Their findings lead to preparation of an antibody that reacted with human globulins (e.g. a family of human proteins) and used this reagent to agglutinate antibody-coated RBCs. This reagent was named as antihuman globulins and the procedure is termed as the antiglobulin (AHG) test. The **AHG test was also called as the Coombs test**, in honor of Coombs (one of the investigators) who first developed the test for laboratory use in 1945.

Before the discovery of antiglobulin test, only "complete" IgM antibodies that agglutinate saline-suspended red cells were detected. The introduction of the antiglobulin test helped to detect the presence of incomplete antibody (IgG antibodies capable of sensitizing red cells but incapable of causing agglutination of the red cells and/or complement on the RBC membrane [complement-sensitized RBCs]). Thus, the **antiglobulin test detects IgG antibodies and complement proteins that have attached to red cells either in vitro or in vivo** but do not produce visible agglutination. This has gained its usefulness in the discovery and characterization of many new blood group systems. **This test is used for many blood banking testing protocols and provides important information.**

ANTIHUMAN GLOBULIN REAGENTS

The antiglobulin test is the **most important test in blood bank** and performed using a **reagent called antihuman globulin** (Fig. 9.1). AHGs are obtained from immunized nonhuman species. Presently, there are clonal AHG reagents that are made by developing a cell line that will produce an antibody to a specific human protein.

Types of Reagents

Two types of AHG sera (reagents) are available for antiglobulin tests namely: (1) **polyspecific AHG** and (2) **monospecific AHG**. Various polyspecific AHG and monospecific AHG reagents are mentioned in Table 9.1. Use of these reagents depends on the application (direct or indirect) and whether for detecting

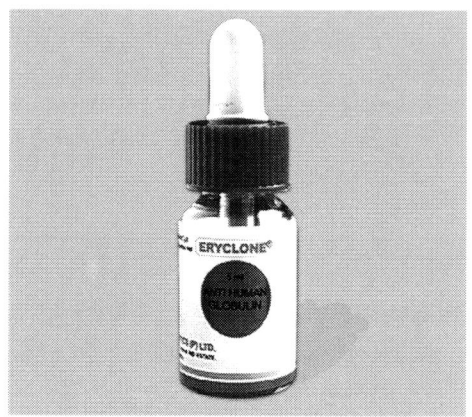

Fig. 9.1: Antihuman globulin (AHG) reagent.

RBC sensitization by IgG, complement, or both. The presence of either IgG or C3d gives rise to a positive direct antiglobulin test (DAT) that indicates the red cells were sensitized in vivo as a result of an immune response to a foreign antigen.

Apart from antibodies, the reagent contains buffers, stabilizers, and bacteriostatic agents.

Polyspecific (Broad-spectrum) AHG Reagents

Polyspecific AHG reagents contain **antibodies to both IgG molecules** (i.e. contain **anti-IgG**) **and complement components** (i.e. contain **anti-C3d, anti-C3b**). Therefore, it **detects both IgG and C3d** molecules on red cells.
- The majority of red cell antibodies are noncomplement-binding IgG. Hence, it is necessary that **anti-IgG should be an essential component of any polyspecific reagent**.

Table 9.1: Summary of various polyspecific AHG and monospecific AHG reagents.

Polyspecific (Broad-spectrum) AHG reagent (contains anti-IgG and anti-C3d)	Monospecific AHG reagent (contains either anti-IgG or anti-C3d/C3b)
Polyclonal: • Rabbit polyclonal anti-IgG and anti-C3d • Rabbit polyclonal anti-IgG/Murine monoclonal blend anti-C3d/anti-C3b *Monoclonal:* Murine monoclonal anti-IgG, anti-C3d and anti-C3b	*Polyclonal:* • Rabbit polyclonal anti-IgG • Rabbit polyclonal anti-C3d • Anti-IgG heavy chain *Monoclonal:* • Murine monoclonal anti-IgG • Murine monoclonal anti-C3d, anti-C3b
Use in DAT	Use in antibody screening/identification, differential DAT

- **Anticomplement antibodies** (anti-C3b and anti-C3d) are also essential. However, if plasma is used, only anti-IgG is necessary because ethylenediaminetetraacetic acid (EDTA) prevents complement activation.

Monospecific AHG Reagents

Monospecific AHG reagents contain **only one antibody specificity**. Monospecific reagents may be IgG, IgM, IgA or complement components such as C3b or C3d (i.e. anticomplement). Antibodies against heavy chains of IgG, IgM and IgA and are called as anti-γ, anti-μ and anti-α. They are useful in defining the immunochemical characteristics of antibodies. Commonly used monospecific AHG reagents—anti-IgG and anti-C3b-C3d.
1. **Anti-IgG:** Anti-IgG reagents contain antibodies specific for the Fc fragment of the gamma heavy chain of the IgG molecule (refer Fig. 1.4) without any anticomplement activity. Monospecific antibodies may also be available for IgG subclasses.
2. **Anticomplement:** Anticomplement reagents (e.g. anti-C3b, anti-C3d reagents) are reactive against only the designated complement components without any activity against human immunoglobulins. Monospecific anticomplement reagents are often a blend of monoclonal anti-**C3b** and monoclonal anti-**C3d** products (anti-C3b + C3d).

Preparation of Antihuman Globulin

The classic method of producing AHG reagents is by **injecting animals** (usually rabbits) **with** purified **human antibody (obtained from a large pool of normal sera) molecules** (human IgG) **and complement proteins**. In these animals, the injected proteins (human antibody molecules—IgG) are recognized as foreign antigens. They **stimulate the animal's immune system to produce antibodies to human antibody molecules and complement proteins**.

Polyspecific Antihuman Globulin

Polyspecific AHG can be produced using **polyclonal or monoclonal antibodies**. These two processes of antibody production differ from one another. Their usage has different advantages and disadvantages. This polyspecific AHG may be polyclonal or monoclonal. Commercially, several reagent preparations are available for polyspecific products derived from either polyclonal or monoclonal antibody sources.
- *Polyclonal AHG production*:
  - **Conventional polyspecific antiglobulin reagents** are prepared by immunizing one colony of rabbits (Fig. 9.2) with purified human immunoglobulin (IgG) antigen and another colony with human C3 antigen. The immunogen (IgG antigen) used is obtained from serum of many donors and pooled IgG antigen thus obtained has the heterogeneity of IgG molecules. These heterophilic IgG molecules are used to immunize rabbits. Injected proteins are recognized as foreign antigens by animal. It stimulates the animal's immune system **to produce antibodies to human antibody molecules and complement proteins**. The anti-IgG produced from many immunized rabbits is pooled together. The polyclonal reagents, prepared is used for routine test, are **capable of detecting the many different IgG antibodies**. This is an advantage of using anti-IgG of polyclonal origin for antiglobulin serum. Separate blends of the anti-IgG and anticomplement antibodies are prepared. These antibodies (e.g. anti-IgG, antibody to the C3d component) are used as reagents and are called as **antihuman globulins**. Polyclonal antibodies contain a mixture of antibodies from different plasma cell clones.
- *Monoclonal AHG production (Fig. 9.3)*: The monoclonal antibody technique is **useful in producing high-titer antibodies with well-defined specificities to IgG and to the fragments of C3**. Hybridoma technology (refer pages 63, 64) may be used to produce monoclonal antiglobulin serum. Monoclonal antibodies are derived

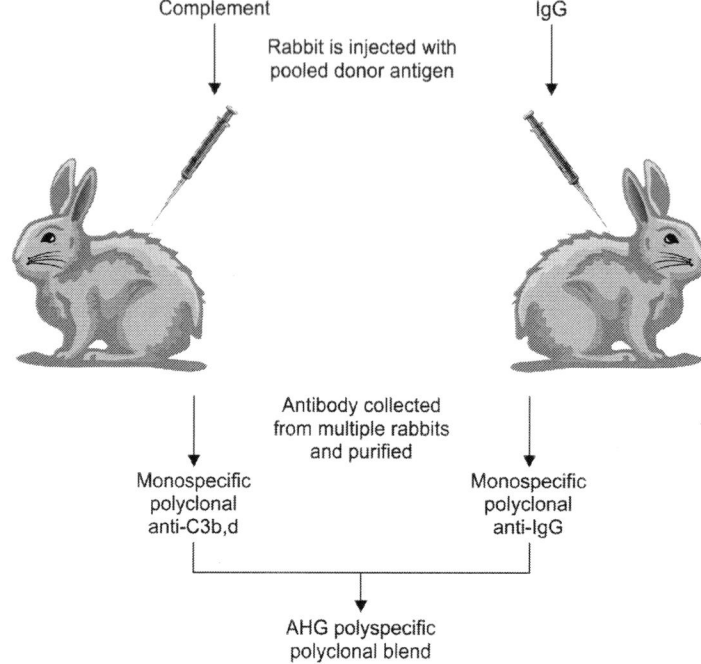

Fig. 9.2: Polyclonal antihuman globulin (AHG) reagents preparation by conventional method. It is prepared by injecting pooled donor antigen to rabbits. In rabbit, it produces a broader spectrum of reactivity, but the source of antibody is limited to the life span of the inoculated animal. Polyspecific AHG may be prepared by combining (blending) polyclonal anti-IgG with either polyclonal or monoclonal anticomplement components.

from one clone of plasma cells and recognize a single epitope.

Monoclonal antibody is produced by immunizing the laboratory animals, usually mice, with purified human globulin. After a suitable immune response, mouse spleen cells containing antibody-secreting lymphocytes (plasma cells) are obtained, these antibody-secreting lymphocytes are fused with myeloma cells and result in **"hybridomas"**. The antibodies produced by hybridoma are screened for the required specificity and affinity. Then the antibody-secreting clones are either propagated in tissue culture or by inoculation into mice, in which case the antibody is collected as ascites. The clone of hybridoma cells produces antibody molecules which are identical in terms of antibody structure and antigen specificity.

Advantage: Once an antibody-secreting clone of cells is produced, antibody with the same specificity and reaction characteristics will be available indefinitely. Thus, a consistently pure and uncontaminated AHG reagent can be produced.

Monoclonal antibodies to human complement components anti-C3b and anti-C3d may be blended with polyclonal anti-IgG from rabbits. This will provide a potent reagent that gives fewer false-positive reactions as a result of anticomplement.

Monospecific Antihuman Globulin

Monospecific AHG can be produced in similar manner as that for polyspecific AHG. However, it contains only one antibody specificity (e.g. anti-IgG or anti-C3d). Monospecific AHG reagents are prepared by separating the specificities of the polyspecific AHG reagents. Commercially, **anti-IgG** and **anti-C3d** are

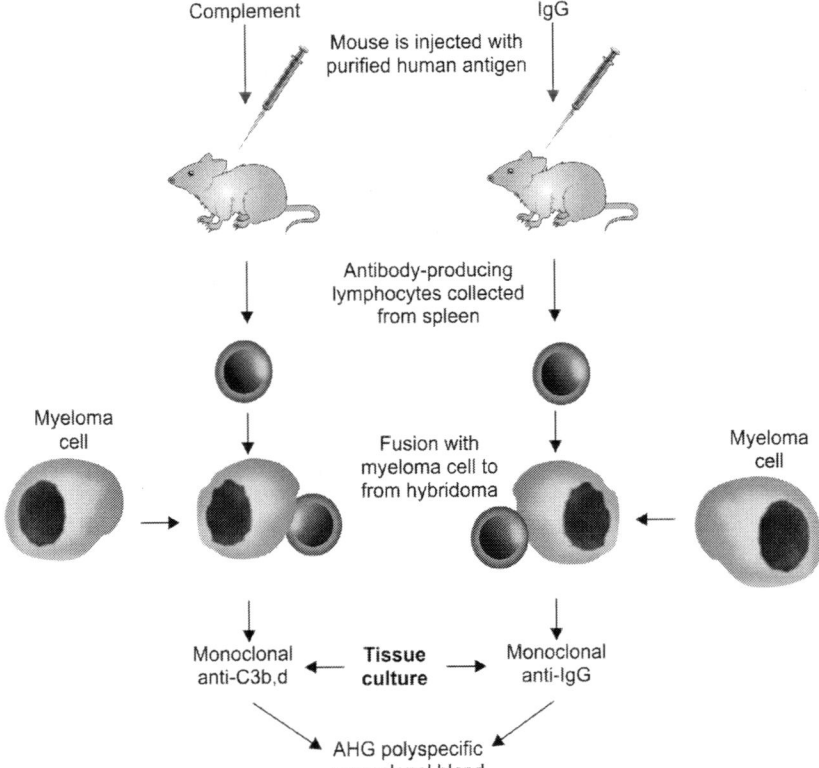

Fig. 9.3: Preparation of monoclonal AHG reagents by hybridoma technology. In hybridoma technology, the antibodies last longer than the polyclonal source, because the hybridoma can live indefinitely. A monoclonal blend may be manufactured by blending monoclonal anti-C3b, monoclonal anti-C3d, and monoclonal anti-IgG.

available as either **polyclonal** or **monoclonal** product.

- **Monospecific anti-IgG** contains antibodies to human gamma chains. Often monospecific anti-IgG is labeled heavy-chain specific. This means that the antiserum contains antibodies specific for the gamma heavy chains of the IgG molecule. If the products are not having this label, they may contain antibodies that react with immunoglobulin light chains. Immunoglobulin light chains are either kappa or lambda type and are common to all immunoglobulin classes (e.g. IgG, IgM, and IgA).

  Uses: Apart from their use in the **investigation of a positive DAT**, anti-IgG reagents are used for **antibody detection, antibody identification**, and **crossmatching procedures**.

- **Anti-C3b and anti-C3d monospecific reagents:** They **do not react with human immunoglobulin molecules**. These reagents **specifically detect complement proteins that attach to the red cell surface**. These compliments get activated by the complement's classical pathway (refer Fig. 1.15). Activation of the complement pathway can cause destruction of red cell in vivo through either intravascular hemolysis or extravascular hemolysis. To detect any complement proteins bound in vivo, a reagent needs specificity for the C3d fragment. The **C3d fragment of complement** is usually the **only protein that remains attached to the patient's red cells**.

  Differential DAT: If the DAT (direct antiglobulin test) is positive with polyspecific antiglobulin reagents, it is necessary to identify/investigate the cause of positive test. To find out the cause, differential DAT is performed. In this test, monospecific anti-IgG and monospecific anti-C3d/anti-C3b reagents (Table 9.2) are used to determine the cause of a positive DAT.

IgG-Sensitized Red Cells (Coombs Control Cells or Check Cells)

A **control system is needed when an antiglobulin test is** interpreted as **negative**. The **control system consists of red cells with attached IgG antibodies** (IgG-sensitized red cells). The addition of IgG-sensitized red cells to negative AHG tests **is needed for antibody detection and crossmatch procedures**. This IgG-sensitized red cell control is called to as check cells or Coombs control cells. IgG-sensitized red cells are used as an additive system for negative antiglobulin tests to control the possibility of false-negative results. **When, AHG test is negative, the addition of IgG-sensitized red cells should react with the AHG reagent and produce agglutination**. To interpret the result as negative, agglutination should be present after the addition of control cells. If no agglutination is observed in an antiglobulin test, it may be due to three potential reasons. Hence, check whether the test cells were sufficiently washed, whether AHG is added and AHG reagent was potent.

Preparation of IgG-sensitized Red Cells

- Prepare 5% suspension of Rh-positive red cells.
- Add IgG anti-D serum (diluted with normal saline).
- Mix equal volumes of above two.
- Incubate mixture at 37°C for 30 minutes.
- Wash red cells three times with normal saline and decant after last wash. They are now ready for use in the antiglobulin tests.

Note:
- Coombs control cells are any Rh+ve cells coated with IgG.
- Only O+ve cells coated with IgG can be used in the indirect antiglobulin test (IAT).
- Extent of dilution of IgG-anti-D serum is determined by titration. The dilution of anti-D should be such that it coats the red cells but does not agglutinate them.

PRINCIPLES OF THE ANTIGLOBULIN TEST

In certain diseases or conditions, an individual's blood may contain IgG antibodies. These antibodies can bind to antigens on the RBC surface membrane. **IgG antibodies are** called as **incomplete antibodies. Red cells coated with complement or IgG antibodies do not agglutinate directly when centrifuged**. These red cells are said to be sensitized with IgG or complement. The **sensitized red cells** (coated with incomplete antibodies [IgG] or complements) either in vivo as in DAT or in vitro as in IAT **can be agglutinated by the additional antibody termed as AHG reagent**. The AHG binds to IgG antibodies or the C3b or C3d component of complement coating the red cells. This form bridges between red cells sensitized with antibody and causes them to agglutinate. The principles involved in the antiglobulin test are given in detail in Box 9.1.

Types of Antiglobulin Test

The AHG test is an essential testing methodology in transfusion medicine. There are two types namely: (1) DAT and (2) IAT. Both tests use the AHG reagents.
- **Direct (Coombs) antiglobulin test (DAT):** In immunohematology, it is used **to detect antibodies or complement bound to RBCs in vivo** or within the body. The patient's cells, after careful washing, are tested for sensitization that has occurred in vivo.

Table 9.2: Differential direct antiglobulin test procedure.

Interpretation	Monospecific anti-IgG	Monospecific anti-C3d
Patient red cells sensitized with IgG only	+	0
Patient red cells sensitized with IgG and C3d	+	+

Antihuman Globulin Test

> **Box. 9.1:** Principles of the antiglobulin test.
>
> - Red blood cells (RBCs) coated with **incomplete antibody (many IgG) or C3 complement cannot directly produce detectable agglutination of RBCs** (hemagglutination), even after centrifugation and the use of enhancement media and techniques such as polyethylene glycol, low-ionic strength saline (LISS), albumin, or enzymes
> - The reactions by these **antibodies can be visualized by using antihuman globulin (AHG) reagents (Coombs reagent).** AHGs bind to human globulins such as **IgG** or **complement, either free in serum or attached to antigens on RBCs.** This is the basis of the AHG test
> - **Direct antiglobulin test:** If the RBCs coated by incomplete antibody or complement are treated with AHG reagent, the antibodies present in AHG sera act as a bridge between RBCs already sensitized with antibody or complement and produce/induce the characteristic latticework of second-stage agglutination of such RBCs
> - **Indirect antiglobulin test:** If incomplete antibodies or compliments are present freely in serum, they are treated with IgG-sensitized red cells. When AHG reagent is added, it causes agglutination
> - The AHG reagents will not detect IgA or IgE antibodies

Sensitization is a process in which immunoglobulin or complement attached to the cells from the immune system (in vivo) or from a test procedure (in vitro).

- **Indirect (Coombs) antiglobulin test (IAT):** It is used in immunohematology **to detect the antibody bound to RBCs in vitro** (or within a test tube) after an appropriate incubation phase. In this test, normal red cells are incubated with a serum suspected of containing an antibody and subsequently tested, after washing, for in vitro-bound antibody. The red cell antibody screen is an example of an IAT.

■ DIRECT ANTIGLOBULIN TEST

Normally, red cells are not sensitized with either IgG or complement in vivo. Pathologically, sensitization of red cells can occur in certain clinical events such as autoimmune hemolytic anemia (AIHA; anemia due to immune destruction of own red cells), HDFN (hemolytic disease of fetus and newborn), a drug-related mechanism, or an antibody reaction to transfused red cells. In such situation, DAT is performed to detect IgG or complement proteins bound to patient cells. A positive DAT (direct antiglobulin test) indicates potential immune-mediated red cell destruction in the body. Red cells attached with IgG or complement are destroyed particularly in the spleen by macrophages belonging to mononuclear phagocytic system. This immune destruction of red cells often leads to anemia.

Procedure/methods of direct antiglobulin test: Direct antiglobulin test (direct Coombs test) **detects antibodies (IgG) and/or complement coated on the surface of patient's RBC membrane due to vivo sensitization.**

Materials Required

- 75 × 12 mm glass test tubes
- Patient's RBCs (test red cells)
- Antihuman globulin reagent
- Normal saline
- Positive control red blood cells (IgG-coated).

Technique (Figs. 9.4 and 9.5)

Blood sample: Patient's RBCs are obtained from either the **fresh blood** (not more than 24 hours old) or blood sample (of choice) **collected in an EDTA tube.** When samples are stored, complement can attach nonspecifically to red cells (in vitro). Blood samples collected in EDTA will prevent in vitro activation of the complement pathway and the test detects only complement proteins that have been bound to the red cells in vivo. If plasma is used, the test will not be detected neither complement proteins, attaching to red cells due to red cell storage, nor complement-dependent antibodies. **Patient's red cells are used in this test.**

1. Prepare a 3–5% suspension of the red cells (in normal saline) to be tested in a clean glass tube.
2. Add one drop of red cell suspension to a clean prelabeled test tube. The patient's

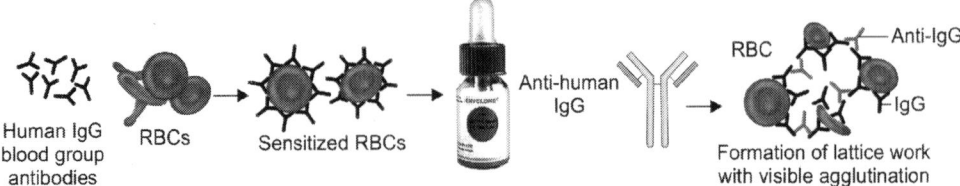

Fig. 9.4: *Antiglobulin test.* This detects IgG molecules and complement protein molecules that are attached (sensitized) to red cells but will produce a visible agglutination reaction only after adding AHG reagent. AHG antibodies present in AHG reagent form a bridge between adjacent RBCs sensitized by human immunoglobulin (IgG) or complement components *(For color version, see Plate 2).*

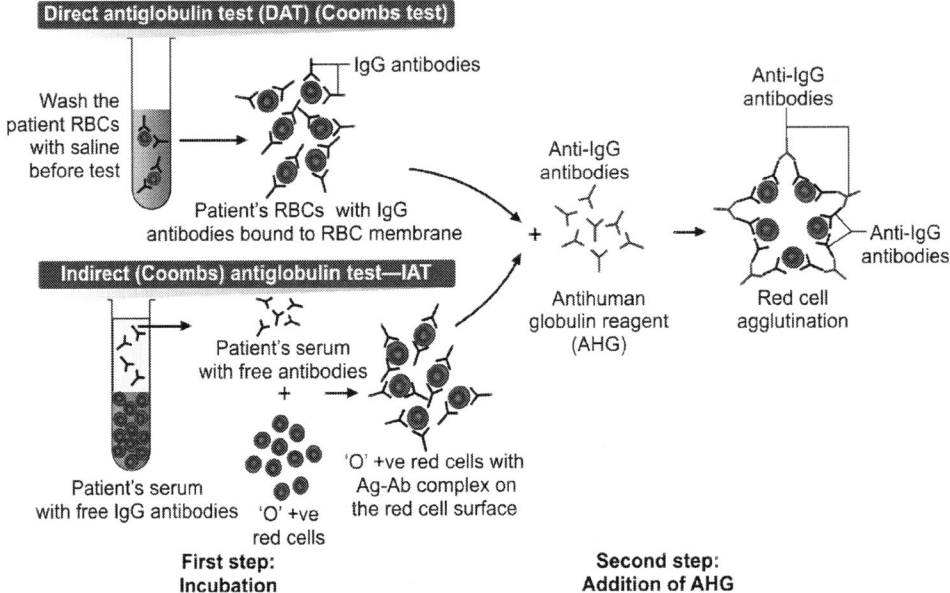

Fig. 9.5: Direct and indirect methods of antiglobulin test (Coombs test) *(For color version, see Plate 2).*

red cells are first washed three or four times with normal (physiologic) saline to remove unbound proteins and decant the final wash completely (refer Note on page 181).
3. Take two drops of polyspecific AHG (anti-IgG + anticomplement).
4. Mix well. Incubation at 37°C is not necessary because the antibody was attached in vivo.
5. Centrifuge at 1,000 rpm for 1 minute.
6. Gently shake the tube and observe for agglutination. If the test result is negative add one drop of control cells.
7. Mix and centrifuge at 1,000 rpm for 1 minute and look for agglutination.
8. If no agglutination is observed, the result is invalid. Repeat the test procedure.

Interpretation
- If **polyspecific AHG reagent** is used, it detects both IgG and complement molecules on the red cell. Agglutination with polyspecific AHG reagent is interpreted as positive DAT (Fig. 9.4). Positive test (agglutination) indicates the presence of IgG antibody, complement molecules, or both bound to the patient's red cells. If there is no agglutination after the addition of polyspecific AHG reagent, it is interpreted as a negative DAT. Retesting with monospecific AHG is unnecessary.

Antihuman Globulin Test

- If test is positive, then to determine which molecule was on the red cell, repeat the test using **monospecific AHG reagents**. Use monospecific AHG reagents specific for IgG and complement separately.

Note:
Washing of red cells with physiologic saline is an essential step to remove any unbound molecules before the addition of the AHG reagent. The washing in antiglobulin test is done by filling of test tubes with saline to mix with the test red cells present in the tube. The saline-suspended red cells are centrifuged. The saline wash is then decanted, and this process is repeated for two to three times. After completing the third or fourth wash, the saline is removed, and the tube is blotted dry to remove most traces of the saline. If the test red cells are not adequately washed, any unbound antibody or complement present in the test can bind to the AHG reagent. This will inhibit its reaction with antibody or complement molecules attached to the test red cells. This effect is called as neutralization of the AHG reagent. Neutralization is the blocking antibody sites that cause a negative reaction. **Neutralization of the AHG reagent is a source of error in antiglobulin testing** and can mask a positive antiglobulin test. To detect potential neutralization, if there are negative reactions, to this tube add IgG-sensitized cells. After centrifugation, a positive reaction should be found to confirm that washing was adequate.

Uses of Direct Antiglobulin Test

The DAT is used (Table 9.3) for the demonstration of in vivo attachment (sensitization/coating) of immune antibodies (IgG) to red cells or the complement component generally C3d.

- **Diagnosis of hemolytic disease of the fetus and newborn (HDFN): Alloimmune hemolytic disease of newborn** in which direct antiglobulin/Coombs test is performed on the newborn baby's red cells from the cord blood. In vivo sensitization is by maternal antibody coating fetal RBCs.
- **Diagnosis of autoimmune hemolytic anemia:** To demonstrate in vivo attachment of antibodies to red cells. In vivo sensitization is by autoantibody coating individual's RBCs.
- **Investigator of drug-induced red cell sensitization.**
- **Investigation of hemolytic transfusion reaction (HTR):** Alloimmune hemolysis following an incompatible transfusion and investigation of HTR. In vivo sensitization is by recipient antibody coating donor RBCs.

Examples of causes of positive test and source of IgG are presented in Table 9.3.

INDIRECT ANTIGLOBULIN TEST

Indirect antiglobulin test (indirect Coombs test) **detects the presence of incomplete (IgG) antibodies and/or complement in the patient's serum. Patient's serum is used for this test.** Indirect antiglobulin test (IAT). is used for demonstrating in vitro antibody binding to RBCs. Many laboratories use monospecific anti-IgG in antibody detection and identification tests and in crossmatch procedures.

Two-stage procedure: Indirect antiglobulin test is a two-stage procedure.
1. **First incubation step:** In this first stage, a **plasma of patient is incubated** at body temperature **with a red cell source** (O Rh+ve red cells). This allows the

Table 9.3: Examples of causes of positive direct antiglobulin test.

Condition	Cause	Source of IgG
Hemolytic disease of the fetus and newborn (HDFN)	Coating of fetal red cells with IgG	Maternal antibody crossing the placenta
Autoimmune hemolytic anemia	Coating of patient red cells by IgG or C3	Patient autoantibody (own antibody)
Drug-induced	IgG-drug complex attached to red cells	Immune complex formed with drug
Transfusion reaction	Coating of donor red cells with IgG	Antibody from recipient (patient)

attachment of IgG antibodies present in the patient's serum/plasma to specific red cell antigens. The red cell suspension is washed with physiologic saline to remove unbound antibody or complement proteins.

2. **Second step:** After saline washing of red cell, the **AHG reagent is added** to the test and **centrifuged**. If agglutination occurs, the test is interpreted as a positive IAT. A positive IAT indicates a specific reaction between an antibody in the serum/plasma of patient with an antigen present on the red cells. If there is no agglutination, the test is interpreted as a negative IAT.

Materials Required

- 75 × 12 mm glass tubes
- Patient's (test) serum
- Reagent "O" Rh-positive RBCs
- Antiglobulin reagent
- Normal saline
- Positive control (IgG-coated red cells).

Technique (see Fig. 9.5)

- Take **two drops of patient's serum** in a test tube labeled as "T". (The sample should be fresh for detecting complement-binding antibodies, otherwise fresh AB serum should be added to it).
- **Add one drop of 2–4% suspension of reagent "O" Rh+ve cells** to the tube.
- **Incubate** the tube with mixture at 37°C for the time period indicated for the assay being performed (from 15 to 60 minutes). During this time, the reagent "O" Rh+ve RBCs are coated with (IgG) antibodies (if present) in the patient's serum.
- If indicated in the procedure, centrifuge and examine the serum for hemolysis or the cells for agglutination. Agglutination or hemolysis at this stage indicates presence of saline reacting antibody.
- If no hemolysis or agglutination is seen, **wash the sample three to four times** in normal saline to remove the excess of free antibodies (in the case of inadequate washings of the red cells, negative results may be obtained). Decant the last wash completely by removing the supernatant.
- **Add two drops of antiglobulin** (AHG) reagent (polyspecific or monospecific anti-IgG) to the washed cells in each test tube. Mix and incubate at 37°C for 10 minutes.
- **Centrifuge** at 1,000 rpm for 1 minute.
- Gently shake the tubes and look for agglutination using optical aid.
- Record the result.
- If the test is negative, add one drop of control cells (IgG-coated cells).
- Mix and centrifuge at 1,000 rpm for 1 minute.
- Look for agglutination. If no agglutination is seen, the test is invalid and whole test procedure is repeated.

Note: Autocontrol should be run with the IAT.
Steps and their purposes in IAT are listed in Table 9.4.

Interpretation

- **Positive:** Agglutination of RBCs indicates the presence of IgG antibodies or complement in the patient's serum and test is reported as positive for IAT.
- **Negative:** If there is no agglutination, the test is interpreted as a negative IAT. It indicates that there is no IgG antibodies or complement in the patient's serum.

Uses of Indirect Antiglobulin Test

The IAT has wide application in blood transfusion serology. In immunohematology, it is used in testing both patient and donor samples. Antiglobulin test is used to detect the presence of incomplete antibodies and complement-binding antibodies in the serum after coating on red cells in vitro. Indirect antiglobulin reaction phase is used as a procedure such as antibody screening, antibody identification, crossmatching, and antigen typing. Reaction phase is observation of agglutination at certain temperatures, after incubation, or after addition of AHG. IAT uses are as follows:

- **Hemolytic disease of newborn:** Mother's serum is tested to detect anti-Rh antibody.
- **Crossmatching for blood transfusion:** To detect incompatibility of recipient's serum with donor's cells.

Table 9.4: Steps and their purposes in indirect antiglobulin test.

Step	Purpose
Incubate RBCs with antisera	Allows time for antibody molecule in test serum to get attached to RBC antigen
Performing a minimum of three saline washes	Removes free globulin molecules
Adding antiglobulin reagent	Forms RBC agglutinates (RBC Ag + Ab + anti-IgG)
Centrifuge	Speeds agglutination by bringing cells close to each other
Examine for agglutination	Interprets test as positive or negative
Grading of agglutination reactions	Determines the strength of reaction
Adding antibody-coated RBCs to negative reactions	Checks for neutralization of antisera by free globulin molecules (Coombs control cells are D-positive RBCs coated with anti-D)

- **Phenotyping of red cell antigens** using known antisera
- Titration of anti-Rh antibodies
- **Screening and identification of unexpected antibodies in serum**
- **Compatibility testing**
- Crossmatching
- **Detection of red call antigens using specific antibodies reacting only in antiglobulin test** Fy^a, Fy^b, K, JK^a, JK^b, etc.

Various applications for DAT and IAT techniques are presented in Table 9.5.

Comparison of DAT and IAT procedures is presented in Table 9.6.

ALTERNATIVE METHODS TO THE TUBE TEST

In the conventional tube method for AHG testing, enhancement media (refer pages 66, 67) such as low-ionic strength saline (LISS), polyethylene glycol (PEG), polybrene, and albumin can be used. Only advantage of tube method over gel and solid phase is the reagents used have low cost.

Antiglobulin tests may be performed using by several other methods. These procedures may be semiautomated or fully automated.

Gel Test/Gel Card Method

This is **more sensitive** for detecting antibodies than conventional tube technique of antiglobulin test. The **gel test** is a process which detects RBC antigen-antibody reactions by means of using a chamber filled with polyacrylamide gel. The gel acts as a trap and free unagglutinated RBCs form pellets in the bottom of the tube, whereas agglutinated RBCs are trapped (Fig. 9.6A) in the tube for hours. Hence, negative reactions appear as pellets in the bottom of the microtube (Fig. 9.6B), and positive reactions are fixed in the gel. The washing is required in tube technique, and not in the gel method. (Details are mentioned on pages 78-81)

Types of gel test: There are three different types of gel tests namely: (1) neutral, (2) specific, and (3) antiglobulin.

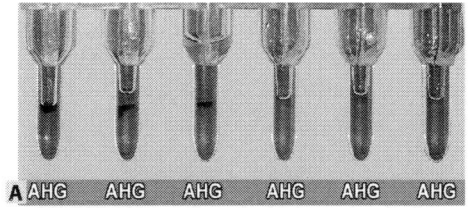

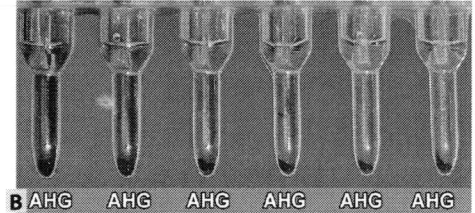

Figs. 9.6A and B: Antiglobulin (AHG) test by column agglutination technique (CAT) using glass microbeads matrix. All shows 6 microtubes (vertical columns): (A) Shows 3 microtube in the left with agglutination of red cells at the top indicating positive AHG and right three are blank tubes; (B) All 6 microtubes show formation of red cells button at the bottom of each tube and indicates no agglutination indicating negative AHG.

Table 9.5: Applications for direct and indirect antiglobulin techniques.

Applications	Purpose/Mechanism	Inference
DIRECT ANTIGLOBULIN TEST (DAT)		
Investigation of hemolytic transfusion reactions (HTRs)		
Alloimmune hemolysis following an incompatible transfusion	A positive DAT is the first evidence of a hemolytic reaction after transfusion	Positive DAT may be due to IgG and/or C3d depending on the antibodies responsible
• Recipient alloantibody and donor antigen	To detect circulating donor red cells, which might have been sensitized with recipient antibody	Alloantibodies in the recipient of a transfusion react with antigen on donor RBCs
• Donor antibody and recipient antigen	To detect antibody in the plasma of the donor with antigen on the recipient RBCs	Antibodies present in donor plasma react with antigen on RBCs of a transfusion recipient
Diagnosis of hemolytic disease of the fetus and newborn (HDFN)		
Diagnosis of HDFN	To detect maternal alloantibodies (IgG) that have crossed the placenta to sensitize fetal red cells. DAT is performed on the newborn baby's red cells from the cord blood	DAT is positive due to the presence of IgG; occasionally, C3d positive if ABO antibodies involved
Diagnosis of autoimmune hemolytic anemia (AIHA)		
Warm autoimmune hemolytic anemia—WAIHA (IgG and/or C3)	To detect in vivo attachment/reaction of autoantibody to patient's own red cells	*Warm autoantibodies:* DAT is positive due to IgG
Cold agglutinin syndrome—CAS (C3)	Cold-reactive IgM autoagglutinin binds to RBCs in peripheral circulation (32°C). IgM binds complement as RBCs return to warmer parts of circulation; IgM dissociates, leaving RBCs coated only with complement	*Cold autoantibodies:* DAT may be positive due to C3d only
Paroxysmal cold hemoglobinuria—PCH (IgG)	The IgG autoantibody reacts with RBCs in colder parts of body, causes complement to be bound irreversibly to RBCs, and then elutes at warmer temperature	DAT is positive
Investigation of drug-induced hemolysis		
Investigation of drug-induced hemolysis	To detect antidrug/red cell antibodies and/or subsequent activation of the complement system	DAT may be positive due to IgG, C3d, or both, depending on the mechanism involved
INDIRECT ANTIGLOBULIN TEST (IAT)		
Antibody detection (or antibody screening)	To detect clinically significant IgG alloantibodies in the recipient	Recipient IgG antibodies bound to reagent screening cells
Antibody identification	To specifically identify antibodies detected by reagent screening cells or by donor red cells	Recipient IgG antibodies bound to reagent cells from a panel of 10–12 donors
Crossmatching for blood transfusion	To detect compatibility/incompatibility of recipient's serum with donor's cells. To detect antibodies that may have been missed by the antibody screen because of absence of the corresponding antigen or presence of a dosing antibody	Recipient IgG antibodies bound to donor red cells
Red cell antigen typing using known antisera	To type patient or donor red cells for antigens that can be detected by IgG antisera reactive only by the antiglobulin test (e.g. weak D test)	Specific binding of reagent IgG antibodies to red cells positive for the corresponding antigen

Antihuman Globulin Test

Table 9.6: Comparison of direct antiglobulin test and indirect antiglobulin test procedures.

Features	Direct antiglobulin test	Indirect antiglobulin test
Component detected	Detects IgG and complement-coated red cells	
Occurrence of IgG attachment to red cells	Within the patient's body	During the incubation step of test
Procedure	One-stage procedure	Two-stage procedure
Incubation step	No need for incubation step	Requires an incubation step before the addition of antiglobulin reagent
Examples of uses	Hemolytic disease of the fetus and newborn, hemolytic transfusion reaction, autoimmune hemolytic anemia, etc.	Used as a reaction phase of several tests in immunohematology (e.g. antibody screen and antibody identification panel)

- **Neutral gel:** It does not contain any specific reagent. It acts only by its property of trapping agglutinates. This is mainly used for antibody screening and identification with enzyme-treated or untreated RBCs and reverse ABO typing.
- **Specific gel tests:** In this test, a specific reagent incorporated into the gel. It is used for antigen determination.
- **Gel low-ionic antiglobulin test (GLIAT):** In this test, AHG reagent is incorporated into the gel. It may be used for the IAT or the DAT.

The gel technology for AHG testing has gained popularity than the conventional tube testing using saline. It is less labor intensive than conventional tube testing (including saline, LISS, and PEG), it can be standardized for both procedure and endpoint grading and it can be automated. A few disadvantages (refer page 82) of the gel method are: (1) the increased cost of instrumentation and reagents, (2) the need to stay proficient with alternative methods for backup, and (3) the increased likelihood of detecting unwanted autoantibodies.

Solid-phase adherence tests: Solid-phase technology (refer pages 82, 83) can be used as a manual or automated method for use in IAT. Similar to gel technology, solid-phase technology is more likely to detect weakly reactive antibodies than the LISS tube method. The solid-phase method is more sensitive at detecting the anti-D than the gel method.

Advantages and disadvantages of various testing methods for antiglobulin test are presented in Table 9.7.

SOURCES OF ERROR IN ANTIGLOBULIN TEST

Problems in antiglobulin test can result in either false-negative results or false-positive results. All efforts must be made to avoid any such possible source of error for accurate and precise result.

Causes of false-positive and false-negative tests are listed in Table 9.8.

QUALITY CONTROL FOR ANTIGLOBULIN TEST

Quality Control of the Antiglobulin Reagents

The quality control of antiglobulin reagents should be carried out following the exact technique and all reagents should be used according to the manufacturer's instructions. The validation of a new antiglobulin reagent should be assessed for the following qualities of the reagent:

- **Specificity:** The reagent should only agglutinate red cells sensitized with antibodies and/or coated with significant levels of complement components.
- **Potency of anti-IgG by serological titration**
- **Specificity and potency of anticomplement antibodies:** A polyspecific reagent should contain controlled levels anti-C3c and anti-C3d to avoid false-positive reactions or a suitable potent monoclonal anti-C3d. The content of anti-C4 should be little or nil. To assess these qualities,

Table 9.7: Advantages and disadvantages of various testing methods for antiglobulin test.

Advantages	Disadvantages
Conventional tube testing (CTT)	
• No additives • Reduced cost • No reactivity with autoantibodies • Ability to assess multiple phases of reactivity	• Long incubation • Least sensitive • Needs highly trained staff • Many steps in procedure • Fewer method-dependent antibodies (Abs) detected
Gel method	
• More sensitive DAT method • No washing steps • No need for check cells • Stable endpoints • Small test volume • Enhanced anti-D detection • Can be automated	• Warm auto-Abs enhanced • Mixed-cell agglutination with cold Abs • Increased costs • Increased need for additional instrumentation • Increased chances of detected unwanted Abs • Requires to maintain backup method
Solid-phase technology	
• No need for check cells • Stable endpoints • Small test volume • Enhanced anti-D • Increased sensitivity for all Abs • Can be automated	• Increased sensitivity for all Abs • Detects unwanted Abs • Warm auto-Abs enhanced • Increased costs • Increased need for additional instrumentation

Table 9.8: Sources of error causing false-positive and false-negative results in antiglobulin testing.

False-positive	False-negative
Due to specimen error • Improper specimen (refrigerated, clotted) may cause in vitro complement attachment • Using a serum sample for a DAT (use EDTA, acid-citrate-dextrose [ACD], or citrate-phosphate-dextrose [CPD] anticoagulated blood) **Due to technical errors** • Overcentrifugation and over-reading causes red cell button packed so tightly on centrifugation that nonspecific clumping cannot be dispersed • Over incubation with enzyme-treated cells • Centrifugation after the incubation phase when PEG or other positively charged polymers are used as an enhancement medium • Improper use of polyethylene glycol (PEG) or polycation enhancement reagents • Inadequate resuspension of cell button • Bacterial contamination of cells or saline used in washing • Dirty glassware with particles or contaminants **Due to errors in blood sample itself** • Direct agglutination before adding AHG reagent caused by strong cold agglutinins in patient • Rouleaux formation • Small fibrin clots in the test tube may trap cells and mimic agglutination • Cells with a positive DAT will yield false-positive indirect antiglobulin test	**Due to specimen error** • Excessive heat or repeated freezing and thawing of test serum • Serum: Cell ratios are not ideal • Low pH of saline **Due to reagent** • Antihuman globulin (AHG) reagent failure or AHG reagent that has lost potency (improper reagent storage) • Contamination of AHG by extraneous protein (i.e. glove, wrong dropper) **Due to faults in technique** • Failure to add AHG reagents, test serum, or enhancement medium not added • Improper or inadequate washing of cells before the addition of AHG reagent. This causes neutralize AHG reagent by unbound human serum globulins • Failure to wash additional times when increased serum volumes are used • Delay or interruption of washing (elution of weakly attached antibody) • Serum: cell ratio too low • Failure to add test serum or enhancement reagents • Under centrifugation • Resuspension of cell button too vigorous • Early dissociation of bound IgG from RBCs due to interruption in testing • Early dissociation of bound IgG from RBCs due to improper testing temperature (i.e. saline or AHG too cold or hot) • Cell suspension either too weak or too heavy **Due to errors in blood sample itself** High concentration of IgG paraproteins in test serum

it needs red cells specifically coated with C3b, C3bi, C3d and C4.

Quality Control of the Antihuman Globulin Test

Two types of quality control RBCs are normally used to standardize antiglobulin sera and to confirm true-negative antiglobulin reactions.
1. RBCs coated with IgG: To sensitize RBCs with IgG usually Rh antibodies are used.
2. RBCs coated with C3b and/or C3d.
   - To prepare RBCs coated with C3b, whole blood is incubated in LISS or with human anti-Lea or anti-I.
   - To prepare C3d-coated RBCs, C3b-coated cells are incubated with fresh serum or trypsin to split C3b→C3d.

IgG or complement-coated control cells should give a 1+ to 2+ reaction (Table 9.9) when tested with anti-IgG or anti-C3b + C3d.

Quality control red cells used for the antiglobulin test are called as *check cells* or *Coombs control cells*.

Table 9.9: Agglutination grading system.

Grading	Macroscopic appearance
1+	Many small clumps; reddish background
2+	Many medium clumps; pink background
3+	Many large clumps; clear background
4+	One clump; clear background

Sensitivity of the Antihuman Globulin Test

Antiglobulin test is extremely sensitive. However, a negative test does not rule out the possible presence of antibodies on RBCs. About 200–500 IgG or C3 molecules bound per red cell are needed for detection by antiglobulin antibodies. A negative reaction can be observed when there are small quantities of bound IgG and C3. AHG sera may also show greater activity against some subclasses of IgG than against others. Thus, certain AHG sera may produce negative results with RBCs coated by a particular IgG subclass.

SUMMARY

- The antiglobulin test detects incomplete antibodies (IgG) and/or complement protein molecules that have attached (sensitized) to red cells but have not resulted in a visible agglutination reaction.
- AHG reagents used in antiglobulin test may be polyspecific or monospecific.
- There are two types of antiglobulin/Coombs test namely: (1) direct, and (2) indirect.
- In direct antiglobulin test (DAT) patient's red cells are used and it detect in vivo sensitization of RBCs with IgG antibody or complement molecules. Certain clinical conditions that can result in a positive DAT include HDFN (hemolytic disease of fetus and newborn), HTRs (hemolytic transfusion reactions), and AIHAs (autoimmune hemolytic anemias).
- The IAT (indirect antiglobulin test) detects in vitro sensitization of RBCs. In IAT, patient's serum is tested. This test requires an incubation step for sensitization. The IAT is commonly used in antibody screens, antibody identification, testing of donor and recipient compatibility and RBC phenotyping. It is useful in HDFN where the mother's serum is tested for the presence of antibodies.
- Apart from conventional tube methods, there are other methods such as gel technology and solid-phase testing available to use in AHG testing. They can be performed as semiautomated or fully automated method.
- EDTA sample is preferred to collect blood samples for the DAT to avoid in vitro complement attachment associated with refrigerated clotted specimens.
- There are multiple sources of error that can be introduced into the AHG procedure. These can cause false-positive or false-negative AHG test results. Their recognition and prevention help in the correct interpretation of the AHG test result.

SELF-ASSESSMENT EXERCISE

Write short notes on:
- Antiglobulin test and their uses
- Write notes on use, principle and interpretation of direct and indirect antiglobulin test
- Quality control in antiglobulin reagents

CHAPTER 10

Antibody Detection (Screening) and Identification

CHAPTER OUTLINE

- Basic concepts in red cell antigen expression
- Types of antibodies in transfusion medicine
- Antibody detection (screening)
- Antibody identification
- Interpretation (evaluation) of panel results
- Complex antibody identification
- Considerations following antibody identification

INTRODUCTION

It is very essential to **carry out the antibody screen tests** in **pretransfusion and prenatal period**. There are two steps involved:
1. **Antibody screening/detection**: Screen to **find out whether any antibodies** (unexpected) **are detected** against red cell antigens.
2. **Antibody identification**: If antibody is detected then **determine the specificity of antibody**. Determining the specificity of antibodies, or antibody identification, requires the knowledge of blood group system antigen and antibody characteristics discussed in previous chapters (Chapters 3 to 5). It is also necessary to know about the reagents used to enhance or eliminate reactions. Clues during antibody identification are most often slight (subtle) and hard to explain (elusive). Hence, the process must be methodical and accurate. If there is a single antibody (with one specificity), it is easy to identify. However, each sample is often unique and may require several different approaches to come to a conclusive identification. Proficiency and confidence in antibody resolution usually require experience and an understanding of basic theoretical concepts involved.

The above two steps should be done in all patients who need blood transfusion or in antenatal patients. In transfusion, it is necessary to carryout antibody screen to detect clinically significant antibodies in both the blood donor and transfusion recipient.

Advantages: It helps to find compatible blood for patients who have developed unexpected antibodies. In antenatal patients, the antibody detection and identification have two purposes namely: (1) to **find a compatible blood** (if needed), and (2) aids in **prediction** and possibility of severity of **hemolytic disease of fetus and newborn** (HDFN). The purpose of antibody screens and identification are presented in Box 10.1.

Box 10.1: Purpose of antibody detection (screening) and identification.

Performed to detect antibodies in:
- **Recipients**
  - Patients requiring transfusion
  - Pregnancy: Prenatal testing for obstetric patients to evaluate the risk of hemolytic disease of fetus and newborn (HDFN) in the fetus and to assess the mother's candidacy for Rh-immune globulin (RHIG) prophylaxis
  - Patients with suspected transfusion reactions
- **Donors**
  - Blood and plasma donors
  - To evaluate the compatibility of hematopoietic progenitor cell (HPC) and bone marrow donors with the intended transplant recipient

BASIC CONCEPTS IN RED CELL ANTIGEN EXPRESSION

Antibody identification depends on the reaction of serum or plasma with red cells of known antigen expression. The antigen expression is variable and its basic knowledge is necessary to interpret reaction in antibody identification.

Zygosity and Dosage

Dosage: The reactive strength of some antibodies varies because of dosage.
- A cell with **homozygous** antigen expression is from an individual who inherited only one allele at a given genetic locus. Certain antibodies (e.g. those of the Kidd system) may be detected only when tested against red blood cells (RBCs) expressing one allele (homozygous). Therefore, the cell surface has a "double dose" expression of that antigen when an individual is homozygous for the gene that encodes the particular antigen. Antibodies that react more strongly with cells having homozygous antigen expression are said to show **dosage** (Box 10.2). Some antibodies more strongly reactive with red cells having "double-dose" expression of the antigen.
- A cell with **heterozygous** antigen expression is from an individual who inherited two different alleles at a locus. In individuals who are heterozygous for the gene, the red cells may express fewer antigens and therefore, they may react weakly or nonreactive with the corresponding antibody.
- Alloantibodies vary in their tendency to demonstrate dosage. Many antibodies to antigens in Rh, Duffy, MNS, and Kidd blood groups demonstrate dosage.
- The cells with **homozygous** expression for most of the antigens may be frozen in glycerol for subsequent use. They **react better** with their corresponding antibodies due to increased number of antigen sites. It increases the possibility of **detecting weak or dose-dependent antibodies.**

Variation with Age

- Some antigens (e.g. I, P1, Le^a) show variable expression on red cells in different adults which is not due to zygosity.
- Some antigens show different expression on cord/neonate red cells compared to adult red cells of same individual.
- Antigen expression on cord/neonatal red cells may be absent, weaker or stronger than that of adult red cells (Table 10.1)

Changes with Storage

- During storage, some red cell antigens (e.g. Fy^a, Fy^b, M, P1) may deteriorate more rapidly than other and the rate of deterioration varies in different individuals. Storage of red cells in freezer may cause deterioration of some antigens.
- **Storage medium:** The pH and other features of the storage medium can affect the rate of antigen deterioration. For example, Fy^a and Fy^b antigens may be weakened when a low pH and low ionic strength medium is used.
- **Nature of specimen:** Antigens on red cells from **clotted blood samples** usually **deteriorate more quickly than** those blood samples **collected in citrate anticoagulants**.

Box 10.2: Common blood group systems with antibodies that show dosage.
- Rh (except D)
- Kidd
- Duffy
- MNSs
- Lutheran

Table 10.1: Examples of antigen expression on cord red blood cells.

Examples of antigens	Antigen expression on cord red blood cells
Le^a, Le^b	Negative
I, H, P1, Lu^a, Lu^b	Weak
i, Lw^a, Lw^b	Strong

TYPES OF ANTIBODIES IN TRANSFUSION MEDICINE

Naturally Occurring Antibodies

These can present naturally in the circulating plasma and are produced without any RBC stimulation. They may be produced as a result of exposure to environmental sources. These include pollen, fungus, virus, and bacteria, which have structures similar to some RBC antigens. The naturally occurring anti-A and anti-B (ABO blood group system antibodies) are the only red cell antibodies commonly found in the serum of plasma of human beings. The only naturally occurring/expected blood group antibodies in a patient's sample are ABO antibodies, which follow Landsteiner's law (refer page 69).

Unexpected (Irregular) Red Cell Antibodies

The term unexpected refers to **all antibodies other than ABO blood group system antibodies** (i.e. naturally occurring anti-A and anti-B). In other words, except anti-A and anti-B, all other antibodies are called as unexpected (irregular) red cell antibodies. They are called as "unexpected" because of their relative rarity. The **antibody detection methods in transfusion mainly focus on "irregular" or "unexpected" antibodies** than the "expected" antibodies of the ABO system. The detection of unexpected antibody in the screen of a patient or donor initiates the antibody identification process. This may be seen like detective work in blood bank test. The two categories of unexpected antibodies are:
1. **Alloantibodies:** These are antibodies produced by an individual to an antigen which the individual lacks. Because these antibodies are directed to a non-self-antigen, they are called alloantibodies. The blood sample of patients or donors may contain alloantibodies.
   a. **Immune alloantibodies:** The primarily important **unexpected antibodies** are the **immune alloantibodies.** They are produced when the red cells carrying corresponding antigens enter into an individual, who normally lacks the antigen (e.g. anti-D). The immunization to RBC antigens occurs due to exposure to foreign red cell antigens. This exposure **occurs during** previous **transfusion** of red cells, **transplantation, pregnancy** or delivery (exposure to fetal cells), **needle sharing or injections of immunogenic material.** Detection of these preformed red cell antibodies in a patient or donor is essential to provide a safe red cell product for transfusion purposes.
   b. **Passively acquired antibodies:** Antibodies formed in one individual may be passively transmitted to other individuals. This may occur from donor plasma-containing blood components, injected intravenous immunoglobulin (IVIG), passenger lymphocytes in transplanted organs or HPCs. These are known as passively acquired antibodies.
2. **Autoantibodies:** These are antibodies produced against an antigen expressed on one's own antigen (e.g. against own RBCs antigens). These antibodies are usually reactive with most reagent red cell and autologous (own) red cells. Autoantibodies are usually formed by a disease process or medication.

Clinically Significant Antibodies

Definition: Clinically significant antibody is defined as **an antibody** that is frequently **associated with HDFN, hemolytic transfusion reactions or a notable decrease in the survival of transfused red cells**.

Clinically significant antibodies cause decreased survival of RBCs having the target antigen. These antibodies are **usually IgG antibodies and react at 37°C or that react in the antihuman globulin (AHG) phase of the indirect antiglobulin test**.

Significance: The presence of naturally occurring, passive and autoantibodies may complicate the detection and identification of clinically significant antibodies. After detection of an antibody, an antibody identification panel is performed to determine its type (allo and/or auto) and the specificity of the antibody (or antibodies) present. Once identified, the antibody's possible clinical significance should be assessed. The degree of clinical significance can vary among antibodies of same specificity. For example, some may cause destruction of incompatible blood within minutes or hours, whereas others may reduce the survival of red cells by only few days, and still may not significantly shorten the survival of red cells. Some antibodies are well known to cause HDFN, whereas others may give only a positive direct antiglobulin test (DAT) without any clinical evidence of HDFN.

ANTIBODY DETECTION (SCREENING)

The detection of antibodies against RBC antigens or **antibody screening is critical step in pretransfusion compatibility testing**. It is one of the main tools for investigating potential hemolytic transfusion reactions and immune hemolytic anemias. It helps in detecting and monitoring patients who are at risk of delivering infants with HDFN.

Purpose of antibody screen: To **detect any potentially clinically significant antibody in a donor's or recipient's blood** sample. Normally, only a small percentage of the healthy population (from 0.02% to 2%) has detectable red cell antibodies whereas in individuals receiving chronic transfusion (e.g. sickle cell anemia) 14–50% of them may reveal red cell alloantibodies.

Indications: Antibody screens are performed to detect antibodies in certain individuals as listed in Box 10.3.

Box 10.3: Indications for antibody screening.
- Patients who require transfusion
- Patients with suspected transfusion reactions
- Women who are pregnant or after delivery
- Blood and plasma donors

Reagents for Antibody Detection

Reagent Group O Red Cells (Screening Cells)

The RBC reagents or screening cells are used in antibody screen (antibody detection) tests. The antibody screening/detection is performed on a patient's/recipient serum. This procedure finds whether antibodies with specificity to red cell antigens are observed in patient and donor samples.

Panels: The RBC reagents or screening cells are always **obtained from donors of group O**. They are commercially supplied as **sets of two-vial or three-vial** samples of reagent single-donor red cells. Each panel consists of red cells with particular antigens of most clinically significant red cell antibodies. A **set of two specially selected group OR_1R_1 (R_1) and OR_2R_2 (R_2) cells are widely used.** Each vial in these sets (of 2 or 3) consists of the red cells obtained from a single donor. Also, a product containing pooled screening group O red cells obtained from two donors in equal proportions is commercially available.

Group O donors are selected because in individuals with **group O phenotype have neither A nor B antigens and will not interfere in the detection of antibodies to other blood group systems**. Hence, group O red cells do not react with ABO antibodies present in patient or donor serum or plasma. Serum or plasma from any ABO type may be used in the antibody screen test without interference from the ABO antibodies. Reagent RBCs used for antibody screening should have a negative DAT to prevent false-positive reactions in the IAT phase used for antibody screening.

- **Unpooled screening group O red cells:** Tests for antibodies on recipient specimens (e.g. specimens of a patient are going to receive a transfusion) should be performed using unpooled screening group O red cells. This is because it **provides maximum sensitivity even for weakly reactive antibodies**. On the contrary, pooled red cell reagent reduces the ability to detect a weakly reactive antibody. It is best if the

Donor no.	Genotype	Rh							MNSs				P1	Lewis		Lutheran		Kell		Duffy		Kidd	
Panel	Cell	D	C	E	c	e	f	c^w	M	N	S	s	P1	Le^a	Le^b	Lu^a	Lu^b	K	k	Fy^a	Fy^b	Jk^a	Jk^b
1	I R1R1	+	+	0	0	+	0	0	+	+	0	+	0	+	0	0	+	+	+	+	0	+	+
2	II R2R2	+	0	+	+	0	0	0	0	+	+	0	+	0	+	0	+	0	+	0	+	+	0

Fig. 10.1: Typical panel of commercial screening group O red cells. It shows profile of antigen phenotypes of each donor used in the screening cells.
(+ = the antigen is present on the screening cell; 0 = the antigen is absent on the screening cell)

manufacturer provides screening red cells from donors that are homozygous (with double-dose expression) for the common antigens.
- **Pooled screening cells** can be used in **screening donors for red cell antibodies.**

Preservation of cell panel: Commercial screening RBCs for tube testing are suspended **preservative solution/diluent at a concentration between 2% and 5%.** This preservative diluent maintains the integrity of the antigens and prevents hemolysis. They can be directly used. Washing of red cells before use is not necessary unless the preservative solution is likely to interfere with identification of antibody.

Storage: The vial must be stored at **2–8°C** when not in use. For long-term storage, the cells of cell panel are frozen in small aliquots by adding cryoprotective agents (e.g. glycerol or sucrose). They are frozen at -80°C in deep freezer or in liquid nitrogen at -196°C. When required, the individual aliquots of different panel of cells may be thawed for antibody screen and identification.

Antigram or antigenic profile of reagent cells: Each lot of reagent screening O group red cells comes with an accompanying antigenic profile, or antigram, of each donor. Antigram is a chart that shows the antigenic makeup (profile of antigen phenotypes) of each cell (donor cell used in the manufacture of commercially supplied panel). The reagent cells are selected from different donors of known phenotype. Screening sets of cells are prepared so that they contain all antigens to the most commonly encountered blood group antibodies. Thus, the antigenic profile should be capable of detecting most clinically significant red cell antibodies. Within the set, there should be one cell that is positive for each of the following antigens: C, E, c, e, M, N, S, s, P1, Le^a, Le^b, K, k, Fy^a, Fy^b, Jk^a, and Jk^b. Typical panel of screening cells is shown in the Figure 10.1. For example, in Figure 10.1, the first panel shows red cells with antigens D, C, e, C^w, M, N, s, Le^a, Lu^b, K, k, Fy^a, Jk^a, and Jk^b.

Precaution: Reagent red cells **should be refrigerated when not in use** and **should not be used after expiry date.** As the screening cells approach the end of their dating period, there may be diminished reagent reactivity due to antigen deterioration. Hence, these screening cells should not be used beyond their expiration date. There may be signs of significant hemolysis, discoloration, or agglutination due to contamination and they should not be used.

Enhancement reagents/media or potentiators (discussed on pages 66, 67).

Antiglobulin Reagents
(Refer Pages 174-7)

Most antibody detection and identification studies include indirect antiglobulin test (IAT) phase. The anti-Ig used may be either AHG specific to human immunoglobulin G (IgG) or a polyspecific reagent that contains anti-IgG and anticomplement.
- A **polyspecific reagent** may more readily detect antibodies that bind complement. This is because a single IgG molecule can deposit multiple molecules of complement. It may be helpful to detect low-level IgG antibodies due to its complement activation. It is necessary to use serum rather than plasma for complement binding. This is because the anticoagulant in plasma binds calcium making it not available for complement activation. This

complement binding is advantageous in some instances such as detection of certain JK system antibodies.
- Antihuman globulin reagents are more sensitive and avoid unwanted activities from in vitro complement binding by cold-reactive antibodies.

Specimen Requirements

Both serum and plasma can be used for antibody testing. However, for testing complement, only serum should be used. Depending on the test methods used, a 5–10 mL of whole blood is enough for simple antibody specificities. However, more whole blood may be needed for complex studies. When autologous red cells are tested, blood should be collected in EDTA, which avoids problems associated with in vitro uptake of complements by red cells.

Methods for Antibody Detection (Screening)

The antibody screen in the patient is performed to detect antibodies that are **directed toward common or high-prevalence antigens**. It will neither detect antibodies to antigens of low prevalence, nor will it detect antibodies bound to the red cells of the patient if an *autocontrol* is not performed along with the antibody screen.

All methods used for antibody detection and identification are based on the principle of hemagglutination (tube or column agglutination systems) or red cell adherence (solid phase). Antibody screening cells are group O reagent red cells. These reagent red cells are tested with the patient's serum to know whether an unexpected antibody is present in patient's serum or plasma.

Primary method: Antibody screening should be carried out by an IAT as the primary method for the detection of IgG antibodies. In antibody screening, the patient's serum or plasma is incubated at 37°C with antibody screening (reagent red) cells and an **IAT is performed**.

Additional methods (e.g. two-stage enzyme or Polybrene) may also be used. But these are inferior for the detection of some clinically significant antibodies and should not be used alone. Vast majority of antibodies reactive only by enzyme technique are of no clinical significance.

For liquid-phase techniques, it is recommended to use red cells suspended in low ionic strength saline (LISS), rather than in standard normal ionic strength saline (NISS), because LISS increases the speed and sensitivity of detection of many potentially clinically significant antibodies. However, it is doubtful whether there is improved sensitivity by addition of PEG.

Liquid-Phase Techniques—Tubes and Microplates

Tube tests techniques

It is still used as primary method for antibody screening in developing countries. Tube testing offers flexibility to test different phases and option to use a variety of enhancement media (and thus provides varying degrees of sensitivity). It requires little specialized equipment.

Procedure of tube method (Fig. 10.2)

In conventional test tube methods, one volume 3–5% screening reagent cells and two volumes patient serum are taken (i.e. average ratio of serum to cells is about 50:1). The different phases (Fig. 10.2) in the procedure of tube method are as follows:
1. **Immediate spin phase**: The test may include an immediate spin phase to detect antibodies reacting at room temperature. This phase is not required and is optional. It may lead to the detection of clinically insignificant cold antibodies.
2. **Incubation (37°C) phase**: During incubation phase, IgG molecules sensitize any RBCs that possess the target antigen, coating those RBCs with antibody. The tube is incubated at 37°C with an enhancement medium (to increase the degree of sensitization) for the time specified by the manufacturer. With LISS-suspension techniques, it is necessary to maintain a high serum: cell ratio, without affecting the ionic strength. Equal volumes

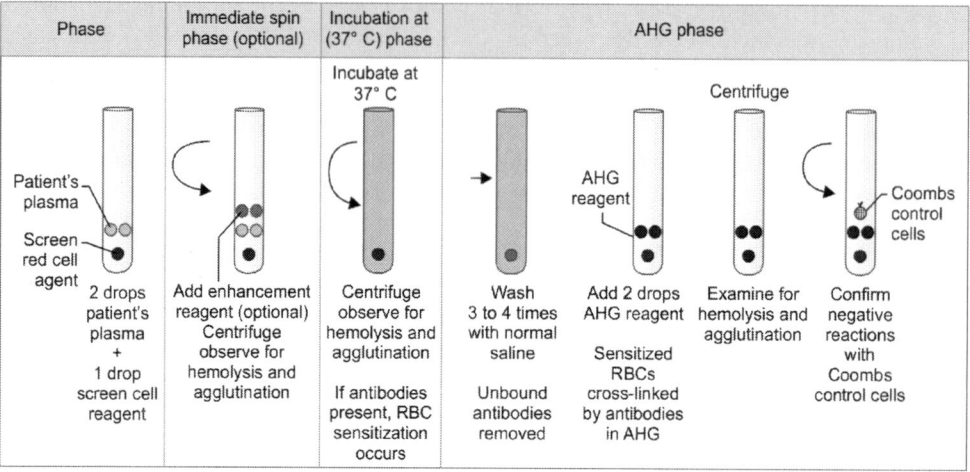

Fig. 10.2: Various phases and steps involved in the tube antibody screen test.

of serum and 1.5–2% cells suspended in LISS will have a serum: cell ratio of > 60:1. This will have optimal sensitivity. They are centrifuged and examined for hemolysis or agglutination.
- To observe for hemolysis, the tube is carefully removed from the centrifuge so that the there is no dislodgement of the RBC button. The supernatant is observed for pink or red discoloration.
- To observe for agglutination, the tube is gently tilted or rolled to dislodge the cell button. The degree of agglutination should be assessed only after all of the RBCs have been dislodged from the bottom of the test tube.

3. **AHG phase**: Then the screening cells are washed three to four times with 0.9% saline to remove all antibodies that remain unbound. Add AHG reagent (also known as Coombs' serum) to the tube for final detection of IgG alloantibodies. The tubes are centrifuged and examined for hemolysis and agglutination.
   - **Hemolysis:** In this phase, hemolysis may appear as a loss of cell button mass.
   - **Agglutination:** The red cells should be examined using a careful "tip and roll" procedure to prevent disruption of weak agglutinates. Reading aids (e.g. a light box or concave mirror) may also be used with this technique.
   - If **the RBCs are coated with IgG antibodies**, the anti-IgG antibody in the AHG reagent will create a bridge between sensitized RBCs. This will form an **observable agglutination**.
   - If there are **no antibodies directed against** any of the antigens present on the **screen cell RBCs**, the RBCs will not be sensitized. There will be **no agglutination.** In all negative tests, Coombs' control cells (also known as *check cells*) should be added to confirm the negative result.
   - **Grading:** Depending on the enhancement media used, the agglutination reactions may be observed macroscopically only or may need a microscopic examination. The degree of reactivity is graded as 0 (no agglutination present) to w+ (agglutination barely visible to the naked eye) to 4+ (one solid agglutinate).

Autocontrol and Direct Antiglobulin Test

In antibody identification, the autocontrol and the DAT can provide important and useful information regarding antibody specificity. They help in determining whether the patient's antibody is directed against his or her red cells or against transfused cells, in the case of a recent transfusion.

- **Autocontrol**: This tests the patient's serum with his or her own red cells and includes the potentiator used in the antibody screen or panel. The autocontrol is usually incubated with the antibody identification panel. The control is read in the reaction phases appropriate for the potentiator.
- **Direct antiglobulin test**: It is performed on the patient's cells without serum and potentiator or an incubation step.

It is optional to perform autocontrol routinely with the screen. However, it is preferable to perform a DAT only if the screen is positive.

Potentiators are commonly used in both antibody screening and identification procedures. They increase the speed and sensitivity of the antibody attachment to the red cell antigen. (They are discussed on pages 66, 67).

Alternative Methods in Antibody Screen and Identification Procedures

Alternative methods (e.g. solid-phase, gel technology) are also used for routine screening

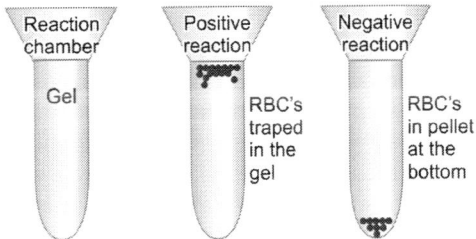

Fig. 10.4: Gel method for antibody screening.

and antibody identification procedures. Each method has limitations and advantages.

Column agglutination technologies: It utilizes the differential migration of RBC agglutinates through a small microtube filled with buffered dextran acrylamide size exclusion gel column (Figs. 10.3 and 10.4). Refer page 78 of Chapter 4, ABO blood grouping for principles and features of column agglutination techniques.

Solid-phase adherence tests: Another alternative to tube tests for alloantibody detection is indirect solid-phase adherence test systems. For details refer page 82.

Interpretation of Antibody Screening Tests

The results obtained when the panel cells are tested against the patient's plasma are

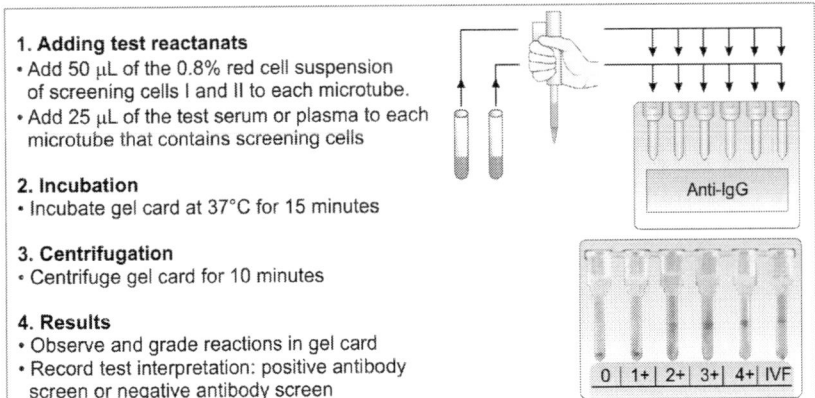

Fig 10.3: Different steps in Gel Test Antibody Screen (IAT). First 0.8% suspensions of screening cells and patient serum or plasma are added to the microtubes of Anti-IgG Card. The gel card is incubated for 15 minutes at 37°C. Then the gel card is centrifuged for the reaction to take place. After centrifugation, the gel card is observed for agglutination reactions. The agglutination reaction is graded from 4+ to 0, depending on the position of the red cells in the gel microtube.

compared to the antigram to determine the identity of antibody (ies) in the specimen. Presence of agglutination or hemolysis at any stage of test during antibody screening indicates that the test is positive (i.e. antibody is present). In such cases, it is necessary to identify the antibody by further tests. However, evaluation of the antibody screen results (and autologous control, if tested at this time) can give clues and give direction for the identification of the antibody or antibodies.

Evaluation Steps

The following evaluation steps should be considered:

1. **Phase and Reaction**

    Different blood group antibodies commonly show characteristic reaction patterns during IAT test. Therefore, close examination during different phases of tests may give useful information in evaluating the cases where screening is positive for antibodies.
    - **Direct agglutination** of the cells **in enrichment media namely albumin or LISS** after **37°C incubation**: Usually indicates the presence of **Rh antibody**.
    - **IgM antibodies** (e.g. anti-I, anti-P1, and Lewis antibodies) have a wide thermal range. IgM antibodies react best at room temperature or lower. They can cause agglutination of saline-suspended RBCs (immediate spin reaction), **in enrichment medias such as albumin or LISS**. However, these reactions **usually become much weaker after conversion to the IAT**. Of the commonly encountered antibodies, anti-N, anti-I, and anti-P1 are usually IgM type.
    - Except rare exceptions, **in vitro hemolysis of reagent cells after 37°C indicates** the presence **of Lewis, Kidd, Ii, P, PP1Pk, or Vel antibodies**.
    - **Majority of IgG antibodies** (except Rh) will **not be detected until after washing** and **conversion to the IAT**. IgG class react best at the AHG phase. Antibodies directed against Rh, Kell, Kidd, Duffy, and Ss antigens are usually IgG.
    - Lewis and M antibodies may be IgG, IgM, or a mixture of both.
    - **Reactions of different screening cells in multiple phases or with varying strengths** usually are **due to more than one antibody**.

2. **Result of the Autologous Control**

    In autologous control (refer page 92), the patient's RBCs are tested against the patient's serum or plasma in the same way as the antibody screen.
    - **Positive antibody screen and a negative autologous control**: It indicates the presence of an alloantibody.
    - **A positive autologous control**: It indicates the presence of autoantibodies or antibodies to medications. If the patient has been recently transfused (i.e. in the previous 3 months), the positive autologous control may be due to alloantibody coating circulating donor RBCs.

3. **Number of Screen Cell Sample Reacted and Strength and Phase of Reaction**
    - **Number of screen cell sample reacted:** In following situations, more than one screen cell sample may be positive.
        - Patient with multiple antibodies
        - When a single antibody's target antigen is found on more than one screen cell.
        - Patient's serum containing an autoantibody.
    - **Strength and phase of reaction:**
        - **Single antibody**: If all screen cells yield a positive reaction at the same phase and strength, it is probably due to a single antibody.
        - **Multiple antibodies**: They most likely react with screen cells at different phases or strengths.
        - **Autoantibodies:** They are suspected when the autologous control is positive.

4. **Hemolysis and Mixed-Field Agglutination**
    - Some antibodies (e.g. anti-Le[a], anti-Le[b], anti-PP1Pk, and anti-Vel) cause in vitro hemolysis.

Table 10.2: Antibody screening (Worksheet for laboratory).

Sl. No.	Name	Age	Sex	Patient MRD No./ Donor Unit No.	Reagent Cells	Technique						Signature
						Room temperature Saline	37°C Saline	37°C Albumin	I stage Enzyme	Saline	LISS*	
					OI							
					OII							

*LISS, low ionic strength solution.

- Mixed-field agglutination is found with anti-Sd^a and Lutheran antibodies.

5. **Differentiate between True Agglutination and Rouleaux Formation**
   In case of positive antibody screening, before starting extensive workups, it is recommended to investigate the patient's diagnosis, review methodologies, and obtain a new sample.
   Antibody screening (Worksheet for laboratory) is presented in Table 10.2.

False-Positive Reactions

A positive antibody screen is observed when there is prior exposure to red cell antigens from pregnancy or transfusions. Recognition of false-positive reactions and its potential causes is equally important as the detection of clinically significant antibodies. False-positive reactions that appear like an agglutination can cause unnecessary testing and delay if transfusions. Causes of false-positive reactions are listed in Box 10.4.

Rouleaux: Nonspecific aggregation of RBCs is called as rouleaux. Rouleaux are one of the most commonly encountered anomalous serologic reactions. Its formation, though not a significant finding observed during antibody screening tests, is **confused with antibody-mediated agglutination upon macroscopic examination**. Rouleaux are not observed in the IAT phase of testing because the washing

Box 10.4: Causes of false-positive reactions.

- Rouleaux
- Antibodies to preservatives
- Fibrin
- Contamination of the sample
- Presence of cryoprecipitate from frozen samples
- Polyethylene glycol (PEG) (if the reactions are read at 37°C)

steps remove the majority of plasma proteins responsible for rouleaux formation.

- **Causes of rouleaux formation:** Rouleaux formation is an invitro phenomenon that may occur with serum of **patients having altered albumin-to-globulin ratios** (e.g. multiple myeloma) or from **patients who were given high-molecular-weight plasma expanders** (e.g. dextran). It may be difficult to detect antibodies by direct agglutination in a test serum that has rouleaux-producing proteins.
- **Characteristics of rouleaux:** Following features helps in differentiating between rouleaux and agglutination:
  - Red cells in rouleaux have a **"stacked coin" appearance** when examined **under microscope**.
  - **Rouleaux are seen in all tests containing the patient's serum,** including the autologous control and the reverse ABO grouping.
  - Rouleaux **do not interfere with the AHG phase of testing**. This is because

of the washing of the patient's serum before the addition of the AHG reagent.
- Unlike agglutination, rouleaux are **dispersed by the addition of one to three drops of saline** to the test tube.

Limitations of Antibody Screening Tests

Antibody screening tests are designed to detect as many clinically significant antibodies as possible and to avoid detecting insignificant antibodies. When a three-cell screen set is used, a negative result in all three cells indicates that there are no clinically significant antibodies. However, **antibody screen will not detect antibodies in following situations**:
- It **cannot detect antibodies when their titer is dropped below the level of sensitivity** for the screening method used.
- It **cannot detect antibodies directed against low-prevalence (low-frequency) antigens** that are not present on any of the RBCs in the screen cell set.
- If none of the screen cells have homozygous expression of the target antigen, the **antibodies showing dosage may not be detected**.

Factors influencing the sensitivity: Several factors may influence the sensitivity of the antibody screen. These include cell-to-serum ratio, temperature and phase of reactivity, length of incubation, and pH (refer pages 11-5).

ANTIBODY IDENTIFICATION

Agglutination or hemolysis at any stage of antibody screening test **indicates that the screening test is positive** (i.e. red cell antibodies are present in the serum of a blood recipient). This indicates the need for antibody identification studies to identify the specificity of antibody detected. **Determination of the specificity of a red cell antibody** in blood banking is called **antibody identification**. This **needs reagent red cell antibody identification panels** and is performed only when the antibody screen test is positive. Patient or donor serum/plasma is tested with the reagent (antibody identification panel) cells to identify the specificity of an antibody to red cell antigens.

Reagents for Antibody Identification (Antigen Identification Red Cell Panels)

Features of Initial Antibody Identification Red Cell Panels (Reagents)

- The **serum or plasma is tested against an antibody identification panel.**
- The **main difference between antibody screening and antibody identification is the number of panel cells used** for testing. Antibody screening is generally performed using two to four different donor cells (panel cells), while **antibody identification uses cells from a larger number of donors**. Generally, an antibody identification panel cells consists of a collection of **11-20** (depending on the manufacturer) **group O RBCs** (packaged in sets) with known antigen composition and various antigen expression. However, if the initial testing does not provide a clear reactivity pattern, additional cells must be tested and/or other antibody identification methods must be used.
- Each **reagent red cell sample in the panel** is **obtained from a different donor**.
- The phenotypes of the **reagent red cell should have diverse pattern of antigen expression**. This diverse pattern of antigen expression should be possible to distinguish one antibody from another. It should be distributed in such a way that **single common alloantibody specificities can be clearly identified** and most others can be excluded. A reagent red cell panel must **possess** the majority of the **most inherited red cell antigens** and must be able to **identify most commonly frequently/encountered clinically significant alloantibodies** (e.g. anti-D, anti-E, anti-K, and anti Fy^a). The panel should include reagent red cells with homozygous expression (double-dose antigen expression) of common antigens that show dosage. Thus, it should include

cells with homozygous (double-dose antigen) expression of Rh, Duffy, Kidd, and MNSs antigens.
- The reagent red cells are selected in such a way that **positive and negative reactions will result when the reactivity of all panel cells is considered.**
- Patterns of reactivity for most examples of single alloantibodies should not overlap with any other. For example, all the K⁺ red cells should not be the only ones that are also E⁺.
- Each panel/set of commercial panels of screen cells should be **accompanied by an antigen profile sheet** specifying which antigens are present in each vial of cells and provide a place to record reactions **(refer Fig. 10.5)**. Similar to the screen cells used in antigen detection, the profile sheet for identification panel is lot-specific and should not be interchanged with that of another panel. The profile sheet usually indicates the presence of rare cells, which are positive for low-prevalence antigens or negative for high-prevalence antigens.
- **Source**: Usually, red cell samples are **commercially available**. However, the panel of red cells for antibody screening may also be prepared in the blood bank laboratory from regular local donor population or staff members by doing full phenotyping of all O Rh positive and O Rh negative donors/staff members. Except in special circumstances, the panel cells belong to blood group O. This allows to test serum or plasma of any ABO blood group.
- **Method**: For the initial identification of antibody, the same methods and test phase as in antibody detection or cross match should be performed using commercial red cell reagent panel.
  - Tube-testing protocols have greater flexibility for reading at different phase of the test namely immediate spin, room temperature, 37°C and IAT. The gel-column and solid-phase methods involve a single reading of the test at the IAT phase.
- **Use of enhancement media** may be helpful in enhancing the detection of certain antibodies (e.g. anti-M, -N, -P1, -I, -Le^a, or Le^b).
- **Expiry date**: After the expiry date, the panel cells should not be used as sole source for antibody identification. However, after initial identification with the in-date reagent cells, red cell reagent with expired date can used to exclude or confirm uncommon specificities.
- They are stored as reagents for antibody detection (refer page 191).
- The antibody detection should not be performed using pooled reagent cells.

Note: The antigen extended-profile sheet lists the phenotypes of the red cells. Correct panel sheet should be used and should not be interchanged when interpreting results. This is because the combination of red samples is different for each lot of reagent (profiles are lot-specific).

Antibody panel in antibody **identification** is given in Box 10.5.

Abbreviated identification panel:
- If the history suggests that the patient had previously detected to have an antibody, the known antibodies should be considered when selecting reagent red cells for the antibody identification test. For example, if the patient previously had anti-e, testing the patient's serum with commercial reagent red cells panel in

Box 10.5: Antibody panel in antibody identification.

- Group O RBCs
- Available in sets ranging from 10 to 20 vials
- Best to test using same enhancement media used in the screen
- Panel antigen profiles are lot-specific. Hence, use the correct one.
- *Autocontrol*: Optional to perform not normally done with screen
  o Patient's RBCs tested against patient's own serum in the same manner as the antibody panel
  o Helps determine whether alloantibody or autoantibody specificity exists

which 9 of 10 red cell samples are e-positive is not helpful. Hence, it is better to test selected panel of e-negative red cells to find out any newly formed antibodies. It is not needed to test or confirm for anti-e in such patients because regardless of reactivity to anti-e, only e-negative blood unit will have to be selected for transfusion.

- If the patient's red cell phenotype is known, it is necessary to select those reagent cells which detect the antibodies that are potentially likely to form. For example, if the patient's Rh phenotype is C-E+c+e, it is not necessary to select red cell reagent cells to exclude anti-E and anti-c. This is because the individual is not expected to form these antibodies (i.e. anti-E and anti-c) in which the individual is having antigen E and c. Exceptions is those individuals who have weak or altered (partial) Rh antigens and those in which Rh phenotype is predicted by DNA testing rather than serology.

Autologous Red Cell Phenotype

It is necessary to determine the phenotype of an individual's autologous red cells by serology or genotyping. This is because the antibody maker's red cells are expected to lack antigens which produce alloantibodies. Determining a phenotype autologous red cell may not be always simple. Recent transfusions or immunoglobulins coating the red cells may cause difficulty in determining the correct phenotype unless techniques are used to rectify these issues. These techniques include separation of autologous cells or removal of bound albumin. Red cell genotyping (molecular extraction of DNA from white cells) is the best method to get valid phenotype and avoids interference from circulating donor cells or Ig-coated patient red cells.

Three types of reagent red cells are used for routine testing (Box 10.6).

Preanalytic Phases of Antibody Identifcation

Preanalytic phases of antibody identification are outlined in Box 10.7.

Box 10.6: Reagent red cells used for routine testing in blood bank.

- A_1 and B cells in ABO serum testing
- Screening cells to detect red cell antibodies
- Panel cells to identify red cell antibodies

Box 10.7: Preanalytical steps involved in antibody identification.

Preanalytic information: It requires examination of the patient's history.
- Age, sex, race
- *Medical history:*
  - Previous antibody identification
  - History of pregnancy
  - History of prior transfusion
- Diagnosis and disease
- Drug (medication) and biological therapies
- Reason for transfusion (transfusion need) or blood products
- *Sample volume:* Know whether the volume of sample provided is sufficient to complete the evaluation.

Patient History

It is helpful to find out the antibody identification process. Before beginning the antibody identification, patient's medical history should be considered. Information regarding the patient's age, sex, race, diagnosis, transfusion and pregnancy history, medications, and intravenous solutions may provide valuable clues in antibody identification studies. This is particularly in complex cases.

History of Previous Red Cell Exposure

Usual exposure to foreign red cells may occur during transfusion and pregnancy: It will help to know whether the patients were exposed to "non-self" RBCs via transfusion or pregnancy. It is uncommon for patients to produce clinically significant alloantibodies unless the individual has been transfused or pregnant. Women are more likely to develop alloantibodies because of exposure to foreign (i.e. fetal) red cells during pregnancy. Infants < 6 months usually do not produce alloantibodies but newborns may have passive antibody derived from mother.

Transfusion: If there is history of previous transfusion, it is important to know whether the transfusion was during the past 3 months.
- In a patient **transfused within the past 3 months**, a positive DAT result may be due to a delayed hemolytic transfusion reaction. *Autoadsorption* (refer page 212) can be performed if the patient has not been recently transfused (in the preceding 3–4 months).
- If the **transfusion is recent**, the results of antigen-typing the patient's RBCs must be interpreted carefully. This is because positive reactions may be due to the presence of donor RBCs remaining in the patient's circulation. Positive reactions caused by donor RBCs usually show mixed-field agglutination. *Alloadsorption* (refer page 212) must be used if the patient has been recently transfused. If the laboratory is not informed about the recent transfusion and autoadsorption is performed, it is possible the persisting transfused antigen-positive cells could adsorb alloantibody, making it not detectable in tests of the adsorbed sera.
- **Naturally occurring antibodies** (e.g. anti-M, anti-Le^b) should be **suspected in patients with no history of transfusion or pregnancy**.
- History of previous antibody identification. The reason for checking for previous antibodies is that antibodies do not always persist for the person's lifetime.

Diagnosis and Disease

Some diseases may be associated with red cell antibodies.
- **Anti-I:** It may be associated with cold agglutinin syndrome, Raynaud phenomenon, and infections with *Mycoplasma pneumoniae*.
- **Anti-i:** May be associated with infectious mononucleosis.
- **Autoantibody anti-P:** Paroxysmal cold hemoglobinuria associated with syphilis in adults and viral infections in children may show autoantibodies anti-P especially by Donath-Landsteiner test.
- **Warm antibodies**: May be seen in autoimmune hemolytic anemia, systemic lupus erythematosus, multiple myeloma, chronic lymphocytic leukemia or lymphoma.
- **Passive antibodies**: May develop in patients who have undergone solid-organ or HPC (hematopoietic progenitor cell) transplants that originated from the donor passenger lymphocytes.

Drug (Medication) and Biological Therapies

For example, IVIG, Rh-immune globulin (RhIG), and antilymphocyte globulin may passively transfer antibodies such as anti-A or anti-B, anti-D, and antispecies antibodies, respectively. This will result in the presence of an unexpected serum antibody.

Autoantibodies: The patient's history is important when the autologous control or DAT is positive. Certain infectious and autoimmune disorders may be associated with RBC autoantibodies, and some medications can cause positive DATs. Patients with *autoantibodies* require adsorption to look for underlying alloantibodies.

As with any testing, it is important to complete the preanalytic phase to ensure laboratory qualification processes for reagents and equipment, including preventive maintenance before the first sample is processed for the day.

Analytical Phase

Initial Panel

Once antibody is detected in the pretransfusion antibody screen, it should be followed by testing the serum or plasma against a panel of reagent red cells to identify the specificity of antibody/ies. This antibody detection panel, similar to the antibody screening cells, consists of group O reagent red cells with phenotypes for most common antigen specificities. Manufacturers prepare antibody detection panels with various antigen configurations, which may include 10, 11 (Fig. 10.5), 15, 16, or 20 cells and be considered extended antibody screens. Initial testing of the antibody detection panel cells uses the same potentiators as those in the

Manual of Transfusion Medicine

Donor	Cell no.	D	C	c	E	e	Cw	K	k	Kpa	Kpb	Jsa	Jsb	Fya	Fyb	Jka	Jkb	Lea	Leb	P1	M	N	S	s	Lua	Lub	Xga
R1R1	1	+	+	0	0	+	0	0	+	0	+	0	+	+	+	+	0	0	+	+	+	+	+	+	0	+	+
R1r	2	+	+	+	0	+	+	+	+	0	+	0	+	+	0	0	+	0	+	0	+	0	+	+	0	+	+
R1R1	3	+	+	0	0	+	0	0	+	0	+	0	+	0	+	+	+	0	+	0	+	0	+	0	+	0	+	+
R2R2	4	+	0	+	+	0	0	0	+	0	+	0	+	+	0	+	+	0	+	+	+	0	+	0	0	+	+
r'r	5	0	+	+	0	+	0	0	+	0	+	0	+	0	0	0	+	+	0	+	+	0	+	+	0	+	0
r"r"	6	0	0	+	+	0	0	0	+	0	+	0	+	+	0	0	+	0	0	+	0	+	0	+	0	+	+
rr K	7	0	0	+	0	+	0	+	+	0	+	0	+	+	0	0	+	0	+	+	0	+	0	+	0	+	+
rr	8	0	0	+	0	+	0	0	+	0	+	0	+	+	+	0	0	+	0	+	0	0	+	0	0	+	+
rr	9	0	0	+	0	+	0	0	+	0	+	0	+	+	0	+	0	0	+	+	+	+	0	+	0	+	0
R1r	10	+	+	+	0	+	0	0	+	0	+	0	+	+	0	+	+	0	+	+	+	0	0	+	0	+	+
R0	11	+	0	+	0	+	0	0	+	0	+	+	+	0	+	0	+	+	0	0	+	0	+	+				
Patient cells																											

Fig. 10.5: Antibody identification panel sheet.
(+ = antigen present in the red cell panel; 0 = antigen is not present in the red cell panel).

antibody screen. An autocontrol is included with the panel, especially if not routinely tested with the antibody screen.

Test with RBCs of known phenotype: Antibody identification is accomplished by first testing the patient's serum or plasma against an extended panel of additional reagent RBCs of known phenotype (i.e. RBCs possessing known antigens) by the IAT technique. The antibody identification test method should be as sensitive as that used for antibody detection.

Autologous control (autocontrol) and DAT: The autologous control (autocontrol) is an important part of the antibody identification and should always be included as part of the testing. The autologous control (autocontrol) is performed by using serum or plasma and autologous red cells and testing under same conditions as testing against reagent red cells. This will help to differentiate whether autoantibody, alloantibody, or both are present. It is not the same or equivalent to a DAT.

- **Autocontrol negative:** Indicates that the serum reactivity is **most likely due to alloantibodies.**
- **Autocontrol positive:** Reactivity in the autocontrol due to in vitro phenomenon may be caused due to incubation and the presence of enhancement reagents.

If the autocontrol is found to be positive in the antiglobulin phase, a DAT should be done. **DAT test** is useful to confirm or rule out prior in-vivo sensitization of the patient's cells.

- **If the DAT result is positive**, then it is necessary to interpret it with careful attention to the transfusion history. **Examine the DAT** closely for the appearance of **mixed-field agglutination.**
  - If patient has an alloantibody and was **recently transfused**, the alloantibody may get attached to a minor population of transfused donor RBCs. The positive DAT may be due to coating of donor red cells with alloantibody. It causes classic mixed-field agglutination. This is the **first sign of a developing immune response.** This usually produces clinically significant delayed hemolytic transfusion reaction.
  - In a **massively transfused patient**, only a **small percentage of cells** may be **DAT-positive.**
  - Positive test may be due to autoantibodies or drugs.
- **If the DAT result is negative**, then it is probably due to the antibodies to a constituent of an enhancement medium or autoantibodies that are reactive only in the presence of enhancement

medium. Warm autoantibodies and cold autoantibodies such as anti-I, -IH, or Pr may react in IAT when certain enhancement media are used. Hence, it is necessary to repeat IAT using another enhancement medium.

The immunohematologist then compares the pattern of positive and negative serum reactions against the antigen phenotype pattern on the printed worksheet that accompanies each panel to find a match.

INTERPRETATION (EVALUATION) OF PANEL RESULTS

The results of antibody identification are recorded for each phase and negative reactions are confirmed with check cells (IgG-sensitized reagent red cells). It is followed by and evaluation of panel results which should be carried out in a systematic step-by-step method as discussed below. This will ensure that antibody is properly identified and to avoid missing antibody specificities that might have been masked by other antibodies. Antibodies generally fall into the following categories:

- **Single antibody specificity**: It has a pattern which is easily identified with a panel following the rules of interpretation. Confirmation of the specificity can be done by identifying that the patient or donor is negative for the corresponding antigen.
- **Multiple antibodies**: It needs the use of carefully selected cells and additional techniques such as enzymes. It needs a good understanding of antibody characteristics of various blood groups.
- **Antibodies to high-frequency antigens**: It should be suspected if all panel cells are positive.
- **Antibodies to low-frequency antigens**: They are usually found with other antibodies. Identification needs additional cells for testing.
- **Weak IgG antibodies**: They can be enhanced by using different potentiators, increasing the serum-to-cell ratio, or increasing incubation time.
- **Cold alloantibodies**: They are usually clinically insignificant.
- **Autoantibodies:** They may be cold or warm type. They should be suspected if the autocontrol or DAT is positive. Adsorption and elution techniques (refer pages 213-4) are usually performed to identify the antibody on the red cell and the alloantibody in the serum.

General Assessment of Positive and Negative Reaction

It is the first step of the interpretation process. Results of antibody detection are interpreted as positive or negative depending on the presence or absence of reactivity. This reactivity may be in the form of **hemagglutination or hemolysis in serum tests or red cell effacement in solid phase tests.** Both positive and negative reactions are equally important in antibody identification. They provide general idea of the specificity (ies) present in the sample.

- **Positive reactions**: Their phase and strength can be compared to the antigen patterns of the panel red cells to help to suggest specificity.
- **Negative reactions:** They support the specificity suggested by the positive reactions.
- A single common alloantibody usually gives a clear pattern with antigen-negative and antigen-positive reagent red cells. Exclusion of antibodies must be done to ensure that all antibodies have been properly identified. After evaluating each negatively reacting cell, examine the remaining antigens to see if the pattern of reactivity matches a pattern of antigen-positive cells (inclusion technique).
1. **Identify the reaction strength of positive reaction:** The strength of the antibody reaction is a clue to the number of antibodies present. Check whether all of the positive cells react to the same degree. Carefully **grade the positive reactions** which may help in identification of antibody. The strength of the reaction indicates the amount of antibody available

to participate in the reaction. However, it does not indicate the significance of the antibody.
- **Stronger reaction:** Antibodies such as anti-K, anti-D, anti-E, anti-e, anti-c, and anti-C are commonly stronger than anti-Fy^a, anti-Fy^b, anti-Jk^a, anti-Jk^b, anti-S, and anti-s.
- **Antigen dosage**: The strength of the reaction also varies with the antigen dosage. A stronger reaction may be due to dosage (i.e. panel cells with homozygous antigen expression react more strongly than cells with heterozygous antigen expression). In some cases, weak antibodies may not even react with heterozygous antigen expression.
- **Reactions of varying strengths suggest the presence of more than one antibody**. A cell having more than one of the target antigens may react more strongly than a cell having only one of the target antigens.
- Some antigens with variable expression may also produce strong reaction. Few antigens such as I, P1, Le^a, Le^b, Vel, Ch/Rg, and Sd^a antigens are expressed more strongly on some RBCs than on others. The antibodies to these antigens may react more strongly with one panel cell than another.

2. **Identify the phase of positive reaction:** Reaction of positive cells and its relation to phase:
    - **Single versus multiple phases**:
        - If the reactions of certain cells occur at one phase and different cells at another phase (i.e. reaction at different/multiple phases) may indicate more than one (multiple) antibody and a combination of IgG and IgM antibodies.
        - Cells which react at multiple phases may be a sign of an antibody showing dosage. The cells with homozygous antigen expression react at an earlier phase than those with heterozygous antigen expression.
    - **Phase of reactivity** (Table 10.3)**:** The phase or reaction temperature at which agglutination is found is an indication that the antibody is IgG or IgM. Thus, it may provide a clue in establishing the clinical significance of an antibody.
        - **Immediate spin phase (room temperature** or colder): **IgM antibodies** are usually not significant and usually react at the immediate spin phase (room temperature).
        - **37°C incubation phase**: Some potent IgG antibodies, such as D, E, and K, may be detected following the 37°C incubation.
        - **Antiglobulin phase: IgG antibodies** are clinically significant and are usually detected during the **AHG** (antiglobulin) **phase**.

3. **Matching of serum reactivity (matching the pattern) with any of the remaining specificities:** The next step in panel interpretation is to look at the reactions that are positive. Match the pattern. If there is only a single alloantibody, the pattern of reactivity usually exactly matches a pattern of antigen expression.

Table 10.3: Phase of reactivity for common antibodies in transfusion medicine.

Phase	Antibodies	Immunoglobulin class	Clinically significant
Immediate spin phase (room temperature)	Cold autoantibodies (I, H, IH); Le^a, Le^b; M, N; P$_1$; Lu^a	IgM	No
37°C incubation	Potent cold (IgM) antibodies (mainly those causing hemolysis); Some warm antibodies, if high in titer (e.g. D, E, and K)	Usually IgG that activate complement	Yes
Antiglobulin (AHG) phase	Rh antibodies; Kell; Duffy; Kidd; S, s; Lu^b; Xg^a	IgG	Yes

Antibody Detection (Screening) and Identification

4. **Exclude all commonly encountered RBC antibodies:**
   - **Low prevalence antibodies:** The chance of exposure to low prevalence antigens is low and thus the antibodies against them are uncommon. Hence, it may not be necessary to perform additional tests to exclude these specificities.
   - **High prevalence antibodies:** These are commonly observed antibodies and it is important to test selected cells that will rule out the presence of these antibodies.
5. **Result of the autologous control (Autocontrol):** The autocontrol reveals whether the antibody is alloantibody or autoantibody specificity. In autocontrol, the patient's red cells are suspended with the patient's serum. It is incubated with the panel cells and is read at the same phases as the panel. In the interpretation or worksheet, the autocontrol is usually included at the end of the panel, indicated on the panel as "patient cells."
   - **Positive reactions** are due to autoantibody. Autoantibodies may be classified into cold autoantibody or warm autoantibody type, depending on the optimal reaction temperature. The autocontrol and DAT help determine whether an autoantibody or alloantibody is present.
     - Usually, a **positive autocontrol or positive DAT (Table 10.4) indicates an autoantibody or an antibody produced against recently transfused red cells**.
     - A positive **autocontrol and the negative DAT** indicate a **false-positive result**. The **potentiator may be the cause of false-positive** results. In such situation, the panel should be repeated using a different type of potentiator or no enhancement solution.
     - Negative reactions are caused by alloantibody.
     - The presence of autoantibodies may mask the presence of alloantibodies,

Table 10.4: Interpreting a positive direct antiglobulin test.

Condition	Specificity	Serum antibody
Transfusion reaction	IgG	Specific alloantibody
Autoimmune disease • Warm antibody • Cold antibody and pneumonia	IgG (C3) C3	Reacts with all cells at antihuman globulin phase Reacts with all cells at colder temperatures
Drug interaction	IgG (C3)	Serum may be nonreactive
Clot tube stored at 4°C	C3	None
Hemolytic disease of the fetus and newborn (HDFN); maternal antibodies on infant's red blood cells (RBCs)	IgG	Alloantibody or ABO antibody from mother on blood cells

and complicates the process of antibody identification.

Interpretation of a positive DAT is presented in Table 10.4.

6. **Ruling out:** Panel cells that give negative reactions (0) with all tested phases are used to rule out antibodies.
   - If an **antigen-antibody reaction did not occur**, the antibody did not react with the antigen on the panel red cell and **it can be eliminated as a possible antibody**.
   - **Caution**: Panel cells that are heterozygous, particularly in the Duffy, Kidd, and MNS system, should not be ruled out. This is because the **antibody might have been too weak** to react **or is exhibiting dosage**.
   - Continue ruling out using the panel cells that gave a negative reaction.
7. **Confirm the suspected antibody (Rule of three):** Antibodies identification involves performing tests and making a conclusion based on antibody reaction patterns. Conclusive antibody identification requires testing the patient's serum with at least three antigen-positive (red cells that

react) and three antigen-negative (red cells that do not react) cells (also known as the 3 and 3 rule). This "rule of three" should be met. Rule of three is confirming the presence of an antibody by demonstrating three cells that react and three that do not react. This will ensure that the pattern of reactivity is not the result of chance alone. If there were not enough cells in the panel, additional cells from another panel would be selected for testing. This panel is known as a selected cell panel.

8. **Confirm that the patient lacks the antigen corresponding to the detected antibody:**
   - Individuals cannot produce allo-antibodies to antigens present on their own RBCs. Hence, the last step in antigen identification studies is to test the patient's RBCs for the corresponding antigen. If a negative result is expected it is an additional evidence that identification results are correct.
   - If the patient's RBCs are positive for the corresponding antigen, it indicates that the antibody identified is wrong or due to a false-positive result.
   - Antigen typing may be helpful to resolve complex cases as it may eliminate possible specificities.
   It is not possible to do extend typing on all patients with antibodies. However, it can be useful, especially in patients who chronically receive transfusions and are at risk for alloimmunization. This category of patients includes those with sickle cell disease or thalassemia.
   Important guidelines and concepts for interpretation and evaluation of a panel in antibody identification are outlined in Table 10.5.

Antibody Exclusion and Initial Specificity Assessment

The first step in the interpretation of panel results is to exclude antibodies that could not be responsible for the reactivity seen. Such method is called as "cross-out," "rule-outs," or "exclusion" method. To perform exclusions or "rule-outs," note the RBCs that gave a negative reaction (nonreactive) of the patient's sample with the red cells that expresses the antigen in all phases of testing. The antigens on these negatively reacting red cells are probably not the antibody's target.

Once the results of all panels have been recorded, the antigen profile of the first nonreactive red cells is examined on the antigen worksheet. If an antigen is present on the red cell and the patient sample was not reactive with it, the presence of the corresponding antibody may be excluded tentatively. Generally, this rule-out technique is to be performed only if there is homozygous expression of the antigen on the cell. This avoids excluding a weak antibody that is showing dosage. However, there are few low-prevalence antigens that are rarely expressed homozygously. These include K, Kp^a, Js^a, and Lu^a. After all of the antigens for the red cell sample have been crossed out, the same process is done with the other nonreactive red cell; additional specificities are then excluded. In most circumstances, this process leaves a group of antibodies that have not been excluded.

- **Exclusion of clinically significant allo-antibodies** should be done at least for antigens namely: D, C, E, c, e, K, Fy^a, Fy^b, Jk^a, Jk^b, S, and s.
- Then evaluation of red cells that are reactive is done. If the antigen pattern exactly matches the test reactivity, this is most likely identifying the specificity of the antibody. Additional testing may be required to eliminate remaining specificities that were not excluded.

Selected Red Cells for Exclusion and Confirmation

To confirm or rule out the presence of antibody use selected red cells which either carry or lack the specific antigens. For example, if a pattern reactive red cells fits anti-Jk^a, but the anti-K and anti-S were not excluded, the serum should be tested with selected red cells. Usually, the red cells chosen should have the phenotypes namely: Jk(a-), K+, S-, K-, S+; and Jk(a+), K-, S-.

Table 10.5: Summary of guidelines for interpretation of a panel in antibody identification.

Observe at	Result	Interpretation
Autocontrol	Negative	Alloantibody
	Positive	Autoantibody or drug interaction
		Delayed transfusion reaction in which transfused cells are sensitized with antibody
Reaction phase	Room temperature or immediate spin	Cold or IgM antibody
	Reaction at 37°C	Reaction started at room temperature: May be cold (IgM)
		Reaction not seen at room temperature but noticed at AHG: May be warm (IgM)
	Antihuman globulin (AHG)	Clinically significant warm or IgG antibody
Reaction strength	Single strength	Probably one antibody specificity
	Varying strength	More than one antibody or one antibody showing dosage
Ruling out	Negative reaction	No reaction: Probably antibody to antigen on the panel was not present
		If the antigen on the panel red cells is heterozygous: The antibody may be showing dosage which should be ruled out
	Positive reaction	Never rule out when there is positive reaction
Matching the pattern	Single antibody	Pattern of positivity matches one of the antigens in the panel
	Multiple antibody	If more than one antibody, it is difficult to match to a pattern unless the phases or reaction strength are unique
Rule of three	Three positives	Is the suspected antibody negative with at least three panel cells that are antigen-positive?
	Three negatives	Is the suspected antibody negative with at least three panel cells that do not possess the antigen?
Patient's phenotype	Negative	If the patient does not possess the antigen, it is possible to make antibody
	Positive	Transfused red blood cells (RBCs) are present if patient received a unit of RBCs within last 3 months
		Suspected antibody is not correct

Probability of Accurate Identification

Accurate identification of antibody greatly depends on two factors namely: (1) the antibody having a sufficient titer (i.e. quantity of circulating antibody) to provide reliable positive reaction and (2) antigen strength on test cells must be adequate to provide a consistent target antigen. Conclusive antibody identification needs the sample to be tested against a sufficient number of red cell samples that lack and express the antigen that corresponds with the antibody's apparent specificity.

Consistency of Antibody Identified with Autologous Red Cell Phenotype

Individuals do not produce alloantibodies to antigens they possess (self-antigens). The patient's autologous red cell phenotype is used to support the presumptive antibody identification. The red cells should lack the corresponding antigen. Another way to confirm antibody identification is to test the patient's red cells to ensure they are negative for the antigen corresponding to the identified antibody. This should be performed only if no recent transfusions are given. Donor red cells may remain in the circulation for 3 months and may cause misleading and incorrect results if there are different cell populations. The accurate phenotype of a recently transfused patient may need cell separation techniques to separate transfused and autologous or patient red cells.

Transfusion

Transfusion in the last 3 months: Phenotyping may be complicated in a patient who gives a positive DAT or has been transfused in the last 3 months. When the DAT is positive due to IgG coating the RBCs, typing reagents using the IAT may give invalid results. The IgG coating antibody blocks the antigen sites and prevents the typing serum from reacting. The AHG reagent will react with the coating antibody and gives a false-positive result. The antibody coating should be removed and then freed into a solution to get an accurate phenotype and this process is called elution (refer page 210).

Recent transfusion: Mixed-field reactions are common when phenotyping is performed in recently transfused patients. The donor cells stimulate antibody formation and react with the typing serum, whereas the patient's autologous cells do not react.
- **Reticulocyte typing** can be done to know an accurate phenotype of the patient's autologous cells. In this technique, the patient's RBCs are drawn into microhematocrit tubes and centrifuged. The reticulocytes being less dense than mature RBCs, the patient's reticulocytes form layer on the top of the RBC layer. These reticulocytes can be harvested and used for antigen typing.

Positive and negative control cells: They should be tested on the day of use with each antiserum used for antigen typing.
- **Positive control cell**: It should have heterozygous antigen expression to ensure that the antiserum has the sensitivity to detect small quantities of the antigen.
- **Negative control cell**: The target antigen should be absent in these cells to confirm reactivity with only the target antigen.

Methods of antigen typing:
- **Routine antigen typing**: It is performed using the tube, solid phase adherence, or gel methods.
- **Flow cytometry**: It is used to detect minute quantities of antigens.
- **Molecular methods**: Polymerase chain reaction (PCR) is used to examine DNA for the single-nucleotide polymorphisms (SNPs) that give rise to various RBC antigens. Molecular testing can screen multiple antigens at one time and screen large numbers of donors in a relatively short time. There is no interference of these methods due to a recent transfusion or positive DAT on the RBCs.

Panel interpretation for antibody identification is outlined in Box 10.8).

Additional Techniques (Selected Procedures) for Resolving Antibody Identification

Routinely, the same method is used for antibody detection tests and antibody identification. In certain circumstances, the initial antibody identification panel may not reveal a clear-cut specificity. In such situations, additional testing or alternative techniques and methods are needed or required to resolve complex antibody identification problems. It is to be kept in mind that no single method is enough to detect all antibodies. If routine methods fail to indicate specificity, or the presence

---

Box 10.8: Panel interpretation for antibody identification.

Phase of reactivity:
- IgM reacts best at low temperatures (immediate spin phase)
- IgG reacts best at AHG phase
- Reactions at more than one phase may be due to a combination of IgM and IgG antibodies
- Reaction strength
  - Gives clue to number of antibodies present
  - Varying strengths suggest more than one antibody or dosage
- Autocontrol
  - If negative, suspect alloantibody
  - If positive, suspect autoantibody

of an antibody is suspected but cannot be confirmed, the use of other enhancement techniques or procedures may be helpful. It is necessary to run autocontrol when techniques involving enzyme treatment of red cells, testing at lower temperatures or testing with various enhancement media are used. This will ensure proper interpretation of results.

Selected Cell Panels

- It is the simplest step in which test is performed taking additional cells from a different panel. Such cells selected for testing should have minimal overlap in the antigens they possess.
- Selected cell panels are also useful when a patient has a known antibody and to determine whether additional antibodies are present.

Enzymes

If there is suspicion of multiple antibodies in a sample, treating the panel cells with enzymes may help separate the specificities and help for their identification.

Enzymes used: Ficin and papain are most commonly used enzymes to treat RBCs. Other enzymes used include bromelain, trypsin, α-chymotrypsin or pronase.

Effect (Table 10.6): Enzymes modify the RBC surface by removing sialic acid residues from the red cell membrane and by denaturing, eliminating or removing glycoproteins. This will destroy certain antigens and enhance expression of others (exposing the antigen).

Uses: Two procedures can be used for enzyme treatment.
- **One-stage enzyme test method**: In this, patient serum, enzyme (papain), and red cells are incubated together. Enzymes can be used instead of enhancement media, such as LISS or PEG, in a one-step enzyme test method.
- **Two-stage enzyme test method**: It is a more sensitive method in which the panel RBCs are first treated with enzymes (ficin or papain) and washed. Then the antibody identification panel is performed using the treated cells without other enhancement media in the antiglobulin test. The enzymes destroy some antigens. Hence, it is not possible to exclude all specificities using the enzyme panel alone. Whenever possible, it is advisable to compare the reactivity of the same cells before as well as after enzyme treatment. The following observation may be helpful in antibody identification.
  - Observe which cells reacted positively in the untreated panel but did not react (or gave weaker reactions) with the treated panel.
  - Also observe cells that reacted more strongly or at an earlier phase in the enzyme panel than in the untreated panel.

After enzyme treatment, red cells are retested with the serum to determine whether the antibody (or mixture of antibodies) is still reacting. When using an enzyme-treated cell, observe agglutination only at the AHG phase to avoid false-positive reactions. Because enzymes denature some antigens, it should not be used as the only antibody detection or identification method.

Neutralization (Inhibition) Techniques

There are certain soluble substances in the body and in nature which have antigenic structures similar to RBC antigens. These substances can be found in body fluids such as saliva, urine, and plasma. They can also be found in natural sources or can be synthetically prepared. These can be used to neutralize antibodies (inhibit the reactivity of the antibody) that could mask the presence of underlying non-neutralizable antibodies in serum. The inhibition of the reactivity by these

Table 10.6: Enzyme treatment and their effect on blood group.

Blood group	Reactivity with enzymes treatment
Rh, P1, I, Kidd, Lewis	Antibody reactions enhanced
M, N, S, Duffy	Antigens are destroyed (S and s variable)
Kell	Not affected

soluble substances can help for separation of antibodies or confirmation that a specific or particular antibody.

Method:
- First, the patient's serum is incubated with the neutralizing substance. This allows the soluble antigens in the neutralizing substance to bind with the antibody.
- Then an antibody identification panel is done using this treated serum. The neutralizing substance inhibits reactions between the antibody and panel RBCs.
- However, **it is necessary to run a control** (saline and serum) to prove that the loss of reactivity between the antibody and panel RBCs is due to neutralization and not due to dilution of antibody strength by the added neutralizing substance.

For example, if a suspected anti-P1 does not produce a definitive pattern of agglutination and loss of reactivity after the addition of a soluble P1 substance (that dissolves anti-P1) suggests that the specificity is anti-P1.

Use: This technique is **useful when there is suspicion of multiple antibodies**. Table 10.7 lists sources of some neutralizing substance.

Elution

Elution **frees antibody bound to a RBC** and can be used for several purposes (Box 10.9).

Principle of elution technique is depicted in Figure 10.6. Elution is a method used to release, concentrate, and purify antibodies bound to antigen on sensitized red cells. The

Table 10.7: Examples of sources of neutralization substances for antibodies.	
Antibody	Source of neutralizing substance
Anti-P$_1$	Hydatid cyst fluid, ovalbumin of pigeon eggs (commercially prepared P$_1$ substance is also available)
Anti-Lewis (Le^a and Le^b)	Plasma or serum, saliva (commercially prepared Lewis substance also available)
Anti-Sd^a	Urine
Anti-Chido, anti-Rodgers	Ch and Rg antigens are epitopes on the fourth component of human complement (C4) present is serum
Anti-I	Human breast milk

Box 10.9: Uses of elution techniques.
- To investigate a positive DAT result
- To concentrate and purify antibodies, detect weakly expressed antigens, identify multiple antibodies
- Prepare antibody-free red cells for autologous adsorption studies

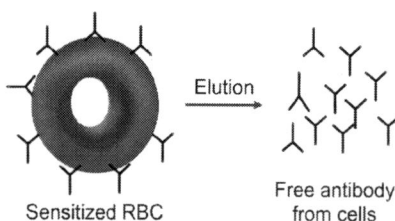

Fig. 10.6: Principle of the elution technique.

extract or the material obtained after removal of antibody from red cells (elution) is called an eluate and is used for antibody identification.

Methods: The methods employed to release the bound antibody are:

i. **Glycine acid:** This lowers the pH. It is rapid and sensitive. However, Kell antigens are denatured during this method, so phenotyping of patient cells cannot be reliably done for Kell.

ii. **Heat freeze-thaw** (physical): Changing the thermodynamics of the antigen-antibody reactions. It is rapid, effective for ABO antibodies and inexpensive. However, it is not sensitive for antibodies other than ABO.

iii. **Ether, methylene chloride, and chloroform:** It is an organic solvent that is sensitive and inexpensive. However, it is hazardous, carcinogenic and inflammable.

Objective: The objective is to recover bound antibody in a usable form. Most critical step in preparing any eluate is the original washing. The washing is performed to remove unbound immunoglobulins. If not washed properly, these antibodies will remain in the test system and will contaminate the final eluate and give false-positive results. As a control, the supernatant obtained after the last wash should be tested in parallel with the eluate to detect the presence of unbound antibody.

The last wash should be nonreactive and if it is reactive, the eluate results will be invalid.

After elution, the serum may be tested against an RBC panel to identify the antibody.
- **Total elution** in which antibody is released and the RBC antigens are destroyed, is usually needed in antibody identification.
- **Partial elution** in which antibody is removed but RBC antigens remain intact, is useful to prepare RBCs for phenotyping and to use in auto adsorption procedures.

Uses: Uses of elution techniques are listed in Box 10.9.

Technical factors: Technical factors influencing the outcome of elution procedures are outlined in Box 10.10.
- **Incomplete washing:** It is necessary to thoroughly wash (six washes in saline) sensitized cells before an elution to prevent contamination of elute with unbound residual antibody. To know the efficacy of washing, the supernatant fluid from final wash should be nonreactive when tested for antibody.
- **Binding of antibody to glass surfaces:** If an eluate is prepared in the test tube that was used during the sensitization or washing phases, antibody that nonspecifically binds to the surface of the test tube may dissociate during the elution. This can be avoided by transferring the red cells used to prepare an eluate to a clean test tube before washing and then to another tube before the elution procedure is initiated.
- **Dissociation of antibody before elution:** IgM antibodies (e.g. anti-A, anti-M) or low-affinity IgG may dissociate spontaneously from red cells during washing phase. This can be minimized by cold (4°C) saline or using wash solution supplied by manufacturer.
- **Incorrect technique:** These include: (1) incomplete removal of organic solvents and (2) failure to correct the tonicity or pH of elute. These may cause the reagent cells used in the test to hemolyze or appear "sticky." If there is stromal debris, it may interfere with reading of test results. Hence, it is necessary to follow correct technique.
- **Instability of elutes:** Elution into saline results in dilution of protein and these are unstable. After preparation, the eluate should be tested as early as possible. Alternatively, stability can be achieved by adding bovine albumin to the final concentration and freezing the preparation during storage. Elutes can also be prepared in antibody-free plasma or 6% albumin.

Adsorption

Adsorption is a **procedure in which red cells (known antigens) are used to remove red cell antibodies from a solution** (plasma or antisera). For example, group A red cells can remove anti-A from solution. Similar to the neutralization technique, antibodies from serum can be removed by adsorption. Absorption method can be used in cases where the coating antibody resists elution. In the adsorption method, the **antibodies from the serum are adsorbed by adding the red cells containing corresponding target antigen.** The antibody in the serum attaches to the membrane-bound antigen on the RBCs. The antibody remains attached to antigen on the red cells and this antigen-antibody complex forms solid precipitates. They can be removed by centrifugation (serum/plasma and cells get separated). The bound antibody to RBCs can be harvested by elusion or we can examine the supernatant adsorbed serum/plasma for antibody (ies) remaining after the adsorption process. Then this absorbed serum/plasma is tested against an RBC panel for the presence of unabsorbed alloantibodies. The adsorbent used is usually RBCs but another antigen-bearing substance may also be used.

Box 10.10: Technical factors influencing the outcome of elution procedures.
- Incomplete washing
- Binding of antibody to glass surfaces
- Dissociation of antibody before elution
- Incorrect technique
- Instability of elutes

- If the patient's RBCs are positive for the target antigen, it indicates that the antibody coating the red cells is absorbed from the diluted antiserum, and the supernatant will react negatively when tested against a cell with heterozygous antigen.
- If the patient's RBCs are negative for the target antigen, the antibody will remain in the antiserum, and the supernatant will be positive when tested against the heterozygous cell.

Commercial reagents for adsorption: These include human platelet concentrate (to adsorb Bg-like antibodies [against erythrocytic B-G antigens] from serum) and rabbit erythrocyte stroma (RESt) (possesses I, H, and IH-like structures and absorbs cold-reacting autoantibodies).

Autoadsorption (Fig. 10.7)

Autoadsorption is attachment of the patient's antibodies to the patient's own red cells and subsequent removal from the serum. Autoantibodies are usually removed through adsorption techniques. Simplest method of adsorption is by using the patient's own RBCs.
- First the autologous red cells are washed thoroughly to remove unbound antibody.
- These cells are then treated to remove any autoantibody coating the RBCs.
- Next, the cells are incubated with the patient's serum for up to 1 hour. Temperature of incubation depends on the thermal range of the autoantibody being removed. Usually 37°C for warm-reacting autoantibodies and 4°C for cold-reacting autoantibodies. The sample is inspected for any evidence of agglutination throughout the incubation period.
- If agglutination appears, it indicates that all the RBC binding sites are saturated with autoantibody. The serum is then harvested and incubated with new aliquots of autologous RBCs.
- When no agglutination is seen during incubation, the harvested serum is tested against the patient's RBCs. If no reactivity is observed, the absorption is complete. The serum now contains only the alloantibody.
- However, if a reaction is observed, it indicates that the autoantibody remains in the serum. Hence, it needs further absorption. About three to six aliquots of RBCs may be necessary for autoadsorption. Some powerful warm autoantibodies may not be removed completely by adsorption and may only diminish the reactivity.

Allogeneic Adsorption

It is the use of blood from a genetically different individual, such as reagent or donor cells that have been phenotyped for common red cell antigens, to remove alloantibodies and autoantibodies.

Homologous Adsorption

If a patient is severely anemic that it is not possible to get enough autologous RBCs to perform an adequate number of adsorptions or when a patient has been recently transfused (donor RBCs in the specimen may adsorb

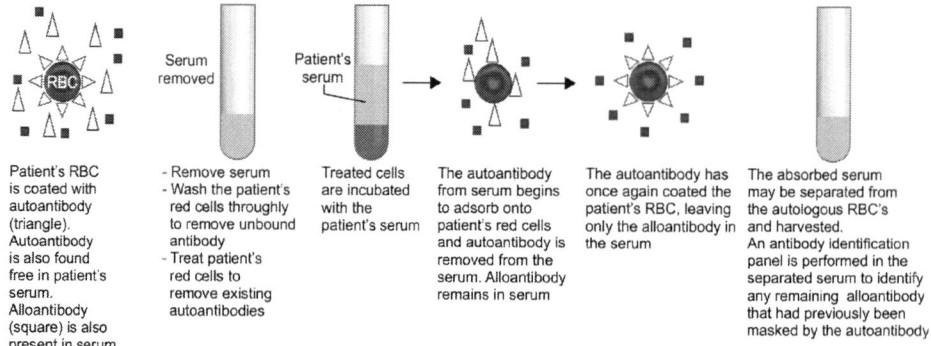

Fig. 10.7: Steps for performing an autoadsorption.

Antibody Detection (Screening) and Identification

alloantibodies), it may be necessary to perform homologous or differential adsorptions instead of autoadsorption. For homologous adsorption, the patient is first phenotyped, and then phenotypically matched RBCs are used for the adsorption in place of autologous red cells.

Differential Adsorption (Fig. 10.8)

When phenotyping the patient is difficult as a result of a positive DAT or recent transfusion, differential absorption can be done. In this method, the patient's serum sample is divided into a minimum of three tubes/aliquots. Each tube/aliquot is adsorbed using a different phenotyped red cell. One cell is usually R_1R_1, one is usually R_2R_2, and the third is usually rr. After adsorption, antibody identification panels are separately performed on each tube/aliquot to determine the specificity. The reactivities seen are compared to reveal underlying alloantibodies.

Uses of adsorption technique are listed in Box 10.11.

Increased Serum-to-Cell Ratio

If the antibodies are present in low concentrations, its reactivity may be enhanced by increasing the volume of serum incubated with a standard volume of red cells. One of the procedures that are widely accepted is to mix 4 volumes (drops) of serum or plasma with one volume of 2–5% saline suspension of red cells and incubate the mixture for 60 minutes at 37°C. The contact between the red cells and antibodies can be promoted by periodic mixing during incubation.

Box 10.11: Uses of adsorption technique.

- Separate multiple antibodies in a single serum
- Remove autoantibody so as to detect or identify underlying alloantibodies
- Remove unwanted antibody (e.g. anti-A, anti-B or both) from serum that can be used as a reagent
- Confirm the presence of specimen on RBCs by their ability to remove antibody of corresponding specificity

Increased Incubation Time

Routine incubation time used for tests varies depending on whether enhancement media is used or not. Usually, it is 10–15 minutes for some enhancement media and 30 minutes for tests without any enhancement media. In albumin or saline tests, extending the incubation time to 30 and 60 minutes often improves the reactivity and clarify the pattern of reactions. When LISS or PEG is used, extended incubation time is contraindicated because of reduction or loss of reactivity.

Combined Adsorption-Elution

Uses: Combined adsorption-elution tests can be used to: (1) separate a mixture of antibodies

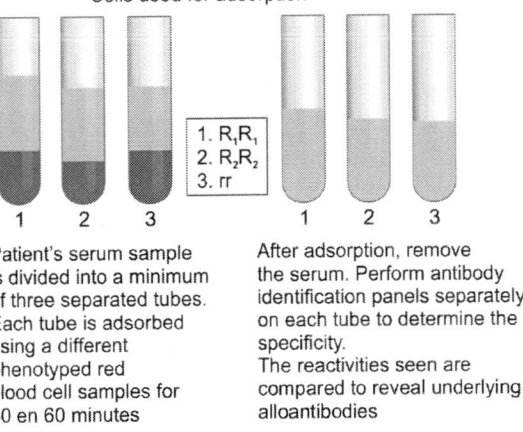

Cells used for adsorption

1. R_1R_1
2. R_2R_2
3. rr

Patient's serum sample is divided into a minimum of three separated tubes. Each tube is adsorbed using a different phenotyped red blood cell samples for 30 en 60 minutes

After adsorption, remove the serum. Perform antibody identification panels separately on each tube to determine the specificity. The reactivities seen are compared to reveal underlying alloantibodies

Fig. 10.8: Steps in differential adsorption.

in a single-serum sample, (2) to detect weakly expressed antigens on red cells, or (3) to identify weakly reactive antibodies.

Method: First incubate the serum with selected red cells and then elute antibody from the adsorbing red cells.

Precautions: The red cells used for adsorption to separate a mixture of antibodies should express only one of the antigens corresponding to the antibody. This is because the eluate will contain only one type of antibody.

Direct Antiglobulin Test and Elution Techniques

Detection of antibodies coating RBCs is important; when investigating there is suspicion of hemolytic transfusion reactions, HDFN, and autoimmune and drug-induced hemolytic anemias. The DAT is performed (refer page 179 and Fig. 9.5) to detect in vivo sensitization of RBCs.

- In the tube method, the **patient's RBCs are thoroughly washed** to remove any unbound antibody, and then **AHG reagent is added**. If there are **IgG antibodies or complement coating the RBCs**, there will be **agglutination**. If neither is present, there will be no agglutination. To validate the negative test, Coombs' control cells are added.
- DAT may also be done by other methods such as solid phase adherence and gel methods.

If IgG antibodies are detected, the next step is to dissociate the antibodies from the RBC surface by elution (refer page 210) so that it can be identified.

Temperature-dependent Methods

The simplest methods involve altering the temperature of the antigen-antibody environment. Heat can be used to remove antibody. After washing with saline, coated RBCs are suspended in an equal volume of saline or albumin. Temperature-dependent elution methods are best for detecting IgG antibodies directed against antigens of the ABO system.

- The gentle heat method is performed at 45°C. It removes the antibody but leaves the RBC intact.
- Elution performed at 56°C is a total elution method. This allows antibody identification.
- The Lui freeze method is also a total elution method. In this method, washed, coated RBCs suspended in saline or albumin is frozen at -18°C or colder until solid. The mixture is then thawed rapidly. This leads to bursting of RBCs and frees the bound antibody.

pH

Changing the pH of the test can change the reactivity of certain antibodies. Change in the pH can enhance reactivity of some and decrease that of other antibodies.

- Reduction of pH by acid elution is a common and relatively quick and easy method for total elution to detect non-ABO antibodies. In this method, the washed antibody-coated cells are mixed with a glycine acid solution at a pH of 3. The low pH disrupts the antigen-antibody bond and releases the antibody into the acidic supernatant. The supernatant is harvested, and the pH is neutralized so that antibody identification testing can take place. Acid elution can also be done using citric acid and digitonin acid.
- When pH is lowered to 6.5, anti-M is enhanced. The pH can be lowered to about 6.5 by taking 1 volume of 0.1 N HCl to 9 volumes of serum or plasma.

Organic Solvents

Several organic solvents such as dichloromethane, xylene, and ether have been used in total elution methods. They act on the lipids in the RBC membrane and reduce surface tension. This reverses the van der Waals forces that hold antigens and antibodies together. Organic eluates are very potent when compared to the temperature-dependent eluates and are best for detecting non-ABO antibodies.

Antibody Detection (Screening) and Identification

Disadvantages: Its procedures are time-consuming, and the chemicals may be health and safety hazardous (may be carcinogenic or flammable). Hence, they are rarely used in the clinical laboratory.

Antibody Titration

After the identification of an antibody, sometimes it is useful to quantify the amount of this antibody (antibody concentration levels). Techniques such as flow cytometry, radioimmunoassay, or enzyme-linked immunoassay may give more precise results. However, these methods are not readily available in most of the laboratories. Hence, in most of the laboratories antibody concentration levels are determined by performing an antibody titration.

In this technique, the titer of an antibody is usually determined by testing serial twofold dilution of the serum containing an antibody. These diluted serum samples are tested against a suspension of selected RBCs that possesses the target antigen. The **titer level** (result) is the reciprocal of the highest (greatest) serum dilution in which macroscopic agglutination (of 1+ or greater) is found. A score may also be given depending on the strength of reactivity. Each reaction is given a value, and the score is determined by adding up each value. After the initial titer is determined, the specimen should be frozen. When new specimens are submitted for determination of titer, the initial titer specimen should also be tested in parallel to control variability among technique (e.g. pipetting, grading reactions) and the relative strength of the target antigen on the cells used in testing. The current specimen's results are then compared with the initial specimen's results. A four-fold or greater increase in titer (reactivity in two or more additional tubes) or an increase in score of 10 or more is considered to be significant.

Precautions: When performing the antibody titers following precautions are necessary:
- **Careful preparation of dilutions** is necessary. Contamination from a tube with a higher antibody concentration can give falsely elevated titer-level results. This problem can be prevented by changing pipette tips between each tube when preparing the dilutions and working or reading from the most diluted tube to the least diluted.
- The **phenotype of the RBCs** used in testing **should be consistent** throughout the series of titer-level studies. If for the initial titer a red cell with homozygous antigen expression was used, then all subsequent titer specimens should be tested against a homozygous red cell.
- The **method used must** also **be consistent**. Titers using the gel method are more sensitive than those using the tube method and give a higher titer level.

Uses of titer-level studies:
- **Prenatal studies**: Useful in **monitoring the obstetric patient who has an IgG antibody** that may cause HDFN. If an antibody titer level during pregnancy increases, it suggests that the fetus is antigen-positive and therefore, there is a risk of developing HDFN. An increasing titer level may indicate the necessity of intrauterine exchange transfusion.
- To **differentiate immune anti-D from passively acquired anti-D due to RhIG** administration. The titer level in RhIG is rarely above 4.
- **Antibody identification**: To **confirm the presence of antibodies that are usually not clinically significant but may mask significant antibodies**. These, previously known as high titer, low avidity (HTLA), are antibodies directed against high prevalence antigens. They are observed at the AHG phase of testing with weakly positive reactions. The weak reactions may persist even with dilutions as high as 2048. Examples of these antibodies include anti-Ch, anti-Rg, anti-Cs^a, anti-Yk^a, anti-Kn^a, anti-McC^a, and anti-JMH.
- **Separating multiple antibodies**: Titration results may suggest that one antibody is reactive at higher dilution than the other antibody.

Obtaining Autologous Red Cell Phenotype

If the patients were transfused in the past 3 months, it may be difficult to determine the patient's red cell phenotype. If a pretransfusion specimen is available, it should be used to determine the phenotype. If pretransfusion sample is not available, the patient's newly formed autologous red cells can be separated from the transfused red cells and then phenotyped. Separation of young red cells by centrifugation is based on the differences in the densities of new and mature red cells. Separation is most successful when ≥ 3 days have elapsed since the last transfusion, which will provide time for new autologous red cell production. New autologous red cell must be isolated from the sample when it is fresh. The technique is ineffective and can often result in false-positive typing if the sample is too old (> 24 hours) or the patient is not producing new red cells.

COMPLEX ANTIBODY IDENTIFICATION

Not all antibody identifications are straightforward.

Multiple Antibodies

When a sample contains two or more (i.e. more than one antibody) alloantibodies, it may be difficult to interpret the results obtained from single panel of red cells. It requires additional techniques to resolve the problem. The following findings may suggest the presence of multiple antibodies.

1. **The observed pattern or reactive and nonreactive red cells does not fit a single antibody:** When the exclusion approach fails to indicate a specific pattern, it is helpful to determine whether the pattern matches two combined specificities. If the reaction pattern does not fit two combined specificities, the possibility of presence of more than two antibodies must be thought of.
2. **Reactivity occurs at different test phases:** When tube tests are performed and reactivity occurs at several phases, each phase along with the strength of reaction should be analyzed separately.
3. **Unexpected reactions** occur when attempts are made to confirm the specificity of a suspected dingle antibody.
4. *A phenotypically similar red cell is nonreactive:* A phenotypically similar red cell is one that lacks the same common antigens as the patient's red cells. When all or nearly all panel red cells are reactive, the simple way to recognize multiple antibodies is to test a phenotypically similar red cell. Absence of reactivity with a phenotypically similar red cell suggests that the alloantibodies are directed at common antigens which are absent from the test red cell.

Multiple Antibody Resolution

Reactivity without Apparent Specificity

Difficulties in the interpretation of antibody identification tests may be due to zygosity (i.e. copy number-refer page 189), variation in the expression of antigens and other factors. When the reactivity of the serum is very weak and/or the pattern of reactivity and cross-out process have excluded all probable possibilities, alternative approaches are needed. These are as follows:

Alternate Test Method

Depending on original method used, it may be necessary to either enhance antibody reactivity by using a more sensitive method or to decrease the sensitivity of the method to avoid detection of unwanted and clinically insignificant reactivity. Examples of more sensitive methods include PEG, enzymes, increased incubation time, or increased serum-to-cell ratio. Methods to inactivate certain antigens on the reagent red cells may also be helpful (e.g. enzyme treatment for antigens Fy^a and Fy^b). Adsorption or elution methods to separate antibodies selectively adsorb and isolate unknown reactivity, and elution of unknown reactivity from adsorbing cells can concentrate the antibody.

Optimal Phase or Temperature for Antibody Was Not Tested

When a weak or questionable positive result is observed at the IAT phase, perform tube tests with readings at immediate spin phase at room temperature or 37°C (if these phases were not included in the original testing). This may make clearly visuality of an antibody that optimally reacts as a direct agglutinin at 37°C or below.

Potential Phenotype Exclusion

If serum reactivity has no apparent specificity, type the patient's red cells by serology or genotyping for common red cell antigens, and eliminate from initial consideration specificities that correspond to antigens on the patient's autologous red cells. This along with other techniques may help in identifying on specificities of the antibodies. Phenotyping may not be possible when the patient has been recently transfused or has had a positive DAT result.

Presence of Antigens in Common

Instead of excluding antibodies to antigens on nonreactive red cells, close observation may identify presence of antigens in common. Typing the patient's red cells to confirm that they do not have the corresponding antigen may also be useful.

If strongly positive results are obtained, the exclusion method should be used with nonreactive cells to eliminate specificities from initial consideration. The strongly reactive reagent cells may be examined for any antigen in common.

The presence of some antigens in common may suppress the expression of other antigens. This can miss weak antibodies or certain red cells to be unexpectedly nonreactive when a suspected antibody fails to show reactivity will all antigen-positive red cells.

Inherent variability

Some antibodies vary markedly in their expression on red cells from different individuals.

Unlisted antigens

A sample may react with an antigen which is not routinely listed on the antigen profile supplied by the manufacturer of the reagent. Though serum studies show clearly reactive and nonreactive test results, such antibodies may not be recognized. In such situations, review additional phenotype information provided with reagent panel or consult the manufacturer. If one cell is unexpectedly reactive, this is most likely to be due to antibody to a low-prevalence antigen.

ABO types of red cells tested

The sample may be reactive with many or all the group O reagent red cells but not with red cells of the same ABO group as the autologous red cells. Such a reaction pattern occurs mostly with anti-H, anti-IH, or anti-Le^{bH}. Group O and A$_2$ red cells have more H antigen than A$_1$ and A$_1$B red cells, which express very little H. Thus, sera containing anti-H or anti-IK strongly react with O group reagent cells, whereas autologous A$_1$ or A$_1$B red cells or donor red cells used for cross matching may be weakly reactive or nonreactive.

Warm Autoantibodies

When the patient's sera contain warm-reactive autoantibodies, it may be reactive with almost all red cells tested. Majority of warm autoantibodies are IgG type and IgM, warm autoantibodies are unusual, but they may cause severe and often fatal autoimmune hemolytic anemia. If a patient with warm autoantibodies needs transfusion, it is necessary to detect any clinically significant alloantibodies. Solid-phase and gel-column methods and use of PEG, enzymes, and LISS (to a lesser extent usually enhance warm-antibodies. If such tests are nonreactive, it can exclude common alloantibody specificities and same procedure can be used for compatibility testing without the need for adsorptions.

If such tests remain reactive, adsorption is needed to rule out alloantibodies.

Cold Autoantibodies

Cold autoantibodies may be clinically benign or pathological. All potent cold autoantibodies that are reactive with all red cells (including patient's own) at room temperature or below can create problems. This is especially so when the reactivity persists above room temperature and in IAT phase of antibody identification. In such cases, it is difficult to detect and identify potential clinically significant alloantibodies that are masked by cold autoantibody reactivity. The detection of cold autoantibodies depends on the test method employed. Gel-column method may give a mixed-field appearance even though there is only one cell population. Solid-phase minimizes their detection. There are different approaches to test sera with potent cold autoantibodies. Once the presence of cold autoantibodies is confirmed, these should be removed to detect the underlying and potentially clinically significant antibodies. These may be achieved as follows:

- Omit the room-temperature and/or immediate-spin phase of testing if it was performed.
- Use anti-IgG instead of polyspecific AHG reagent for IAT phase of antibody identification.
- Cold auto- or allogeneic adsorption of the patient's serum or plasma to remove autoantibodies but not alloantibodies.

Delayed Serologic/Hemolytic Transfusion Reactions

Definition: Delayed transfusion reactions are the development of a new alloantibody in a patient following transfusion. It results in laboratory evidence (serologic) or laboratory and clinical evidence (hemolytic) of the destruction of incompatible transfused red cells that were compatible at the time of infusion.

If the patient has been transfused in the last 3 months and autocontrol is positive in the IAT phase, there may be antibody-coated donor cells in the patient's circulation. It results in a positive DAT that can show mixed-field reactivity. An elution should be performed, especially when tests on plasma or serum are inconclusive. It is rare for transfused red cells to make the autocontrol positive at a phase other than IAT, but this can occur, especially with a newly developing or cold-reacting alloantibody. If the DAT result does have a mixed-field appearance and the plasma or serum is reactive with all cells tested, a transfusion reaction caused by an alloantibody to a high-prevalence antigen should be considered.

Antibodies to High-prevalence Antigens

If all reagents red cells are reactive in the same test phase and with uniform strength but the autocontrol is nonreactive, an alloantibody to a high-prevalence antigen should be considered. Antibody to a high-prevalence antigen can be identified by testing selected red cells of rare phenotypes and by typing the patient's autologous red cells with antisera to high-prevalence antigens. Chemically modified and/or enzyme-modified red cells (e.g. DTT-treated or ficin-treated red cells) can give characteristic reactivity patterns that help limit possible specificities.

If red cells negative for a particular high-prevalence antigen are not available, red cells that are positive for the lower prevalence antithetical antigen can sometimes be helpful.

Antibodies to Low-prevalence Antigens

If a sample is reactive only with a single donor or reagent red cell sample after alloantibody exclusions are complete, an antibody to a low-prevalence antigen should be suspected. This can be identified by testing a panel of reagent red cells that express low-prevalence antigens with the serum. Alternatively, one reactive red cell sample can be tested with known antibodies to low-prevalence antigens.

CONSIDERATIONS FOLLOWING ANTIBODY IDENTIFICATION

After the detection and identification of unexpected red cell antibodies, next step is to determine the clinical significance. This is followed by providing an effective transfusion of red cell component or to identify the need for further monitoring for HDFN.

Significance of Identified Antibodies: To predict the clinical significance of the unexpected antibody, two factors should be taken into consideration namely: (1) phase in which the antibody is identified and (2) its specificity.

- Antibodies that are reactive at 37°C and in an IAT or both are potentially clinically significant.
- Antibodies that are reactive at room temperature or below are usually not clinically significant.

Subsequent Antibody Identification in Patients with a Known History of Antibodies: After a clinically significant antibody is detected, the patient should be given red cells negative for the corresponding antigen. It is not usually necessary to routinely repeat the identification of known antibodies in subsequent pretransfusion testing.

Selection of Donor Units for Patients whose Serum Contains Antibodies: When the patient sample contains clinically significant antibodies or the patient has a history of clinically significant antibodies, **RBC units for transfusion must be negative for the corresponding antigen**. Even if the antibodies are not detectable, all future RBC transfusions should be antigen-negative blood to prevent secondary immune response. The crossmatch technique must demonstrate compatibility at the AHG phase.

SUMMARY

- The aim of the antibody screen is to detect unexpected antibodies in the plasma/serum in recipient or donor.
- The antibodies may be classified as immune (due to RBC stimulation in the patient), passive (transferred to the patient through blood products or derivatives), or naturally occurring.
- Antibodies may also be classified as alloantibodies (i.e. against foreign antigens), or autoantibodies (i.e. against own antigens).
- A clinically significant antibody is one that causes reduced survival of RBCs possessing the target antigen. Clinically significant antibodies are IgG antibodies that react best at 37°C or in the AHG phase of testing. They can cause hemolytic transfusion reactions and HDFN.
- Screen cells are prepared group O RBC suspensions obtained from individual donors who are phenotyped for the most commonly encountered and clinically important RBC antigens.
- Enhancement reagents (e.g. LISS and PEG) are solutions added to serum and cell mixtures in the IAT to promote antigen-antibody binding or agglutination.
- Coombs' control cells are RBCs coated with human IgG antibody. They are added to all AHG-negative tube tests to ensure that washing step was adequately performed and that the AHG reagent is present and functional in the test system.
- Apart from tube testing, alternative methods such as gel and solid phase adherence methods are available. These alternative methods may be automated to increase efficiency.
- The antibody exclusion method rules out possible antibodies based on antigens that are present on negatively reacting cells.
- The aim of the antibody identification is to know the specificity of the antibody (if discovered during antigen screening).
- The process of alloantibody identification and resolving complex autoantibody problems becomes easier with experience.
- The DAT detects RBCs that were sensitized with antibody in vivo. Elution methods help to free antibody from the red cell surface and allow antibody identification.
- In each type of antibody problem, a methodical process should be followed to take into account important clues and reach an accurate conclusion.

SELF-ASSESSMENT EXERCISE

Long essay on:
- Discuss advances in antibody screening and compatibility testing

Write short notes on:
- Importance of antibody screening in blood transfusion
- Antibody screening in blood transfusion therapy
- Importance of antibody screening in blood transfusion

CHAPTER 11

Pretransfusion and Compatibility Testing

CHAPTER OUTLINE

- Steps in pretransfusion testing
- Pretransfusion testing in special circumstances

INTRODUCTION

Pretransfusion testing also referred to as **compatibility testing,** refers to set of **procedures** (serologic and nonserologic protocols) **required before blood is issued as being compatible**. A compatibility testing is an entire quality process **composed of many procedures**. The compatibility testing involves many steps and designed to provide the safest blood product possible for the recipient of the transfusion. The compatibility procedures in the broader sense in transfusion service include proper record keeping, accurate donor and recipient identification, sample collection and handling, actual serologic testing of the recipient specimen before transfusion and crossmatching. Compatibility testing is a term often considered synonymous and confused with crossmatching. **Crossmatching (crossmatch test) is one of the components of compatibility test that is performed** prior to release of red blood cells for transfusion. The compatibility testing begins with the transfusion request and ends with the transfusion of blood product to the recipient. In current blood banking, the crossmatch is only one element of what is referred to as pretransfusion (compatibility) testing.

Purpose of pretransfusion testing: To select blood and its components such that

- The transfused red blood cells (RBCs) should have an acceptable survival rate when transfused.
- There should not be significant destruction of recipient's own red cells, i.e. prevent an immune-mediated hemolytic transfusion reaction. There should be no adverse reactions from transfused blood.

Pretransfusion testing will confirm ABO compatibility between component and the recipient and detect most clinically significant unexpected antibodies.

None of the current pretransfusion testing (including compatible crossmatch) can guarantee neither normal survival of transfused RBCs in the recipient's circulation nor always avoid adverse responses to transfusion. The benefits of RBC transfusion should be weighed against the potential risks. A careful and meticulous in vitro testing and compatible units sometimes can undergo hemolysis in the patient.

STEPS IN PRETRANSFUSION TESTING

Pretransfusion compatibility testing protocol with different steps are outlined in Box 11.1.

Request for Transfusion

All requests for transfusion (blood and blood components) must be accompanied by a

Box 11.1: Pretransfusion testing protocol.

- A request to perform testing and prepare components for transfusion (blood or blood products).
- Recipient blood sample collection:
  ○ Patient's identity: Accurate identification of patient (recipient)
  ○ Acceptable blood sample: Proper sample collection, labeling and handling
- Check and review the patient's previous blood bank records, if any.
- Pretransfusion testing of recipient's blood specimen:
  ○ ABO grouping and Rh typing
    – ABO forward testing: Recipient red blood cells with anti-A and anti-B
    – Rh testing: Recipient red blood cells with anti-D and a Rh control, if needed
  ○ Test for detection of unexpected/irregular antibodies (antibody screen): Recipient serum (plasma) with screening cells. Antibody identification (if possible)
  ○ Review and comparison of previous records with the present for blood type and unexpected antibodies
- Donor
  ○ RBC unit testing: ABO group confirmation and Rh type confirmation for Rh-negative RBC units
  ○ ABO reverse testing: Recipient serum (plasma) with A_1 cells and B cells
  ○ Donor red cell unit selection: Selection of ABO and Rh compatible donor blood that is compatible with the transfusion recipient. It should be free from blood transmissible infections and unexpected allogeneic irregular antibodies
- **Crossmatch**: Crossmatch of recipient's sample with donor units:
  ○ Selection of crossmatch procedure:
    – Serologic
    – Computer or electronic
  ○ Selection of blood for transfusion
  ○ Performance of a crossmatch: Recipient serum with donor red blood cells
- Proper labeling of blood or blood components of donor before use with the recipient's identifying information and issue
- Reidentify recipient before transfusion
- Carefully observe recipient's vital signs during and after transfusion
- Monitor post-transfusion hematocrit and hemoglobin levels for efficacy of transfusion

request form (Box 11.2). The request form must be complete, accurate, and legible. It must contain the information about the patient and should be signed by the doctor in-charge of the patient or any authorized person. The request form is in effect a prescription.

The details given in request form should match with the details on blood sample received.

Incomplete request form should not be accepted. Always record the time of receiving the request form. A new sample of blood must be asked, if the earlier blood transfusion was given more than 3 days back.

- **Terms used to define the priority of testing:** "STAT" (at once), "ASAP" (as soon as possible), or "routine"
- **Patient location in the hospital:** It can also help determine urgency for testing priority; for example, a location of emergency room (ER) or operating room (OR).
- Accurate identification of patient (recipient) and recipient's acceptable blood sample is necessary.

Recipient Blood Sample

Safe and accurate pretransfusion testing begins with the patient's (recipient's) blood sample.

Identification of Patient (Recipient) and of Blood Sample, and Labeling Requirements

Proper collection: The sample of blood for pretransfusion testing should be collected after proper identification of recipient (patient) by the patient's physician (doctor in-charge of the patient). Accurate patient identification is very important for the safety of patient. The blood sample should be properly collected in a clean dry screw cap test tube/vial/vacutainer (in case the tests are done by automation).

> **Box 11.2:** Request form with information to be provided along with blood sample.
>
> - Date
> - Full name of patient
> - Date of birth/age
> - Gender/sex and weight
> - Hospital registration number (ID No)
> - Ward and bed no.
> - Patient's address
> - Clinical diagnosis
> - Patient's blood group (if known)
> - Presence of any antibodies
> - History of previous transfusion or any previous transfusion reaction
> - Obstetric history (in female)
> - Number of blood units required
> - Number and type of blood components/products required including any special needs (e.g. irradiation) or special processing required (e.g. volume reduction)
> - Indications for transfusion
> - Date and time of the proposed transfusion (i.e. when blood component is required)
> - Type of request (priority indicator): STAT (at once)/ASAP (as soon as possible), routine/emergency/group and screen, transfuse on date, preoperative, standby, etc.
> - Name and signature of the physician/authorized health professional requesting the blood

Proper labeling: The collected sample should be properly labeled using an undetachable legible and indelible label. The label should bear sufficient information with accurate patient details. The label must provide the following details of patient (recipient), i.e. patient's (recipient's) first and last name, age, gender, unique identification number (e.g. hospital no), ward/bed, and date of collection, etc. To prevent a possible sample mix-up, never use prelabeled tubes for blood collection.

Errors during collection of blood: The **major cause of transfusion-associated fatalities** and greatest threat to safe transfusion therapy are **due to clerical error**.

- The most common cause of error is **misidentification of the recipient** when the blood sample is drawn or when the transfusion is given to the recipient. Other causes include mix-up of samples during handling in the laboratory.
- This results in incorrect ABO groupings and transfusion of ABO incompatible blood. The hemolytic transfusion reactions are due to misidentification of patients or sample labeling errors.
- For patient identification, many laboratories use electronic identification system that uses machine-readable information. For example, Bar-coding technology helps in avoiding possible errors.

Confirm sample linkage (sample and the requisition form) and acceptability of blood specimen: Laboratory personnel while receiving the pretransfusion sample in the laboratory must match and confirm that the information provided on the sample label and the information on the requisition form are in agreement. A new sample must be obtained if there is any doubt.

Sample Needed

Pretransfusion testing needs **recipient red cells and either serum or plasma**. Plasma is preferred over serum, because clotted serum may contain small fibrin clots with trapped red cells which may produce false positive results. Hemolyzed or lipemic samples may create difficulties in visualizing agglutination during crossmatching.

Sample Collection Tubes

Plain tubes without anticoagulant and tubes with ethylenediaminetetraacetic acid (EDTA) are most commonly used. In case of emergencies, it is not necessary to wait for a blood specimen to clot, especially when most crossmatches are performed at immediate-spin (IS).

Age of Sample

Pretransfusion samples collected for testing should reflect the current antibody status of a patient. Hence, it should be collected **within 3 days** (day of collection is day 0) **of the scheduled transfusion,** if:
- The patient/recipient has been transfused with blood or components containing RBCs within the preceding 3 months, or
- The patient/recipient has been pregnant within the preceding 3 months, or
- The history of previous transfusion or antibody is uncertain or not available.

Many laboratories prefer a 3-day limit for all pretransfusion testing samples. Patient samples and a segment from the donor unit used for crossmatching must be stored for at least 7 days after transfusion. This is required for necessary investigation in case there is transfusion reaction.

If there is no history of recent pregnancy or transfusion and no current or past unexpected antibodies, the sample may be kept and reused. This will be useful for preoperative testing before a patient's surgical procedure and crossmatching at the time of need. In case where patients are repeatedly transfused, new samples may be required for these patients (e.g. every other day).

Appearance of Collected Sample

- **Hemolyzed sample**: If the serum or plasma is hemolyzed during the collection process it should not be used and a fresh sample should be collected. Various mechanical causes of hemolysis include the use of small-gauge needles, trauma to a vein, the forcible emptying of blood into the tube, or the further addition of blood to a partially clotted sample. The hemolysis caused by mechanical trauma may mask the detection of antibody-induced hemolysis (a positive reaction in some examples of ABO, P1, Lewis, Kidd, or Vel system antibodies).
- **Diluted samples:** Samples diluted with intravenous fluids are also not acceptable. In diluted samples, there are chances of missing a weak antibody or there may be false-positive reactions caused by the molecules in the intravenous fluid.
- **Patients with intravenous fluid infusion**: In these patients, the blood should be collected from below an intravenous site, preferably from a different vein and ideally from the other arm. In situation where the intravenous site is the only site for drawing blood, the intravenous catheter should be turned off and flushed with saline. Then the first 5–10 mL of blood is to be discarded and the sample is collected.

Checking the Patient's Previous Record

It is necessary to perform a record check for the patient before any pretransfusion testing. If the patients have history of transfusion, their previous records (Box 11.3) must be checked (if possible). Any inconsistencies or problems must be investigated and resolved before proceeding with transfusion.

Pretransfusion Testing of Recipient Blood

Pretransfusion testing on the recipient's (patient's) sample includes the determination of the patient's ABO and Rh typing, an antibody screen, and a crossmatch (Table 11.1). ABO, Rh grouping, and antibody screening of the patient's serum can be done in advance or at the same time as the crossmatch. A record must be maintained of all results obtained in testing patient samples. Accurate medical

Box 11.3: Previous details of a patient who has history of transfusion.

- Discrepancies in previous ABO and Rh blood group
- Presence of clinically significant antibodies
- Any problem encountered during earlier blood grouping/typing and compatibility testing
- Any transfusion reaction

Table 11.1: Various tests performed in pretransfusion testing.

Test	Components used
ABO forward (front) typing	Recipient red blood cells with anti-A and anti-B
Rh typing	Recipient red blood cells with anti-D and a Rh control, if needed
ABO reverse (back) typing	Recipient serum (plasma) with A_1 cells and B cells
Antibody screen/detection	Recipient serum (plasma) with screening cells
Crossmatch	Recipient serum with donor red blood cells

history including information on medications, recent blood transfusions, and previous pregnancies are very helpful.

The terms ABO phenotype, ABO type, and ABO group are used to describe the detectable ABO red cell antigens. They are used interchangeably in the blood bank.

Testing methods: Pretransfusion testing may be done **by traditional tube method or using semiautomated or automated tests** that use column agglutination, microplate solid-phase or hemagglutination-microplate techniques.

ABO Grouping

To transfuse an ABO and Rh compatible blood, determination of the patient's (recipient's) correct ABO group and Rh are the most important pretransfusion serological tests.

Method (refer pages 71-74): ABO grouping can be performed in tubes, using column gel technology or solid-phase RBC adherence. ABO grouping of patient's samples must be performed by using forward and serum grouping methods.
- In forward grouping or front typing, patient's red cells are tested with anti-A and anti-B reagent.
- In reverse or back typing, patient's serum or plasma is tested against group A_1 and group B reagent red cells.
- If the results of ABO forward and reverse grouping do not agree, additional testing must be done to resolve the discrepancy.
- If immediate transfusion is necessary before resolution of the patient ABO group, patient should receive group O Rh-negative red cells.
- Donor red cells must be ABO compatible with recipient's plasma.

Rh Typing (Refer Pages 106-9)

- Rh typing of the recipient is performed using **recipient's red cells which are tested for D antigen** using commercially available anti-D reagents.
- Tube tests should be performed according to the manufacturer's directions using a suitable control to avoid a false-positive interpretation. These controls must be run in parallel when Rh typing tests are performed on patient samples to avoid wrong designation of Rh-negative patients as Rh-positive.
- If the Rh type of the recipient cannot be determined and immediate transfusion is necessary, Rh-negative blood should be given. However, most monoclonal or monoclonal blend anti-D reagents react at room temperature and do not require the use of a control.
- The test for weak D (D^u) is unnecessary when testing transfusion recipients as there is no harm by giving Rh (D) negative blood to these patients. Female patients with weak D are considered Rh-positive and may receive Rh-positive blood during transfusion. On direct testing, if individuals are Rh-negative they should receive Rh-negative blood, and those Rh-positive should receive Rh-positive blood. There are those in the blood bank community who prefer complete Rh typing of all recipients to conserve Rh-negative blood for Rh-negative patients.

Repeat testing of donor blood: Blood bank is responsible for confirming the correct ABO labeling of all donor blood (whole blood or RBCs). It is **mandatory to retest ABO and Rh typing on all units labeled "negative."** For example, if an Rh-negative unit is mislabeled as Rh-positive, and transfused to a Rh-positive individual, it may not produce clinical harm. However, if an Rh-positive unit was mislabeled Rh-negative and if it is transfused to an Rh-negative recipient, it will produce an immunization to the D antigen. Retyping is performed by preparing a red cell suspension of the donor blood from a segment attached to the donor bag. Records of these repeat tests must be maintained for 5 years.

Antibody Screening (Detection) and Identification of Irregular (Unexpected) Antibodies

The recipient's serum or plasma must be screened for clinically significant unexpected/irregular antibodies. This should be done before doing crossmatching to select compatible blood. In general, clinically significant unexpected antibodies (Table 11.2) refer to antibodies that are reactive at 37°C or in the antihuman globulin (AHG) test. These antibodies are known to cause hemolytic disease of the fetus and newborn (HDFN), hemolytic transfusion reaction or unacceptably short survival of transfused RBCs. Antibodies reacting at 37°C and/or in the antiglobulin test are more clinically significant than cold reacting antibodies. Antibody screening (detection) and identification of irregular (unexpected) antibodies are discussed in detail in Chapter 10.

Unexpected alloantibodies form as a result of exposure to a foreign RBC antigen. This occurs by allogeneic transfusion of RBCs, pregnancy or transplantation. Its incidence depends on the patient's ability to respond to that exposure. The transfused donor RBCs should have best survival rate in the patient's (recipient's) circulation and the risk of hemolytic transfusion reaction should be reduced. This is achieved by detection of unexpected antibodies. Antibody screening tests detects the presence of all potentially clinically significant alloantibodies in the recipient's serum or plasma. If antibodies are detected during the screening tests, further tests are necessary to identify and also determine potential clinical significance. The results of these tests will help in deciding whether there is a need to select antigen-negative units for transfusion.

Before transfusion, the recipient's **ABO group and Rh typing** must be performed. It is also necessary to test for unexpected antibodies to red cell antigens (e.g. antibody screen) before transfusion of whole blood, RBCs, and granulocytes. Results obtained by current sample should be compared with precious transfusion service records to identify any discrepancies between the two.

CROSSMATCH TESTING (CROSSMATCHING)

The term crossmatch is a crossway mixing of donor and recipient blood components. In crossmatching, the serum or plasma from the recipient is mixed with red cells from the donor. A crossmatch is only one part of pretransfusion (compatibility) testing (refer Box 11.1).

Crossmatching is routinely done only with donor products containing red cells, hence must be performed for red cell transfusions. **Hemolysis or agglutination at any phase or step** of the crossmatch process **indicates that the antibodies present in the recipient** interact with donor red cell antigens and a mismatch between donor and recipient (Table 11.3). A crossmatch is considered as compatible when there is neither agglutination nor hemolysis in testing and the donor unit is acceptable for transfusion purposes. A crossmatch is considered as incompatible when either agglutination or hemolysis

Table 11.2: Clinical significance of 37°C-reactive antibodies.

Usual	Unusual
ABO	Bg (HLA)
Rh	Ch/Rg (complement C4)
Kidd	Le^b
Duffy	JMH
S, s, U	Xg^a
P	

Table 11.3: Interpretation of crossmatch.

Appearance	Interpretation
Neither agglutination nor hemolysis	Compatible
Agglutination or hemolysis	Incompatible

is present in testing and the donor unit is unacceptable for transfusion purposes.

Crossmatch is needed on any blood component containing ≥ 2 mL of red cells. Crossmatch should be performed before whole blood, RBC transfusion, and granulocyte and platelet transfusion.

AABB definition of crossmatch: It is a technique that "shall use methods that demonstrate ABO incompatibility and clinically significant antibodies to red cell antigens and shall include an antiglobulin test." Again, an exception is provided. If there are no clinically significant antibodies were detected in the current sample or in the patient's past records, (if there is no history/record of previous detection of such antibodies) an IS (immediate spin) crossmatch is allowed to fulfill the requirement of detecting ABO incompatibility.

Main purposes of the crossmatch testing: The objective is to select donor units that can provide maximal benefit to the patient. The crossmatch test is carried out to ensure that there are no antibodies present in patient's serum that will react with donor cells when transfused. There are mainly two purposes for the crossmatch namely—(1) to prevent life-threatening or uncomfortable transfusion reactions and (2) maximize survival of transfused red cells in vivo. These purposes are fulfilled in the following ways:

- The crossmatch acts as a double-check for any ABO errors caused by misidentification of patient or mislabeling of a donor unit. Thus, it acts as a final check of ABO compatibility between donor and patient.
- If the recipient has a clinically significant antibody in the serum or has a history of antibody, the crossmatch provides a second means of detecting antibody and checks the results of the antibody screen.

Types of crossmatch testing: Two types namely—(1) major cross match (patient's serum + donor's cells) and (2) minor crossmatch (donor's serum + patient's cells). Minor crossmatch has now been given up in most blood bank laboratories because donor samples are screened beforehand, for common irregular type of antibodies.

Crossmatch techniques: Usually, the method selected for crossmatch is the same as that used for the antibody screen. The various crossmatch techniques are listed in Fig. 11.1 and Box 11.4. A crossmatch can be done by two main methods: hemagglutination (tube and gel testing) and solid-phase red cell adherence.

Crossmatch procedures: The crossmatch procedure must be performed using the recipient's serum or plasma and donor red cells taken from a segment originally attached to the blood product bag. Segment is a sealed piece of integral tubing from the donor unit bag that contains a small aliquot of donor blood. It is used in the preparation of red cell suspensions for crossmatching.

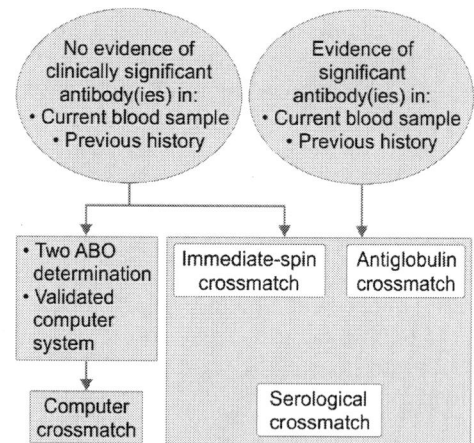

Fig. 11.1: Comparison of various types of crossmatch namely computer, immediate-spin, and antiglobulin crossmatch requirements.

Box 11.4: Crossmatch techniques.

- **Serological crossmatch**
  - Immediate spin (IS) technique
  - Saline room temperature technique
  - Albumin/low ionic strength solution (LISS) addition technique at 37°C
  - Indirect antiglobulin technique
- **Non-serological crossmatch:** Computer/electronic crossmatch

Serological Crossmatch Techniques

Major serological crossmatch test consists of testing the patient's (recipient's) serum with donor RBCs. The routinely used two serological methods are **immediate-spin (IS) crossmatch**, and an **indirect antiglobulin test (IAT) crossmatch**. In both these serologic crossmatch procedures, the recipient's serum or plasma is tested with the red cells from the donor unit. Only these two serological, i.e. the IS and IAT methods and one nonserologic method namely the "computer" crossmatch is discussed here.

Major serologic crossmatch needs 37°C incubation, followed by conversion to the IAT. This protocol was followed before the transfusion of whole blood or packed RBCs. However, in 1984, this requirement was eliminated by the AABB Standards as long as—the current antibody screen on the patient is completely negative and there is no past history of clinically significant antibodies. For patients who meet these criteria, an abbreviated procedure was followed to detect ABO incompatibility. This may consist of an IS crossmatch or an electronic crossmatch.

Principles of Serological Testing

The pretransfusion testing is performed to detect in vitro red cell antigen and antibody reaction by observing for either agglutination or hemolysis. Agglutination is a reversible reaction and has two stages (refer page 11) namely:
1. Sensitization (in which antibody binds to red cell antigen) and
2. Agglutination (in which the sensitized red cells are bridged and macroscopically appear as lattice).

The antiglobulin phase or Coomb's test detects bound red cell antibodies that do not produce direct agglutination. This test uses AHG sera which attaches to and causes agglutination of red cells sensitized with human globulins.

Immediate-Spin (IS) Crossmatch

This is the simplest serologic test to detect most ABO incompatibility in which the recipient's serum or plasma is mixed with donor's red cell suspensions and centrifuging immediately (i.e. immediate spin). Then observe it for agglutination. It may be performed for recipients with no evidence of clinically significant antibody or antibodies in the current sample (i.e. antibody screen is nonreactive) and if there is no history of unexpected antibody (or no previous records of such antibodies). **Absence of hemolysis or agglutination indicates ABO compatibility**. This serologic test is used to detect ABO incompatibility and is enough to rule out any ABO grouping error. In this method, there should not be any delay in the centrifugation step or reading the reaction.

Advantages: IS crossmatch procedure requires less turn-around time, work load, and reagent cost compared to full AHG crossmatch.

Disadvantages: This method **does not detect all ABO incompatibilities** and is inadequate for detection of clinically significant IgG type of antibodies.

False reactions: It may be observed in the presence of other IS-reactive antibodies (e.g. autoanti-I) or in patients with hyperimmune ABO antibodies. False reactions may also be seen when the procedure is improperly done (e.g. delay in centrifugation or reading), when rouleaux is observed, or when infants' specimens are tested. Adding EDTA to the test system may prevent some of the false-positive reactions, thus improving the sensitivity of the IS crossmatch.

Procedure for immediate-spin crossmatch (Fig. 11.2):
- Take two drops of patient's serum/plasma in a prelabeled glass test tube.
- Add one drop of 3–5% saline of suspension of donor red cells. Cells usually are washed once to remove any anticoagulant or plasma protein which may interfere with the testing.
- Mix the contents and incubate for 5–10 minutes for IS method or for 45–60 minutes for saline room temperature technique.
- Immediately centrifuge the tube at 1000 rpm for 1 minute (IS method). While in

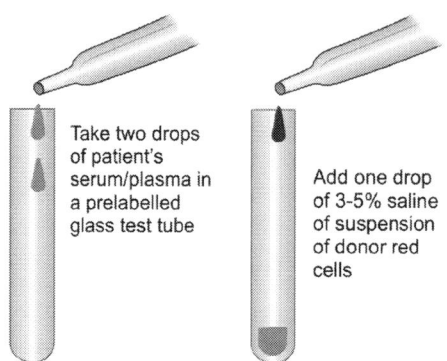

Fig 11.2: Immediate-spin (IS) Crossmatch. Patient/recipient serum is crossmatched with donor red cells and it is called as major crossmatch. In minor crossmatch, the donor's serum is crossmatched with patient's/recipient's red cells. Antibody screen testing on donor samples has replaced the minor crossmatch.

case of saline room temperature technique, centrifugation is optional.
- Gently dislodge the cell button and examine the tube for the presence or absence of hemolysis or agglutination.

This procedure has come to be known as the abbreviated or IS crossmatch.

Interpretation:
Positive test: If hemolysis or agglutination is present at this stage, the test is considered as reactive/positive. If the IS crossmatch is reactive, consider the following:
- The unit selected may be **ABO incompatible** and the unit is **not considered acceptable for transfusion** (crossmatch is incompatible).
- The patient's serum may show **rouleaux formation**. If the antibody screen does not have an IS phase, the rouleaux may be undetected.
- The patient may have autoantibodies or alloantibodies that were not detected in the antibody screen.
- The test tube may have been contaminated.

Negative test: If there is **no hemolysis or agglutination**, test is considered as nonreactive/negative and the **unit is considered acceptable for transfusion** (compatible).

If results are negative, proceed with indirect antiglobulin test crossmatch mentioned below.

The Indirect Antiglobulin Test Crossmatch

If the current pretransfusion antibody screening tests detect clinically significant antibody, or a history/record of patient indicates the previous detection of such antibodies, a 37°C incubation phase and an antiglobulin crossmatch must be performed. In the indirect antiglobulin crossmatch, compatibility between recipient serum and donor red cells is tested by the antiglobulin method. An IAT crossmatch may also be performed for patients who do not demonstrate clinically significant antibodies (antigen-negative units). The procedure of antiglobulin crossmatch begins in the same manner as the IS crossmatch.

Use of enhance media: Many enhancement media may be used to enhance antigen-antibody reactions. The enhancement media includes albumin, low ionic strength solution (LISS), polyethylene glycol, and polybrene (refer pages 67, 68). After IS cross match, the test is continued by incubation at 37°C (the incubation time depends on the choice of enhancement solution and is usually 15-minute room temperature), and finishes with an antiglobulin test. The antiglobulin reagent used may be monospecific (IgG) or polyspecific (IgG and bC3d).

To increase the sensitivity of test, usually an **AHG reagent containing both anti-IgG and anticomplement is used** for the final phase of this crossmatch method. It is advisable to run an auto control, in which the patient's own cells and serum are tested in parallel with the crossmatch test. Results of the autocontrol helps in clarification of positive results in the crossmatches and are discussed on page 92. **Indirect antiglobulin test is widely used in crossmatching technique** as it detects majority of incomplete antibodies.

Crossmatching by gel or solid-phase red cell adherence methods perform only by antiglobulin phase.

In the tube method, the antiglobulin crossmatch procedure usually includes three phases. These are—(1) an IS phase, (2) a 37°C incubation phase, and (3) an antiglobulin phase. Enhancement media used in the antibody screen are usually added to the crossmatch tubes in conditions where the antibody was detected.

Method of antiglobulin crossmatch (indirect antihuman globulin technique)
- Mix equal volumes (1-2 drops) of patient's serum and donor's cells.
- Incubate mixture at 37°C for 1 hour.
- Centrifuge 1000 rpm for 1 minute.
- Discard supernatant.
- Wash the red cells with large volumes of normal saline 4 times and decant the last wash completely. Prepare 5% suspension.
- Mix 1 drop each of 5% cell suspension and add one drop of AHG reagent.
- Incubate at room temperature for 5 minutes.
- Centrifuge the tube at 1000 rpm for 1 minute and look with optical aid for hemolysis or agglutination by tilting the tube.
- Record the results.

The crossmatch procedure can be done in one test tube or in separate tubes for all techniques. Albumin and LISS can be used with AHG test to increase the sensitivity.

Interpretation of crossmatches:

Negative: If there is **no hemolysis or agglutination at all phases of testing, test is interpreted as nonreactive, negative or compatible.** The units are considered acceptable for transfusion.
- If the test is negative, add one drop of control IgG-coated red cells. Centrifuge again at 1000 rpm for 1 minute.
- Look for hemolysis or agglutination. If no agglutination, the test is invalid, repeat the procedure.

Positive: If hemolysis or agglutination is detected at any phase of testing, it is interpreted as positive or incompatible. When an IAT crossmatch is positive, consider the following:

- The unit selected may be ABO incompatible and is not considered acceptable for transfusion.
- The unit may have a positive direct antiglobulin test.
- The patient may have an antibody to a low incidence antigen that was not present on the screening cells.
- The patient may be developing an additional antibody.
- The test system might have been contaminated.

Antiglobulin crossmatch by column agglutination technology using **glass microbeads** matrix is presented in Figure 11.3.

Non-Serological Crossmatch

Computer /Electronic Crossmatch

An electronic crossmatch (EXM), also called the computer crossmatch or computer-assisted crossmatch, is a non-serologic method of crossmatching. ABO compatibility may also be verified by computer electronic crossmatch. It uses logic tables located in a laboratory information system (LIS) to detect ABO incompatibilities between a patient and a donor. The recipient's plasma is not physically tested against the donor cells. In computer crossmatch, the computer compares donor unit information and patient ABO group and Rh type. Similar to the IS crossmatch, the electronic crossmatch can be used as sole crossmatch method only if the recipient has no present/current or previously detected, clinically significant antibodies or any history of alloantibodies. It may be performed when only the detection of ABO incompatibility is required, provided the following criteria are met.

The computer used must:
- Be validated on-site and this establishes the validity of the system.
- Contain logic to prevent the release of ABO-incompatible donor units.
- Contain the donor unit information (i.e. donor number, the name of the component, the ABO group and Rh type of the unit, and

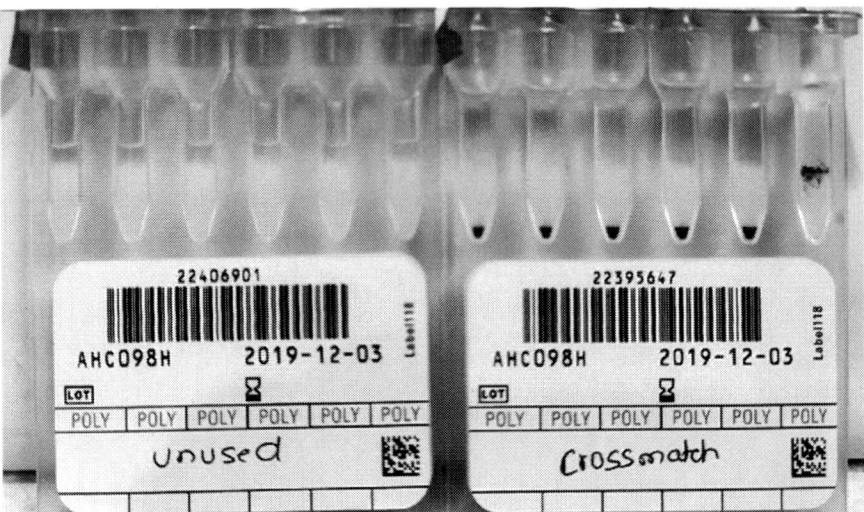

Fig. 11.3: AHG crossmatch by column agglutination technique (CAT) using glass microbeads matrix. Left half of the figure shows 6 microtubes (vertical columns) in a blank card before test. The right half of figure shows 6 microtubes of which first 5 microtubes show formation of red cells button at the bottom of each tube and indicates no agglutination and thereby these 5 samples have compatible crossmatch. The 6th extreme right microtube shows agglutination of red cells at the top indicating that the 6th sample is not compatible crossmatch.

Box 11.5: Advantages of the computer crossmatch.	Box 11.6: Limitations of the major crossmatch.
<ul><li>Increased time efficiency and less time-consuming</li><li>Decreased workload</li><li>Less volume of sample is needed on large crossmatch orders</li><li>Reduced human error</li><li>Reduced exposure of laboratory personnel to blood sample</li><li>Potential for a centralized transfusion service</li><li>**Non-serological crossmatch:** Computer/electronic crossmatch</li></ul>	<ul><li>Antibodies that may not be detected includes:<ul><li>Those which exhibit dosage</li><li>Antibodies reactive only at room temperature. However, this is of no concern because such antibodies are considered clinically insignificant</li></ul></li><li>Cannot detected all:<ul><li>ABO grouping errors in the potential recipient or donor</li><li>Rh grouping errors in the potential recipient or donor</li><li>Clinically significant antibodies</li></ul></li><li>No assurance about:<ul><li>Normal survival of transfused red blood cells</li><li>Complete absence of any adverse reaction in recipient</li></ul></li></ul>

the ABO confirmation tests performed on the unit).
- Contain the recipient ABO group and Rh type.
- Have a method to verify the correct entry of data.

Advantages of the computer crossmatch is presented in Box 11.5.

Crossmatching for newborn: Mother's serum (because newborn's lack their own antibodies) + Donor's cells.

Limitations of Crossmatch Testing (Box 11.6)

The crossmatch testing does not guarantee a successful transfusion outcome. The risks of transmission of virus, allergic reactions, and white blood cell reactions can occur. A recipient could have a negative antibody screen result and an incompatible crossmatch. A negative antibody screen means that the recipient's serum contains no antibodies that react with the screening cells by the method used. However, it does not guarantee that the recipient's serum is free from clinically significant red cell antibodies. A compatible crossmatch also does not guarantee the

> **Box 11.7:** Causes of missed antibodies in compatibility testing.
>
> - Corresponding antigen is absent from screening cells
> - Weak antibody
> - Antibody is not detectable by a routinely employed method
> - Antibody history is unknown

optimal survival of transfused red cells. Non-life-threatening transfusion reactions such as hives, low-grade fever, chills, and itching can also occur.

Causes of missed antibodies in compatibility testing are listed in Box 11.7.

Main objective of the crossmatch test is to detect the presence of antibodies in the recipient's serum (including anti-A and anti-B), which can cause destruction of transfused RBCs. When the crossmatch test shows a positive result, it indicates incompatibility. The recipient should not receive a transfusion until the cause of the incompatibility has been determined. The determination of the cause of the incompatibility may be arrived by review of the results of the autocontrol and antibody screening test.

Causes of Positive Results in the Serologic Crossmatch

The various causes of a positive result in the serologic crossmatch test include the following:

1. **Incorrect ABO grouping of the patient or donor:** Immediately repeat ABO grouping, especially if strong incompatibility is seen in a reading taken after IS. The samples' identity should be rechecked with the original patient sample and the donor bag should be used for retesting.
2. **An alloantibody in the patient's serum reacting with the corresponding antigen on donor RBCs:** The autocontrol tube will be negative except in the patient who has been recently transfused with incompatible RBCs. If the antibody screening test is positive, antibody identification panel studies will help in identification of antibody specificity. Then select the units lacking the antigens for compatibility testing (refer page 219).
   - If red cells of **all donors tested are incompatible** with the patient's serum and also **antibody screening test is positive**, suspect antibody directed **against an antigen of high incidence** or **multiple antibodies** in the patient's serum.
   - If **antibody screening test is negative** and **only one donor unit is incompatible**, then the antibody in patient's serum is likely be directed against an **antigen of low incidence** that is present on that donor's RBCs.
   - If antibody screening test is negative, patient's serum may contain either naturally occurring antibody (e.g. anti-A_1) or passively acquired ABO agglutinins. Anti-A, anti-B or anti-A, B may be passively acquired after transfusion of non-ABO-specific blood products (e.g. platelets) or after organ or bone marrow transplantation. Check the serum grouping of patients to confirm the presence of unexpected reaction with anti-A_1 with known A_1 cells. Also, check the patient's history for any transfusion and transplant.
3. **An autoantibody in the patient's serum reacting with the corresponding antigen on donor RBCs:** This can be solved by running an autocontrol which will be positive. Panel adsorption and elution studies will help to identify if there are also alloantibodies. Auto adsorption of the patient's serum to remove autoantibody activity may be helpful. It is followed by compatibility testing using the auto absorbed serum.
4. **Prior coating of the donor RBCs with protein:** It can result in a positive AHG test.
5. **Abnormalities in the patient's serum:**
   - **Rouleaux formation:** It is characterized by sticking together RBCs on their flat sides that gives and appearance

of stacks of coins when viewed with microscope. It may occur when there is an imbalance in the normal ratio of albumin and gamma globulin (A/G ratio), as in diseases such as multiple myeloma and macroglobulinemia. The rouleaux formation will affect all tests, including the autocontrol. Strong rouleaux may mimic true agglutination. Rouleaux are prominent after 37°C incubation but they disappear after thorough washing before the AHG test.
- **Plasma expanders:** The presence of high-molecular-weight dextrans or other plasma expanders may produce false-positive results. Saline replacement may be useful to resolve the problem.
- **Antibody against additives in the albumin reagents**: These may rarely cause false-positive results in compatibility tests. This occurs when the patient has antibodies to the stabilizing substances (e.g. caprylate) added to the albumin reagents. This problem can be resolved by using caprylate-free albumin solutions in testing.
6. **Contaminants in the test system:** These may produce false-positive compatibility test results. Contaminants include dirty glassware, bacterial contamination of samples, chemical or other contaminants in saline, and fibrin clots.

Various causes of positive pretransfusion tests are listed in Box 11.8.

Testing the Donor Sample

These tests are performed on blood sample obtained in an attached segment on the

---

Box 11.8: Various causes of positive pretransfusion tests.

Negative antibody screen, incompatible immediate-spin crossmatch
- Donor red cells are ABO incompatible
- Anti-A_1 is the serum of an A_2 or A_2B individual
- Rouleaux formation
- Passively acquired anti-A or anti-B
- Contaminant in the test system

Negative antibody screen, incompatible antiglobulin crossmatch
- Positive direct antiglobulin test on donor red blood cells
- Antibody reacts only with RBCs having strong expression of a particular antigen (e.g. dosage) or variation in antigen strength
- Alloantibody in recipient to a low-incidence antigen on the donor red cells
- Passively acquired anti-A or anti-B

Positive antibody screen, compatible crossmatches
- Antibodies dependent on reagent red cell diluent
- Antibodies demonstrating dosage and donor red cells are from heterozygotes (i.e. expressing a single dose of antigen)
- Donor unit is lacking corresponding antigen
- Contaminant in the test system

Positive antibody screen, incompatible crossmatches, negative autocontrol
- Alloantibody (ies) directed toward antigen on donor red blood cells

Positive antibody screen, incompatible crossmatches, positive autocontrol, negative direct antiglobulin test (DAT)
- Antibody to a substance/ingredient in enhancement media or enhancement dependent autoantibody
- Rouleaux formation

Positive antibody screen, incompatible crossmatches, positive autocontrol, positive DAT
- Alloantibody present in recipient who has been transfused and causing either a delayed serologic or hemolytic transfusion reaction
- Passively acquired autoantibody (e.g. intravenous immune globulin)
- Cold or warm-reactive autoantibody
- Rouleaux present

donor unit taken from the donor at the time of collection. The tests that are performed include ABO grouping and Rh typing (including a test for weak D) and tests intended to prevent disease transmission. A screening test for unexpected antibodies to RBC antigens should be done on samples from donors who have a history of transfusion or pregnancy.

Selection of Appropriate Donor Units

Blood and blood components must be selected to suit to need of each individual patient. Following points must be kept in mind while selecting donor units for transfusion.

ABO group-specific: In almost all cases (or whenever possible), the first choice for transfusion is blood and blood components of the patient's (recipient's) own ABO group and Rh type. This is defined as ABO group-specific (ABO-identical blood).

Alternatives:

- **Alternate ABO compatible blood:** When group specific blood and blood components of the patient's (recipient's) ABO blood group is not available or some other reason precludes their use, use alternate ABO compatible blood. The donor units selected should not contain any antigen against which the recipient has a clinically significant antibody. However, blood and blood components that do not contain all of the antigens carried on the patient's own RBCs can be used. For example group A- or B-packed RBCs can be safely transfused to a group AB recipient.

- **Different ABO group:** In situations when ABO compatible blood is not available, a recipient can be given only packed RBCs of a different ABO group. The whole blood is incompatible and cannot be administered because whole-blood plasma contains preformed ABO antibodies. For example, whole blood of a donor with group A cannot be transfused into a recipient with group AB, because the plasma of the group A whole blood contains anti-B antibodies.
  - In patient with AB group, group A blood as an alternate source is preferred over B group blood, as anti-B in group A is weaker than anti-A in B group.
  - Packed O group RBCs can be safely transfused to all patients. However, it depends on availability of group O blood and used only in special circumstances. If ABO group-specific blood is not available or is in low supply, alternative blood groups that can be transfused are summarized in Table 11.4.
  - It is advisable not to change from group A to group B blood or vice-versa, when more than one unit is given in a continuous transfusion.

Rh types: Select the blood of same Rh (D) type as that of patient, particularly in female patients who are of child-bearing age.

- **Rh-negative blood:** It **can be given to Rh-positive patients**. However, Rh-negative blood should be conserved for use in Rh-negative recipients. If the Rh-negative unit

Table 11.4: Donor ABO group selection for transfusion of RBCs.

Patient's (recipient's) blood group	First choice (ABO group–specific)	Alternative Blood Group (given as packed cells)	
		Second choice	Third choice
O	O	None	None
A	A	O	None
A_2 with anti-A_1	A_2 with anti-A_1	O	None
B	B	O	None
A_1B	A_1B	A or B	O
A_2B	A_2B	A or B	O
A_2B with anti-A_1	A_2B with anti-A_1	A_2 or B	O

is near expiration, the unit should be given rather than wasted.
- **Rh-positive blood**: It **should not be given to Rh-negative female** patients of childbearing age. If there are no preformed anti-D in the recipient's sera, and if Rh (D) negative blood is not available, it is acceptable to transfuse Rh-negative male patients and female patients beyond menopause with Rh-positive blood. About 80% of Rh-negative patients produce anti-D if they receive 200 mL or more of Rh-positive blood.

Antigen-negative RBCs: If patient has unexpected antibody, identify the antibody if possible and then select the corresponding antigen negative blood for crossmatch. It is not necessary to give antigen-negative RBCs for patients if their sera contain antibodies which are reactive only below 37°C. This is because in vivo these antibodies do not cause significant destruction of RBC. Providing antigen-negative donor units for transfusion to recipients with blood group antibodies may be difficult, expensive, and unnecessary.

Before compatibility testing, donor units should be visually examined for unusual appearance and correct labeling. If the donor units show abnormal color, turbidity, clots, incomplete or improper labeling or any leakage, it should not be used.

Donor ABO group selection for transfusion of RBCs is presented in Table 11.4.

In general, oldest units should be used first. There are following exceptions for this and fresh blood should be given in following situations:
- **Massive transfusion**: It is transfusion of blood in which equal to or more than patient's volume is transfused within 24 hours. Patients receiving massive blood transfusion should be given fresher blood available.
- **Exchange transfusion** in neonates should also receive fresh blood (less than 5 days old).
- Patients of thalassemia and sickle cell anemia should also receive relatively fresh blood.

- **ABO hemolytic disease of fetus and newborn:** Group O red cells of the same Rh (D) type as that of the baby should be selected.
- **Rh hemolytic disease of fetus and newborn:** Rh (D) negative blood of the same ABO group as that of the baby is used, if it is same as that of the mother or if it is compatible with mother's blood. Once the baby's ABO group is not compatible with mother's ABO group then O Rh (D) negative blood is selected and matched with the mother's serum.

Tagging, Inspecting, Issuing, and Transfusing Blood Products

- After the completion of compatibility testing, the suitable unit or units for transfusion are selected. A tag is attached to each donor unit. The donor unit tag must contain the patient's full name and identification number, name of the component, donor number, expiration date, ABO and Rh typing of the unit and interpretation of the crossmatching test. Check the unit tag information against the unit label and the expiration date. Visually inspect the unit for discoloration, clots, or other abnormal appearance. The visual check of the donor unit before issue is an important step. Bacterial contamination of units or traumatized donor units can be detected by visual check.
- Patient identification is very important for safe transfusion. Patient's details should match exactly with the information on the unit tag. If the issued blood product is not to be used immediately for transfusion, it may be returned to the blood bank for storage. Unmonitored refrigerators should never be used for storage of blood products.

PRETRANSFUSION TESTING IN SPECIAL CIRCUMSTANCES

Usually pretransfusion testing should be performed as per the standard operating procedure.

Emergencies

In certain situations, such as in trauma, the recipient may need the transfusion of RBC components prior to the completion of pretransfusion testing. It is necessary that adequate pretransfusion samples should be collected before transfusion of any donor blood. This will help to carryout subsequent pretransfusion testing, if necessary.
- In case of an **emergency**, blood can be issued after performing the **patient's** and donor **ABO and Rh grouping** followed by crossmatch by IS technique. Then the ABO group-specific blood can be given.
- In **extreme emergencies, there may be no time to obtain and test a pretransfusion** sample or even before a patient blood specimen is available. If the ABO and Rh types of the patient are not known, **group O Rh-negative packed cells can be transfused** to tide over the situation.
- In an **Rh-negative patient**, if large amounts of blood are likely to be necessary, a decision should be made rapidly whether the demands of Rh-negative blood can be met with. Rh-positive blood cells can be given if the patient is a man or is a woman beyond child-bearing age. Injections of Rh immunoglobulin to prevent formation of anti-D may be given after the crisis has been resolved. Accurate records must be maintained regarding all units issued in the emergency. Subsequently after issue of blood, pretransfusion testing should be done as per the protocol, and any incompatible result should be reported immediately to the recipient's physician.

Transfusion of Non-Group-Specific Blood

Sometimes as an extreme emergency donor unit of an ABO group other than the recipient's own type might have been transfused. For example, group A recipient is given large volumes of group O RBCs. In such cases, freshly drawn serum sample of the recipient should be tested for the presence of unexpected anti-A or anti-B before giving any additional RBC transfusions.
- If the freshly drawn serum sample is compatible with donor RBCs of the recipient's own ABO group, ABO group-specific blood may be given for the transfusion.
- If the serologic crossmatch shows incompatibility, additional transfusions should be of the alternative blood group. For example, if a patient with group B has been transfused with a large number of units of group O packed cells, the serum of recipient may contain adequate amounts of anti-B. This will cause a positive reaction in an IS crossmatch. For any additional transfusions, such individuals should be given group O units.

Compatibility Testing for Transfusion of Plasma Products

Compatibility testing procedures are not needed for transfusion of plasma products. However, when large volumes of plasma and plasma products need to be transfused, a crossmatch test between the donor plasma and patient RBCs may be done. The main purpose for crossmatch is to detect ABO incompatibility between donor and patient; therefore, an IS crossmatch is sufficient. Plasma, platelets, and cryoprecipitate do not contain red cells and do not need to be crossmatched.

Intrauterine Transfusions

Blood used for intrauterine transfusion must be compatible with maternal antibodies capable of crossing the placenta.
- **If the ABO and Rh groups of the fetus have been performed** and if there is no fetomaternal ABO or Rh incompatibility, **group-specific blood** may be given.
- **If the ABO and Rh groups of the fetus are not known**, then group O **Rh-negative RBCs** should be used for the intrauterine transfusion. The group O Rh-negative cells must not contain any antigens against which the mother's serum contains

unexpected antibodies (e.g. anti-K1, anti-Jka). Crossmatch testing is performed using the mother's serum sample.

Neonatal and Pediatric Transfusions

Indications: Neonatal RBC transfusion is given because of anemia of prematurity, HDFN, or iatrogenic blood loss.

Blood for an exchange or regular transfusion of a neonate and infants younger than 4 months of age have unique test requirements. The blood must be compatible with any maternal antibodies that have entered the infant's circulation and are reactive at 37°C or AHG. As long as the ABO and Rh groups are not involved in the fetomaternal incompatibility, blood of the infant's ABO and Rh group can be used.

- An initial pretransfusion specimen from the infant must be tested for ABO and Rh groups. The ABO group is determined by testing a sample of infant's RBCs only with anti-A and anti-B reagents. The expression of A and B antigens is usually weaker in this age group, so that testing with anti-A,B can also be performed and will help in discriminate a group O from a non-group O.
- The naturally occurring anti-A and anti-B are not usually demonstrated till 6 months of age. Hence, a reverse type (i.e. testing of the infant's serum with reagent RBCs) is not performed.
- **Antibody screen:** Antibody detection testing can be done using the serum of the mother, the infant's serum (e.g. cord serum), or an eluate prepared from the infant's RBCs. If the red cells selected for transfusion are not group O, the infant's serum or plasma must be tested to demonstrate the absence of anti-A (using A_1 cells) and anti-B. This testing should include an antiglobulin phase. The maternal sample may be used because antibodies detected at this age are passively acquired from the mother. There is also difficulty in obtaining an adequate sample volume from an infant.
- During any one hospital admission, if the infant received only ABO-compatible and Rh-compatible transfusions and had no unexpected antibodies in the serum or plasma, there is no need to repeat pretransfusion ABO/Rh tests.
- When there are clinically significant antibodies (including anti-A and anti-B) present in the serum, the red cells that lack the corresponding antigen must be selected for transfusion until the antibody is no longer demonstrable in the infant's serum.

For both intrauterine and infant (less than 4 months old) transfusions, fresh blood or blood should not be older than 7 days should be used.

Interpretation of Infant's Antibody Screen Results

- **If the antibody screen is negative:**
  - **When group O RBCs are selected for transfusion:** A crossmatch and additional testing are usually not needed
  - **When other than group O RBCs are selected for transfusion**: An initial **crossmatch** that **includes an antiglobulin phase is needed**.
- **If the antibody screen is positive**: **Antibody identification studies** are done by testing **either the mother's or infant's serum**. If clinically significant antibodies are identified, the selection of antigen-negative units or units compatible by antiglobulin crossmatch is needed till the passively acquired antibody is no longer demonstrated.

Massive Transfusions

Definition: Massive transfusion is defined as emergent transfusion in a relatively short time frame (within 24 hours) in which the amount of whole blood or packed cell components transfused (> 10 RBC units) equals or exceeds the patient's total blood volume. Thus, it is the replacement of one total blood volume in 24 hours or the replacement of 50% of the blood volume in 3 hours. It can be ongoing blood loss of 150 mL/minute. It may require either a transfusion of 8–10 RBC units to an adult patient in less than 24 hours, or as the acute transfusion of 4–5 RBC units in 1 hour.

Conditions that require massive transfusion: Large-volume blood is usually lost due to trauma but may occur due to gastrointestinal hemorrhage (e.g. chronic liver disease), ruptured aortic aneurysms, obstetric emergencies, and some surgical procedures such as liver transplantation.

Management of massive bleeding: (1) Prevent or treat hypovolemic shock, (2) maintain adequate oxygen-carrying capacity, (3) maintain oncotic pressure, (4) prevent coagulopathy, and (5) avoid adverse effects of transfusion.

Initial patient evaluation: It should include medical history (about liver, kidney, cardiovascular, and hematologic diseases), history of previous transfusions or problems during pretransfusion testing, any evidence of microvascular bleeding, complete blood count (CBC), and coagulation profile (PT, APTT, fibrinogen, thromboelastography).

Guidelines: In massive transfusion, the patient's circulation contains mainly donor blood. Hence, the purpose of the crossmatch is somewhat diminished. Frequently an abbreviated crossmatch may be done which reduces the amount of testing that is normally performed. Most blood banks switch to an IS or electronic crossmatch, even in a patient with known RBC alloantibodies. Special attention is required for patient and sample identification to avoid transfusion errors. The compatibility testing procedure may be shortened or eliminated and technical manual guideline includes the following:

Patient (recipient) having a clinically significant unexpected antibody: If time permits, all transfused units should be tested for absence of the corresponding antigen in the donor.

- In patients requiring massive transfusion, serum antibody is typically dilution with large volumes of donor blood/plasma and other fluids transfused, the antibody in the patient's serum is undetectable in vitro.
- Red cell can be transfused if estimated blood loss is more than 15% of blood volume (i.e. about 1000 mL in an adult) occurs with ongoing bleeding. Transfusion can be started with group O uncrossmatched RBCs. If the patient's Rh type is not known, Rh (D)-negative RBCs are used for transfusion, especially for females with child-bearing age.
- If antigen-positive units are infused, a rapid rise in antibody titer level followed by delayed hemolytic (destruction of donor RBCs) transfusion reaction in patients with alloantibodies may develop. However, it is better to transfuse antigen-untested units rather than to withhold transfusion till the test results are obtained. The basis is to give the patient a chance for survival and then to treat the immune-mediated anemia induced by massive transfusion of antigen-untested units.
- Coagulopathies may develop during massive transfusion due to dilution, consumption, and/or dysfunction. Consumptive coagulopathies may occur with disseminated intravascular coagulation (DIC), burns, brain injury, hyperthermia, and sepsis. Coagulation studies reveal prolonged PT and APTT, low fibrinogen and platelet counts, and the presence of fibrin degradation products or D-dimers.
- Once the patient is stabilized, the routine crossmatch procedure is done within 24 hours of the massive transfusion event.

Complications of Massive Transfusion (Table 11.5)

Massive blood replacement may produce metabolic complications, coagulation abnormalities, immune hemolysis, and air embolism. These complications are related to transfusion volume and infusion rate. Patient-related comorbid factors such as resuscitation maneuvers, underlying disease, severity and duration of hypotensive shock, and hypothermia may further contribute to the metabolic and coagulation abnormalities. These complications include:

Table 11.5: Complications in massive transfusion.

Complication	Causes	Treatments
Microvascular hemorrhage	Dilution and consumption of coagulation factors and platelets Hypotension	Platelets Fresh frozen plasma to control deficiencies of coagulation factors Control hypotension
Citrate toxicity	Decrease in ionized calcium due to anticoagulants in blood products	Slow the rate of infusion If severe calcium replacement is needed
Hypothermia	Rapid infusion of blood products	High-flow blood warmers

Metabolic complications

Metabolic complications can depress cardiac function. These complications include:

i. **Citrate toxicity**
   Pathophysiology: In massive transfusion, large volumes of citrated blood components can **raise the plasma citrate level** especially in the presence of liver disease and **citrate can bind calcium** resulting in **hypocalcemia**. In individual with normal liver function, citrate is rapidly metabolized and these symptoms are transient.
   - **Hypocalcemia:** If the transfusion rate exceeds about 100 mL/minute, a clinically significant drop in ionized calcium may occur. There is accumulation of citrate and this citrate toxicity will result in hypocalcemia. Hypocalcemia is more likely to cause clinical manifestations in patients who are hypothermic and in shock. The symptoms of hypocalcemia include tingling, shivering, light-headedness, tetany, muscle cramps, spasm, and hyperventilation.
     - **Treatment:** It can be treated by supplementing calcium. Hypocalcemia may be exacerbated if there is liver disease, hypotension, and hypothermia. Monitoring the corrected QT interval in the ECG is useful. Measurement of total calcium is not very useful because it may not indicate the actual level of ionized calcium.

ii. **Hyperkalemia and Hypokalemia**
   Pathophysiology
   - **Hyperkalemia:** During storage (1–6°C), packed red blood cells gradually leak the intracellular potassium into the plasma or additive solution of the blood component. This potassium is rapidly diluted and redistributes into cells and rarely causes any problems in the recipient. However, hyperkalemia can produce problems when a large volume of packed red blood cells is rapidly infused in neonates/premature infants and patients with cardiac, hepatic, or renal dysfunction. The transient hyperkalemia due to massive transfusion depend on the patient's acid-base balance, ionized calcium levels, and rate of infusion of the packed red blood cells.
   - **Hypokalemia:** Hypokalemia is more frequent than hyperkalemia after massive transfusion. This is because potassium depleted donor red cells reaccumulate potassium ion intracellularly and citrate metabolism causes further movement of potassium into cells in response to consumption of protons.

   Treatment and prevention: Usually there is no necessity for treatment or preventive measures for both hyperkalemia and hypokalemia, provided that the patient is adequately resuscitated from the underlying condition that necessitated massive transfusion. Extreme hyperkalemia or hypokalemia can compromise the myocardial function. Hyperkalemia can be reversed by slowing the transfusion rate and by maintaining the acid-base balance in the patient.

iii. **Hypothermia:** Hypothermia can induce metabolic and hemostatic derangements. Hypothermia can be prevented by infusion of prewarmed resuscitation fluids and refrigerated blood components or using high-flow blood warming devices. Proper procedure should be followed for the use of blood warmers, because overheating may lead to hemolysis and serious often fatal transfusion reactions.
iv. **Acid-base disorders:** During rapid transfusion of RBCs, a moderate reduction in arterial pH may be found.
v. **Metabolic alkalosis:** It is common after massive transfusion. During massive transfusion, the rate of citrate delivery may exceed the liver's capacity for its clearance. The metabolic by-product of citrate is bicarbonate. The bicarbonate accumulation may cause, metabolic alkalosis. Rarely, hypomagnesemia-associated myocardial depression can be found with severe citrate toxicity. These complications are seen in patients with liver failure.

Coagulation (hemostatic) abnormalities

Hemostatic abnormalities in massive transfusion include dilutional coagulopathy, DIC, and liver and platelet dysfunction.

Pathophysiology: Coagulopathy can develop especially when lost blood is replaced by RBCs and crystalloids. Coagulopathy in massive transfusion is usually due to: (1) dilution of platelets and clotting factors as patients lose hemostatically active blood (hemodilution) and (2) reduction in the enzymatic activity as the core body temperature lowers if a blood warmer is not used. Coagulopathy may be secondary to DIC. Mortality rate associated with hemostatic abnormalities ranges from 20 to 50% and results from hypothermia, metabolic acidosis, and coagulopathy. Microvascular bleeding (MVB) is characteristic of coagulopathy associated with increasing transfusion volume. MVB increases with platelets counts below ~50,000/µL. Coagulation abnormalities include:

- Thrombocytopenia
- Hypofibrinogenemia
- Reduced levels of coagulation factors
- Tissue injury may disrupt the procoagulant-anticoagulant balance, leading to DIC.
- Risk of bleeding secondary to a combination of platelet and coagulation factor consumption and secondary fibrinolysis.

Treatment and prevention: Transfusion-related adverse events during massive transfusion can be avoided through careful patient monitoring. This monitoring includes observing for the development of sign and symptoms, changes in laboratory values (e.g. platelet counts, partial thromboplastin time [PTT], fibrinogen level as clinically indicated), and the appropriate use of medications and blood components. Prophylactic replacement of hemostatic components depending on the volume of RBCs or whole blood transfused can prevent the development of bleeding diathesis. *Antifibrinolytic* agents may be useful in controlling massive bleeding from trauma.

Air embolism

- It can occur if blood is infused under pressure in an open system or by entry of air into central catheter while containers or blood administration sets are being exchanged. The minimum volume of air needed in an adult to produce a fatal air embolism is about 100 mL.
- **Symptoms** include cough, dyspnea, chest pain, and shock.
- **Treatment:** If there is suspicion of air embolism, the patient should be placed on the left side with head down to displace the air bubble from the pulmonary valve.

Autoimmune Hemolytic Anemia

When autoantibody is present in the recipient, it can cause special problems in pretransfusion testing. Following should be kept in mind:

- It is necessary to make sure that there is a need for transfusion.
- Use of auto-absorbed serum may be necessary for pretransfusion testing.
- Alternative pretransfusion testing may be indicated when cold autoantibody is present.
- If clinically significant alloantibodies have been excluded, it is not crucial to know the specificity of the autoantibody.

Crossmatching in case of autoimmune hemolytic anemia:
- Autoantibodies are detected by DAT
- Transfuse least incompatible blood as determined by titration.

Transfusion strategies: These include—(1) infuse a small volume of donor RBCs with close monitoring of the patient, (2) use warmer blood if it is due to cold autoantibodies, and (3) use leukocyte-reduced blood to minimize possible adverse reaction.

Specimens with Prolonged Clotting Time

Difficulties may arise when testing blood samples from patients with prolonged clotting times due to coagulation abnormalities associated with disease or medications (e.g. heparin). When a partially clotted serum is added to saline-suspended screening or donor RBCs, a fibrin clot may form spontaneously. In such samples, complete coagulation can be accelerated by adding thrombin. One drop of thrombin, 50 U/mL to 1 mL of plasma is usually enough to induce clotting. In patients on heparin anticoagulant, adding a small amount of protamine sulfate can counteract the effects of heparin.

Preoperative Autologous Blood

Autologous transfusion (refer Chapter 19 pages 411-3) is the removal and storage of blood or components from a donor for the donor's possible use at a later time. It is usually performed during or after an elective surgical procedure.
- ABO and Rh groups of the units must be determined.
- Tests for unexpected antibodies and tests designed to prevent disease transmission are not required. Tests for unexpected antibodies in the recipient's serum or plasma and a crossmatch are optional.
- Units must be labeled "For autologous use only."

SUMMARY

- Most of the fatal transfusion reactions are caused by clerical errors.
- Samples and forms from recipients (patients) must contain patient's full name and unique identity number.
- Sample must be collected within 3 days of before transfusion.
- Perform ABO grouping, Rh typing, and antibody screening on patient. Check patient records (history) for results of previous tests.
- Crossmatch is used to prevent issue of an ABO-incompatible red blood cell component.
- Three methods used to perform pretransfusion tests are tube, gel and solid phase. Usually, IS or antiglobulin crossmatch are performed based on current or historical serologic results.
- In case of emergencies, select uncrossmatched, group O, Rh negative packed RBCs.
- No compatibility testing is required for plasma products units.
- Visual check for the physical condition of the blood product is performed prior to transport, upon receipt, prior to issue and prior to administration.
- During transfusion, patients should be monitored throughout the procedure for signs and symptoms of a transfusion reaction.

SELF-ASSESSMENT EXERCISE

Write short notes on:
- Precompatibility testing before blood transfusion
- Crossmatching
- Neonatal and pediatric transfusions
- Massive transfusion
- Pretransfusion testing of donor blood
- Problems in pediatric blood transfusions
- Massive blood transfusion and its management
- Describe briefly the complications of massive blood transfusion. What precautions can be taken to prevent the complications
- Hemostatic defects associated with massive blood transfusion

CHAPTER 12

Blood Components and their Preparation

CHAPTER OUTLINE

- Whole blood
- Blood components
- Preparation of blood components
- Red blood cell components
- Platelet components
- Plasma components
- Granulocyte concentrates

INTRODUCTION

Nowadays, a single unit of whole blood is usually separated into different components and whole blood is rarely used for transfusion directly. It may be useful in trauma where there is heavy blood loss. Labile coagulation factors in whole blood decreases on storage and platelets may activate and develop storage lesions. Hence, the whole blood is collected into sets having multiple connected bags. The blood withdrawn first enters the primary bag, where it is mixed with anticoagulant-preservative solution.

In the present era, with the development of plastic blood bags with integral tubing, high-speed refrigerated centrifuges, deep freezers and cell separators, it is now easier and practical to separate blood components. By separating the blood components, a single blood donation can provide transfusion therapy to multiple patients. These components that can be prepared from a single unit of whole blood include packed red cells, platelet concentrates, cryoprecipitate, fresh frozen plasma (FFP), and cryoprecipitate, etc. Other products such as derivatives of plasma (e.g. immune serum globulin) can also be used in various diseases or conditions. These components can be used individually to help more than one patient with many purposes. Thus, red cells can be transfused to an anemic patient and plasma for a burns patient. This also ensures that only the required components are transfused. With the availability of more advanced chemical techniques (plasma fractionation), various plasma derivatives or fractions can be made.

Advantages of using components are outlined in Box 12.1.

Blood collection set (Fig. 12.1): Whole blood is collected from a donor into a **plastic collection bag** containing anticoagulant (primary bag) and also includes a number of **satellite containers** (also called as satellite bags). These satellite bags are integrally attached to the main collection (primary) bag with hollow tubing. Satellite bags become the storage

Box 12.1: Advantages of using components.

- Economical: One unit of blood can be separated into different components and is used in different patients according to their need.
- Ensures optimal use of blood resources. Thus, only the required component need be transfused and other components are preserved for other patients.
- Avoids potential hazards from other unwanted components to the recipient.
- Minimizes the cardiac overload.
- Minimizes the hazards of whole blood transfusion.

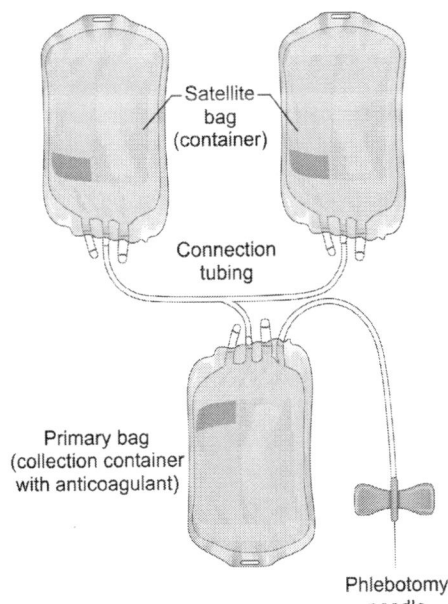

Fig. 12.1: Blood collection set with primary and two satellite bags.

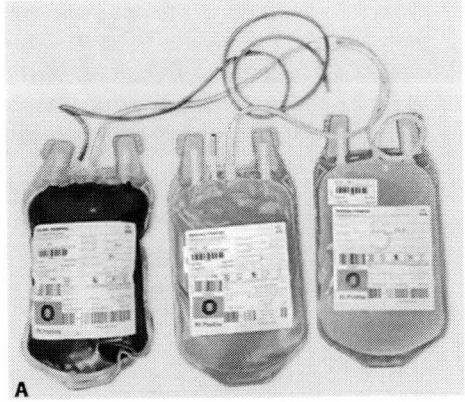

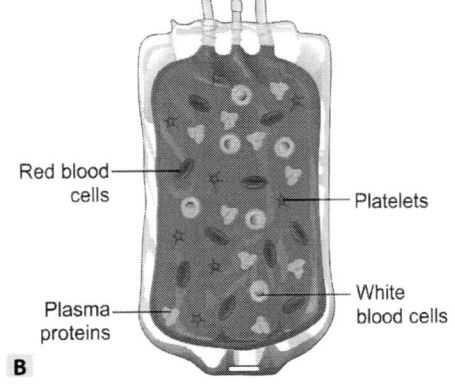

Figs. 12.2A and B: (A) Whole blood collected (first bag on the left) in a triple bag; (B) Various contents of whole blood (diagrammatic) *(For color version, see Plate 2)*.

containers for the blood components prepared from the donation. The entire blood collection set is sterile on the inside and the satellite bags allow whole blood to be separated into individual blood components in a closed system. A closed system ensures that there is no entry of foreign contaminants from the outside environment (e.g. bacteria) into the system.

WHOLE BLOOD

Whole blood is the unmodified component, drawn from a donor. It consists of RBCs, leukocytes, platelets, and plasma proteins (Figs. 12.2A and B) with the anticoagulant-preservative solution.

Amount of anticoagulant-preservative: Whole blood is collected in an aseptic manner with a ratio of 14 mL of anticoagulant preservative solution per 100 mL of whole blood. A unit of whole blood is approximately 450 mL of blood and 63 mL of anticoagulant-preservative (or 350 mL of blood and 49 mL of anticoagulant). Whole blood provides both oxygen carrying capacity and blood volume expansion.

Before the advent of the technology for preparation of the blood component, whole blood was the only blood product available. In the 1960s, the glass bottles used as a collection medium were replaced by plastic bags and it became possible to separate whole blood into its components.

Disadvantages: Whole blood transfusions can produce **circulatory overload** in patients who need only oxygen-carrying capacity from RBCs. Within the first 24 hours of storage, there is **loss of viable platelets** and **decrease in the amount of labile coagulation factors**. Presently, whole blood is considered a raw material rather than a transfusion medium and whole blood was replaced with RBCs.

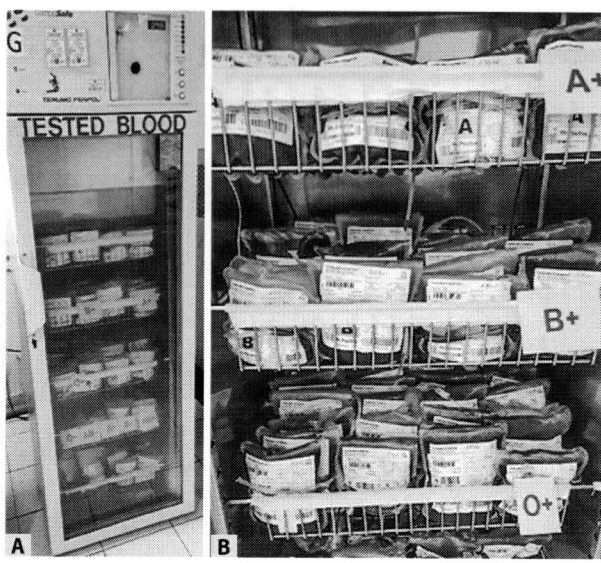

Figs. 12.3A and B: (A) Monitored refrigerator used in blood center; (B) Blood bags stored inside the refrigerator.

Storage: Whole blood is stored in a monitored refrigerator (Figs. 12.3A and B) at 1°C to 6°C to reduce red cell's utilization of adenosine triphosphate and to preserve their viability.

Shelf-life: Whole blood should be at least 70% at the end of a shelf-life of 35 days (if collected in citrate phosphate dextrose adenine [CPDA]-1) or 21 days (if collected in CPD). After storage of blood for 10 days, all predonation 2,3-diphosphoglycerate content in red cells is lost, but up to 50% of it is regenerated in the recipient within 8 hours after transfusion. Additive solutions cannot be added to whole blood to increase the storage period.

Indications for whole blood are given in Box 12.2. It is mainly indicated to provide both oxygen carrying capacity and increase the blood volume in an actively bleeding patient with greater than 25% blood loss. Nowadays, whole blood is rarely available, and RBCs and plasma have become the standard transfusion for most cases of active bleeding in trauma and surgery. ABO must be identical to the recipient and cross matched before transfusion. If whole blood is not available, RBCs may be administered with crystalloid solutions to restore both oxygen-carrying capacity and blood volume. For exchange transfusions in infants, reconstituted whole blood (RBCs reconstituted with group AB FFP from a different donor) is used.

Fresh Whole Blood

Fresh blood means blood that is stored for less than 24 hours. There are no valid indications for fresh blood transfusion because:
- Processing of donor blood cannot be completed within 24 hours. This includes ABO and Rh typing, antibody detection, and testing for common diseases transmitted through blood (hepatitis B and C, HIV, syphilis, and malaria).
- It carries the risk of transfusion transmitted diseases.
- A single unit of fresh whole blood will not help patients with specific component deficiency.

Hemoglobin level after transfusion: Transfusion of whole blood increases the hemoglobin by about 1 g/dL or the hematocrit by about 3%.

Box 12.2: Indications for whole blood.

- Acute loss of blood with hypovolemia
- Exchange transfusion in neonates (blood should be less than 5 days old)
- No red cell concentrates available

- One unit of whole blood (about 350 mL) will increase the hemoglobin level by 0.75 g/dL in an adult patient of about 60–70 kg, who is not bleeding.
- In pediatric patients, transfusion of 8 mL/kg of red cell will increase the hemoglobin by 1 g/dL.

BLOOD COMPONENTS

Various blood components and plasma derivatives are listed in Table 12.1 and Flowchart 12.1.

Main uses of various blood components are presented in Table 12.2.

Precaution needed: For safe and adequate therapy following should be adhered to:
- Separate the components within 6–8 hours from the time of blood collection
- Component separation has to be done in a closed system by using multiple (double, triple or quadruple) plastic bags so that separation is done in a closed system. Separation is done under the laminar air flow bench and sterility is maintained.
- If transfer bags are used, always use a sterile connecting device (SCD).

Table 12.1: Various blood components and plasma derivatives.

Blood components	Plasma derivatives
• Red cells concentrate or packed red blood cells (PRBCs) • Leukocyte poor red cell concentrate • Platelet rich plasma (PRP) • Platelet concentrates • Granulocyte concentrates • Single donor plasma • Fresh frozen plasma (FFP) • Cryoprecipitate • Cryo-poor plasma	• Albumin • Plasma protein fraction (PPF) • Factor VIII concentrate • Fibrinogen • Immunoglobulins • Other coagulation factors

Table 12.2: Main uses of various blood components.

Various blood components	Main uses
Red cell concentrates	To restore tissue oxygenation
Platelets	To treat bleeding due to thrombocytopenia
Fresh frozen plasma (FFP)	Coagulation factor deficiencies
Cryoprecipitate	As a source of fibrinogen
Factor VIII and von Willebrand factor	Deficiency of factor VIII and von Willebrand factor
Specific factor concentrates	Specific factor deficiency

Flowchart 12.1: Various components that can be prepared from blood.

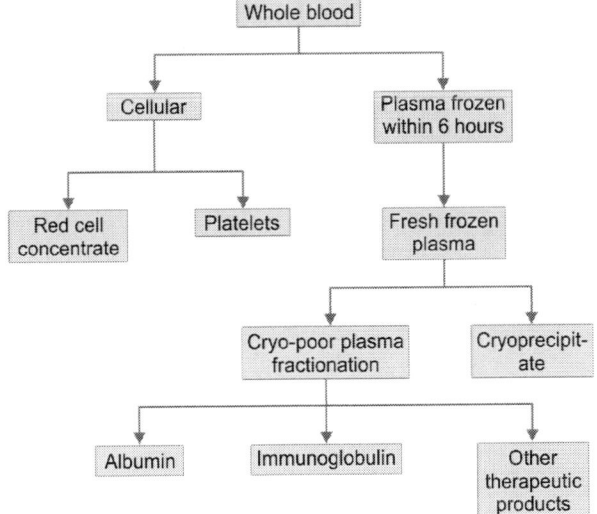

Blood Collection for Components

1. Select a healthy donor and clean the venepuncture site to minimize bacterial contamination.
2. Prevent activation of the blood coagulation system; blood must be collected rapidly with a single venepuncture and with minimal trauma to the tissues.
3. Frequent, gentle mixing of the blood with the anticoagulant should be done during blood collection.
4. All the satellite bags must be accurately identified, numbered, labeled as coming from the original unit.
5. Process all the blood bags within 4–6 hours of phlebotomy.
6. Balance all blood bags accurately before centrifugation.

Plastic closed bag system used for preparation of blood components from whole blood is diagrammatically shown in Figure 12.4.

PREPARATION OF BLOOD COMPONENTS

The whole blood should reach the component laboratory as soon as possible. To get the maximum benefit of the products, it is necessary to separate within 6 hours. Aseptic technique is important during the preparation of components.

Separation of components can be done while the other laboratory tests on the blood are being carried out such as grouping and screening for hepatitis B, venereal disease research laboratory (VDRL), anti-HIV and anti-HVB. Thus, the blood need not be held in component laboratory for longer in the blood center than for processing of whole blood.

Centrifugation

Separation of components from the original whole blood unit is performed by using centrifuge. It requires high-speed centrifuges which can accommodate four or six units of whole blood. The separation of various blood components is based on the specific gravity or weight of each individual blood constituent. When a tube of anticoagulated blood is centrifuged, distinct layers develop (Fig. 12.5). The blood components such as red blood cells (RBCs), platelets, and plasma have different specific gravities. The specific gravity of RBCs is 1.08–1.09, platelets is 1.03–1.04 and plasma is 1.02–1.03. Hence, these components are separated from one another by using differential centrifugation. The heavier RBCs will move to the bottom of the collection bag because they are the heaviest component. The lighter plasma components occupy the top. Between these two prominent layers is a smaller layer composed of white blood cells (WBCs) and platelets (the buffy coat/layer). Apheresis technology (Chapter 13) uses this same principle for separating blood components.

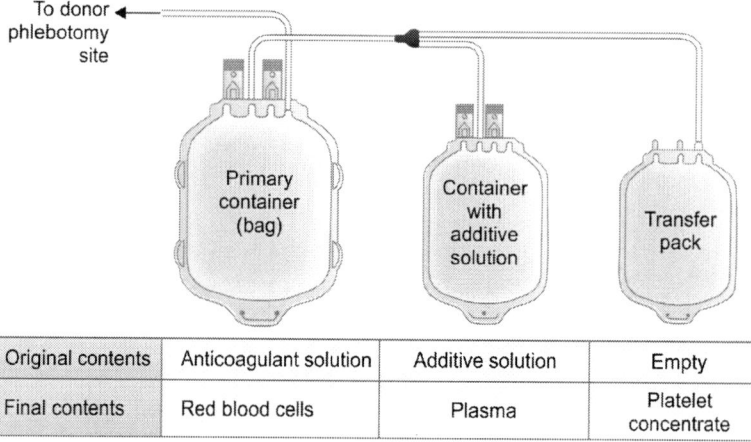

Fig. 12.4: Plastic closed bag system used for preparation of blood components from whole blood (diagrammatic).

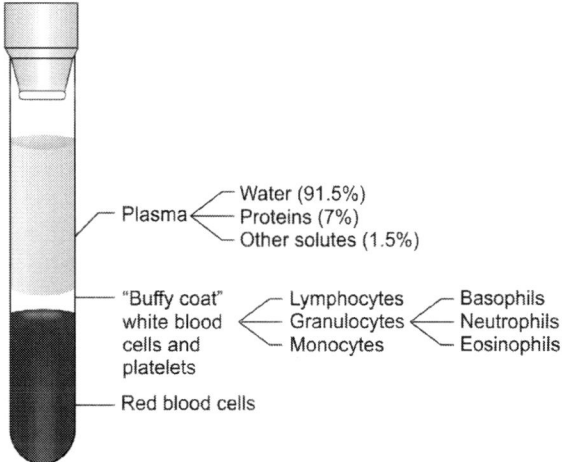

Fig. 12.5: Various layers in a sedimented blood sample.

Refrigerated centrifuge: It is used for centrifugation of blood. Important variables in centrifugation are: (1) Rotor size, (2) speed of the centrifuge (revolutions per minute [RPM] or relative centrifugal force [g-force]) and (3) duration of spin. Types of spins used in various component preparations with their speed and duration are mentioned in Table 12.3.

Quality control: Each centrifuge used for preparing blood components is calibrated for optimal time and speed for each component to be prepared. Quality control measures should be performed to evaluate the products and determine whether the centrifugation parameters are set for maximum product yield. Centrifuges should be properly validated and maintained. A **short centrifugation time at a low RPM is usually called a light spin**, whereas a **longer spin time at a higher RPM is called a heavy spin.**

It is very essential that the contents in **opposing cups of the centrifuge must be equal in weight**. If not so, it impairs not only efficiency of centrifuge but also may cause damage to the rotor. For balancing, plastic or weighted rubber disks and large rubber bands or stoppers are used. The balanced cups are carefully placed diagonally opposite in the cold centrifuge.

The whole blood is dealt differently depending upon the components required. First the platelet rich plasma (PRP) is removed and then the additive solution is added to the concentrated red cells for optimum preservation of red cells. There are many devices which semi-automatically separate whole blood, but are in limited use.

Equipment and consumables used for preparation of blood component are listed in Box 12.3.

Whole blood can also be separated into components using apheresis (Chapter 13).

Table 12.3: Types of spins used in various component preparation with their speed and duration.

Type of spin	Speed and duration of centrifugation
Heavy spin (longer spin, high RPM and concentrates component)	
• Packed red cells • Platelet concentrates	5000 x g for 5 minutes
• Cell free plasma • Cryoprecipitate	5000 x g for 7 minutes
Light spin (short time and low RPM)	
Platelet rich plasma (PRP)	2000 x g for 3 minutes

RED BLOOD CELL COMPONENTS

Red Cells Concentrate or Packed Red Blood Cells (PRBCs)

Description of component: Red blood cells are the cells remaining after removal of the most of the plasma from whole blood. The fluid portion of the unit (about 130 mL) is mainly the additive preservative solution, though about

> **Box 12.3:** Equipment and consumables used for preparation of blood component.
>
> **Equipment**
> - Suitable refrigerated centrifuges for blood component preparation
> - Blood bank refrigerator
> - Deep freezer
> - Double pan balance
> - Hand sealer, roller and cutter
> - Dielectric sealer
> - Plasma extractor/expressor
> - Platelet rotator/agitator with incubator
> - Thawing bath
> - Cryo-bath
> - Laminar flow cabinet
> - Aluminum canisters
> - Sterile bag to bag connecting device
>
> **Consumables**
> - Blood collection bags (double/triple/quadruple/special bags with additives)
> - Transfer bag
> - Bag to bag connectors
> - Plastic cover for blood bags

20 mL of plasma remains from the original unit of whole blood.
- In a unit of 450 mL of whole blood, plasma constitutes approximately 200–250 mL and the red cell constitutes about 190 mL of red cells (450 mL × 42% hematocrit). It has a hematocrit of about 60%.
- In a unit of 350 mL of whole blood, plasma constitutes 150–175 mL.
- Their final hematocrit value should be less than 80% (70–80%). This blood component is usually called "packed red cells" or "packed cells." It has the same oxygen carrying capacity as whole blood.

Additive system: In whole blood with additive solution (refer pages 165, 166 and Table 8.4), RBCs contain even less plasma but hematocrit is between 55% and 65% because of the added additive solution. PRBCs can be prepared at any time during their shelf-life, but additive solution (AS) should be added within the first 72 hours of storage.

Methods of Separation of Red Blood Cells

Packed red cells are obtained by **centrifugation or sedimentation** of the whole blood and the plasma is transferred to another bag.

Centrifugation

Usually the red cells and plasma are separated **within 8 hours of collection**. This is because if the plasma is to be used as a source of factor VIII, it must be kept in the freezer before 8 hours after collection. When the red cells have to be prepared within a few hours after collection, it is performed by centrifugation. This is because, it is usually done as part of a large scale operation, and speed is important. The centrifugation conditions (time and speed) are determined by the method being used to prepare the platelets or plasma. Steps involved in centrifugation are:

1. **Collection:** Blood is collected in double/triple CPDA bags or special bags with additive solution (e.g. ADSOL [adenine, dextrose, sorbitol, sodium chloride and mannitol] or SAG-M [saline, adenine, glucose and mannitol solution]). Weigh and balance each blood unit.
2. **Heavy spin:** Load blood units into a swinging bucket apparatus (Figs. 12.6A and B). Balance each unit (an assortment of rubber weights is usually used). After balancing, the bags of whole blood are centrifuged at 5000 x g for 5 minutes (heavy spin) with a temperature setting at 40°C in a refrigerated centrifuge. If also preparing platelet concentrates, the initial spin will be light (2–3 minutes at 3,200 rpm).
3. **Plasma expresser (Fig 12.7):** After the centrifuge has stopped completely, place the blood unit/bag carefully onto a plasma expresser and release the spring. This allows the plate of the expressor to contact the bag. About 4/5th of plasma is expressed into the attached satellite or transfer bag. If special bags with additive solution are used, the maximum amount of plasma is separated into the satellite bag and the additive solution is transferred into the primary bag containing the red cells. If there are more than one satellite bags attached, apply hemostats to one of the bags so that the plasma will flow into only one bag. Remove the appropriate amount of plasma by using a scale. Usually, 230–256 g of plasma will produce a hematocrit level between 70% and 80%. If additive solutions

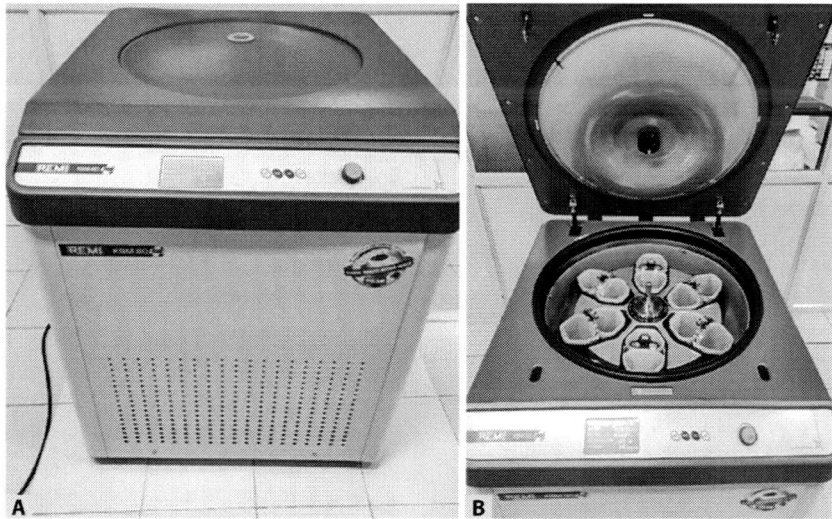

Figs. 12.6A and B: (A) Refrigerated centrifuge; (B) Interior of refrigerated centrifuge shows swinging buckets for holding blood bags.

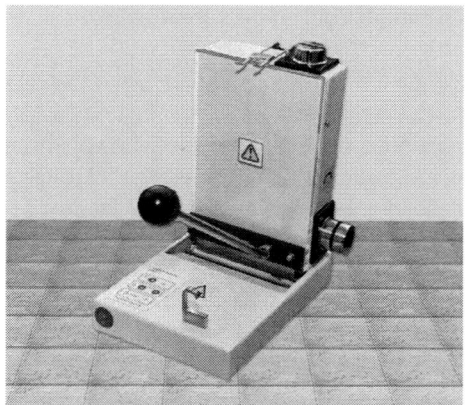

Fig. 12.7: Plasma expresser.

are to be added to the red cell product, almost all of the plasma may be removed (90–95% hematocrit).

4. **Sealing**: After the removal of appropriate amount, the tubing between the primary bag and satellite bag (transfer bag) is sealed by a dielectric heat sealer (refer Fig 7.6) or a hand sealer.
5. **Labeling**: Donor number of the satellite bag should be same as on the primary bag. The bag containing the RBCs is labeled as PRBCs.

Whole blood separated into plasma and red cells is diagrammatically depicted in Figure 12.8.

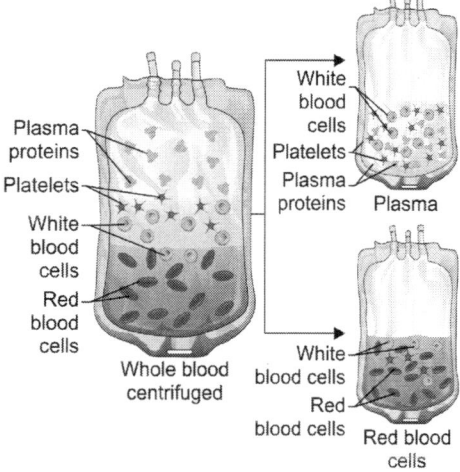

Fig. 12.8: Whole blood separated into plasma and red cells.

Shelf-life and storage

- PRBCs are stored in the refrigerator/cold room at temperature **4°C** (1–6°C).
- Depending on the anticoagulant-preservative solution used, PRBCs have the same shelf-life for **21–42 days** same as whole blood from which they are prepared. However, once the hermetic seal (sealing which makes a given object airtight) is broken during processing, the red cells must be used within 24 hours. The plasma

is stored depending on the product desired (FFP, liquid plasma, etc.).
- Red cells should be refrigerated until the time of the transfusion to prevent the risk of bacterial proliferation within the pack at room temperature. **If the red cells have been out of refrigeration for 30 minutes or longer, they cannot be returned to stock in blood center.** A unit of red cells should be **infused within a maximum period of 4 hours.**
- If **bags with additive** (refer page 165) solution (combinations of saline, adenine, phosphate, bicarbonate, glucose, and mannitol provide better red cell viability during storage) **shelf-life is 42 days.** Red cells and red cells in additive solution can be used interchangeably. However, **red cells in additive solution are not recommended for exchange or massive transfusions in neonates.** During storage, red cells undergo senescence changes similar to aging in vivo. These senescent RBCs in transfused red cells are rapidly cleared by the spleen.
- The end of the storage period is called as the expiration date or the "outdate."
- When blood is transported to the recipient for transfusion, it may be allowed to warm to 10°C. If it is not utilized, it is still be suitable for return to the blood center and reissue to other patients.
- The maximum storage time allowed for RBCs is defined by the requirement for recovery of 75% of transfused cells 24 hours after transfusion.

Sedimentation method
If the original unit of whole blood is not used to prepare platelets or FFP, the red cells can be separated from the plasma at any time during the storage period of the blood. Then the unit of whole blood is kept in an upright position in the refrigerator and allowed to remain undisturbed for several hours till the red cells settle down (sediment). The supernatant plasma can be expressed from the bag into a satellite bag or transfer bag. When sedimentation method is used, the red cells will not be as concentrated as in centrifugation method. Thus, this red cell unit **has a lower hematocrit** and **less plasma is recovered**. The plasma is valuable as a source for production of plasma derivatives. Hence, to recover the maximum amount of plasma, sedimentation is not usually used to separate whole blood into its components. However, sedimentation method can be used when centrifugation method is not available (e.g. in developing countries).

Quality control (Frequency: 4 units/month)
The most important quality requirement of PRBCs is survival of RBCs in circulation of normal recipient. The post transfusion survival of red cells should not be less than 75% after 24 hours. The volume of PRBCs should be 280 ± 60 mL (when prepared from 450 mL whole blood). Packed call volume (hematocrit) should be 0.70 ± 0.05 (65–75%). **PRBCs need crossmatching before transfusion.**

Indications for Use of PRBCs (Box 12.4)
RBCs in the blood contain hemoglobin, which transports oxygen to the tissues. Transfusion of PRBCs increases the mass of circulating red cells in conditions where there is impaired tissue oxygenation due to acute or chronic blood loss (e.g. hemorrhage, anemia). In the packed red cell unit, the hematocrit is between 55% and 65%. Since, the volume is only 200 mL; there is less risk of volume overload.

Features of PRBCs are presented in Box 12.5.

Box 12.4: Indications for use of packed red blood cells (PRBCs).

Anemia
- Hemolytic anemia especially in aplastic crisis
  - β-thalassemia major
  - Sickle cell anemia in sequestration crisis
- Hypoplastic anemia: Aplastic anemia and anemia of chronic renal disease
- Severe anemia of any cause to reduce the chances of circulatory overload
- Hypovolemia due to hemorrhage (trauma)
- Blood loss during surgery: Patients undergoing cardiac, orthopedic, and other surgeries
- Other causes: Oncology patients undergoing chemotherapy or radiation therapy, end-stage renal disease, premature infants, and neonates

Blood Components and their Preparation

Box 12.5: Features of packed red blood cells (RRBCs).

- **Purpose:** To increase O_2 transport to tissues.
- Each unit of packed RBCs should raise the hemoglobin (Hb) by 1 g/dL and the hematocrit (Hct) by 3%.
- **Advantages:**
  - Packed RBCs have less volume and a higher Hct than does the whole blood.
  - Blood group antibodies are less in PRBCs. Thus, nonspecific blood namely O negative can be transfused to patients with other groups.
  - Plasma proteins are less in PRBCs. Hence, chances of anaphylactic reaction are minimal.
- **Disadvantage:** *Yersinia enterocolitica*, a pathogen that thrives on iron, is the most common contaminant of stored blood.

Effect of PRBCs transfusion on hemoglobin and hematocrit level in the recipient: One unit of PRBC will increase the average hemoglobin concentration and hematocrit in an average-sized adult (70 kg) by about 1 g/dL and 3%, respectively. In order to prevent unnecessary transfusion, the requirement of PRBCs should be based on clinical assessment rather than the level of hemoglobin or hematocrit. The level of 7.5 g/dL is taken as transfusion trigger for surgical and patients with leukemia.

Transport and Shipping

Similar to whole blood, PRBCs must be transported in a manner that ensures **temperature between 1°C and 10°C**. If a unit of PRBC is taken out from 5°C storage and left at room temperature of 25°C, the temperature of the unit reaches 10°C in 30 minutes. However, smaller units (pediatric units) become warm more quickly.

During transport and shipping, wet ice and secure bagger is needed to maintain temperatures. An appropriate volume is placed on top of the units within the cardboard box or insulated container.

Leukodepleted (Leukocyte-reduced) Blood Products (Components)

The leukocytes are one of the cellular components present in blood. When blood is transfused, the leukocyte present in the blood components, particularly in RBCs and platelet concentrates (PCs) cause adverse effects. These include febrile nonhemolytic transfusion reaction, immunization to leukocyte (particularly human leukocyte antigen [HLA]) antigens with subsequent refractoriness to platelet transfusions, transmission of leukocyte-associated viruses, graft versus host disease (GVHD) and immune modulation. To prevent or minimize these adverse reactions many methods have been devised to reduce the concentration of leukocytes in cellular components (leukocyte-reduced components/universal leukocyte reduction). However, **leukocyte reduction does not prevent post-transfusion GVHD.**

Leukoreduction or leukodepletion is done for RBC and platelet therapy. In many hospitals, the use of leukocyte-reduced RBCs has become standard practice.

Definition of leukodepletion: It is the **process by which leukocytes are removed from the blood collected** from a donor. In leukocyte poor RBCs, **at least 70% leukocytes should be removed** and the loss of red cells should be less than 20%.

Indications for transfusion of leuko-reduced blood components are listed in Box 12.6.

Method of leukoreduction: Leukocytes are removed by using commercially available **leukocyte reduction filters**. Filtration is the most effective method for leukoreduction, has consistent performance and there is only minimal loss of red cells or platelets. Specific

Box 12.6: Indications for transfusion of leuko-reduced blood components.

- To prevent or reduce febrile nonhemolytic transfusion reactions (FNHTR)
- Neonatal transfusions
- Prevention of HLA (human leukocyte antigen) alloimmunization
- Hematological malignancies
- Transplant recipients
- Platelet refractoriness in multitransfused patients
- Prevention of transmission of leukotropic viruses such as cytomegalovirus (CMV) and Epstein-Barr virus (EBV).

leukocyte depleting filters are available. Most effective leukoreduction filters used for leukodepletion are made up of cellulose acetate or cotton wool polyester.

Categories of Leukocyte Reduction

There are two major categories of leuko-reduced RBCs: prestorage and poststorage.

Prestorage leukocyte reduction

It is leukocyte reduction done by filtration at the time of component manufacture. In this method, multiple layers of polyester or cellulose acetate nonwoven fibers are used to trap leukocytes and platelets. But it allows RBCs to flow through. These filters result in a leukocyte-reduced product with normal shelf-life and meet the requirement for 85% retention of original RBCs.

Leukocytes should be removed early in the prestorage period. This is because during storage, leukocytes degranulate, fragment or die, releasing substances that may cause febrile and allergic transfusion reactions. Special type of blood collection bags with leukocyte filter have been developed to prepare prestorage leuko-depleted blood component. There are also special prestorage leukocyte-removing filters which provide ≥ 99.9% removal of leukocyte to meet the 5×10^6 requirement. They have multiple layers of synthetic nonwoven fibers that selectively retain white cells and allow red cells and/or platelets to flow through. Benefits of prestorage leukodepletion are listed in Box 12.7.

Methods of prestorage leukoreduction:
There are three methods for prestorage leukoreduction:
1. **Using inline filters integral to the collection set:** Inline filter attached to the whole blood unit and filtered via gravity. The leukocytes from whole blood are removed without removing platelets. RBCs and plasma can then be prepared.
2. **After the separation of plasma from red cells:** In this, first plasma is removed from the whole blood unit. Then the packed red cells are passed through an in-line reduction filter.
   In both the above methods, random-donor platelets cannot be prepared. This is because of trapping of platelets in the filter.
3. Sterile docking device is attached to a leukocyte reduction filter to a unit of RBCs, which is allowed to flow via gravity.

Poststorage leukocyte reduction (bedside filtration)
In this, leukocyte reduction is done during transfusion at the bedside. It is used in most of the developing countries.

Methods of poststorage leukoreduction: In poststorage leukoreduction, leukocytes are removed in the blood center before issuing blood or at the bedside before transfusion or when the unit is transfused. In this system standardization of leukocyte removal is difficult to attain. Its disadvantages are listed in Box 12.8.

Frozen Red Blood Cells

Frozen RBCs are the **cells which are stored in the frozen state** at optimal temperatures in the presence of a cryoprotective agent. RBCs

---

Box 12.7: Benefits of prestorage leukodepletion.

- Better control of process and quality assurance
- Less incidence of febrile nonhemolytic transfusion reaction (FNHTR)
- Less incidence of alloimmunization
- Reduction in the risk of transmission of cytomegalovirus (CMV)
- Less chance of bacterial contamination of blood components
- Improved chance of finding an organ transplant match, if needed
- Reduced storage lesion effect
- Reduced risk of transfusion-related acute lung injury (TRALI)

Box 12.8: Disadvantages of poststorage leukocyte reduction.

- Bedside variables which are uncontrollable, e.g. flow rate, blood temperature, filter clogging, etc.
- During storage, leukocytes degranulate or die, releasing cytokines
- Adequate training of staff is difficult
- Number of RBCs/platelets filtered is variable
- Evaluation of quality is difficult

can be frozen for long-term preservation to maintain rare units or to extend the availability of autologous units. **Freezing and storing at or below −65°C, extends storage up to 10 years** from collection. Red cells must be frozen within 6 days of collection. To prepare RBC units for freezing, **glycerol is commonly used as a cryoprotective agent.** This agent protects red cells from freezing injury. It prevents dehydration of red cells and formation of ice crystals, which causes cell hemolysis. Glycerol is slowly added to the unit till a final glycerol concentration of 40% weight per volume is achieved. The blood unit is transferred to a polyolefin or polyvinyl chloride bag and placed in a metal or cardboard canister to prevent breakage at low temperatures. Units can subsequently be stored at −65°C for up to 10 years from the date of collection.

Uses of frozen RBCs: They are used mainly **for storage of rare RBC types and prevention of nonhemolytic febrile transfusion reaction** due to leukocytes, platelets, and plasma (because excessive washing during deglycerolization removes them).

Deglycerolized Red Blood Cells

Before transfusion, thawing of frozen red cells in 37°C dry warmer or water bath and removal of cryoprotective agent by washing must be performed. This is done to avoid osmotic hemolysis when the red cells are transfused. The **process of removal of glycerol cryoprotectant from frozen red cells** by washing red cells in a series of saline solutions of decreasing osmolarity is called deglycerolization. To draw the glycerol out of the red cells, saline solutions of 12% and 1.6%, followed by 0.9% normal saline (that contains 0.2% dextrose), are used. The dextrose in the 0.9% normal saline provides nutrients to the red cell during post-transfusion period. This process of deglycerolization is usually **performed on an instrument called blood cell processor.** Most of the plasma, platelets and leukocytes are removed during the freezing, thawing or during deglycerolization. Because the process of glycerolization and deglycerolization involves entering the blood unit, the system is considered "open." Hence, the deglycerolized RBCs must be transfused within 24 hours. As a visual check of the supernatant from the final wash, the deglycerolized RBCs helps to confirm that sufficient glycerol is removed and the hemolysis is minimal. Presently, automated system for addition of glycerol to RBCs and its removal from RBCs (deglycerolization) in a closed system is also available.

Use of deglycerolized RBCs: This is the **process before using frozen RBCs for transfusion.**

Washed Red Cells

Washed red cells are the red cells remaining after washing with a solution used to remove almost all of the plasma. Red cells can be washed by adding normal saline to the red cells in an ordinary bag, centrifuging them and removing the supernatant. They **can be washed manually or by using semiautomated washing devices** such as those used for deglycerolization. In automatic blood cell processor used for deglycerolizing frozen RBCs approximately 1000–2000 mL of 0.9% saline is used for washing red cells. The washed red cells may contain a variable number of leukocytes and platelets. There is usually some loss of red cell (about 15–20%) during the washing step, and the washed red cell unit may contain a fewer red cells than a standard unit. The washed red cells have a **storage period of 24 hours**. It is no longer considered an effective method of removing leukocytes.

Indications: Washed red cells may be indicated for patients:
- Who react to the small amount of plasma proteins that may be present in a unit of RBCs. These reactions may be allergic, febrile or anaphylactic.
- With IgA deficiency requiring a transfusion having clinically significant anti-IgA.
- Who need intrauterine or neonate transfusions.

Red Blood Cells Irradiated

Blood components that contain viable donor T lymphocytes in cellular blood components (RBCs and platelets) when transfused may cause transfusion-associated GVHD in the recipient (especially in severe immunosuppressed patients). The consequences of GVHD include fever, skin rashes, hepatitis, diarrhea, suppression of bone marrow, and infection, and it is fatal in more than 90% (high mortality) of affected patients. This can be prevented or reduced if the **lymphocytes of donor are inactivated** before transfusion. This can be achieved by irradiation of blood.

Factors that determine a patient's risk for transfusion-associated GVHD include: (1) whether the patient is immunodeficient and if so degree of immunodeficiency and (2) the degree of HLAs matching between donor and recipient.

Indications for irradiated blood components (Box 12.9): The donor's T lymphocytes are responsible for transfusion-associated GVHD. Gamma irradiation of cellular blood components prevents proliferation (multiplication) of donor's T lymphocytes. RBCs that have been leukocyte reduced by filtration do not prevent GVHD because some leukocytes still remain in the RBCs component.

Method of irradiation: Irradiation of blood components can be performed with gamma rays/irradiator (cesium-137 or cobalt-60 radioisotopes), linear accelerators, UV-A irradiation, and non-radioisotope equipment (X-rays). Prophylactic gamma irradiation of dose between 15 and 25 Gy (i.e. 1500–2500 rads) is effective. It can cause 90% reduction of T lymphocyte population and abolish mitogen-induced blast transformation. It does not damage either RBCs or platelets.

Expiration date: RBC components that have been irradiated expire on their originally assigned expiry date or 28 days from the date of irradiation whichever is earlier. Platelet expiration date does not change with irradiation.

Apheresis red blood cells (Discussed in Chapter 13).

PLATELET COMPONENTS

Introduction

Normal platelet function and adequate numbers of circulating platelets are necessary for the formation of primary hemostatic plug. The process of hemostasis involves different steps namely platelet adhesion, activation, aggregation and secretion. Main functions of platelets are listed in Box 12.10.

Sources of platelet: Two main sources of platelets for transfusion are as follows:
1. Platelet concentrate may be **obtained from whole blood by centrifugation of platelet rich plasma (PRP) and removal of platelet-poor plasma.** The source may be either a single donor or pooled plasma.
2. Platelets can also be obtained from a single donor **by platelet apheresis.**

Principle: PRP is separated from whole blood by "light spin" centrifugation and the platelets are concentrated by "heavy spin" centrifugation. The supernatant plasma is subsequently removed. Platelet concentrates are prepared from blood units that have not been allowed to cool below 20°C.

Preparation of donor: Aspirin and alcohol ingestion may affect platelet function for 3 days

Box 12.9: Indications for irradiated blood components.

- Congenital immunodeficiency syndrome
- Recipients who are undergoing bone marrow transplant or progenitor cell transplantation
- Premature newborn
- Patients with hematological malignancies
- Patients with solid malignant tumors receiving extensive chemotherapy
- Fetuses receiving intrauterine transfusion
- Patients receiving exchange transfusion
- Immunocompromised recipients

Box 12.10: Main functions of platelets.

- Maintains vascular integrity
- Initial arrest of bleeding by forming platelet plug (primary hemostatic plug)
- Stabilizes the hemostatic plug and contributes to the process of formation of fibrin (secondary hemostatic plug)

after ingestion. A donor who has taken aspirin within this period should not be accepted for platelet preparation.

Method of Preparation of PRP and Platelet Concentrate

It can be prepared by three methods:
1. Using refrigerated centrifuge
2. Buffy coat removal method for preparation of platelet concentrate
3. Apheresis machine (cell separators)

1. *Using refrigerated centrifuge*
   Step 1: To prepare PRP
   a. Whole blood collected to prepare platelet concentrates must be obtained by a **single nontraumatic venepuncture.** Appropriate volume of blood is collected in double or triple/ADSOL triple or quadruple blood collection bags containing appropriate anticoagulant solution (CPDA).
   b. Whole blood collected is kept at room temperature (20–22°C) before and during platelet preparation (i.e. during separating PRP from red cells till processing). The **separation must be performed within 6–8 hours of collection of the whole blood. Do not refrigerate** and blood should not be chilled at any time before or during platelet separation.
   c. Set the centrifuge temperature at 22°C. **Centrifuge the blood bags** after accurate balancing at 20–24°C **using a light spin** (2000 x g for 3 minutes) to separate PRP. This should separate most of the RBCs but leave most of the platelets suspended in the plasma. Platelet preparation should be done using a closed and multibag system.
   d. **Express the PRP** (Figs. 12.9A and B) **into the first satellite bag** intended for platelet storage. Transfer the red cell additive solution into the red cells in the primary bag. Sufficient plasma must remain on the RBCs to maintain a 70–80% hematocrit level.
   e. Seal the tubing between the primary bag (containing RBCs) and the two satellite bags by dielectric sealer and

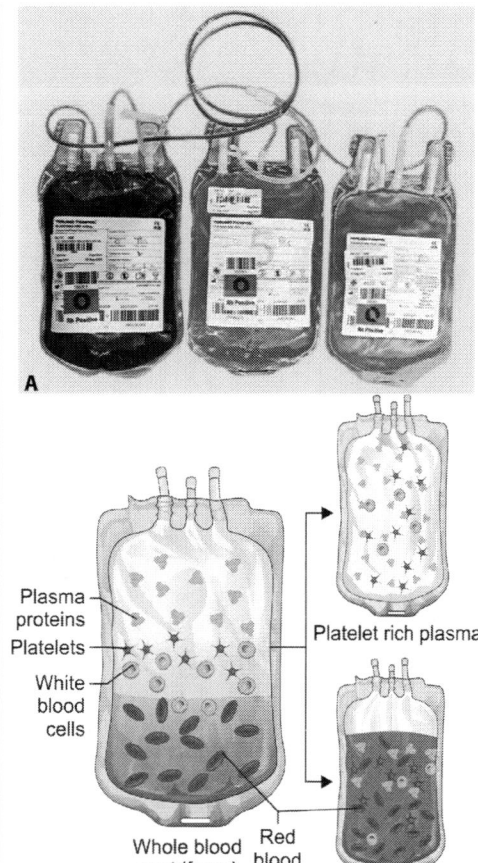

Figs. 12.9A and B: (A) Packed red cells in first bag (on left) and platelet rich plasma in second bag; (B) Platelet rich plasma produced from whole blood (diagrammatic) *(For color version, see Plate 3).*

   separate the primary bag. Disconnect the primary bag containing the RBC and store at 2–6°C (4°C).
   f. Platelet rich plasma may be used as such or processed further to prepare platelet concentrates and FFP. PRP should be used with ABO compatibility.

Step 2: To prepare platelet concentrate from PRP (Flowchart 12.2).
   a. Balance the bag containing PRP and recentrifuge the bags (contain PRP) at 22°C using a heavy spin (at 5000 x g [3,600 rpm] for 5 minutes). This will separate the platelets from the plasma.
   b. The supernatant platelet poor plasma is expressed into the second satellite/

Flowchart 12.2: Preparation of platelet concentrate by of platelet-rich plasma (PRP) method.

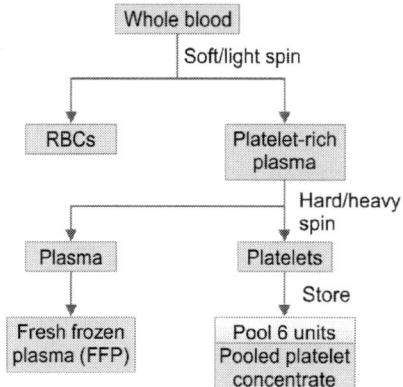

transfer bag (if triple bag is used). Leave about 50–70 mL of plasma with the platelet concentrate to maintain the pH at 6.2 or higher for the entire storage period. Seal the tubing between the bags and separate the bags.

c. This **entire process is traumatic to the concentrated platelets.** Hence, platelet concentrate **should be kept undisturbed for 1–2 hours at 20–24°C** (air-conditioned room) or till all platelet clumps have been resuspended in the residual plasma. If not allowed to rest, the platelets may aggregate irreversibly and not be functional. Make sure that the platelet button is covered with the plasma. If required, gentle manipulation can be done. Weigh the plasma bag, and determine and record the volume on the bag.

d. Place the plasma in a protective container and freeze. The plasma should be frozen in such a way that evidence of thawing can be determined. Before freezing, make sure that any tubing segments and the transfusion ports of the bag are tucked in or placed in such a manner as to prevent or minimize possible breakage. Freezing produces some sort of indentation into the bag. This is visible as long as the plasma remains frozen. The freezing container is important because the plastic bag becomes quite brittle when frozen at low temperatures and can crack or break easily. Properly label the frozen plasma. The plasma can be stored as FFP, single-donor plasma frozen within 24 hours (PF24), or liquid recovered plasma. Shelf-life is 12 months when stored at –18°C or lesser temperature.

e. After completion of 1 hour when the platelet concentrate (Figs. 12.10A and B) has rested, resuspend the platelets by gently agitating the platelet bag by hand to allow uniform resuspension. Label (mentioning the volume, expiration date) and store at 20–22°C in a platelet

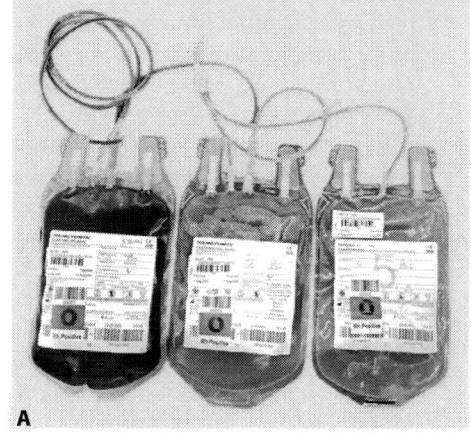

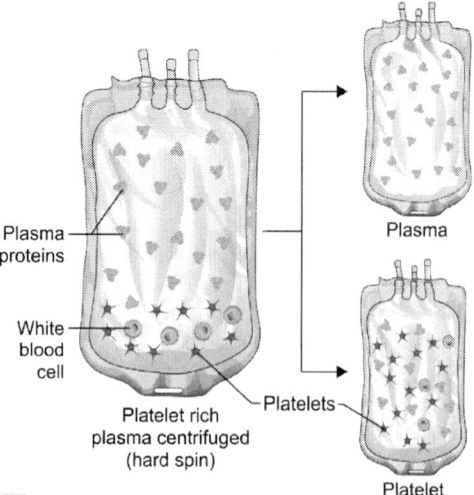

Figs. 12.10A and B: (A) Packed cells (First from left), platelet poor plasma (second from left) and platelet concentrate (third from left); (B) Production of platelet concentrates from platelet rich plasma (diagrammatic) *(For color version, see Plate 3).*

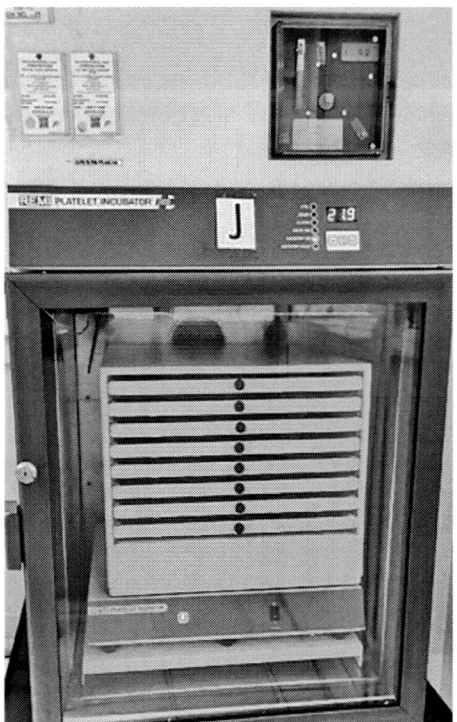

Fig. 12.11: Platelet agitator and incubator.

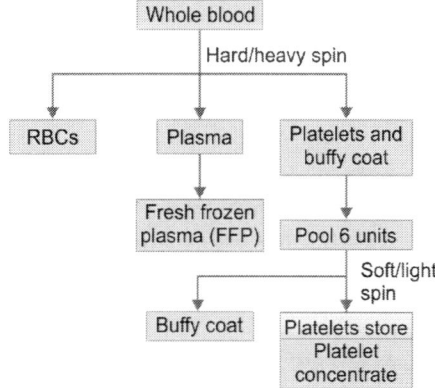

Flowchart 12.3: Preparation of platelet concentrates by buffy coat (BC) method.

agitator and incubator (Fig. 12.11) to maintain gentle agitation during storage. **Platelet concentrate shelf-life is 5 days** from the date of blood collection. The day of preparation is considered as zero day. If the system is opened, transfusion must be done within 6 hours.

2. ***Buffy coat removal method for preparation of platelet concentrate***
   Centrifugation spin profiles used for separation of the buffy coat are different from those used in conventional PRP method for preparation of blood component. In this first spin is hard spin for separation of 3 layers in a single step. The second spin is soft spin followed by separation of platelet concentrate.

   Methods: Platelet concentrate from buffy coat may be prepared by two methods:
   i. One-unit platelet concentrate from single buffy coat
   ii. Pooled platelet concentrates from pooling of 4 to 5 buffy coats (Flowchart 12.3).

Advantages of platelet concentrate of buffy coat over PRP-derived
- Improved and standardized with minimal contamination by red blood cells.
- Enhanced platelet quality and better in vivo survival.
- Several platelet suspension media can be used (e.g. plasma, platelet additive solution, PAS).
- When PAS is used as suspension media, plasma yield is higher which can be used for other purposes.
- Lower leukocyte contamination.
- Standardization of preparation by using automated devices (e.g. optisystem)

Advantages of pooled platelet concentrate by buffy coat method
- Pooling helps in providing high dose of platelet concentrate equivalent to those obtained by apheresis.
- Platelet additive solution can be used with more plasma yield which can be used for other purposes.
- Ready to use platelets.
- Easier inactivation of pathogens can be done.

Platelet extraction from pooled buffy coat:
It needs a buffy coat pooling set. These sets are integrated systems used for increase the quality of platelets obtained from buffy coat method. Each set is designed to pool together v4 to 6 buffy coats. Normally, buffy coat contains all the platelets, white blood cells and few red blood cells.

Buffy coat pooling set: It has 5 to 6 tubing connected together to a pooling container. The buffy coat residues of identical ABO groups are pooled into the pooling container. The plasma in these buffy coats is very negligible in amount. One unit of plasma or platelet additive solution is added to these pooled buffy coats. The pooled platelets are subjected to soft centrifugation (refer Flowchart 12.3) and platelet concentrate is transferred to the storage container. The platelet concentrate is leuco-depleted as it passes through the leuco-depletion filter.

3. *Apheresis of platelets:* It is discussed in Chapter 13.

The official term for **platelet** concentrates component is platelets. **Platelet concentrates** are prepared **from whole blood** are usually called as **random-donor platelets (or platelet concentrates)** to distinguish them from **single-donor platelets produced by apheresis**. These are platelets suspended in plasma or platelet additive solution. Various constituents of platelet additive solutions include sodium chloride, potassium chloride, magnesium chloride, sodium citrate, sodium phosphate buffer, sodium acetate, and sodium gluconate. Platelet concentrates prepared from a unit of whole blood must contain at least 5.5×10^{10} platelets per unit and should raise the platelet count by about 5000 µL in a recipient weighing 75 kg. Though there is no required volume, these units usually contain a volume of about 50 mL to maintain viability and function during storage.

ABO and Rh Compatibility

ABO: Platelets have ABO antigens on their surface. Hence, it is advisable to use ABO matched platelets whenever possible. But there is no necessity to delay transfusion in order to obtain ABO compatible platelets.

Rh: Platelet do not express Rh antigen (i.e. D antigen is not detectable on platelets). Therefore, if platelets from D-positive donor are given to recipients with anti-D, there will be normal post-transfusion survival of platelets. But the platelet units may contain up to 0.5 mL of visibly apparent RBCs. They may cause alloimmunization in a D negative recipient to red cell antigens. Hence, it should be avoided in immunologically normal D-negative females of childbearing age and transfuse Rh negative individuals with platelets only from Rh negative individuals. An alternative is to use immunoprophylactic dose of Rh immune globulin (RHIG) injection. In infants, avoid administration of plasma that is incompatible with the red cells of infants.

Storage and Shelf-life

Platelets are **stored at 22–24°C** (room temperature) **in a platelet agitator and incubator (Fig. 12.11)**. Platelets stored at refrigerator temperature (1–6° C) have greatly diminished post-transfusion survival. The purpose of continuous gentle agitation on a platelet agitator is that the gentle agitation will keep the platelets in suspension and prevent clumping and encourages gas exchange. Horizontal agitation of 70/min is preferred to vertical agitation.

Platelets can be **stored for 72 hours or for 5 days** depending upon the quality of the storage bags (first day, i.e. day of preparation is taken as zero day. Day 1 starts at 12 am of the next day). At the end of storage, the pH of the platelet concentrates must be 6.0 or higher.

Transport and Shipping

During transport, platelets should be maintained at 20–24°C. Use a well-insulated container without added ice designed to keep the temperature at 20–24°C. Filter-filled envelops or newspapers can be used as insulators. For very long distances or more than 24 hours of travel, double insulated containers may be used.

Quality Control

- All platelet products must be inspected before the release and issue. If the units show excessive platelet aggregates, it should not be used for transfusion.
- Platelet count must be $> 5.5 \times 10^{10}$ platelets per unit/bag in 75% of the units tested. A minimum of four bags must be tested per month. It is necessary to select units

on random basis for quality control after routine storage of 24 hours. At least in a month, 2% of platelets prepared should be subjected to quality control.
- The pH of the bag must be 6.2 or greater at the end of the permitted storage period.
- Bags must be held against a light source and gently tapped to see if there is a "swirling" appearance. This swirl phenomenon correlates well with adequate platelet viability.

Indications for platelet concentrate are given in Box 12.11.

Transfusion of platelets is done to control or prevent bleeding associated with critical reduction in the numbers of circulating platelet or functionally abnormal platelets. Platelet transfusions are not usually useful or indicated in conditions where there is destruction of circulating platelets caused by autoimmune disorders (e.g. idiopathic thrombocytopenic purpura, heparin-induced thrombocytopenia, or thrombotic thrombocytopenic purpura [TTP]).

Each unit of platelets usually increases the platelet count by 5,000–10,000/μL in a 70 kg adult. Usual dose of thrombocytopenic patients with bleeding is 6–10 units of platelet concentrate. Normally, transfused platelets circulate with a lifespan of only 3–4 days. Hence, frequent transfusions may be needed in patients requiring platelets.

Box 12.11: Indications for platelet concentrate.

Bleeding due to:
- Thrombocytopenia, when platelet count is less than 20,000/mm³
  - Chemotherapy or radiation therapy or drug induced
  - Leukemia
  - Marrow infiltration, e.g. leukemia, carcinoma
  - Dilutional (e.g. massive transfusion with stored blood)
  - Hypoplastic anemia
  - Viral disease associated (e.g. dengue)
- Abnormal platelet function
- Disseminated intravascular coagulation (DIC)
- Recipients of hematopoietic progenitor cell transplants for a period after transplant
- Patients with postoperative bleeding
- Organ transplant patients (e.g. liver transplants)

Box 12.12: Causes of platelet refractoriness or poor response to platelet transfusions.

Immune: HLA alloantibodies, platelet alloantibodies, and autoantibodies
Nonimmune: Splenomegaly, drugs, sepsis, active bleeding and disseminated intravascular coagulation (DIC)

Efficacy of platelet transfusion: Evaluation of the effectiveness of platelet transfusions is important to determine whether the patient is refractory or unresponsive to the platelet transfusions (Box 12.12). It is assessed either by performing platelet count at 1 hour and 24 hours after transfusion or by clinical assessment.

Corrected count increment (CCI): It determines the increase in platelet count adjusted for the number of platelets transfused and the size of the patient. Platelet counts should be performed before transfusion and within 1 hour after transfusion. CCI is assessed by the following formula:

$$CCI = \frac{\text{Post-transfusion platelet count} - \text{Pre-transfusion platelet count}}{\text{Number of platelets transfused} \times 10^{11}} \times \text{body surface area (BSA) m}^2$$

For example, if a patient with a body surface area of 2 m² is transfused 4×10^{11} number of platelets and initial platelet count of 15,000/μL and post-transfusion count was 55000/μL. Then

$$CCI = \frac{55000 - 15000}{4} \times 2 = 20000/\mu L$$

Corrected count increment value of less than 5000/μL at 10 minutes to 1-hour post-transfusion in a clinically stable patient indicates a refractory state to platelet transfusion. Platelets do not require crossmatching before transfusion but should be ABO compatible with the recipient's red cells whenever possible.

Pooled Platelets

To achieve a therapeutic dose of platelets in a recipient, platelet concentrates obtained by whole blood centrifugation are pooled for transfusion in adults. Pooling of platelets is done by transferring the platelet concentrates (usually 6-8 units for an adult) into a transfer set (single bag), while taking care not to contaminate the ports. An approximate dose is 1 unit per 10 kg of patient body weight, yielding pools of 6-10 platelets. This platelet pooling method creates an "open system." This in turn reduces the expiration of the pooled product to 4 hours from the start of pooling. The pooled platelets must be stored at 20-24°C with gentle agitation till one transfusion. The pooled unit must be provided with a unique pool number and must be placed/written on the label. Units selected for pooling must ABO compatible because there will be some RBCs in each unit.

Platelets are given either as pools of 4 to 6 prepared random donors (RDs) or as single-donor apheresis platelets (SDAPs) from a single donor.

Platelets Leukocytes Reduced

Leukocyte reduction can be done by using apheresis devices and leukocyte reduction filters (refer pages 251, 252). It prevents recurrent febrile nonhemolytic reactions and HLA alloimmunization in patients who need long-term platelet support or transplantation. Similar to leukocyte reduced RBC products, leukocyte removal before storage reduces cytokines and the potential febrile reactions. Leukocyte-reduced platelets can prevent CMV infection.

Salient features of platelet transfusion are presented in Box 12.13.

■ PLASMA COMPONENTS

Plasma is separated from red cells by centrifugation of the whole blood. The red cells are used as packed red cell component. Plasma may be used to replace the lost plasma proteins in cases of extensive burns.

Coagulation: It is a process that involves a series of biochemical reactions that use circulating coagulation factors present in the plasma and convert plasma into an insoluble gel through conversion of fibrinogen to fibrin. Apart from coagulation factors, it needs phospholipids and calcium. Impairment of the coagulation system may occur, either due to decreased synthesis of the coagulation factors or consumption of the factors. Defects in the plasma clotting factors may be due to congenital or acquired conditions. Plasma also contains albumin, immunoglobulins, and other proteins essential for metabolism.

Fresh Frozen Plasma

Introduction: Blood components containing coagulation factors can be prepared either from units of whole blood or from plasma by large-scale fractionation.
- **Whole blood-derived components** used to replace coagulation factors include FFP, FP-24, plasma and cryoprecipitate.
- **Plasma-derivative** products are factor VIII, factor IX, antithrombin III (AT III), prothrombin factor complex, and fibrinogen concentrates.

Definition: FFP is plasma separated from whole blood (refer Figs. 12.12 and 12.15A) along with anticoagulant, placed at −18°C or lower (frozen) within 6-8 hours after collection.

Contents of FFP: FFP contains **maximum levels of all labile** (V and VIII) **and nonlabile clotting factors** and includes albumin, protein C and S, and antithrombin. FFP is an acellular component and does not transmit intracellular infections (e.g. CMV).

Shelf-life: FFP has a shelf-life of **12 months** (1 year) from the date of collection of blood. Plasma is separated from whole blood and frozen for extended preservation. In the liquid state at refrigerator temperatures, plasma losses labile clotting factors (particularly factors VIII and V). The labile factors do not store well at temperatures greater than −18°C.

Box 12.13: Salient features of platelet transfusion.

- Purpose is stop significant bleeding due to quantitative (thrombocytopenia) or qualitative platelet defects (e.g. aspirin).
- Platelets have HLA antigens and ABO antigens on their surfaces. They do not have Rh antigens.
- Each unit of platelets transfused should raise the platelet count by 5,000–10,000 cells/mm^3. If there is increase in the count, it is most likely being consumed (e.g. DIC).

Method of Preparation

1. Blood is collected in a collection unit (double/triple, CPD/CPDA) with integrally attached satellite bag(s). It should be obtained by clean, single venepuncture with proper mixing of blood with anticoagulant during its collection from the donor.
2. Balance the bags by using dry balancing materials (e.g. rubber disk or larger rubber bands).
3. Centrifuge the bags soon after collection using a heavy spin 5000 x g for 5 minutes. The refrigerated centrifuge should be set at a temperature of 4°C.
4. Place the primary bag containing the centrifuged blood on a plasma extracter and place the attached bag on a weighing scale adjusted to zero. Express the plasma into the satellite bag and weight the plasma.
5. Seal the transfer tubing with a dielectric sealer at two places.
6. Label the transfer bag with the unit number and blood group before it is separated from the primary bag. Record the volume of plasma on the label.
7. Cut the tubing between the two seals.
8. Place plasma at –20°C or lower within 6 hours of collection from the donor.

Contents of triple bag namely packed red cells, fresh frozen plasma (FFP) and platelets are shown in Figure 12.12.

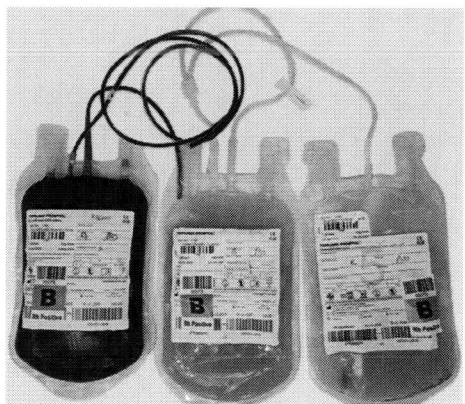

Fig. 12.12: From left to right-packed red cells, fresh frozen plasma (FFP) and platelets *(For color version, see Plate 4)*.

Volume and constituents: FFP from a whole blood donation of 450 mL measures 175–200 mL. It contains 70–80 units/dL of factor VIII, factor IX, von Willebrand factor (vWF), and other plasma coagulation factors.

Factor activity: One unit of factor activity is defined as the amount present in one mL of fresh normal plasma with one-tenth part citrate as an anticoagulant.

Storage and Shelf-life

- Fresh frozen plasma **should be rapidly frozen** (snap freezing) by any of the following methods by placing the bag: in a dry ice ethanol or dry ice-antifreeze bath; between layers of dry ice; in a blast freezer or, in a mechanical freezer maintained at –65°C or lower.
- FP should be **stored at –18°C or lower.** If temperature is maintained between 15–18°C, it has a **shelf-life of 12 months** from the date of the whole blood collection. **FFP frozen and maintained at –65°C can be stored up to 7 years.**

Methods to check on inadvertent thawing of FFP during storage: Any one of the following methods can be used.

1. Place a rubber band around the bag of plasma. After freezing, remove the rubber band which will produce an indentation. This indentation disappears if there is thawing.
2. Press a tube into the bag during freezing which will leave an impression on the bag. It disappears if the unit thaws.
3. Freeze the plasma bag horizontally but store it upright. The air bubbles trapped along the bags will accumulate in the uppermost broad surface during freezing. In the upright position, if there is thawing of the plasma the bubbles move to the top.

Quality control of FFP are given in Table 12.4. A minimum of 4 bags per month need to be tested.

Indications for fresh frozen plasma: FFP is indicated in patients with **bleeding with deficiencies of multiple coagulation factors.** These include **secondary to liver disease,**

Table 12.4: The quantity of constituents that should be present in a bag of FFP.

Constituents	Quantity
Factor VIII	0.7 units/mL
Fibrinogen	200–400 mg
Stable coagulation factors	200 unit
Volume	200–250 mL

DIC, and dilutional coagulopathy resulting from massive blood transfusions. FFP can be used for the treatment of deficiencies of factors II, V, VII, X, or XI because usually there is no specific component therapy available for these factors. FFP can be used **to reverse the warfarin effect** if this must be done more quickly than could be achieved by giving vitamin K. The various indications for FFP are presented in Box 12.14. FFP is not used as a volume expander or as a source of nutrition.

Laboratory parameter used for indication of FFP is Pt/PTT > 1.5 x normal.

Transport and Shipping of FFP

Fresh frozen plasma **must be transported in a frozen state**. This is achieved by using any of the following methods:
- Dry ice in well insulated containers. The dry ice can be layered at the bottom of the container, between each layer of frozen component and on top.
- Standard cartons lined with insulating material such as plastic air bubble packaging.
- Dry packaging fragments.

Thawing FFP for Transfusion

Before transfusion, both FFP and FP24 must be thawed (refer Fig. 12.15B) at 37°C. FFP is thawed by two methods namely—in a water bath or—in an FDA-approved microwave device.
- **Thawing in water bath** (Fig. 12.13): In this method, units of FFP and PF24 are thawed before administration at temperature between 30°C and 37°C for approximately 20–30 minutes. In this method, utmost care must be taken to prevent contamination of the entry ports with water. For this, the FFP bag should be either wrapped in a

Box 12.14: Indications for fresh frozen plasma.
- Management of patients anticoagulated with warfarin who are bleeding or require emergency surgery: Patients on anticoagulant drug therapy namely coumarin anticoagulants-warfarin sodium and dicumarol. Coumarin inhibits the activity of vitamin K dependent coagulation factors. FFP is used for the reversal of coumarin drug effect.
- Replacement of isolated coagulation factor deficiencies.
- Antithrombin deficiency (congenital or acquired), deficiency of protein C and S.
- Correction or prevention of bleeding complications in patients who have severe liver disease with multiple factor deficiencies.
- Vitamin K deficiency.
- Management of patients with disseminated intravascular coagulation (DIC) when the fibrinogen level is less than 100 mg/dL.
- Dilutional coagulopathy.
- Thrombotic thrombocytopenic purpura (TTP).
- Secondary immunodeficiency associated with severe protein-losing enteropathy.
- Abnormal coagulation assays resulting from massive blood transfusion.
- Management of bleeding in patients who need coagulation factors II, V, X or XI, when the concentrates are not available or are not appropriate.
- Replacement solution for therapeutic plasmapheresis for the treatment of TTP and hemolytic uremic syndrome (plasma cryoprecipitate reduced can also be used).
- Management of patients with rare specific plasma protein deficiencies.

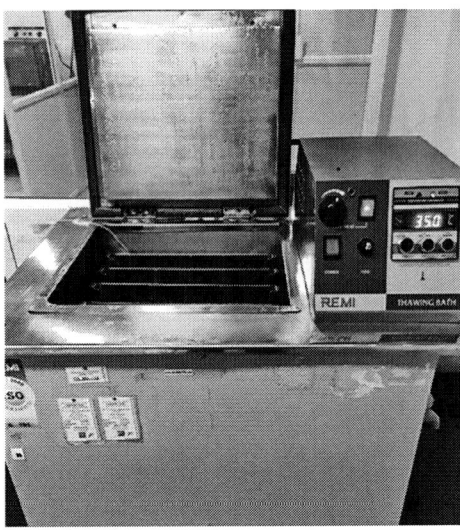

Fig. 12.13: Thawing bath.

plastic protective overwrap or care should be taken to keep the bag in an upright position, with the entry ports above the water level. Water baths with an agitator hastens the thawing process.
- **FDA-approved microwave ovens:** They are specially designed for plasma thawing and can be used as per the manufacturer's instructions. Standard microwave ovens should not be used because they denature plasma proteins.

FFP Thawed (Fig. 12.14): After thawing, the unit is known as "FFP Thawed". It should be transfused immediately or stored between 1 and 6°C for not more than 24 hours. Expiration time and date must be mentioned on the label.

Thawed plasma: FFP is thawed in a closed system and if it is not used within 24 hours, it is relabeled as "thawed plasma." Thawed plasma can be stored at 1–6°C and transfused up to 5 days after thawing. Though it is similar to FFP, there is some reduction in factor V and a clinically significant reduction in factor VIII. Hence, thawed plasma should not be used for replacement of labile coagulation factor VIII. It can be used in burns patient, as a volume expander, and to make albumin and globulin.

Dose: The dose of FFP or PF24 depends on the clinical condition and the underlying disease process. If coagulation factor replacement is necessary, the required dose is 10–20 mL/kg (3–6 units in an adult). Crossmatching is not needed, but the plasma should be ABO compatible with the patient's red cells.

24-hour plasma (FP24/PF24)

This is plasma separated and frozen at –18°C between 8 and 24 hours after collection (phlebotomy) of blood (fozen plasma at any time within 24 hours of collection—FP24). It contains all the stable proteins found in FFP, normal amounts of factor V but only an average of about 55–75% factor VIII. FP24 is often used interchangeably with FFP. It can be stored at –18°C up to 12 months from the date of collection.

Plasma and Liquid Plasma

Plasma can be separated from whole blood at any time during storage up to 5 days after the expiration date of the whole blood. This blood product is not usually available because there are only few indications for the use of plasma. Plasma is mainly used for the production of albumin, immunoglobulins or laboratory reagents.
- **Plasma:** If plasma is stored at –18°C or lower, this can be used up to 5 years after the date of collection.
- **Liquid plasma:** If not frozen, it is called "liquid plasma" which is stored at 1–6°C and transfused up to 5 days after the expiry of the whole blood from which it was prepared.

Solvent–detergent (SD) Plasma

It is being increasingly used in clinical practice because of lower risk of transmission of lipid-enveloped viruses (e.g. HBV, HCV, and HIV) than standard FFP. Solvent-detergent plasma is prepared by treatment of fresh plasma with a combination of the **solvent** tri-n-butyl phosphate (TNBP) and the **detergent** Triton X-100 which inactivates lipid envelope viruses. However, they retain most of the coagulation factor activity. It can transmit nonlipid envelope viruses (e.g. parvovirus or HAV) and thrombotic complications associated with its use have led to withdrawal of SD plasma.

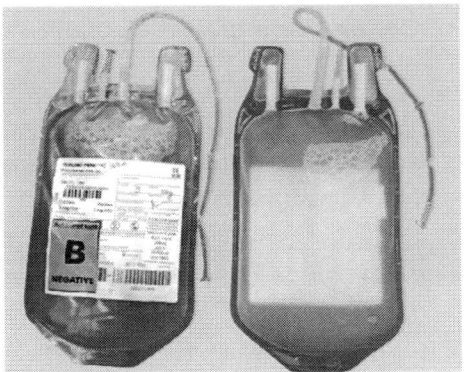

Fig. 12.14: Appearance of thawed fresh frozen plasma (FFP) in a blood bag (front and back view).

Single Donor Plasma or AHG Poor Plasma

It is the plasma separated from an outdated blood or plasma from which antihemophilic factor (AHG) has been removed. It contains all stable coagulation factors. It is used for replacement of prothrombin and replacement of volume.

Cryoprecipitated Antihemophilic Factor

Cryoprecipitated antihemophilic factor (AHF) **also known as cryoprecipitate or simply CRYO.**

Definition: It is the **cold insoluble portion of plasma** (Fig. 12.15C) **that precipitates or remains after FFP is thawed** (melted) between 1 and 6°C refrigerator temperatures.

Content: It is a concentrate of high molecular weight plasma proteins that precipitate in the cold. These plasma proteins include vWF, **factor-VIII (AHF), fibrinogen and factor-XIII.** It contains approximately 50% of the factor VIII and 20–40% of the fibrinogen present in the original plasma unit.

Method of Preparation

1. Blood is collected in a collection unit with two integrally attached satellite bags (triple CPD/CPDA).
2. Fresh frozen plasma is separated as mentioned above on pages 260-2. The plasma is rapidly frozen by using either blast freezes or mechanical freezers capable of maintaining temperature of –65°C or lower. FFP intended for cryoprecipitate preparation can be stored for up to 12 months at –18°C or lower. The cryoprecipitate may be prepared at any time during these 12 months.
3. Allow the FFP to thaw at 1–6°C by placing the collected unit bag in a 1–6°C circulating or thawing water bath or in a refrigerator overnight. The bags should be covered by a plastic overwrap, if thawed in a water bath. Overnight thawing process leads to formation of a plasma protein precipitate (rich in factor VIII) in the form of white flakes of varying sizes.
4. Remove the bags and centrifuge at 5000 x g for 5 minutes at 4°C (heavy spin). When the plasma has a slushy consistency, separate liquid plasma from the cryoprecipitate by one of the procedures below:
   - Hang the bag in an inverted position and allow the separated plasma to flow rapidly into the transfer bag. This leaves the cryoprecipitate adhering to the sides of the primary bag. Promptly separate the cryoprecipitate from the plasma to prevent the cryoprecipitate from dissolving and flowing out of the bag. Leave 10–15 mL of supernatant plasma in the bag for resuspension of the cryoprecipitate after thawing. Refreeze the cryoprecipitate immediately.
   - Place the thawing FFP in a plasma expresser when approximately one-tenth of the contents are still frozen. Keep the bag in an upright position, allow the supernatant plasma to flow slowly into the transfer bag, using the ice crystals at the top as a filter. The cryoprecipitate's paste will adhere to the sides of the bag or to the ice. Seal the bag when about 90% of the cryoprecipitate poor plasma has been removed and refreeze the cryoprecipitate immediately.

Salient features of cryoprecipitate are presented in Box 12.15.

Storage and Shelf-life

- Once separated from FFP, cryoprecipitate is refrozen within 1 hour of preparation and is stored at –18°C or lower preferably –30°C for up to 12 months (1 year) from the

---

Box 12.15: Salient features of cryoprecipitate.

- Purpose is to treat coagulation factor deficiencies involving fibrinogen or factor VIII (e.g. DIC).
- Cryoprecipitate contains fibrinogen, factors VIII and XIII.
- Desmopressin acetate is used instead of cryoprecipitate in treating mild hemophilia A and vWD.

date of blood collection (not from the date of preparation).
- Thawed cryoprecipitate must be stored at room temperature. If pooled, it should be used within 6 hours of thawing, if indicated for replacement of factor-VIII. Pools of thawed individual units must not be refrozen.

Thawing of Cryoprecipitate

Principle: Cryoprecipitate should be rapidly thawed at 30–37°C. Once thawing is completed, it should not remain at this temperature.

Procedure:
- Thawing is performed in a circulating water bath at 37°C or specially designed dry heat devices. Cover the bag with a plastic overwrap to prevent contamination with unsterile water or use a device to keep the containers upright with the ports above water.
- Carefully and completely, resuspend the thawed precipitate either by kneading it into the residual 10–15 mL of plasma or by adding about 10 mL of 0.9% sodium chloride and gently resuspend it.

Quality Control

Composition of bag of cryoprecipitate is presented in Table 12.5.

Samples from at least four donor units should be tested every month. For pooled CRYO units there should be quality control evaluation of at least two containers per month.

ABO compatibility: Cryoprecipitate contains ABO antibodies. Hence, ABO compatibility should be considered when the infused volume will be large relative to the recipient's red cell mass.

Transport and shipping: It is same as that for FFP mentioned on 262.

Indications for Cryoprecipitate (Box 12.16)

Main uses of CRYO are for patients with deficiencies of factor XIII and fibrinogen. Currently, viral inactivated factor VIII concentrates are available for treatment of hemophilia A, von Willebrand disease, and factor VIII:C deficiency. Hence, CRYO is less commonly used for correcting or preventing bleeding in these patients. Currently, CRYO is the only concentrated fibrinogen product available and is used mainly as a source of fibrinogen. It is used to treat patients with congenital or acquired fibrinogen defects.

Dose: The dose of cryoprecipitate for factor VIII depends on the nature of bleeding and severity of factor VIII deficiency. Each unit of factor VIII per kg increases plasma factor by 2%. Presently, recombinant factor VIII is available and is the treatment of choice for hemophiliacs.

Plasma Cryoprecipitate Reduced

As already discussed above (on page 262) when FFP is thawed, there is cold insoluble portion of plasma (cryoprecipitate) as well as remaining plasma. **After removing the cryoprecipitate from FFP, the remaining plasma** unit can be **refrozen** (Fig. 12.15D). **This product is relabeled as "Plasma, Cryoprecipitate**

Table 12.5: Composition of bag of cryoprecipitate.	
Constituent	Amount
Volume	10–15 mL
Factor VIII	80–120 IU/concentrate (minimum of 80 IU)
Factor XIII	20–30% of original
Fibrinogen	150–250 mg/concentrate
von Willebrand factor (vWF)	40–70% of original FFP
Fibronectin (opsonic glycoprotein)	55 mg

Box 12.16: Indications for cryoprecipitate.

- Hemophilia A (deficiency factor VIII)
- von Willebrand disease (deficiency vWF)
- Hypofibrinogenemia: Congenital or acquired fibrinogen deficiency
- Acquired factor VIII deficiency, e.g. DIC, massive transfusion
- Topical/local use as a hemostatic agent: To prepare fibrin glue or fibrin sealant which is used during surgery as a topical source of fibrin
- Deficiency of factor XIII

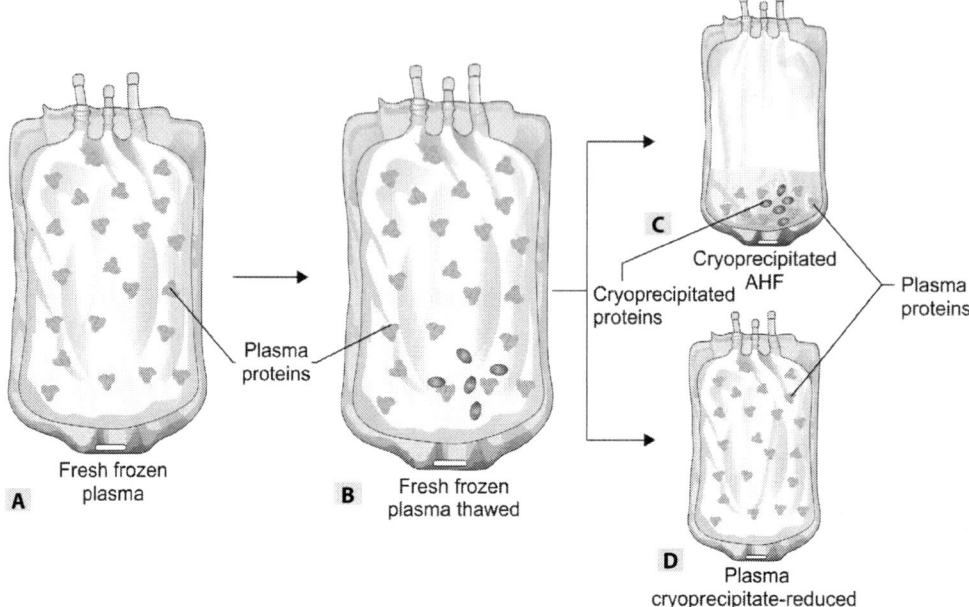

Figs. 12.15A to D: Production of cryoprecipitate, plasma cryoprecipitate-reduced from fresh frozen plasma.

Reduced" [CRYO-poor plasma (CPP)]. The refreezing of plasma must be done within 24 hours of the thawing.

Storage: It is stored at −18°C or lower for 1 year from the date of collection. It has to be thawed before transfusion. Once thawed for use, CPP has a 5-day expiration date and should be stored at 1–6°C.

Content: The plasma cryoprecipitate reduced (CPP) contains **ADAMTS13**. Hence, it is **used** mainly used in **the treatment of TTP** where there is reduction of ADAMTS13 protein. Albumin and coagulation factors II, V, VII, IX, X, and XI remain in the same concentrations as in FFP.

Cryoprecipitated Antihemophilic Factor, Pooled

Cryoprecipitated AHF can be pooled into a transfer bag to obtain a therapeutic dose of AHF.

Pooling of cryoprecipitate: Pooling is done under laminar flow.
- **Thawing:** The cryoprecipitate packs are separated depending on ABO group and arranged in lots of 4 or 5. It is necessary to overwrap to prevent contamination of the ports. They are placed in a water bath containing fresh, clean tap water at 25–30°C for 15 minutes. The temperature should not be exceeded. After allowing time for proteins to dissolve, remove the packs from water bath and try them by wiping. If the unit contains fibrin appearing as insoluble strands, discard the unit.
- Place each lot of four or five thawed cryoprecipitate along with the appropriate transfer bag in the laminar flow cabinet. Laminar flow should be switched on 10 minutes before use, so that ultraviolet light sterilizes the area. Make sure that that the door of the cabinet is closed since UV light is dangerous to the naked eye.
- Switch off UV light and start the cabinet motor to filter the air. Open the door of the laminar flow cabinet and start pooling. Pool by inserting a medication injection site into the port of each bag.
- **Pooling:** Cryoprecipitate from each bag of each batch is passed into a labeled

CRYO are to be transfused, it is necessary to select ABO-compatible units. Crossmatching is not necessary when transfusing CRYO components. Cryoprecipitated AHF can also be pooled after separation from FFP. Pooling of units is performed by a closed system using a sterile collection device.

Storage: It can be stored frozen for 1 year.
- After thawing, the closed-system pooled CRYO should be stored at 20–24°C and must be used within 6 hours.
- If the CRYO was pooled in an open system, it should be used within 4 hours of first entry and should be stored at room temperature until transfusion.

Labeling: The number of units in the pool should be mentioned on the label, and a unique number should be given to the pooled product. A record must be maintained about the number of units in the pool.

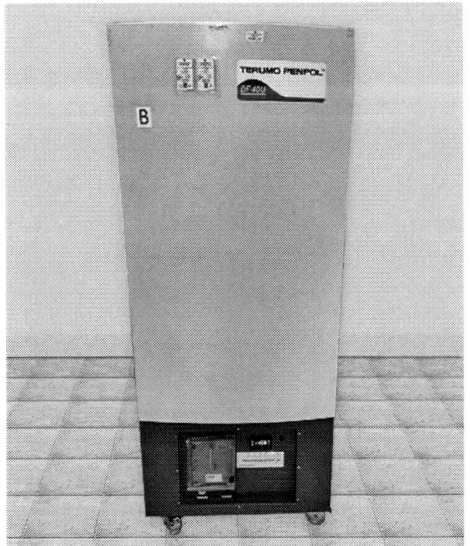

Fig. 12.16: Deep freezer (–40°C).

transfer pack via the outlet port through a filter (plastic). The contents of bags can be rinsed with 10–15 mL of 0.9% sodium chloride while pooling. After removing air from the transfer pack, tie a knot in the tubing. Discard the filter after each batch and double seal the tubing. Mention the particulars such as group, batch number, expiry date, HBsAg-negative, HIV-negative, and anti-HCV negative on each pool. Place these cartoons in deep freezer (Fig. 12.16) in different sections according to the blood group.
- After completion of the pooling process, all the equipment (scissors, forceps) and laminar flow is wiped with alcohol. Close the doors of the cabinet and switch on the UV light for 10 minutes.

It is important to note that factor VIII is heat labile and cryoprecipitate pooling should be performed under strict aseptic condition. It should be frozen immediately to prevent growth of bacteria and loss of labile coagulation factors.

Dose: It varies depending on the patient's condition, weight, and level of the factor needed for replacement. This formula is same as that for CRYO (refer page 264). If large volumes of

Fibrin Sealant from Cryoprecipitated Antihemophilic Factor

CRYO can also be used to prepare a topical hemostatic solution to control bleeding during surgery and other various procedures. This solution contains 1–2 units of CRYO mixed with thrombin. It is applied locally to the bleeding surface by layering, mixing, or spraying. Fibrinogen present in the blood at the site of bleeding is converted to fibrin by the action of thrombin present in the fibrin sealant, its fibrin clot formed at the site stops bleeding.

Algorithm to the approach to the diagnosis of bleeding disorder based on screening laboratory tests (Flowchart 12.4).

Transfusion Treatment of Coagulopathies

Several components are used to treat deficiencies in and abnormalities of coagulation factors. Three types of plasma-derived blood components commonly used platelet products, fresh frozen plasma (FFP), and cryoprecipitate. Blood components used in bleeding disorders are presented in Table 12.6.

Flowchart 12.4: Algorithm to the approach to the diagnosis of bleeding disorder based on screening laboratory tests.

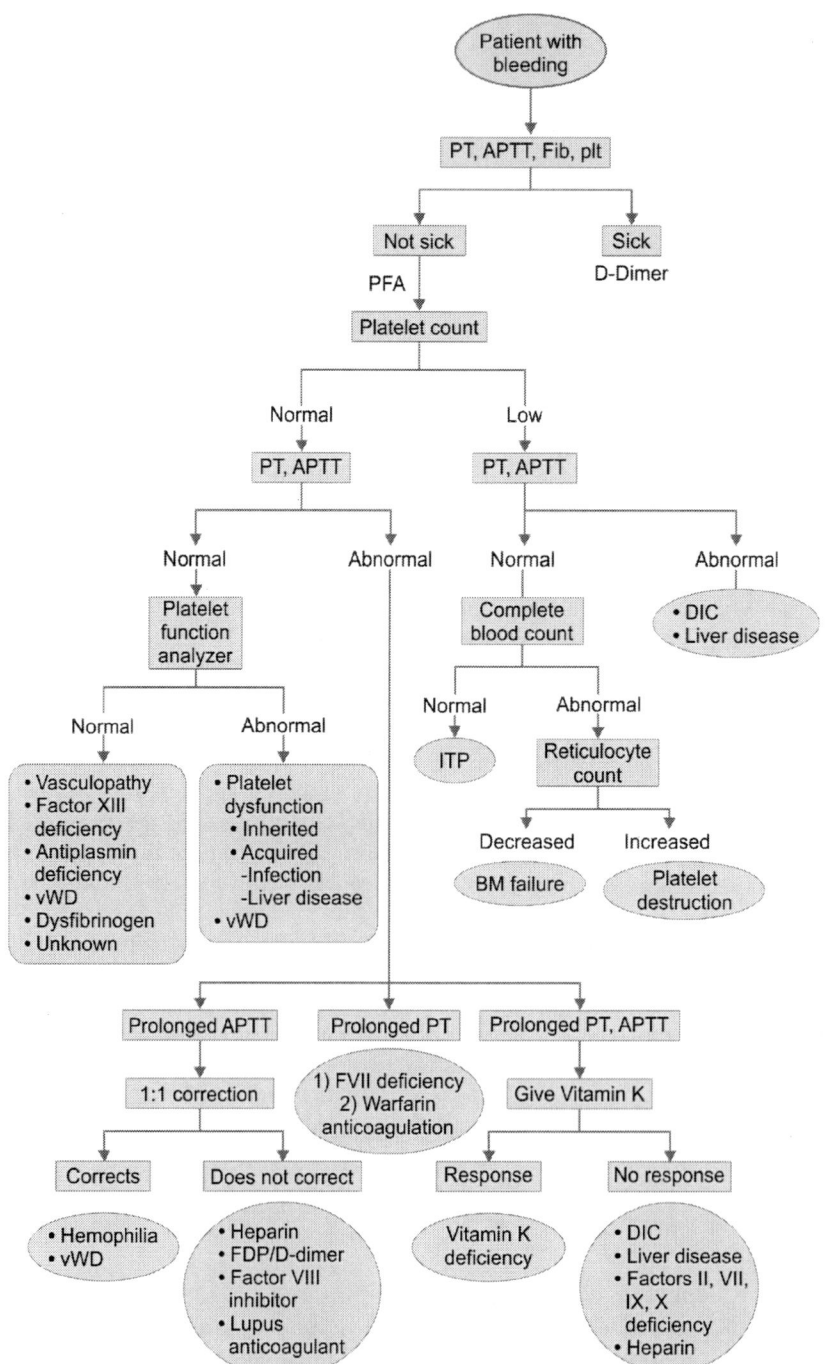

(DIC: disseminated intravascular coagulation; FDP: fibrin degradation products; Fib: fibrinogen level; PT: prothrombin time; APTT: activated partial thromboplastin time; vWD: von Willebrand disease; ITP: immune thrombocytopenic purpura)

Blood Components and their Preparation

Table 12.6: Blood components used in bleeding disorders.

Component	Use in bleeding/coagulation disorder
Platelet: Improve hemostasis; provide functional platelets	**To treat or prevent bleeding in thrombocytopenic patients or patients with dysfunctional platelets** • Thrombocytopenia, when platelet count is less than • 20,000/cu mm (e.g. chemotherapy or radiation therapy or drug induced; leukemia, marrow infiltration [e.g. leukemia, carcinoma]; dilutional [e.g., massive transfusion with stored blood]; hypoplastic anemia; viral disease associated [e.g. Dengue]) • Abnormal platelet function • Disseminated intravascular coagulation (DIC)
Fresh-frozen plasma (FFP): Improves hemostasis; provides all coagulation factors	**To treat or prevent bleeding due to coagulopathy:** • When multiple coagulation factors are deficient (e.g. liver disease, disseminated intravascular coagulation [DIC] and dilutional coagulopathy) • Massively transfused patients • Coagulation factor deficiency if no specific factor concentrate is available • When rapid reversal of warfarin is required **To provide functioning proteins:** • Thrombotic thrombocytopenic purpura (TTP) • In patients with rare, specific protein deficiencies **Replacement fluid in therapeutic plasma exchange**
Cryoprecipitate: Provides Factors VIII, XIII, von Willebrand factor(vWF), fibrinogen, fibronectin	**Replacement of fibrinogen** (in fibrinogen deficiency) **or less often Factor VIII** (Hemophilia A-when factor VIII concentrates are not available) **or von Willebrand factor** (dysfunctional (type II) or absent (type III) von Willebrand disease) Also used **prior to surgery when patient is known to have dysfibrinogenemia** Disseminated intravascular coagulation (DIC)

Summary of preparation of various blood components (Fig. 12.17): The process of preparation of various blood components varies depending on the type of collection bag and uses. Details of leukocyte are discussed on pages 270-2.

- After the collection of **whole blood unit**, it is **centrifuged at a light spin**. The **PRP is pushed through the attached tubing into an empty satellite bag**. The RBCs remain in the original/primary bag. The tube between the plasma and red cells is heat sealed and cut.
- If the collecting bag type used has an additive system, the additive solution is added to the RBCs in the primary bag. Prestorage leukocyte reduction can be performed at this step. The **primary bag containing RBCs are sealed and split from the remaining** bags. Theses RBCs refrigerated at 1-6°C.
- The **PRP** (expressed from primary bag into satellite bag) unit is **centrifuged again at a heavy spin**. This **produces sedimentation of the platelets** to the bottom of the bag. **All but about 50-70 mL of plasma is removed from the platelets** in PRP to **another satellite bag**. The additional plasma (50-70 mL) that remains with the platelets is needed to maintain a pH of 6.2 or higher during the storage period. The satellite bag **containing platelets is sealed** and allowed to "rest" for at least 1 hour. Then they are **stored on a rotator** that maintains continuous gentle agitation. Platelet concentrates are stored at 20-24°C for a maximum period of 5 days.
- The plasma that had been expressed into another empty satellite attached bag can be processed as follows:
  – **Fresh frozen plasma:** Plasma frozen within 8 hours of collection and stored at or below –18°C for up to 1 year or stored at or below –65°C for 7 years. FFP contains all coagulation factors, i.e. labile coagulation factors (factors V and VIII) and stable factors (i.e. factor II, fibrinogen, ADAMTS13, etc.).
  – **Plasma frozen within 24 hours of phlebotomy (PF24):** Contains similar coagulation factors as FFP. However, labile factor VIII levels are reduced and

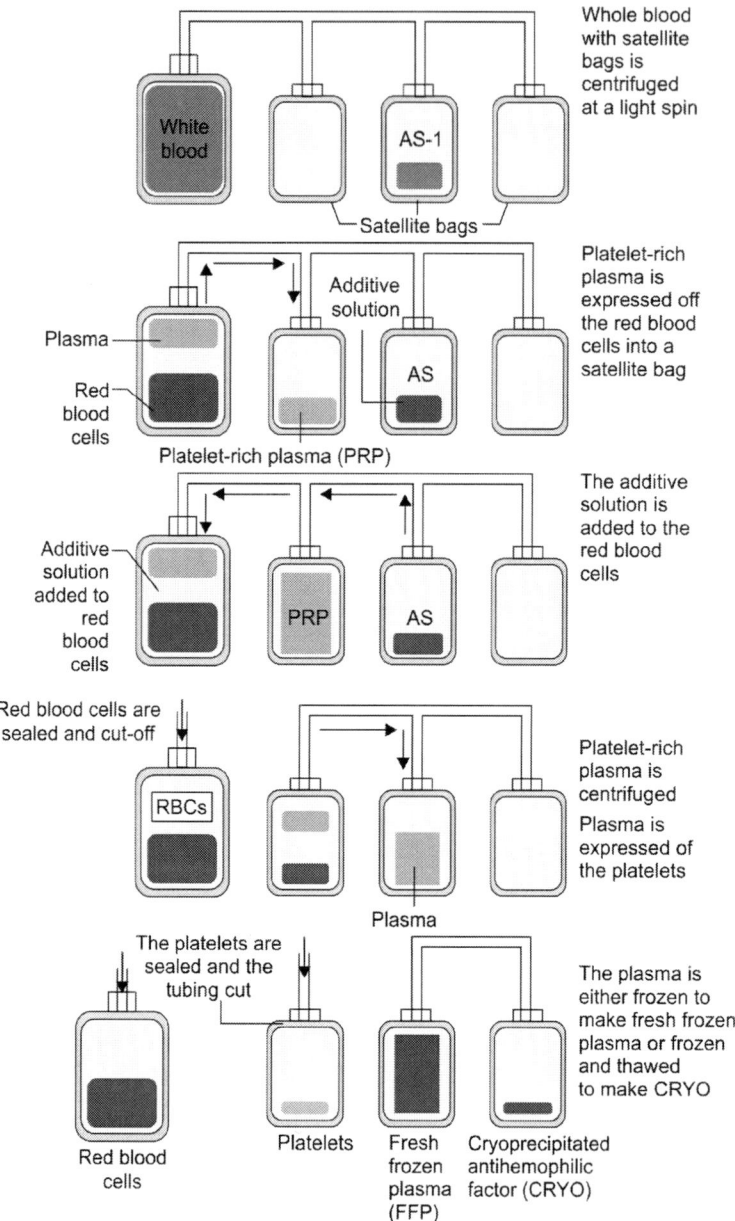

Fig. 12.17: Summary of preparation of various blood components.
(AS: additive solution; CRYO: cryoprecipitated antihemophilic factor; PRP: platelet rich plasma; RBCs: red blood cells)

factor V may be variable compared with FFP. PF24 is stored at or below –18°C for up to 1 year. PF24 is also called FP24. Various components and their shelf-life and storage are presented in Table 12.7.

GRANULOCYTE CONCENTRATES

Granulocyte transfusion is not frequently employed, because it is preferable to administer the growth factors for myelopoiesis like granulocyte colony-stimulating factor

Blood Components and their Preparation

Table 12.7: Various components and their shelf-life and storage.

Component and indications	Shelf-life and storage
Packed red blood cells (PRBCs)	
• To compensate the loss of blood after surgery • To treat severe anemia	42 days in the refrigerator (SAGM) 35 days (CPDA)
Fresh frozen plasma (FFP)	
• To correct a deficiency in coagulation factors • To treat shock from burns or massive bleeding	1 year in the freezer
Platelet concentrates	
• To treat or prevent bleeding due to low platelet levels • To correct functional platelet problems	5 days at room temperature (20–24°C)
Cryoprecipitate	
To correct fibrinogen deficiencies	1 year in the freezer

(G-CSF)/granulocyte-macrophage colony stimulating factor (GM-CSF). But it is indicated when granulocyte count is less than 500/mm³ (agranulocytosis), and to combat infections (in neonatal sepsis and chronic granulomatous disease).

Methods of preparation (granulocyte concentrate) are given in Box 12.17.

Single Unit Leukopheresis in Plastic Bags

The granulocyte pool in the body is divided into those in the circulating system (40%) and those in extracirculatory system (60%).

Gravity leukopheresis: Harvesting buffy coats from whole blood units is lengthy and cumbersome process. Gravity leukopheresis, a method of extraction of leukocytes from whole blood, is a modification of single unit apheresis procedure. In this process, to obtain high yield of granulocyte from a single unit, hydroxyethyl starch (HES) solution is added to the whole blood unit in the ratio of 1:8 within 24 hours of collection. Hydroxyethyl starch causes aggregation of red cells and thereby helps in the complete sedimentation of RBCs. After

Box 12.17: Methods of preparation of granulocyte concentrate.

- Single unit leukopheresis
- Leukopheresis (refer chapter 13) by:
   - Continuous flow centrifugation
   - Semicontinuous (intermittent) flow centrifugation
- Filtration leukopheresis

mixing, the mixture is placed in upright position in a plasma extractor for 1 hour for gravity sedimentation. Then plasma and buffy coat are separated into transfer bag. This transfer bag is centrifuged at 5000 x g for 5 minutes at 22°C temperature. After centrifugation, 90% of plasma is expressed back to red cells. This leaves behind granulocyte concentrate with about 20 mL of plasma. This method can yield 1.25×10^9 granulocyte from single blood unit. Granulocytes can also be prepared by apheresis.

Storage: Granulocytes may be stored at room temperature for up to 24 hours. However, it is desirable to transfuse as soon as possible after collection.

Indications for Granulocyte Transfusion

The availability of better antimicrobial agents and availability of hematopoietic growth factors (e.g. G-CSF), the necessity of granulocyte transfusion has decreased. However, it may be used in certain situations as listed in Box 12.18.

Complications of granulocyte transfusion are given in Box 12.19.

Apheresis granulocytes contain a large number of viable lymphocytes. If transfused

Box 12.18: Indications for granulocyte transfusion.

- Bone marrow with myeloid hypoplasia
- Patients with granulocyte dysfunction
- Profound neutropenia with an absolute count below < 500 polymorphs/μL
- Gram negative septicemia and antibiotic therapy of at least 48 hours which has been proved unsuccessful
- Septicemia in neonates unresponsive to appropriate antibiotics because granulocytes of neonates are not capable of effective phagocytosis

> **Box 12.19:** Complications of granulocyte transfusion.
>
> - Severe pulmonary reactions
> - Granulocytes can transmit CMV
> - Febrile reactions
> - If not irradiated, can cause graft versus host disease.

to a severely immunocompromised patient, these viable lymphocyte increases the risk of developing GVHD. Hence, the product should be irradiated before transfusion. Irradiation does not affect the function of granulocyte. Even if the sedimenting agents are used, granulocyte preparations contain a significant number of RBCs. This granulocyte component resembles a diluted RBC rather than a platelet concentrate. Hence, compatibility test should be performed because the apheresis granulocyte product contains more than 2 mL of RBCs.

SUMMARY

- Whole blood can be separated into RBC, platelet, and plasma components.
- Whole blood units should be stored at 1–6°C and units meant for platelet production should be stored at 20–24°C until platelets have been removed.
- Each blood product is prepared and stored to optimize its purity and potency.
- PRBCs are prepared by separating the RBCs from the plasma. Each unit of packed RBCs should raise the Hb by 1 g/dL and the Hct by 3%.
- In leukocyte-reduced RBCs, the absolute leukocyte count is less than 5×10^6.
- Platelets are used to stop medically significant bleeding either due to thrombocytopenia or qualitative platelet defects.
- Platelets have HLA antigens and ABO antigens on their surfaces but have no Rh antigens.
- Each unit of platelets should raise the platelet count by 5,000–10,000 cells/mm³.
- Random-donor platelets should have at least 5.5×10^{10} platelets; single-donor platelets must have at least 3×10^{11} platelets. They have a shelf-life of 5 days.
- Fresh frozen plasma is used for the treatment of multiple coagulation deficiencies (e.g. DIC and cirrhosis) or treatment of warfarin over anticoagulation if bleeding is life-threatening. FFP must be prepared within 8 hours of collection and is stored at –18°C for 12 months.
- Cryoprecipitate is prepared from FFP and contains fibrinogen, factors VIII, XIII.
- Cryoprecipitated AHF is prepared from FFP. Cryoprecipitated AHF contains coagulation proteins that precipitate out of plasma in the cold. These proteins are factor VIII, fibrinogen, factor XIII, von Willebrand factor and fibronectin.

SELF-ASSESSMENT EXERCISE

Write short essays on:
- Blood components, their preparation in blood center and uses of blood components in blood center.
- List the blood components available for clinical use and indications for their use.
- List the blood components. Describe preparation, methods of their preservation/storage and indications/uses of blood components.
- Different blood components and their importance in transfusion therapy.
- Principles and uses of blood component separation.
- Applications and preparation of blood components.
- Discuss various blood components and their clinical implications (uses in clinical practice).
- Discuss various blood components used in transfusion therapy (component therapy).
- Therapeutic indications of various blood components.
- Blood component therapy in clinical medicine.
- Blood components.
- Transfusion of blood components.
- How do you ensure safety of donors and patients during processing and storage of blood components?
- What are the indications for platelet transfusion? Discuss factors affecting the recovery and survival of platelets after transfusion.
- Leucodepleted blood components.

(Contd...)

(Contd...)

- Indications for leucocyte free blood transfusion.
- Leukocyte free blood transfusion.
- Significance of selective and universal leukoreduction.
- Leucodepletion.
- Rationale of leucodepletion of blood products.
- Irradiated blood components and their use.
- Platelet transfusion.
- Platelet concentrate.
- Discuss single donor platelets versus random donor platelets.
- Preparation, storage, indications and utility of platelet transfusions.
- Fresh frozen plasma.
- Preparation and indications for fresh frozen plasma.
- Use of plasma and its derivatives in clinical practice.
- Cryoprecipitate.
- Preparation of cryoprecipitate and its uses.
- Algorithm to use of blood components therapy in bleeding disorders.

CHAPTER 13

Apheresis

CHAPTER OUTLINE

- Methods of apheresis
- Donor cytapheresis
- Donor plasmapheresis
- Therapeutic Apheresis
- Donor/patient complications common to all apheresis procedures

■ INTRODUCTION

"Apheresis" is a term derived from Greek word, which means "to separate" or "to take away."

Definition: Hemapheresis (or simply apheresis) is the process of removing normal (from donor) or abnormal (from patient) blood constituents from circulating blood. The whole blood is removed from donor/patient and passed through an apparatus that separates out one (or more) particular blood constituent. Then the desired (or unwanted) components are retained and the remaining constituents are returned to the donor/patient's circulation. By using sophisticated automation, an apheresis procedure can be performed on either a blood donor or a patient. It represents a significant advance in blood component collection and the treatment of specific diseases.

Types of Apheresis

Apheresis procedures can be broadly divided into two categories, namely, **cytapheresis** and **plasmapheresis**.

1. **Cytapheresis**: In this cellular elements/component of blood are removed. It can be selective with removal of
   - Red blood cells (erythrocytapheresis): If the red blood cells removed during an erythrocytapheresis are replaced with donor red blood cells in a therapeutic procedure, this is termed as a *red blood cell exchange*.
   - Platelets (plateletapheresis): When a plateletapheresis procedure is performed as a therapeutic procedure, it is termed as a *thrombocytoapheresis*.
   - White blood cells (leukocytapheresis or leukapheresis).
   - Lymphocyte (***lymphocytapheresis***).
2. **Plasmapheresis**: It is the method of collection of plasma by apheresis and the plasma fraction is removed. In this procedure, the whole blood is withdrawn from the donor/patient, centrifuged, and separated into components (plasma and cellular components). The plasma is diverted into a collection bag and all the cellular components (RBCs, platelets, and WBCs) are returned to the donor/patient. Plasmapheresis removes and discards less than 15% (500 mL) of the total plasma volume and does not require replacement fluid.
   - Therapeutic plasma exchange (TPE): If during a plasmapheresis procedure, more plasma is removed and is replaced by plasma or plasma protein fraction (albumin) to replace the lost plasma proteins, the procedure is termed as a *therapeutic plasma exchange (TPE)*. Therapeutic plasma exchange is the

most common form of therapeutic apheresis and is used to treat different diseases. The objective is **to remove some particular constituents from patient's circulation**. These include cells, plasma, or plasma constituents and replaced with normal plasma, crystalloids, or colloids.

The terms **plasmapheresis** and **plasma exchange** are not equivalent, even though they are commonly used in this way.

Donor and Therapeutic Apheresis

1. **Donor apheresis:** Apheresis performed on a donor **to collect a specific blood component** is called donor apheresis. It may be **donor cytapheresis or donor plasmapheresis.**
2. **Therapeutic apheresis:** Apheresis performed on a patient **to remove a particular blood component** for therapeutic purposes is termed therapeutic apheresis. It may be **therapeutic cytapheresis or therapeutic plasmapheresis.**

Advantages over Whole Blood Collection

- Instead of collecting only a single unit of whole blood from a donor, apheresis permits collection of a larger volume of specific components such as platelets or red blood cells.
- It increases the ability to produce the optimal components for patients and prevents wastage.
- As a therapeutic procedure, it permits the removal of disease-causing or unwanted cellular or plasma constituents from a patient.
- Apheresis is also used to harvest stem cells from the peripheral blood of donors and patients. This avoids the need for extraction of stem cells from the bone marrow.

Indications for Apheresis (Box 13.1)

> **Box 13.1:** Indications for apheresis.
>
> **Donor apheresis:** To collect various components for transfusion purposes:
> - Platelets—plateletapheresis
> - Leukocytes—Leukapheresis or leukocytapheresis
> - Plasma—plasmapheresis (the process of removing plasma)
> - Red blood cells—erythrocytapheresis
> - Peripheral stem cells (PBSCs) also called hematopoietic progenitor cells (HPC): HPC apheresis.
>
> **Therapeutic apheresis:** To remove pathological components like cells, plasma, or plasma constituents
> - Thrombotic thrombocytopenic purpura
> - Goodpasture syndrome
> - Guillain-Barré syndrome.

Principle of Component Separation (Fig. 13.1)

Centrifugal force is applied to whole blood and this separates the various components according to their specific gravity (density). The most dense component (red blood cells) layers moves farthest from the axis of rotation and the least dense component (plasma) layers lies closest to the axis of rotation, with components of intermediate density forming layer in between. In apheresis, blood is removed through venipuncture from an individual, usually with a large-bore

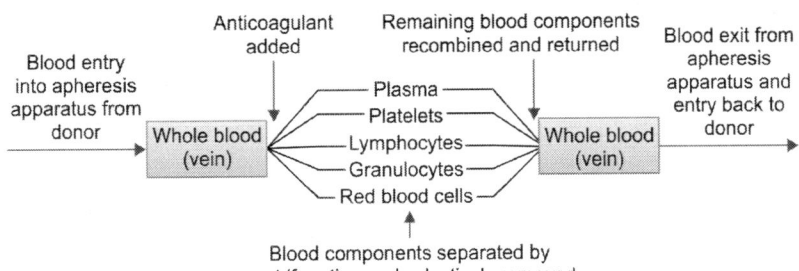

Fig. 13.1: Basic principles of apheresis.

needle. Then the blood is mixed with an anticoagulant, and transported directly to the separation device. This device is usually a machine with a centrifuge bowl or belt. In the apheresis machine, blood is separated into specific components. After the separation of component, whichever (or any) component required is withdrawn. The remaining portions of the blood are then mixed and returned to the donor or patient.

Physiology of Apheresis

Apheresis collection of a blood component (therapeutic or nontherapeutic purposes) is different than the routine collection of a unit of whole blood. Apheresis involves removing whole blood from an individual, manipulating the removed blood, and subsequently reinfusing portions of the blood. Thus, it is natural that apheresis can have varying impact on the human body who undergoes apheresis.

Anticoagulation: Citrate is used as the primary anticoagulant in apheresis procedures. Citrate binds to calcium ions in the blood and inhibits the calcium-dependent coagulation cascade. Citrate is mixed with the blood immediately as it is removed from the donor's (or patient's) vein. The anticoagulated blood then enters the apheresis machine.

Fluid shifts: During the process of an apheresis, removal of blood into the extracorporeal circuit changes in intravascular volume. During donor apheresis, the total volume of components collected may be more than the whole blood donation. If additional fluid is not infused during the apheresis, the donor may develop hypotension due to the depletion of intravascular volume.

Cellular loss: For both donor and patient apheresis, the purpose is to remove a specific cellular component. This decreases the circulating levels of the specific cells removed/harvested. However, it may also affect the other cellular components. The lost cellular component depends on the equipment used for collection and the specific component being collected.

METHODS OF APHERESIS

Apheresis can be performed by either (i) manual method or (ii) apheresis machines. Presently, most apheresis is done using semi-automated instruments, sometimes called blood cell separators.

Steps in apheresis: Various steps are as follows:
- The donor's whole blood is anticoagulated as it is passed through the instrument.
- It is then centrifuged in the instrument and the blood is separated into red cells, plasma, and a leukocyte–platelet fraction.
- The desired fraction or component is removed, and the remainder of the blood is recombined and returned to the donor.

The advantage of apheresis instrument is that several liters of donor blood can be processed. Hence, a larger amount of the desired component can be obtained than from one unit (450 mL) of whole blood.

Manual Method

Apheresis was originally performed manually. The manual method uses refrigerated centrifuge and a specialized plastic bag system. A unit of whole blood is collected from the donor or patient into the plastic bag containing anticoagulant preservative solution. The plastic bag is centrifuged to separate the desired component, which is separated/retained into the satellite bag. The remainder is infused with normal saline/heparinized saline through the same vein from which blood is drawn. The process is repeated.

Advantages: The procedure is simple, inexpensive, and does not require sophisticated equipment.

Disadvantages: The amount prepared/harvested per procedure is lower than the automated devices. This has limited applications.

Apheresis Machines (Fig. 13.2)

At the present time, apheresis is routinely performed with an apheresis (cell-separator) machine. Apheresis instrument is operated only for therapeutic removal of abnormal plasma or collection of plasma. It is not meant for collecting cellular components.

Apheresis machine (blood cell separators): Apheresis is performed using automated technology, and separation is usually achieved by centrifugation. Depending on the procedure and the equipment, the **process can take 30 minutes to 2 hours**. Collection of hematopoietic progenitor cells (HPC) needs longer time.

- Present day, apheresis instrument have a computerized control panel and allows the operator to select the desired component to be collected or removed. On-board optical sensors detect specific plasma–cell or cell–cell interfaces and divert the specific component to a collection bag.
- Currently available apheresis machines use disposable equipment that includes sterile single-use tubing sets, bags, and collection chambers unique to the machine.
- The donor or patient remains attached to the apheresis machine for the entire duration of the procedure.

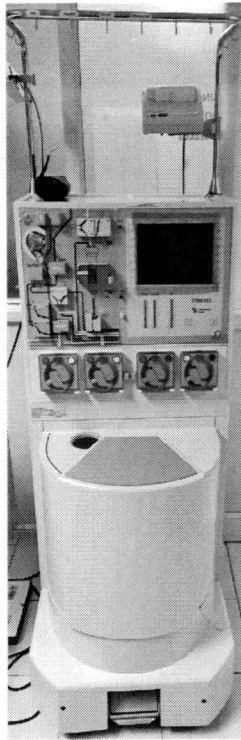

Fig. 13.2: Apheresis (automated cell separator).

by a microprocessor (with software) which controls the blood flow rate, the anticoagulant added to the whole blood entering the system, the centrifuge conditions, the component separation, and the recombination of the remaining components and returning them to the donor.

Principle

- Several different instruments are available for the collection of platelets, granulocytes, lymphocytes, red cells, peripheral blood stem cells (PBSCs), or plasma by apheresis. Many of the apheresis machines used for normal donor apheresis of cellular products **use centrifugal force and differing densities** to separate the various desired blood components. Some require two venipunctures (an outflow and return) and others need only one venipuncture.
- Some are based on the **filtration principle**. Separation by membrane filtration is used

Procedure: The procedure for performing apheresis depends on the blood component to be harvested and the equipment used. Some of the equipment are exclusively meant for plasmapheresis. Procedure **should be followed according to the manufacturer's instruction manual**.

Methods of Centrifugation

Most commonly used instruments utilize one of two methods of centrifugation: intermittent flow centrifugation (IFC) and continuous flow centrifugation (CFC).

Intermittent flow centrifugation (IFC)

In an intermittent flow centrifugation (IFC) procedure, blood is processed in batches or cycles, hence it is termed *intermittent*. IFC procedure can be performed as a single-needle procedure (one arm procedure), i.e. blood is drawn and reinfused after separating the desired component, through the same vein and the same needle (one venipuncture).

This is the major advantage of IFC procedure. This requires a disposable unit consisting of sterile tubing and a bowl. The disposable unit is checked properly before being assembled on the machine. The extracorporeal volume is usually greater with the IFC than with the CFC machines. Hence, it is **advantageous in individuals with small blood volumes,** such as children and elderly individuals, since the additional volume removed may leave the patient hypovolemic during the procedure.

Steps
- Perform venipuncture and connect the donor to the instrument. The operator activates the instrument and the whole blood is drawn from an individual with the help of a pump. To keep the blood from clotting, an anticoagulant-citrate-dextrose (ACD) is mixed with the blood as it is pumped into a disposable centrifuge bowl through the inlet port (Fig. 13.3).
- The centrifuge bowl rotates (spins) at a fixed speed (approximately at 4,800 rpm), and continuously separates the blood components according to their specific gravities. A rotary seal is used, resulting in a closed system.
- The red cells have greater mass/density and get packed against the outer rim of the bowl, followed by the white cells, platelets, and the plasma.
- Once the components are separated, the pump is reversed and the desired component(s) are pumped through the outlet port into a collection bag (Fig. 13.3).
- The undesired components are pumped into a reinfusion bag and returned to the donor/patient, constituting one cycle (or pass).
  - **For platelet collection:** When the platelets reach the exit port, a valve is activated, diverting the flow pathway of the platelets into a separate bag. Thus, platelets are collected in this bag. When the platelets have been collected, the centrifuge stops and also stops the blood flow. Then the pumps get reversed and the plasma and red cells recombined and returned to the donor.
  - **For other components**: The separated components flow from the bowl through the port, with the desired components being harvested into a separate collection bag. The blood components which are not required are automatically returned to the individual. This completes one cycle.
  - **The cycles are repeated several times** till the desired quality of the product is obtained. For example, 6–8 cycles for harvesting good therapeutic dose (yield) of platelets. MCS+ (multicomponent system) is one of the automated machines (cell separators) with minimum operator intervention, as the machine is equipped with optical sensors, which detect plasma cell interfaces and divert components according to the preselected mode.

Multiple component systems (MCS and MCS+) can collect various combinations of platelets, plasma, and red cells. The MCS and MCS+ can collect approximately 4×10^{11} platelets in 90 minutes.

Continuous flow centrifugation (CFC)

In CFC procedure, the blood is withdrawn, processed, and returned to the individual

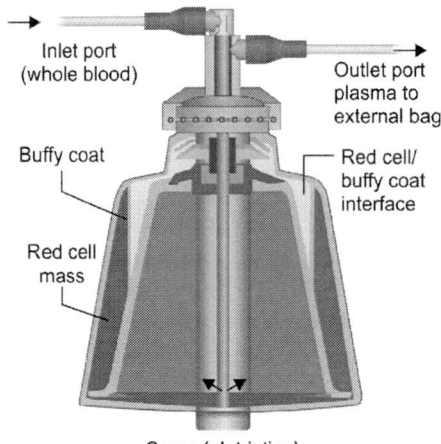

Fig. 13.3: Cross-section of centrifuge bowl and flow pathway of the blood separation in the intermittent flow centrifugation.

simultaneously. In an ongoing manner. This is in contrast to IFC procedures, which complete a cycle before beginning the next one. Because blood is drawn and returned continuously during this procedure, **two venipuncture sites** (venipuncture in each arm, namely, an outflow and return) **are necessary**.

Steps
- The blood is withdrawn from an individual with the assistance of a pump, mixed with the anticoagulant, and collected in a specially designed chamber or belt, depending on the instrument.
- Separation of components is done through centrifugation and the specific component is diverted to be collected in a collection bag.
- The remainder of the blood is reinfused to the individual through second venipuncture/venous site. The CFC has the advantage of speed and small extra corporeal volume. Isovolemic status of the donor is maintained thereby minimizing any fluid loss,

Membrane filtration (separation by membrane filtration)

Membrane filtration technology or filtration technology, which has been widely used in hemodialysis and hemofiltration, can also be used **for both donor and therapeutic apheresis.** It is used to separate blood components and for plasma collection. In this method, components of whole blood are separated depending on size rather than density. The whole blood flows over a membrane containing pores of a specific size (membrane separators). Filtration methods use microporous membranes that are made up of a wide variety of materials and bundles of hollow fibers, arranged either in parallel plates or a flat membrane with specific pore sizes. They utilize pore size to separate cellular components from plasma. In this, the whole blood flows over/across the fibers or membrane containing pores of a defined size. Higher pressure in the blood phase than in the filtrate pushes/allows only plasma constituents smaller than the pore size (component of interest) to pass through the pores of the membrane. These plasma components which pass into the filtrate are collected. Surface properties of the inner membrane surface repel cellular elements in the laminar flow of blood so that platelets are not activated and survival of RBC is not shortened. The remainder of the cellular components/elements is returned to the donor/patient. This technology is useful for the collection of plasma, since sizes of the pores can be varied depending on the requirement to prevent the passage of even small cellular elements. Filtration technique has several advantages over centrifugation, namely, (i) the collection of a cell-free product and (ii) capable of selectively removing specific plasma proteins by varying the pore size.

Combination of centrifugation and filtration

Centrifugation and filtration can also be combined for apheresis. The advantage of the combination of centrifugation and filtration is that the cellular elements cannot clog the pores of the filter. Incorporation of the membrane (affinity columns or filter) that separates plasma from cellular components and cryofiltration to precipitate large molecular substances including IgM antibodies are also available. This helps to selectively remove pathogenic component and return the remaining plasma to the patient. This will prevent unnecessary removal of proteins.

Separation by affinity chromatography

Both centrifugal devices and *membrane filtration* can be used to allow selective removal of specific soluble plasma constituents. This can be done by using the principles of affinity chromatography (Fig. 13.4). In affinity chromatography, a substance with a specific binding affinity is linked to an insoluble matrix. This insoluble matrix specifically binds to its complementary substance from a mixture of materials in suspension or solution. The sorbent, or ligand that is coupled to the matrix, can be a chemical compound. These chemical compounds or ligand include heparin, charcoal, dextran sulfate, protein, antigen, or antibody.

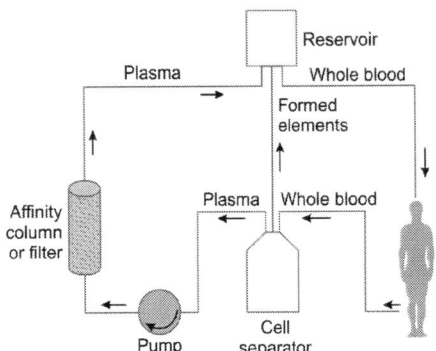

Fig. 13.4: *Affinity chromatography:* It allows selective removal of specific soluble plasma constituent by affinity columns or filters.

Box 13.2: General requirements for apheresis.

- Good equipment
- Well-trained motivated staff having sound knowledge of operation and trouble shooting
- Availability of physician (in case of any complications)
- Informed written consents
- Standard operating manuals in detail.

Immunoadsorption: It uses an antigen or antibody as the ligand, or a protein. These ligands or proteins should have the ability or capacity to remove immune reactants or complementary substances by a mechanism of immunochemistry. The ability to absorb a specific undesirable substance is made specific by the immune mechanism.

General requirements for apheresis are mentioned in Box 13.2.

DONOR CYTAPHERESIS

Donor Selection for Cytapheresis

Cytapheresis is a procedure in which various cells are separated from the withdrawn blood and retained, with the plasma and other formed elements re-transfused into the donor. The cytapheresis procedure takes longer time. Its side effects, the nature of adverse reactions to donation, and the donor medical assessment are different from whole blood donation. The following should be considered:

- **Donor should be normal healthy** and must meet all the donor criteria for whole blood donation.
- The **interval between apheresis procedures should be at least 48 hours**. The amount of blood loss should not exceed 25 mL/week.
- Frequent cytapheresis donor should be tested for plasma protein levels and any evidence of anemia. The **serum protein level should be above 6.9 g/dL**.
- **Donors should be screened** prior to apheresis procedure for all the mandatory **infectious disease markers** as in whole blood donor (refer Chapter 16). The results are valid for 30 days to facilitate repeat directed donations.

For Plateletapheresis

- The platelet count of donor should be adequate (>150,000/µL).
- Donor should not have taken aspirin or any drugs which affect platelet function during the last 48 hours.
- Donor can donate more frequently than whole blood. But interval between donations should be at least 48 hours. Donors should not undergo plateletapheresis more than twice a week or more than 24 times a year.
- If the whole blood unit is collected or if red blood cells are impossible to return to the donor during plateletapheresis, at least 8 weeks should elapse before a subsequent plateletapheresis.
- Test for ABO, Rh, and unexpected antibodies must be done in the same manner as for other blood components.

For Granulocytopheresis

The donors are given steroids and sedimenting agents (e.g. hydroxyl ethyl starch [HES]) to increase granulocyte yield. However, such drugs in donors who are diabetic, hypertensive, or with gastrointestinal ulcer may produce adverse effects.

Donor Plateletapheresis

Definition: It is the process of removal of platelets from a donor with the return of donor red cells, white cells, and plasma to the donor.

This blood component is usually called single-donor platelets or plateletapheresis concentrates. They consist of suspension of platelets in plasma prepared by cytapheresis.

Donor Selection

The donor requirements for plateletapheresis are the same as those for whole blood donation (refer pages 140-7). The time required for return to baseline platelet count following apheresis platelet donation is 4 days in males.

- Donor who has ingested aspirin or piroxicam should be deferred for 2 days before donation and donors who have taken clopidogrel or ticlopidine are deferred from apheresis platelet donation for 14 days after the last dose.
- **Minimum platelet** count required for donation: Donor must have a minimum platelet count of 150,000/µL.

Frequency and Number of Donations

- A donor can donate **twice per week**, but there must be a 2-day interval between apheresis procedures.
- A donor **cannot donate more than 24 times per year**.
- If a donor donates **multiple plateletapheresis products**, such as a double- or triple-platelet product, the donor is **deferred** from additional apheresis donation **for 1 week**.
- After whole blood donation, or after an instrument failure resulting in the inability to return the extracorporeal blood volume, must wait 8 weeks before donating by apheresis.

Time needed for plateletapheresis: Usually requires about 1 ½ to 2 hours and involves processing 4,000–5,000 mL of the donor's blood through the instrument. Platelets obtained by plateletapheresis are processed, tested, and labeled similar to whole blood. This includes ABO and Rh typing and testing for all required transfusion-transmitted diseases.

Storage and shelf life: Platelets obtained by apheresis may be stored for 5 days at 20–24°C on platelet agitator, if it is collected in a closed system. If they are prepared by open system, they should be transfused within 24 hours.

Indications are the same as for platelet concentrates (refer Box 12.11).

Quality control: A unit or bag of plateletapheresis concentrate should contain at least 3×10^{11} platelets in at least 90% of the units tested.

Advantages of Platelets Obtained by Apheresis (Box 13.3)

> **Box 13.3:** Advantages of platelets obtained by apheresis.
>
> - Obtained from a single donor, so less risk of TTD (transfusion transmitted disease)
> - Contains 3×10^{11} platelets per unit and is equivalent to 6 units of platelet concentrate
> - Prevents alloimmunization to HLA (human leukocyte antigen) and platelet refractoriness
> - Can be used to obtain platelets from donors with matched HLA phenotypes
> - Decreased risk of septic platelet transfusion reactions
> - Prestorage leukocyte reduction will delay in alloimmunization to HLA, decreases febrile transfusion reactions, and decreases cytomegalovirus infection.

Anticoagulant citrate dextrose solution used for platelet collection, single donor platelet kit and process of collection of single donor platelets (SDP) are shown in Figures 13.5 to 13.7 respectively.

Donor Leukocytapheresis/Granulocytoapheresis

Granulocyte Transfusions

Definition: Leukapheresis/leukocytapheresis is the process of removal of white cells from a donor with the return of donor red cells, platelets, and plasma to the donor. The specific white cell needed for treating sepsis is granulocyte. This blood component is a suspension of granulocytes in plasma

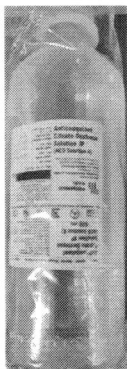

Fig 13.5: Anticoagulant citrate dextrose solution used for platelet collection.

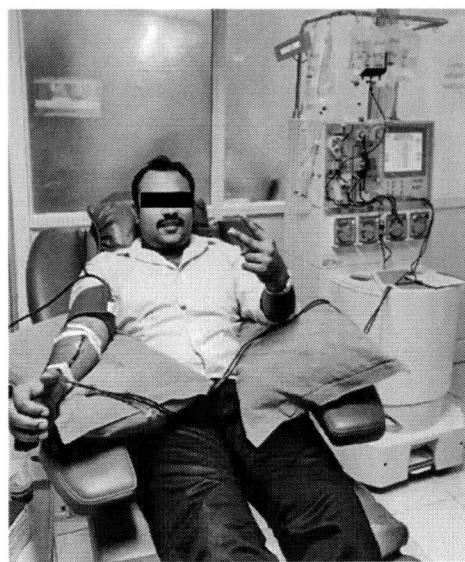

Fig 13.7: Process of collection of single donor platelets.

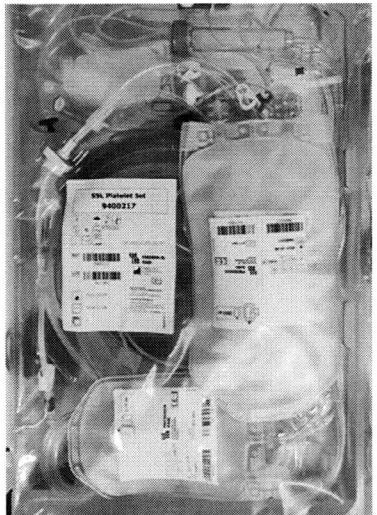

Fig 13.6: Single donor platelet kit.

prepared by cytapheresis and is called granulocytopheresis.

Donor selection: The donor requirements for leukocytapheresis are the same as those for whole blood donation (refer pages 140-7). Significant numbers of red blood cells (greater than 2 mL are present within granulocyte products. Hence, **ABO type of both recipient and donor must be compatible.** Donors must be CMV seronegative. It is necessary that 75% of granulocyte components collected should have a minimum of 1.0×10^{10} granulocytes.

Time needed for leukapheresis: Leukapheresis procedures are **usually more complex and lengthier** than plateletapheresis. The procedure takes **2–3 hours** to process more blood and improve the granulocyte yield. Usually, 6,500–8,000 mL of the donor's blood is processed through the instrument, with removal of about 50% of the granulocytes. The resulting **volume of granulocyte concentrate is about 200 mL**. The granulocytes do not completely separate from the red cells. Hence, granulocyte concentrates usually contain a significant amount of red cells (hematocrit 10% or about 20 mL of red cells). This **necessitates the crossmatching of red cell**.

Shelf life: The maximum shelf life is 24 hours. It has to be stored at 20–24°C without agitation.

Quality control: The granulocyte content in each pack should be at least 1.0×10^{10} in at least 75% of the units tested.

Strategies to increase the granulocyte yield
Increasing the granulocyte count yield of the donor may be achieved by
1. **Treatment of donors with corticosteroids:** It doubles the number of circulating granulocytes. A number of granulocytes are normally present in the marginal, or noncirculating, pool. Steroids either

stimulate bone marrow to increase the cellular output or mobilize them from the marginal pool. Corticosteroid is given to the donor 10 to 12 hours before collection of granulocytes. However, steroids should not be given to diabetic, hypertensive, and patients with peptic ulcer disease.
2. **Hematopoietic growth factors:** Administration of hematopoietic growth factors (e.g. granulocyte colony stimulating factor [G-CSF], granulocyte macrophage colony stimulating factor [GM-CSF]) increases the granulocyte yields up to 10×10^{10} granulocyte/apheresis. Contraindications for the use of G-CSF are inflammatory conditions, gout, and those having risk factors for thrombosis.
3. **By adding sedimenting agent hydroxyethyl starch (HES):** Red blood cells and granulocytes have similar densities and sedimentation rates. This results in poor separation during centrifugation. The addition of sedimenting agents such as hydroxyethyl starch (HES) can improve this separation and thereby increase the granulocyte yield. HES is red cell aggregating agent which induces rouleaux formation among red blood cells. It results in increased red cell sedimentation rate and increased upward flow of plasma during centrifugation and increases separation. HES is available as 6% solution in 9.9% saline. It is added to the input line of apheresis machine in the dose of 170–500 mL for 4–10 liters of blood processing. By this, a total of $7-10^{10}$ granulocytes can be collected in 2–4 hours. Since use of this may result in red cell contamination of granulocytes, it is necessary to use ABO compatible granulocyte concentrate.

For indications of leukapheresis is same as granulocyte transfusion (refer Box 12.18). For complications of granulocyte transfusion refer Box 12.19.

Donor Erythrocytapheresis

RBCs can be collected by apheresis. Usually, it is collected as a double unit (termed as 2RBC or double RBC procedure). A clinical advantage of collecting RBCs by apheresis is that two units from the same donor can be collected and can be given to a single donor. This reduces the donor exposure to one recipient than two.

Criteria for donor selection: Donors must meet the appropriate collection criteria for a whole blood donation.

- *Double red cell donation (2RBC):* Because the volume of RBCs collected during a 2RBC procedure is more than collected for a whole blood donation, the donor **hematocrit must be at least 40% regardless of gender**. The level (hemoglobin or hematocrit) must be determined **by a quantitative method** and not by the use of copper sulfate method. If two units of RBCs are collected by apheresis, the donor can donate (includes RBCs) again only after 16 weeks.
- If one RBC and one plasma and/or platelet unit are collected, the donor can donate another red cell product only after 8 weeks (56 days). These procedures may be performed on both allogeneic and autologous donors.

The RBC apheresis procedure is well tolerated by donors.

Benefits of erythrocytapheresis: A single unit of red blood cells or the equivalent of two units of red blood cells can be obtained by apheresis. Advantages and disadvantages of double red blood cell collections are given in Box 13.4.

Double Red Cell Collection

Automated double red cell collection or red cell apheresis: In this 2 units of red blood cells are collected from a single donor through automation with the help of equipment. This provides high quality of red cells which are leukodepleted in-line with maximum red cell recovery with no additional time. This is very useful in terms of red cell availability, building up of rare group sources, provision of leukodepleted red cell components, time-saving, and reduction in manual errors and variability. It also reduces the risk of transmission of viruses and allo-antigens.

Box 13.4: Advantages and disadvantages of double red blood cell collections.

Advantages:
- Decreased incidence of donor reactions compared with whole blood donation
- Standardized red blood cell dose
- More consistent and controlled component quality
- Decreased donor exposure if a patient receives both parts of a double red cell collection

Disadvantages:
- Stricter donation guidelines for minimum weight, height, hemoglobin, and hematocrit
- Interval between donation should be longer
- More prone for citrate toxicity and device-related complications. Standard operating manuals in detail.

Box 13.5: Various available combinations of blood products.

- *Red blood cell:*
  - With plasma
  - With platelet
  - With plasma, and platelet
  - Double red blood cell
- *Platelet:*
  - Double or triple platelet
  - With single or double plasma
  - Double platelet and single plasma
- *Double or triple plasma*

Neocytopheresis

Neocytes are young RBCs and they are larger and less dense and hence can be separated from the older red cells. These neocytes have longer/improved red cell survival than normal RBCs. It is expensive.

Principle: The neocytes are prepared by the use of automated cell separator based on the principle that young, larger, and less dense red cells are expressed earlier than older cells.

Indications: They are indicated **in patients requiring repeated transfusions**. In patients who need repeated transfusions (e.g. thalassemia major), transfusion of relatively young cells (neocytes) reduces the need for frequent transfusion required and also reduces the rate of iron deposition.

Time needed for apheresis: Neocyte separation take 3–4 hours of donor time.

Multicomponent Apheresis Donation

With currently available instruments, different combinations of blood products can be collected from the same donor. This helps in the optimum utilization of each donor. For example, in a donor with AB group, the maximum amount of plasma can be collected without collecting red blood cells (RBCs are usually not in demand and may become outdated for transfusion). In a donor with O Rh-negative or Rh-positive blood group, a double red blood cell can be collected without collecting plasma (supply of plasma is usually adequate). The various combinations of collections currently available are given in Box 13.5. It is essential that the criteria for selection of donor for each apheresis collections should be applied even for multiple-component collections. For example, a donor for a double red cell collection with a concurrent plasma collection should meet the requirements for a double red cell collection as well as the requirements for frequent or infrequent plasma collection.

Present knowledge of apheresis with newer technology has made it possible to collect very specialized components, as well as the removal of specific plasma constituents.

The number of circulating HPCs can be increased by growth factor (G-CSF or granulocyte-macrophage colony-stimulating factor [GMCSF]) stimulation.

Hematopoietic Progenitor Cell Collection by Apheresis

Hematopoietic progenitor cells (HPCs), also known as *peripheral blood stem cells* (PBSCs), can be collected by apheresis from an autologous or allogeneic donor. Hematopoietic progenitor cells (HPCs) is discussed indetail in chapter are used for autologous or allogeneic transplantation. Apheresis is useful for obtaining progenitor or stem cells for marrow reconstitution in patients with cancer, leukemia in remission, and lymphomas HPCs is discussed in detail in Chapter 24.

DONOR PLASMAPHERESIS

Plasma Products

Types of plasma products: Two types of plasma products are collected by donor plasmapheresis:
1. **Fresh frozen plasma (FFP):** It is the liquid component of whole blood that has been frozen within 6 to 8 hours after collection. The FFP after collection can be divided into multiple units of a volume equivalent to FFP derived from whole blood donations. Alternatively, the entire volume of plasma can be frozen as "jumbo plasma". Advantages of collecting FFP by plasmapheresis jumbo plasma are:
   - **Larger volume** of plasma to be collected from a donor. From a single donor, about 600 to 700 mL of plasma can be collected. Thus, each apheresis unit ("jumbo" plasma) contains plasma volume equivalent to least two whole-blood-derived plasma units. This can be used directly to the patient. The large volume of collection can maximize the production of frequently used or rare products (e.g. AB FFP or IgA-deficient FFP). To collect plasma as **fresh frozen plasma** (FFP) of a particular ABO group, especially group AB.
   - They limit the donor exposure in recipient patients who require large volumes of FFP (e.g. for thrombotic thrombocytopenic purpura [TTP]).
2. **Source plasma:** It is plasma that is subsequently used to commercially manufacture derivative products. These derivative products include albumin, intravenous immune globulin (IVIG), hepatitis immune globulin, Rh-immune globulin, coagulation factor concentrates, and laboratory reagents. Plasma can be collected from donors with high titers of antibodies directed against specific infectious agents. For example, infections by hepatitis B, cytomegalovirus, and varicella zoster. From this plasma, immune globulin can be prepared and these preparations are used in exposed individuals to provide prophylaxis against infectious organisms.

Replacement Fluids for Plasma Exchange

It is necessary to replace the volume of plasma removed by a solution having adequate colloid activity and correct electrolyte composition. Various replacement fluids include crystalloid, 5% albumin, plasma protein fraction (PPF), and fresh frozen plasma (FFP).

Criteria for Plasmapheresis Donors

- Donors must provide informed consent.
- Donors should be observed closely and emergency medical care must be available.
- A qualified, licensed physician knowledgeable in all aspects of apheresis must be responsible for the program.
- Total blood count and total serum proteins should be within normal range. The total serum protein level should not be less than 6.0 gm/dL.
- **Volume:** The maximum amount of plasma which an individual donor donates in one sitting **should not exceed**:
  - 500 mL if the donor's weight is between 50 and 65 kg
  - 900 mL if the donor's weight is more than 65 kg. Adequate replacement fluid (e.g. crystalloid) should be given to donors if the drawn plasma volume is more than 500 mL.
  - The amount of plasma that can be donated within a 12-month period by frequent and infrequent plasma donors, as well as those donors donating multicomponent collections or plateletapheresis varies with weight of the donor. Donors weighing 110 to 175 lb can donate up to 12 L and those weighing more than 175 lb can donate 14.4 L.
- **Frequency:** The donor criteria for plasmapheresis vary according to the frequency of donation. The donors taking warfarin

should be deferred from plasma donation for 1 week following their last dose of medication. This is because their plasma will have decreased vitamin K-dependent coagulation factor activity. Plasmapheresis can be first time, infrequent/occasional or serial.

- **First time donor:** Donors for first time plasmapheresis should be accepted only if they have given blood previously on one or two occasions and age is less than 50 years.
- **Infrequent (occasional) donors:** These donors donate plasma less frequently than every 4 weeks (not more than once in 4 weeks). Donor selection and monitoring in this category are the same as for whole blood donation (refer pages 140-7).
- **Frequent/serial donor** is the donation more frequent than once in 4 weeks (every 4 weeks). The donor requirements are similar to those for whole blood donation. In these donors, the red cell loss should not be more than 25 mL/week and not more than 200 mL/8 weeks. If red cells cannot be reinfused into the donor during the procedure, donors should be deferred for 8 weeks. The total serum protein should be at least 6.0 g/dL and this is estimated before each donation. Donors must also undergo a serum protein electrophoresis or quantitative immunodiffusion every 4 months as well as an annual physical examination by a physician. Frequent plasma donors should not donate more than two within 7 days period with at least 2 days between donations.

THERAPEUTIC APHERESIS

In some diseases, the pathophysiology or symptoms are due to the excessive accumulation of blood cells or plasma constituents. In such diseases, blood cell separators ordinarily used to collect blood components by apheresis from normal donors can also be used therapeutically. The therapeutic apheresis (TA) is based on the following:
- A pathogenic substance present in the blood that contributes to a disease process or its symptoms.
- The substance can be more effectively removed by apheresis than by the body's own homeostatic mechanisms.

Indications of Therapeutic Apheresis

Therapeutic apheresis procedures can be divided into therapeutic cytapheresis and therapeutic plasma exchange (TPE). They has been used to treat a wide variety of illnesses.

Diseases are grouped into four indication categories by the American Society for Apheresis (ASFA) (Table 13.1).

Therapeutic Cytapheresis

Indications are given in Box 13.6.

> **Box 13.6:** Indications of therapeutic cytapheresis.
>
> - **Therapeutic plateletapheresis** is tried in symptomatic thrombocythemia
> - **Therapeutic leukapheresis** is useful in conditions resistant to chemotherapy
>   - Prolmphocytic leukemia
>   - Sézary cell syndrome
>   - Hairy cell leukemia
> - **Red cell apheresis** is used to treat patients with specially sickle cell disease during sickle cell crisis. The goal is to replace RBCs containing Hemoglobin S with a sufficient number of RBCs containing HbA

Therapeutic Plateletapheresis

Thrombocytosis

Definition: Platelet count more than 450,000/cu mm (450×10^9/L) in the blood is known as thrombocytosis. Its causes can be divided into either primary (essential thrombocytosis-ET) or secondary causes. Secondary thrombocytosis, also known as *reactive thrombocytosis (RT)*, accounts for more than 85% of thrombocytosis. Thrombocytosis may produce both thrombotic (predominates) and hemorrhagic complications. Thromboembolic complications are more common in ET and rare in RT (unless provoked by underlying

Table 13.1: American Society for Apheresis (ASFA) Categorization of Apheresis Indications.

Category	Description and Grade
I	Disorders for which apheresis is accepted as first-line therapy, either as a primary standalone treatment or in conjunction with other modes of treatment *Grade 1A:* Strong recommendation with high-quality evidence *Grade 1B:* Strong recommendation with moderate-quality evidence *Grade 1C:* Strong recommendation with low-quality or very-low-quality evidence
II	Disorders for which apheresis is accepted as second-line therapy, either as a standalone treatment or in conjunction with other modes of treatment *Grade 2A:* Weak recommendation with high-quality evidence *Grade 2B:* Weak recommendation with moderate-quality evidence *Grade 2C:* Weak recommendation with low-quality or very-low-quality evidence
III	Optimum role of apheresis therapy is not established
IV	Disorders for which published evidence demonstrates or suggests apheresis to be ineffective or harmful

malignancy or atherosclerosis). Treatments include medications and therapeutic thrombocytapheresis. Therapeutic thrombocytapheresis is reserved as a temporary treatment for patients with symptomatic due to thrombocytosis.

Therapeutic plateletapheresis indications
Thrombocytosis/thrombocythemia: Apheresis in patient with thrombocytosis is performed in symptomatic patients to stabilize their condition until medical management reduces the platelet count. It may be used in preoperative setting to prevent bleeding, and in the treatment of pregnant women. The effects of thrombocytapheresis in thrombocytosis are temporary and last for hours to days, and medical management must be instituted at the same time.

Therapeutic Leukocytapheresis

Hyperleukocytosis
Definition: Hyperleukocytosis is an extreme elevation in white blood cell count. It is defined as a WBC or circulating blast count of over 100,000/µL. The causes include malignant and nonmalignant disease, with the former producing the highest counts. Leukostasis is more common in patients with acute myelogenous leukemia (AML) than with acute lymphoblastic leukemia (ALL).

Symptoms: Hyperleukocytosis can produce neurologic deficits (due to central nervous system leukostasis and CNS hemorrhages) and chest pain (due to pulmonary leukostasis).

Mechanism of action
- Hyperleukocytosis produces **increased viscosity** with changes in blood flow within the microvasculature. Occlusion of the microvasculature in turn results in leukostasis and ischemia.
- The **interactions of adhesion molecules** expressed on the leukemic blasts and endothelial cells may also be responsible for vascular occlusion and endothelial injury.
- **Tumor lysis syndrome:** It most often occurs during the patient's initial chemotherapy. It develops due to the release of massive quantities of intracellular tumor contents from leukocyte which damages the kidneys and/or initiates disseminated intravascular coagulation.

Therapeutic leukocytapheresis indications
The purpose of therapeutic leukocytapheresis in hyperleukocytosis is to decrease the white blood cell count to relieve symptoms and/or prevent tumor lysis syndrome. As with thrombocytapheresis, the indication for treating a patient is the presence of symptoms indicating leukostasis. The leukocytapheresis only temporarily reduces the white blood cell counts. Hence, it is used as an adjunct to therapy and not as a primary treatment modality. The definitive therapy is chemotherapy that

should be started at the same time or shortly after apheresis is initiated. Other indications include prolymphocytic leukemia, Sézary cell syndrome, and hairy cell leukemia. Use of a red cell sedimenting agent, such as HES, may be of benefit during a leukapheresis procedure.

Red Cell Exchange or Therapeutic Erythrocytapheresis

Red cell exchange (RCE) is a form of cytapheresis in which a large number of the patient's red blood cells are removed and the patient's plasma and platelets are returned along with compatible allogeneic donor red blood cells.

Uses: It is most commonly used in the treatment of **sickle cell disease** (SCD) in order to decrease the number of hemoglobin S-containing RBCs. It is especially used for treating or preventing the complications (acute chest syndrome, impending stroke, and unrelenting painful crisis). It may be occasionally used to treat **hyperparasitemia in malaria** and other parasitic infections of red blood cells such as **babesiosis**. Both of these protozoa infect red blood cells, and can produce severe parasitemia. Red cell exchange may be beneficial in patients with the parasite load greater than 10%. However, patients with high parasitemia are often extremely ill and must be closely monitored during the procedure.

Extracorporeal Photopheresis

Extracorporeal photopheresis (ECP) also called **extracorporeal photochemotherapy (ECP) or photopheresis** is a form of leukocytapheresis.

Principle

In this technique, a small percentage of a patient's white blood cells is collected by apheresis. These white blood cells are then treated by incubation with a psoralen compound (which is photoactivable drug). Then these cells are exposed to ultraviolet A (UVA) irradiation within the instrument. These treated white blood cells are then reinfused into the patient. This will result in a disease-dependent immunomodulatory effect that may stimulate or suppress an immune response in the patient.

Indications (Table 13.2)

Table 13.2: Examples of diseases in which extracorporeal photopheresis is effective.

Disease category	Examples
Malignancy	Cutaneous T cell lymphoma (CTCL)
Chronic graft versus host disease (GVHD)	• Mucocutaneous GVHD • Hepatic GVHD
Solid organ transplant rejection	• Heart: acute cardiac allograft rejection • Kidney • Lung (e.g. treatment of chronic rejection characterized by bronchiolitis obliterans syndrome in patients with lung transplantation)
Autoimmune diseases	Systemic lupus erythematosus, rheumatoid arthritis, pemphigus vulgaris, Crohn's disease, psoriasis, scleroderma
Infectious diseases	AIDS-related complex (ARC)
Other diseases	Severe atopic dermatitis

Procedure

Peripheral intravenous line or central venous access is established in the patient. It has three stages, namely, (i) leukocytapheresis, (ii) photoactivation, and (iii) reinfusion.

Leukocytapheresis
- From the veins, 25 mL or 225 mL of whole blood is collected in a Latham centrifuge bowel, where the components are separated by leukocytapheresis. Heparin or acid citrate-dextrose (ACD) may be used as the anticoagulant.
- The buffy coat is retained in a collection bag. The remaining blood components (red blood cells and plasma) after leukocytapheresis are returned to the patient.
- **Preparation of mononuclear cell component suspension**: In this procedure, an intermittent centrifuge is used. Hence, it needs six cycles (12-mL bowl) or three cycles (22-mL bowl) of leukapheresis of

whole blood to collect a 270 mL mononuclear cell count (MNC) suspension. This 270 mL suspension consists of 80 mL of plasma, 90 mL of saline, and 100 mL of MNC (mononuclear cell count).

Photoactivation
- **Adding photoactivable drug**: After completion of the MNC collection, 8-**methoxypsoralen (8-MOP) is added** to the bag.
- **Photoactivation by ultraviolet A (UVA) light**: The MNC suspension is then pumped through a sterile cassette surrounded by UVA bulbs in photoactivation chamber for 30 minutes. The UVA light in the photoactivation chamber irradiates the 8-MOP-containing buffy coat.

Reinfusion of buffy coat
Following photoactivation, the buffy coat is then reinfused into the patient.

Precautions
- **Significant RBCs**: The presence of significant numbers of red blood cells within the leukocytapheresis product will reflect or absorb the UVA irradiation. This results in failure to photoactivation. Hence, it is essential that the hematocrit of the leukocytapheresis product be less than 7%.
- **Excess plasma**: If there is excess plasma in the leukocytapheresis product, it will dilute the white blood cells. This results in fewer passages of each cell through the photoactivation chamber.

Complications: Two complications may develop following photopheresis.
- **Photosensitivity:** Patients undergoing ECP are sensitive to sunlight. Hence, they should avoid direct or indirect sunlight exposure for 24 hours following completion of the procedure. This is by covering exposed skin, using sunscreen, and wearing wraparound ultraviolet (UV) protective eyewear.
- **Leukemogenesis**: This is another possible complication of ECP. This may be due to DNA damage and mutation caused by photoactivation of the 8-MOP. These mutated cells can give rise to hematologic malignancies.

Lymphocytapheresis

Purpose: To remove large quantities of lymphocytes and to generate immunosuppression or immune modulation. It is used for the direct therapeutic manipulation of the patient's cell-mediated immunity. In contrast, the plasmapheresis primarily affects humoral immunity.

Therapeutic Plasma Exchange

Mechanisms of Action of Plasma Exchange

Various mechanisms of action of therapeutic plasma exchange (TPE) with examples of diseases are given in Table 13.3. Of these two most obvious and well-understood mechanisms for the beneficial effects of therapeutic plasma exchange are:
- **Removal of the pathologic** humoral factors/**substance** present in the blood that contributes to a disease process or its symptoms. For example, IgM in Waldenström's macroglobulinemia
- The **replacement of deficient substances/** molecules in the blood by using plasma (e.g. for systemic lupus erythematosus) healthy donors as the replacement fluid. For example, FFP as a replacement source of ADAMTS13 in TTP.

Therapeutic Plasma Exchange Indications (Table 13.3)

Therapeutic plasma exchange (TPE) is indicated for removal of substances
- Too big to be removed by other procedures
- With a long enough half-life to provide a therapeutic period of decreased serum concentration
- That are acutely toxic and resistant to removal by other methods.

TPE combined with immunosuppression: This is helpful to perform successful transplantation of incompatible organ transplants.

Replacement fluids: In TPE, between 1 and 1.5 liters of plasma volume is removed. This volume should be replaced with another fluid. Many replacement fluids are available,

Table 13.3: Various mechanisms of action and indications for therapeutic plasma exchange with examples of diseases.

Mechanism	Examples of diseases
Removal of	
Allo-antibodies	• Hemolytic disease of newborn (HDN) • Anti-Rh antibodies in pregnant women • Neonatal thrombocytopenia • Antibody-mediated transplant rejection
Auto-antibodies • Renal disorders	Goodpasture's syndrome (anti-GBM autoantibodies)
• Neurologic disorders	• Acute inflammatory demyelinating polyneuropathy: Guillain-Barré syndrome (GBS), also known as acute inflammatory • Demyelinating polyradiculoneuropathy (AIDP) • Chronic inflammatory demyelinating polyneuropathy (CIDP) • Myasthenia gravis (acetyl-choline receptor antibodies)
Pathologic antibodies with hyperviscosity syndromes	• Multiple myeloma (due to monoclonal IgG, IgA, or IgD) • Waldenstrom's macroglobulinemia (due to monoclonal IgM)
Immune complexes	• Rapidly progressive glomerulonephritis (RPGN) • Systemic lupus erythematosus (SLE) • Polyarteritis nodosa (PAN) • Rheumatoid arthritis (RA) • Granulomatosis with polyangiitis (formerly called Wegener's granulomatosis)
Toxins in	Hepatic, failure, renal failure, protein-bound toxins or drugs: e.g. Amanita mushroom poisoning, barbiturate poisoning
Proinflammatory cytokines and adhesion molecules	Myasthenia gravis (MG), ANCA + vasculitis, TTP, therapy-resistant sepsis
Replacement of deficient plasma components in hematologic disorders—thrombotic microangiopathies	TTP-thrombotic thrombocytopenic purpura (ADAMTS13 in donor FFP) Hemolytic uremia syndrome (HUS)
Increased sensitivity of lymphocytes and plasma cells to chemotherapy	Acute inflammatory demyelinating polyradiculoneuropathy (AIDP), systemic sclerosis, CNS demyelinating disease
Changes in lymphocyte numbers	AIDS, systemic sclerosis, SLE

each with own advantages and disadvantages (Table 13.4).

Hydroxyl ethyl starch (HES): It is derived from plant starches. It consists of large starch molecules which can be added to saline to produce a colloidal solution. HES will remain in the intravascular space. It can be used in those who require TPE, but whose religious beliefs preclude the use of replacement fluids derived from blood.

- **High molecular weight HES:** It has a half-life of 25.5 hours. So significant amounts of HES can persist after frequent TPE procedures. This can lead to expansion of blood volume and alterations in partial thromboplastin time, total protein, albumin, hematocrit, and fibrinogen.
- **Low molecular weight HES**: It has a shorter half-life. Hence, the changes observed in high molecular weight HES are less common in this HES.

Table 13.4: Advantages and disadvantages of various replacement fluids used in therapeutic plasma exchange (TPE).

Replacement fluid	Advantages	Disadvantages
5% albumin most widely used	• Does not transmit viral diseases • Low risk of reactions	• Hyperoncotic fluid causes net flow of fluid from the extravascular space and results in mild dilutional anemia • Expensive • No immunoglobulins • No coagulation factors
Crystalloid (normal saline)	• Low cost • No risk of disease transmission • Nonallergenic	• No immunoglobulins • No coagulation factors • Hypo-oncotic • Two to threefold more volume is required
Fresh frozen plasma (FFP)	• Relatively inexpensive • Provides physiologic concentrations of coagulation factors, immunoglobulins, and plasma proteins	• Danger of transmission of transfusion-transmitted viral diseases • Transfusion reactions • Need to have an ABO-compatible product • Increase in the frequency of citrate reactions • Reactions to replacement fluids
Plasma cryoprecipitate reduced (cryopoor plasma)	• Iso-oncotic • Reduced high-molecular weight von Willebrand factor and fibrinogen • Normal levels of most other plasma proteins	Same as fresh frozen plasma
Hydroxyl ethyl starch (HES)	• Inexpensive • No risk of transmission of infectious disease • It is an alternative replacement solution for those who have reactions to albumin or FFP	• Allergic reactions • Renal dysfunction • Significant amounts of high molecular weight HES can persist after frequent TPE with its consequences (see text)

Complications of therapeutic plasma exchange are listed in Box 13.7.

Procedures for Selective Removal of Plasma Components

- Each TPE removes about 150 g of plasma proteins (110 g of albumin and 40 g of globulin) to eliminate 1 to 2 g of pathologic substance in the plasma. Repeated TPE can cause bleeding due to loss of coagulation factors and immunodeficiency due to loss of immunoglobulins. If other replacement fluids are used, there will be other risks associated with it. These include disease transmission and allergic reactions.
- To overcome these disadvantages, a number of procedures have been evolved to selectively remove a plasma component, and return the cleansed plasma to the patient's. These procedures will reduce the depletion of normal plasma components and avoid the need for substitution fluids. However, such procedures are more expensive and only few devices are available.

Box 13.7: Complications of therapeutic plasma exchange (TPE).

- Reaction to replacement fluids
- *Vaso-vagal reactions:* Hypotension, bradycardia, syncope, sweating, and rarely convulsions especially in new donors
- Pyogenic reactions
- *Hypocalcemia:* Paresthesia, numbness, and tingling sensation
- Anemia
- Thrombocytopenia
- Hypogammaglobulinemia

Steps involved in selective removal procedures:
- **Separation step**: The cellular elements of whole blood are separated from the plasma.
- **Selective removal**: The plasma is then perfused through the selective removal device. In this, the substance of interest is removed by chemical, physical, or immunologic means.
- **Reinfusion**: The treated plasma is then recombined with the cellular components and reinfused.

Selective removal of low-density lipoproteins apheresis (LDL-apheresis)

It is indicated for the treatment of familial homozygotes as well as heterozygotes hypercholesterolemia (FH) unresponsive to drug therapy.

It is associated with mutations in the hepatic LDL receptor. In this disorder, there is accelerated atherosclerosis due to the inability of the liver to clear LDL cholesterol from the blood. Previously, TPE was used to treat these patients which nonselectively removes both LDL and the cardioprotective high-density lipoprotein (HDL). Lipoprotein apheresis selectively removes LDL while retaining HDL.

DONOR/PATIENT COMPLICATIONS COMMON TO ALL APHERESIS PROCEDURES

Both donor and therapeutic apheresis are safe procedures with minimal complications. Some complications of apheresis apply to all types of procedures. Adverse effects of both cytapheresis and plasmapheresis are given in Box 13.8.

Phlebotomy Related

Vascular access complications include large hematomas, sepsis, phlebitis, and nerve injury/neuropathy (Refer venipuncture under donor collection of whole blood on pages 149-51).

Electrolyte and Acid–base Disturbances

Hypocalcemia: Citrate chelates calcium ions and is used as the primary anticoagulant

---

Box 13.8: Adverse effects of apheresis.

- Vascular access complications (hematoma, sepsis, phlebitis, neuropathy)
- Electrolyte and acid–base disturbances
  ○ Citrate toxicity
  ○ Allergic and anaphylactic reactions
- Hypovolemia, hypotension, and vasovagal reactions
- Hydroxyethyl starch and its associated complications
  ○ *Coagulopathy:* Depletion of clotting factors
  ○ Renal dysfunction
  ○ Depletion of proteins and immunoglobulins
- Air embolus
- Hemolysis
- Circulatory and respiratory distress because of pulmonary edema
- Transfusion-transmitted diseases (refer Chapter 16)
- Lymphocyte loss

---

in both donor and therapeutic apheresis procedures. Its anti-coagulant property is short acting and easily reversible, unlike heparin. In some cases, it may produce hypocalcemia.

Citrate toxicity: Normally, citrate is used as an anticoagulant during apheresis. The administration of citrate solutions to donors, almost as a form of massive autologous transfusion because 4-6 L of their blood is withdrawn, passed through the instrument, citrated, and returned to them during the procedure. Citrate is rapidly and actively metabolized in the body. If the amount of citrate infused is higher than the body's capacity to metabolize, with citrate toxicity, the donor may feel numbness or tingling around the mouth (paresthesias), muscle cramping, tetany, cardiac arrhythmia, etc. It is treated either by decreasing the rate of infusion of returned component or giving exogenous calcium to the donor.

Allergic and anaphylactic reactions: In therapeutic apheresis, allergic and anaphylactic reactions are most often triggered by the replacement fluid. They result from the release of vasoactive substances from mast cells and basophils. These include histamine, leukotriene C4, leukotriene D4, prostaglandin D2, and platelet-activating factor. This causes smooth muscle contraction, increased vascular permeability, and vasodilation. These types of reactions can vary from mild urticaria to life-threatening anaphylactic reactions. Signs and symptoms of these reactions include pruritus, urticaria, erythema, flushing, angioedema, upper and lower airway obstruction, hypotension, shock, nausea, vomiting, and diarrhea.

Allergic reactions can occur in both donors and patients undergoing apheresis procedures. Among donors, reactions can occur in platelet, plasma, and granulocyte donors.

The treatment of allergic and anaphylactic reactions depends on their severity. In donor reactions, the procedure should be stopped.

- **Urticaria** can be treated with oral antihistamines (e.g. diphenhydramine). The same treatment can be given to patients with therapeutic procedures, and the procedure can be restarted following antihistamine administration.
- **Anaphylactic reactions** are life-threatening. The best course of action is to avoid such reactions. Patients with mild reactions should be premedicated with antihistamines. The procedure, whether donor or therapeutic, must be stopped immediately. Vascular access must be kept open using saline.
  - For less severe reactions:
    - **Epinephrine** 0.3 to 0.5 mg can be given subcutaneously and the dose is repeated every 20 to 30 minutes for up to three doses.
    - **Aminophylline** 6 mg/kg may be given if there is bronchospasm.
    - **Volume expansion** with normal saline or lactated Ringer's solution can be given for **hypotension**.
    - **Oxygen**: For respiratory distress.
  - For severe reactions
    - **Epinephrine** 0.5 mg can be given intravenously, with repeated dosing every 5 to 10 minutes.
    - **Dopamine** can be given for hypotension unresponsive to volume.
    - The airway must be kept patent and **endotracheal intubation** may be needed.
  - Donors who have experienced such reactions should be deferred from future donation.

Hypovolemia and Vasovagal Reactions

Hypotension can develop during both donor and therapeutic apheresis procedures. It is especially developed if intermittent flow devices are used. This can be due to two different pathophysiologic mechanisms.

- **In hypovolemia**: The hypotension is due to intravascular volume depletion. This is because too much volume is present within the extracorporeal circuit.
  - **Apheresis donors**: These reactions are not common among apheresis donors, because the amount of volume in the extracorporeal circuit is within the prescribed limits.
  - **Therapeutic apheresis**: The hypovolemia is more likely. There is no prescribed limit on extracorporeal volume during therapeutic apheresis procedures.
- **Vasovagal reaction**: It is the second mechanism causing hypotension during apheresis procedures. In whole blood donors, the factors that predispose to vasovagal reactions include younger age, low weight, and first-time donation. These reactions among apheresis donors increase with age and women (older adults and women), unlike what has been reported with whole blood donors.

Treatment of hypotension and vasovagal reactions: Hypovolemic and vasovagal reactions are treated similarly. The procedure should be temporarily interrupted, and a fluid bolus should be infused (refer page 154 Chapter 7 vasovagal syncope discussed under whole blood donation).

Hydroxyethyl Starch and its Associated Complications

These include coagulopathy, renal dysfunction, and others.

- **Coagulopathy**
  - Removal of plasma from a patient and its replacement of the volume with albumin or some other fluid that does not contain coagulation factors during TPE can cause abnormalities in coagulation. These changes are usually mild, temporary/short-lived and most coagulation factors return to normal levels within 24 to 48 hours.
  - The use of HES as volume replacement or as a sedimenting agent is also associated with reduced coagulation factor levels. HES is cleared gradually from the body. Both high molecular weight HES and low molecular weight HES prolong the partial thromboplastin time (PTT) and reduce the level of fibrinogen. High molecular weight, but not low molecular weight HES is also associated with prolongation of bleeding time.
  - The risk of coagulopathy with HES is dose dependent. High molecular weight HES has a long half-life and this may result in an accumulation of HES over the course of the apheresis procedures. This may lead to coagulopathy especially when multiple collections or therapeutic procedures are performed in a given donor/patient.
- **Renal dysfunction**
  - HES can cause new or worsen the existing renal dysfunction. This is particularly so in critically ill patients. Hence, HES should not be used in critically ill patients with sepsis, patients in the ICU, and patients or donors with pre-existing renal dysfunction unless the benefits outweigh the risks.
- **Other side effects**
  - Persistent pruritus due to deposition of HES in the skin.
  - Marrow and organ failure in a patient undergoing chronic TPE (20 months) with HES.

Air Embolus

- **Cause:** Air embolus is a rare complication of apheresis procedures. It develops when **air enters the venous system** through a **leak in the apheresis** instrument or the **venous access**.
- **Symptoms** of air embolism include dyspnea, tachypnea, cyanosis, tachycardia, and hypotension. All the modern apheresis instruments have sensors that can detect air within the extravascular circuit and stop the procedure.
- **Treatment** of air embolism consists of placing the donor/patient in the Trendelenburg position on the left side. This traps the air in the apex of the right ventricle, away from the pulmonary outflow tract. This in turn improves right ventricular outflow. Over time, the air will dissolve.

Hemolysis

Because blood is pumped through tubing (collapsed or kinked) and centrifuges of various configurations, mechanical hemolysis may develop rarely due to constricted tubing or the geometry of the flow pathways. Hence, it is necessary to carefully observe the plasma collection liner for pink discoloration which indicates hemolysis.

Donation frequency of various apheresis blood components is presented in Table 13.5.

Table 13.5: Donation frequency of various apheresis blood components.

Apheresis component collected	Frequency of donation*
2RBC (double unit of red blood cells)	16 weeks
Plasma (frequent)	Every 2 days (not more than two times in 7 days)
Plasma (infrequent)	Every 4 weeks (not more than 13 times/year)
Platelets, single apheresis unit	Every 2 days (not more than 2 times in 7 days; not more than 24 times in 12 months)
Platelets, double or triple apheresis unit	Every 7 days
Granulocytes	Every 2 days

* Donation frequency will vary, depending on red cell loss and if more than one type of component is simultaneously collected.

SUMMARY

- Apheresis is a procedure in which blood is withdrawn from a donor or patient and separated into its components. One or more of the desired components is retained, and the remaining constituents are recombined and returned to the donor or patient.
- The process of removing platelets is termed plateletapheresis or thrombocytapheresis; removing RBCs is termed erythrocytapheresis and removing leukocytes is known as leukocytapheresis/leukapheresis.
- Removal of plasma from the blood is termed plasmapheresis.
- Apheresis equipment that uses intermittent flow centrifugation (IFC) needs only one venipuncture, in which the blood is drawn and reinfused through the same vein. After the desired component is separated, the remaining components are reinfused to the donor, and one cycle is complete. Apheresis procedures usually require many cycles to reach an acceptable therapeutic endpoint.
- In continuous flow centrifugation (CFC) procedures, two venipuncture sites are needed for the withdrawal process and returning of the blood.
- Membrane filtration technology uses membranes with specific pore sizes. It allows plasma to pass through the membrane whereas the cellular portion withheld.
- Most common anticoagulant used in apheresis is acid citrate dextrose.
- Therapeutic apheresis is indicated to remove a pathological substance, provide an essential or missing substance, alter the ratio between antigen–antibody, or to remove immune complexes in the blood.
- In therapeutic plasmapheresis, the replacement fluids are used to maintain the intravascular volume and oncotic pressure. These fluids include normal saline, FFP, cryo-reduced plasma, and 5% human serum albumin.
- *Complications of apheresis:* These include issues related to vascular access, citrate toxicity, fluid imbalance, allergic reactions, equipment malfunction (hemolysis), and infection.

SELF-ASSESSMENT EXERCISE

Write short essays/notes on:
- Apheresis
- Plateletapheresis
- Plasmapheresis
- Apheresis procedures
- Cytapheresis
- Plateletapheresis and storage
- Preparation to and uses of apheresis platelets
- Apheresis role in blood banking
- Platelet therapy and apheresis

CHAPTER 14

Adverse Effects of Blood Transfusion

CHAPTER OUTLINE

- Hemolysis
- Adverse transfusion reactions
- Immediate/acute transfusion reactions
- Delayed transfusion reactions
- Silent transfusion-related adverse events
- Transfusion-related adverse events in special patient scenarios

Blood transfusion is useful and life-saving when performed with caution and with clear indication. Important complications of transfusion are the development of various adverse reactions. Before going into details of these transfusion reactions, a brief review of hemolysis is done.

HEMOLYSIS

Normal lifespan of red cells is approximately 120 days and premature or increased rate of destruction of circulating RBCs is known as hemolysis.

Types of Hemolysis

The site of destruction of red cells may be extravascular or intravascular. Hence, hemolysis can be divided into **intravascular and extravascular** depending on the site of hemolysis.

Artifactual hemolysis can occur in transfusion medicine due to poor venipuncture technique, prolonged storage of blood, exposure to extremes of temperature, old samples or use of some anticoagulants.

Intravascular Hemolysis

The hemolysis occurs within the circulation with release of red blood cell contents, including hemoglobin directly into the plasma.

Causes

Intravascular hemolysis may be caused by different mechanisms **(Box 14.1)**.

In transfusion medicine

Intravascular hemolysis in transfusion medicine occurs due to the destruction of the transfused donor red cells within the vascular component of the recipient. It is mainly due to IgM antibodies **usually associated with ABO incompatibility** between recipient and

Box 14.1: Causes of intravascular hemolysis.

- Immune (antibody-mediated) mechanism
  - Alloantibodies (anti-A, anti-B, anti-A,B): Complement activation due to binding of antibodies against red cell antigens
  - Autoantibodies, e.g. systemic lupus erythematosus, drug-associated
- Mechanical trauma or injury to RBCs (e.g. trauma by heart valves)
- Infection by intracellular parasites (e.g. malarial parasites, babesiosis)
- Exogenous toxic or chemical injury (e.g. clostridial sepsis, snake venom, lead poisoning).

donor. These antibodies rapidly activate the complement which is responsible for the destruction of donor cells. This is brought out by the naturally occurring (preformed) antibodies, namely, anti-A and anti-B (depending on the blood group).

- **Massive intravascular hemolysis:** This is one of the serious complications which **develop within 1 to 4 hours and with only a few milliliters of incompatible red cells**. The preformed immunoglobulin M (IgM) or IgG **antibodies** (anti-A and anti-B) in the recipient **recognize the corresponding donor red cell antigens**. These antibodies coat transfused donor red cells and form immune **complexes** which in turn **activate complement system**. ABO antibodies of the IgM class activate the classical pathway of complement, and result in intravascular hemolysis. ABO antibodies of the IgG class less commonly activate the complement pathway. IgG antibodies can interact with Fc receptors of mononuclear phagocytes (e.g. spleen) resulting in phagocytosis of red cells.

Consequences of complement activation (refer Fig. 1.15): Complement activation cleaves C3 into C3a (an anaphylatoxin), which is released into the plasma and C3b which binds and coats the red cells. If the complement cascade proceeds to completion, membrane attack complex (MAC), i.e. C5–9 assemble on the red cell surface. In an AHTR (acute hemolytic transfusion reaction), complement functions in three capacities—opsonization, production of anaphylatoxins (vasoactive amines) and red cell lysis (by MAC).

- **Opsonization (Fig. 14.1):** Complement components are produced during complement activation such as C3b (opsonin) and bind to the surface of RBCs. These opsonized RBCs are recognized by phagocytes and result in the phagocytosis of the opsonized red blood cells. These red cells are destroyed by phagocytes (e.g. macrophages in spleen).

- **Vasoactive amines (C3a and C5a)** and **inflammatory mediators (Fig. 14.2):** These are potent inducers of inflammation. They are released into the plasma by complement activation. They are responsible for most of the systemic symptoms. C3a and C5a release histamine and serotonin from mast cells, which cause vasodilation and contraction of smooth muscles of bronchial (bronchospasm) and intestinal muscles.

- **Red cell lysis by membrane attack complex (Fig. 14.3):** The activated lytic membrane attack complex (C5–9) of the complement cascade causes intravascular destruction (hemolysis) of transfused donor red blood cells. **Intravascular hemolysis** results. Liberated hemoglobin is bound by plasma haptoglobin. When

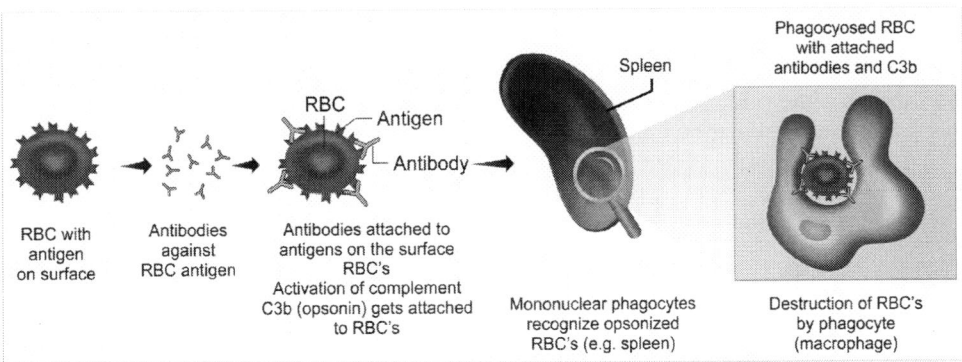

Fig. 14.1: Destruction of RBC by opsonization.

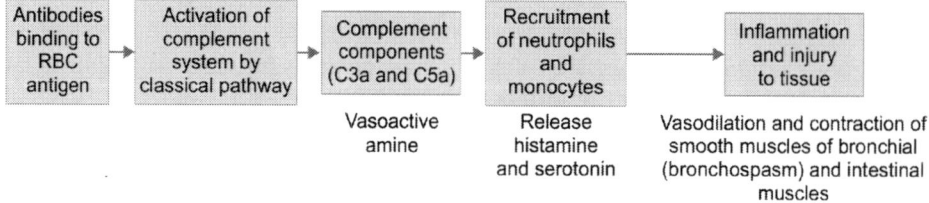

Fig. 14.2: Compliment activation releases vasoactive amines (C3a and C5a) and inflammatory mediators responsible for symptoms of hemolytic reaction.

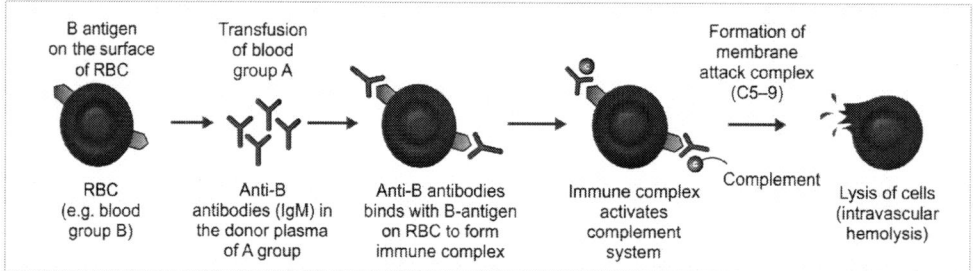

Fig. 14.3: Red cell lysis through lytic membrane attack complex (MAC). Binding of IgG or IgM antibody to an antigen on the red cell promotes activation of complement. This leads to formation of membrane attack complex (MAC) which causes red cell lysis. In this example, transfusion of A group blood to individual with B group is depicted.

the hemoglobin binding capacity of plasma haptoglobin is exceeded, **hemoglobinemia and hemoglobinuria** develop. **Hemoglobinemia and hemoglobinuria** are the hallmarks of intravascular hemolysis. Free hemoglobin released into the bloodstream has cytotoxic and inflammatory effects. C5 is also split into C5a and C5b. C5a is also an anaphylatoxin which is 100 times potent than C3a is also produced as part of the hemolysis.

Consequences (Fig. 14.4)

- **Binding of hemoglobin binds to haptoglobin:** Intravascular hemolysis results in release of hemoglobin and hemoglobin binds to a plasma binding protein called haptoglobin and forms a complex (hemoglobin/haptoglobin complex).
- **Hemoglobinemia:** Haptoglobin is a globulin normally present in concentration of about 1.0 g/L in the plasma. When the amount of released hemoglobin exceeds the hemoglobin binding capacity of haptoglobin, it produces hemoglobinemia (free hemoglobin in plasma).
- **Hemoglobinuria:** With hemoglobinemia, hemoglobin is filtered into the urine and reabsorbed by the renal tubular cells. When the hemoglobinuria exceeds the capacity of reabsorption by tubular cells, it leads to hemoglobinuria.
- **Hyperbilirubinemia:** Hemoglobin/haptoglobin complex is taken up by the hepatocytes and to a lesser extent in macrophages. In these cells, hemoglobin is broken down into heme and globin. Globin is further degraded into amino acids and returned to the amino acid pool. Heme part is split into iron (which is reutilized) and protoporphyrin. Protoporphyrin is converted into bilirubin which binds to serum albumin (unconjugated) and circulates in the blood.
- Conjugation of bilirubin takes place in liver and conjugated bilirubin is excreted via bile into the intestine.
- Conjugated bilirubin is degraded by gut bacteria into various water-soluble colorless compounds, collectively known

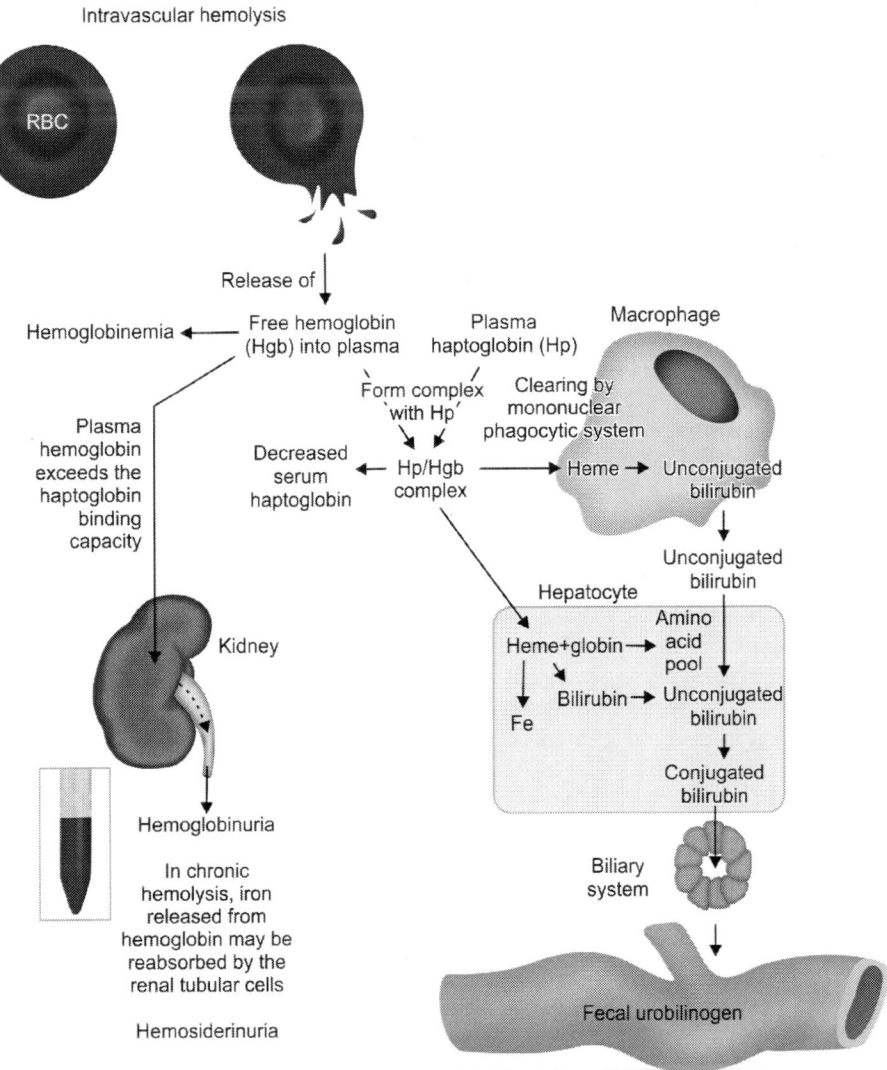

Fig. 14.4: Consequences of intravascular hemolysis.

as urobilinogen. Most of the urobilinogen is oxidized further to stercobilinogen and excreted in feces as stercobilin.
- About 20% of the urobilinogen is reabsorbed from the intestine (ileum and colon), returned to the liver, and recycled directly into the bile again. A small amount of this reabsorbed urobilinogen is found in the blood circulation and is filtered by the renal glomerulus and excreted in the urine as urobilinogen and urobilin.

Note: **Haptoglobins is consumed during intravascular hemolysis** and **its serum values decline with intravascular hemolysis** causing **liberation of hemoglobin into plasma**. Release of free hemoglobin may also occur with artifactual lysis of red blood cells in vitro. These in vitro conditions include poor venipuncture technique, prolonged storage of blood, exposure to extremes of temperature (e.g. freezing of red cells), old samples or use of some anticoagulants.

Extravascular Hemolysis

This type of hemolysis occurs when there is fragmentation of RBCs and with aged (senescent) RBCs. They are **phagocytosed by the macrophages of the mononuclear phagocyte system** (in spleen, liver and bone marrow). The destruction of red cells occurs within the mononuclear phagocytes of the reticuloendothelial (RE) system. The **hemoglobin released from these red cells is not released into free into plasma**. Hence, **hemoglobin is not detected in the plasma**. The hemoglobin is degraded inside the phagocytic macrophages—hence referred to as extravascular hemolysis (macrophage-mediated hemolysis). In extravascular hemolysis, red cells are phagocytosed either because RBCs are rendered "foreign" or become less deformable, which makes their passage difficult in splenic sinusoids. There is **neither hemoglobinemia nor hemoglobinuria** with extravascular hemolysis. However, it may be present when extravascular hemolysis is accompanied by intravascular hemolysis.

Causes
Causes of extravascular hemolysis are presented in Box 14.2.

In Transfusion Medicine
If complement activation does not proceed to completion as in case on non-ABO antibodies, the red cells undergo extravascular hemolysis. In extravascular hemolysis, the red cells coated with C3b and/or IgG are rapidly removed from the circulation by phagocytes. The red cells are destroyed in the spleen.

Box 14.2: Causes of intravascular hemolysis.

- Immune (antibody-mediated) mechanism
- Infection by erythroparasites, e.g. *Mycoplasma*
- Other organisms: Bacteria (e.g. *Clostridium, Leptospira*)
- Fragmentation injury: Secondary to vascular diseases (e.g. hemangiosarcomas), disseminated intravascular coagulation (DIC)
- Inherited RBC disorders: Inherited defect of red cell membrane (e.g. pyruvate kinase deficiency), defects in RBC membrane (e.g. hereditary stomatocytosis)

Activation of coagulation cascade

Antigen–antibody–complement complexes can also initiate the coagulation and fibrinolytic systems. This may occur due to various mechanisms.

- **Activation of intrinsic pathway:** It may be activated by antigen–antibody interaction which activates factor XII (Hageman factor).
- **Activation of extrinsic pathway:** Activated complement, tumor necrosis factor alpha (TNFα) and interleukin-1 (IL-1) may increase the expression of tissue factor. This in turn activates extrinsic pathway of coagulation. This causes life-threatening **disseminated intravascular coagulation** (DIC) and the consequent bleeding.

Consequences (Fig. 14.5)

In the RE system, the destroyed or lyzed senescent red cells release hemoglobin. Hemoglobin is broken down into heme and globin. Globin is further degraded into amino acids and returned to the amino acid pool. Heme part is split into iron (which is reutilized) and protoporphyrin. Protoporphyrin is converted into bilirubin which binds to serum albumin (unconjugated) and circulates in the blood. The remaining steps are the same as in intravascular hemolysis.

Differences between extravascular and intravascular hemolysis are shown in Table 14.1.

ADVERSE TRANSFUSION REACTIONS

Safety measures are usually taken at all steps of the blood collection, donor unit processing, pretransfusion testing, and patient monitoring. In spite of careful precaution and preventive measures, unfavorable adverse effects such as noninfectious complications of transfusions occur (about 2–4% of cases) and are not always preventable. These adverse effects of blood transfusion are **also known as blood transfusion reactions or simply transfusion reactions**.

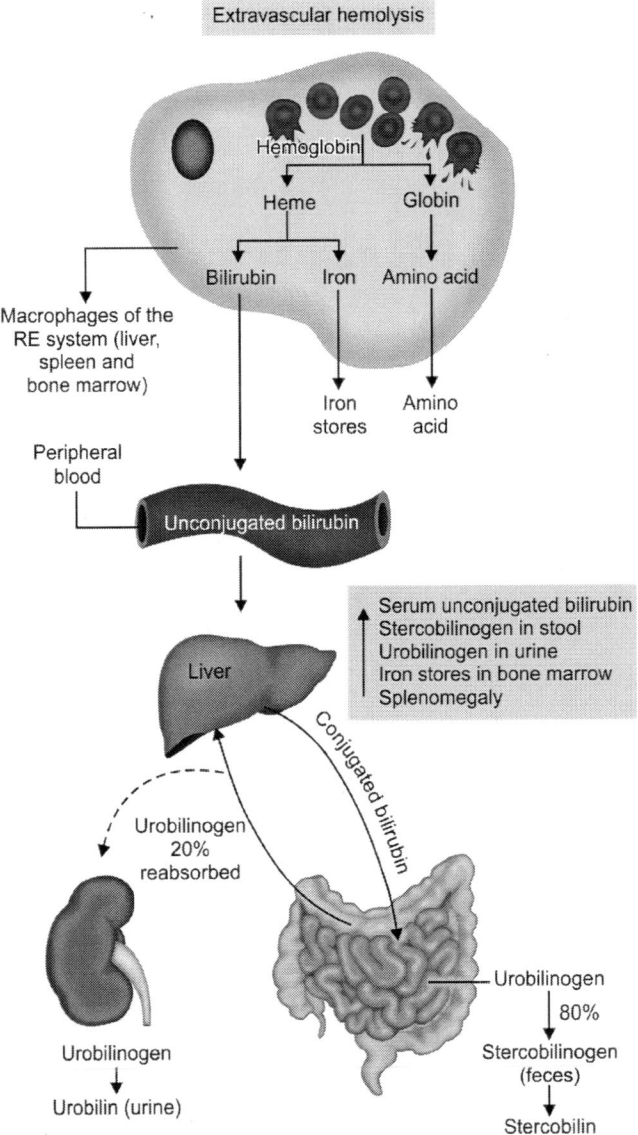

Fig. 14.5: Consequences of extravascular hemolysis.

Definition: An **adverse transfusion reaction** is defined as **any adverse event** (undesirable response/effect or complications related to transfusion) **that occurs in a patient during or after the transfusion** of whole blood, blood components, or human-derived plasma products. It may range from relatively mild to severe and at times can be fatal.

Classification (Box 14.3): Transfusion reactions are a diverse group of adverse reactions to transfusion. They can be categorized into different types.

- **According to the time interval:** Transfusion reactions may also be classified according to the time interval between transfusion and the presentation of adverse effects.

Table 14.1: Differences between extravascular and intravascular hemolysis.

Features	Extravascular hemolysis	Intravascular hemolysis
Site of hemolysis	Mononuclear phagocytes of RE system (spleen, bone marrow)	Within the circulation
Laboratory findings		
• Serum haptoglobin	Normal	Decreased
• Hemoglobinemia	Not seen	Positive
• Hemoglobinuria	Not seen	Positive
• Hemosiderinuria	Not seen	Positive
• Serum bilirubin (unconjugated)	Moderately elevated	Mildly elevated

Box 14.3: Transfusion reaction (complications of blood transfusion).

NONINFECTIOUS COMPLICATIONS
Immediate (acute) reactions
- *Immunological*
  - Acute hemolytic transfusion reactions (AHTRs)
  - Acute nonhemolytic transfusion reactions
    - Febrile nonhemolytic transfusion reaction (FNHTR)
    - Allergic reaction
    - Anaphylactic
    - Transfusion-related acute lung injury (TRALI)
- *Nonimmunological*
  - Non-immune mediated hemolysis
  - Transfusion-associated circulatory overload (TACO)
  - Hypotension
  - Transfusion-associated sepsis (TAS)
  - Metabolic complications (hyperkalemia, hypokalemia, hypocalcemia, hypothermia)
  - Air embolism
  - Physical hemolysis

Delayed reactions
- *Immunological*
  - Delayed hemolytic transfusion reactions (DHTRs)
  - Transfusion associated graft versus host disease
  - Post-transfusion purpura
  - HLA alloimmunization
- *Nonimmunological*
  - Iron overload-transfusion hemosiderosis
  - Citrate toxicity
  - Thrombophlebitis

INFECTIOUS COMPLICATIONS (TRANSFUSION TRANSMITTED DISEASES)
Few of the diseases transmitted by transfusion are:
- Hepatitis (HBV, HCV and HDV)
- HIV (AIDS)
- Malaria
- Cytomegalovirus
- Syphilis

- **Acute (immediate) transfusion reaction:** It is a transfusion reaction with **signs or symptoms occurring during or shortly after transfusion** (within 24 hours of transfusion).
- **Delayed transfusion reaction:** It is a transfusion reaction with signs or **symptoms presenting after 24 hours of transfusion**.
- **According to the pathophysiology/mechanism:** Transfusion reactions may be further classified into:
  - **Infectious and noninfectious** complications (Box 14.3). Noninfectious complications of transfusions are greater risk to patients than infectious diseases.
  - **Immune versus nonimmune.**

IMMEDIATE/ACUTE TRANSFUSION REACTIONS

Definition: *Acute transfusion reaction* is defined as a reaction in which signs and symptoms occur within 24 hours of a transfusion.

Acute Nonhemolytic Transfusion Reactions

Acute transfusion reactions divided according to one of three key presenting symptoms: fever, allergic and pulmonary (Flowchart 14.1).

Acute Hemolytic Transfusion Reaction

A hemolytic transfusion reaction is characterized by the destruction of transfused red cells in the recipient. It results in intravascular

Flowchart 14.1: Acute transfusion reactions divided according to one of three key presenting symptoms: fever, allergic and pulmonary.
(AHTR = acute hemolytic transfusion reaction; FNHTR = febrile nonhemolytic transfusion reaction; TACO = transfusion-associated circulatory overload; TAS = transfusion associated sepsis; TRALI = transfusion-related acute lung injury)

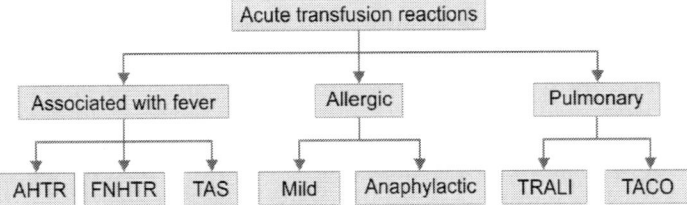

or extravascular hemolysis or a combination of both. Hemolytic reactions are classified as acute or delayed, and both types may stem from immune or nonimmune causes.

Definition: Acute hemolytic transfusion reaction (AHTR) is characterized by **rapid destruction of red cells** (i.e. acute hemolysis) with accompanying presenting **symptoms immediately after or within 24 hours** of transfusion of red cells. The **hemolysis may be due to immune or nonimmune mechanism**.

Immediate Immune-mediated Reactions

Immune-mediated acute hemolytic transfusion reaction is accompanied signs and symptoms mentioned in Box 14.4. **As little as 10 mL of incompatible blood can cause rapid hemolysis**. The severity of symptoms depends on the amount and rate of incompatible blood transfused. The patient's underlying clinical condition can obscure recognition of the reaction.

Pathophysiology
- **Transfusion of ABO incompatible red cells (Flowchart 14.2)**: The hemolysis is due to **interaction of preformed antibodies in the recipient with the donor red cell antigens**. The most severe reactions are associated with transfusion of red cells that have ABO incompatibility with the recipient. This results in **acute intravascular destruction of transfused donor red cells** (intravascular hemolysis). AHTRs are most commonly caused by transfusion of RBC which have an antigen against which the recipient has preformed antibodies. Preformed antibodies in the recipient produce most severe hemolytic reactions.
- **Transfusion of ABO incompatible antibodies:** AHTRs may also occur with transfusion of antibodies. This may occur with minor incompatible apheresis platelets or in donor plasma or intravenous immune globulin (IVIG) infusion into

---

Box 14.4: Signs and symptoms of immune-mediated acute hemolytic transfusion reaction (AHTR).

Symptoms
- Patient typically develops **fever with chills**, nausea, vomiting, diarrhea, pain, dyspnea (chest tightness), tachycardia, hypotension, bleeding and hemoglobinuria.
- Pain during an AHTR is usually localized to the flanks, back, abdomen, chest, head, and infusion site. A subjective feeling of distress is sometimes reported.
- Unexpected bleeding (oozing from infusion site/orifices) epistaxis (nosebleed) may point toward DIC.
- During surgery, hypotension and excessive bleeding may be the only signs of an AHTR.
- Renal failure is a later complication.

Signs
- Hemoglobinemia (red plasma), hemoglobinuria (red urine), increased bilirubin (5–6 hours post-transfusion)
- Hypotension, renal failure, shock, and disseminated intravascular coagulation (DIC).
- Red or dark urine or diffuse oozing may be the only sign in the anesthetized patient.

recipients whose RBCs bear the antigen recognized by those antibodies. This may occur most commonly when group O platelets from donors with high titers of anti-A when transfused to group A recipients. These are **usually not clinically significant or severe**.

Shock

Vasoactive amines, anaphylatoxins, kinins and cytokines mediators are released into the circulation as consequences of intravascular red cell destruction. They produce hypotension with shock. This in turn causes compensatory vasoconstriction and further aggravates organ and tissue damage. Shock is an abnormal condition of inadequate blood flow to the body's peripheral tissues.

Renal Failure

Renal failure due to a severe AHTR is a multifactorial event. It is most prominent in an untreated AHTR. A combination of the vascular collapse due to systemic hypotension, reactive renal vasoconstriction, free hemoglobin (impairs renal function), and the DIC-initiated end organ microthrombi contribute to renal failure. These cumulative effects reduce the blood supply to the renal cortex. The developing renal ischemia may be transient or advance to acute tubular necrosis and renal loss.

Signs and symptoms (Box 14.4): AHTR ranges in severity from fever to death. Severe symptoms of an AHTR can be observed after the infusion of as little as 10 mL of incompatible blood.

Factors that determine the outcome of the incompatible transfusion are:
1. Potency of the anti-A or anti-B (antibodies) in the recipient's in plasma
2. Amount of incompatible blood transfused
3. Rate of transfusion.

Differential diagnosis

Many signs and symptoms of an immune-mediated acute hemolytic transfusion reaction may also be observed in other acute transfusion reactions.
- Fever with or without chills and accompanied hypotension may also be found in transfusion-related **sepsis and TRALI**. However, hemolysis is not associated with TRALI and respiratory difficulty is not a usual symptom of AHTR.
- Fever or chills are more common in **febrile nonhemolytic reaction** but cannot be distinguished symptomatically **from a serious AHTR** without assessing hemolysis.
- **Acute hemolysis** may also develop due to **nonimmune mechanism**.

Fever is the most sensitive initial sign of an AHTR. If there is any rise of temperature of 1°C or more, an immune AHTR is suspected.

Causes of Immune-mediated Acute Hemolytic Transfusion Reaction
- **Clerical error:** Most common cause of AHTRs is ABO incompatibility due to a clerical error.
  - **Improper patient identification at the time of sample collection or transfusion** is the **most common cause** of an acute immune hemolytic transfusion reaction.
  - **Inadequate or wrong labeling** of the recipient's pretransfusion sample, cross-match sample, blood bag, pilot tube. Issue of a wrong blood due to improper checking or transfusion to the wrong recipient.
- **Technical error:**
  - **Errors in blood grouping** of recipient or donor.

Flowchart 14.2: Sequence of events in immune-mediated acute hemolytic transfusion reaction (AHTR).

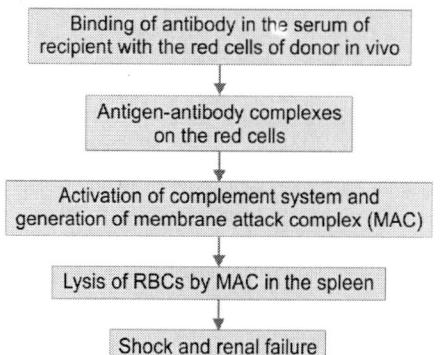

- **Improper technique:** Incompatibility not detected in crossmatching due to improper technique.
- **Failure to detect weak antibodies.**
- **Storage error.**

Preventive measures to control acute hemolytic transfusion reaction are listed in Box 14.5.

Investigation and management of acute hemolytic transfusion reaction are discussed on pages 333-9.

Nonimmune-mediated Hemolysis

During transfusion, if a patient develops hemoglobinemia and hemoglobinuria, it should be first investigated for the possibility of an immune-related response. If no alloantibodies are detected, an investigation into the nonimmune mechanisms of red cell destruction should be initiated. This process **needs examination of the remaining blood in the transfused blood bag**. Accidentally, if a **hemolyzed donor unit** is transfused, the recipient receives free hemoglobin and fragmented red cell membrane. The fragmented red cell may activate complement system and produce a procoagulant state.

Nonimmune hemolysis can also develop following transfusion. It develops **without presence/involvement of any antibodies**.

Box 14.5: Preventive measures to control hemolytic transfusion reaction

- Properly identify the patient while sample is collected for pretransfusion tests
- Properly label the drawn blood sample
- Carefully identify the patient and the blood unit before transfusion
- Use appropriate sensitive techniques for compatibility testing (especially grouping and crossmatching)
- Transfuse only if necessary
- Closely monitor the transfusion
- The time between suspicion of transfusion reaction, investigation, and treatment should be as short as possible. However, avoid undue haste in both serologic evaluation and decision making because human errors are committed most often under pressure.

Most frequently, it **presents as asymptomatic hemoglobinuria**. In acute nonimmune hemolytic transfusion reactions in which asymptomatic hemoglobinuria is the only sign, it is recommended to **maintain adequate hydration**.

Causes of Nonimmune-mediated Red Cell Hemolysis

1. **Exposure of red cells to extreme temperatures** (>50°C or <0°C): Hemolysis can occur when malfunctioning or unregulated improper use of blood warming devices, the use of microwave ovens, or water baths are used. It may also develop if warming occurs during refrigerated storage.
2. **Improper deglycerolization of an RBC unit on thawing**: This complication of transfusion can be prevented by visual inspection of the supernatant of a red cell suspension for evidence of hemolysis after the completion of deglycerolization.
3. **Mechanical or chemical damage with destruction of red cells**: Use of inappropriately small-bore needles for transfusion, patients with mechanical heart valves, excessive pressure, blood salvage equipment improper shipping, and longer duration of storage before issue may cause mechanical trauma to RBCs leading to nonimmune hemolysis of red cells.
4. **Simultaneous infusion of unapproved incompatible solutions**: Only physiological/normal saline may be added to a donor unit (Fig. 14.6). If blood is mixed with nonphysiological solutions (e.g. half-strength saline, 5% dextrose in 0.18% saline, Ringer's lactate, and medications), they may cause osmotic rupture of the red cells. Hyperosmotic or hypo-osmotic fluids mixed with red cells can also cause significant lysis.
5. **Bacterially contaminated blood products**: If they are transfused, they may cause hemolysis.
6. **Intrinsic red cell defect**: For example, sickle cell disease, thermal burns, glucose-6-phosphate dehydrogenase deficiency, and paroxysmal nocturnal hemoglobinuria.

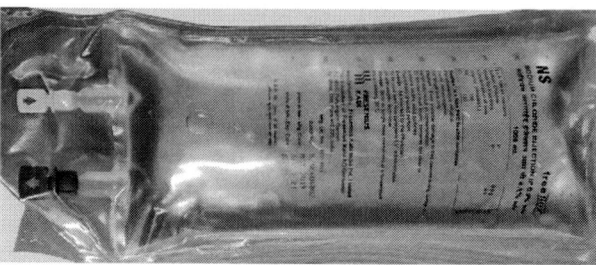

Fig. 14.6: Normal saline.

7. **Blood components stored frozen without additive cryoprotectants** induce the hemolysis of the units.

Clinical signs: These include **hemoglobinemia and hemoglobinuria**. Hyperkalemia may be found in patients with renal failure. Fever may also occur.

Diagnosis: It is established by **finding of RBCs' lysis in the transfused unit**. Exclude other causes of hemolytic transfusion reactions. Check the serum potassium level and obtain an electrocardiogram to assess hyperkalemia.

Complications: Main complications of nonimmune hemolysis are **renal failure and cardiac arrhythmia** due to hyperkalemia.

Management
- If nonimmune hemolysis occurs, the **transfusion should be immediately discontinued**.
- **Maintain intravenous access** and appropriate care similar to immune-mediated hemolysis (refer pages 336-42).
- Urine output should be maintained with hydration unless there is a contraindication such as renal failure.
- The blood bag, together with attached tubing and intravenous fluids, should be saved for further investigation.

Acute Nonhemolytic Transfusion Reactions

Febrile Nonhemolytic Transfusion Reactions

Definition: Febrile nonhemolytic transfusion reaction (FNHTR) is defined as a rise in body temperature of 1°C to 37°C or greater. It is an acute nonthreatening complication of transfusion and occurs during or shortly after transfusion (up to 4 hours after transfusion). It may produce considerable discomfort to the recipient.

Signs and symptoms: The febrile nonhemolytic transfusion reaction is a common adverse effect of transfusion. Apart from **fever,** these are usually accompanied by **chills or rigors**. It can also present with headache, nausea or vomiting, tachycardia, increase in blood pressure, and tachypnea. Symptoms usually occur during the transfusion but they may be delayed for up to 1 hour after the transfusion is completed. Its clinical features are similar to an AHTR and a careful investigation is necessary to rule out hemolysis.

In a patient who is hypothermic at the start of a transfusion, an asymptomatic (without symptoms) rise in body temperature to normal body temperature should not be considered to be an FNHTR.

Pathophysiology of FNHTR
Recipient leukocyte antibodies especially HLA antibodies (antihuman leukocyte antigen) can react with antigens on transfused donor leukocytes (lymphocytes, granulocytes) or platelets leading to FNHTR.

Pyrogens and cytokines: FNHTR may also be due to two different white cell-related mechanisms.
- **Release of endogenous pyrogens:** One mechanism is immune mediated. In this, preformed antibody reacts against white cells in the blood component. It releases endogenous **pyrogens.**

- **Release of cytokines:** The second mechanism is production and release of biologically active pyrogenic cytokines (interleukin-1 [IL-1]) primarily by the white cells/leukocytes present in the transfused component during storage. IL-1 can then cause fever by stimulating prostaglandin E2 production in the hypothalamus.

Laboratory investigations in nonhemolytic transfusion reaction is listed in Box 14.6.

Salient features of febrile nonhemolytic transfusion reactions are presented in Table 14.2.

Diagnosis: Diagnosis of FNHTR is by exclusion. It is important to **rule out a hemolytic transfusion reaction or bacterial contamination of the unit** as the cause of fever.

Prevention
- **Prestorage leukocyte reduction: Some but not all FNHTR can be prevented** by prestorage leukocyte reduction (reduction in the number of white blood cells) in packed red blood cells and stored platelet concentrates before their release of cytokines. Febrile reactions to platelet transfusion can be reduced by using platelet concentrates less than 4 days old.
- **Plasma removal**: It will not **prevent all febrile reactions**. It is equivalent to prestorage leukocyte reduction in prevention of febrile reactions.
- Premedication with acetaminophen may also prevent febrile nonhemolytic reactions.

Treatment/Management
- **Discontinue transfusion** and initiate transfusion traction workup.
- The fever of nonhemolytic transfusion reactions **tends to be self-limited** and usually no treatment is necessary, as fever will resolve within 2 to 3 hours. However, antipyretics, such as acetaminophen (325 to 500 mg) can be given.
- It is **controversial whether to restart the transfusion after a febrile reaction** has been diagnosed and the patient has been treated. The decision to restart the transfusion should depend on the clinical condition of the patient and the results of transfusion reaction testing.

Allergic and Anaphylactic Transfusion Reactions

Definition: It is a type I IgE-mediated hypersensitivity reaction (HSR) against proteins (allergens) present in the donor blood.

Allergic transfusion reactions (ATRs/ALTRs) are acute, immune complications of transfusion. Allergic reactions are the **most common type of transfusion reaction** that

Box 14.6: Laboratory investigations in febrile nonhemolytic transfusion reaction.

No evidence of hemolysis in postreaction sample and is indicated by:
- No red or pink coloration of plasma
- DAT negative
- No increase in bilirubin level
- No hemoglobinuria

Table 14.2: Salient features of febrile nonhemolytic transfusion reactions.	
Clinical signs and symptoms	Fever (temperature increase by >1°C above 37°C), chills, rigors, headache, vomiting
Cause	Antibody to donor leukocytes, cytokines released by leukocytes during storage of blood component
Laboratory tests	DAT-negative, no visible hemolysis
Complications	Nonthreatening, significant discomfort to the recipient
Management	Antipyretics, paracetamol
Prevention	Prestorage leukocyte reduction of blood components

occurs with the transfusion of blood products containing a plasma component.

Pathophysiology of ATR: ATR occurs as a response of recipient antibodies to a soluble allergen present in the donor plasma of blood component. They **can occur with any type of blood component**, including autologous RBCs.

- **Type I hypersensitivity response**: Usually, there is activation of mast cells in the recipient triggered by an allergen (plasma protein) present in the plasma of the blood component. Preformed IgE antibodies in the patient (recipient) interact with the allergen in the donor plasma. The binding of the allergen to the IgE bound to the mast cell (type I hypersensitivity reaction) releases histamine, proteases, and other granule contents from the mast cell.
- ATRs resulting from non-IgE-mediated release of mast cell mediators are called *anaphylactoid*.
- Rarely ATR may be due to selective protein deficiency, classically IgA deficiency. These are caused by anti-IgA in the recipient.

Presenting symptoms (Box 14.7): ATLR can present with a variety of symptoms that can range from minor urticarial effects to fulminant anaphylactic shock and death. Usually, **symptoms occur within minutes** after the transfusion is started. If the symptoms do not occur till >4 hours later, they are probably not related to transfusion.

> **Box 14.7:** Signs or symptoms of allergic reaction following transfusion.
>
> - Urticaria (hives)
> - Pruritus (itching)
> - Localized angioedema
> - Edema of the lips, tongue, and uvula
> - Erythema and edema of the periorbital area
> - Conjunctival edema
> - Maculopapular rash
> - Generalized flushing
> - Hypotension
> - Respiratory distress, bronchospasm
>
> **Definitive characteristics of an allergic reaction**: Two or more of the above signs or symptoms, if observed within 4 hours of transfusion are definitive of allergic reaction.

- **Mild allergic reactions (urticarial response)** to transfusion are common. Symptoms associated with milder reactions can present any time during or after the transfusion.
  - **Cutaneous symptoms**: These are more common and observed in milder reactions. The symptoms include pruritus (itching), urticaria (wheals, hives anywhere in the body), erythema, and cutaneous flushing.
- **Severe reactions (anaphylactoid or anaphylactic response) are rare**. Anaphylactic transfusion reaction is defined as the presentation of **mucocutaneous signs of urticaria and angioedema in combination with involvement of other organ systems** (cardiovascular, respiratory, and gastrointestinal). Angioedema is characterized by rapid swelling of the dermis, subcutaneous tissue, mucosa, and submucosal tissues. Mast cell degranulation is probably triggered by non-IgE mechanisms. The symptoms associated with more severe reactions usually appear shortly after the transfusion has been started and minimal volume has been transfused. Sometimes more severe anaphylactic reactions may be life-threatening. They can present with signs of typical milder allergic reactions and in addition the following symptoms of anaphylactic or anaphylactoid reactions:
  - **Respiratory symptoms:** In about 10% of cases, it presents with pulmonary signs and symptoms (bronchoconstriction/ dyspnea/wheezes/stridor). Loss of consciousness can present with respiratory involvement.
  - **Angioedema**: It presents with periorbital edema and lip swelling. It can involve throat (stridor), tongue, or lungs causing respiratory distress.
  - **Gastrointestinal symptoms** (in 30% of patients)**:** It may produce nausea, vomiting, abdominal pain/cramps, and diarrhea.
  - **Cardiovascular instability**: Hypotension, cardiac arrhythmia, tachycardia, loss of consciousness, shock, and cardiac arrest.

Differential Diagnosis

- **Anaphylaxis versus other causes of shock:** Vasovagal or hypotensive reactions are also associated with hypotension, dyspnea, and/or loss of consciousness and may be mistaken for anaphylaxis. However, symptoms such as urticaria, angioedema, pruritis, and respiratory symptoms such as wheezing or stridor are seen in anaphylaxis and not seen in vasovagal or hypotensive reactions.
- **Anaphylaxis versus asthma or TRALI:** Respiratory symptoms of anaphylaxis may be mistaken for asthma or TRALI. However, the symptoms of allergic reactions such as urticaria, angioedema, and pruritis are not seen in asthma or TRALI.

Treatment/Management

In all allergic reactions, the **transfusion should be discontinued** and intravenous access maintained.

Mild urticarial/allergic reactions: Mild cutaneous reactions usually respond to **intravenous antihistamines** such as diphenhydramine (50 to 100 mg). Once the symptoms disappear, the **transfusion can be usually restarted** and laboratory workup is not necessary. If patients have prior allergic reactions to transfusions, it may be helpful to give antihistamines 30 minutes before transfusion.

Severe urticarial reactions

- **Supportive care:** These include intubation, oxygen, intravenous fluids, and placement of the patient in the Trendelenburg position, should be started promptly.
- More severe reactions may require **epinephrine** (0.5 mg intramuscularly. Pediatric dose is 0.01 mg/kg) and is the first line of treatment for anaphylaxis. It may be repeated every 5 minutes.
- They may be **treated with H_1 and H_2 receptor antagonists and corticosteroids** (e.g. hydrocortisone 100 mg). Steroids may be useful in patients who manifest repeated allergic reactions.
- **If there is upper airway involvement**, prompt **intubation** may be needed. Oxygen may be administered if there is dyspnea. **Restarting the transfusion is not advisable** in more serious reactions associated with airway involvement.
- **Concentration of cellular blood components**: In patients who develop repeated or significant allergic reactions, transfusing the concentration of cellular blood components may be beneficial. Concentration of cellular blood components is prepared by removal of most of the plasma or by the washing of red cells and platelets.
- In patients with **proven absolute IgA deficiency**, anti-IgA testing should be done. Patients **with known anti-IgA antibodies** must be transfused with **blood components and intravenous immunoglobulins deficient in IgA.** These patients may be transfused red blood cells and platelets that are washed to remove sufficient amounts of IgA to prevent reactions.
- Patients with haptoglobin deficiency can develop similar anaphylactic transfusion reactions due to IgG or IgE antihaptoglobin. Salient features of allergic transfusion reactions are presented in Table 14.3.

Transfusion-related Acute Lung Injury

Transfusion-related acute lung injury (TRALI) is an acute transfusion reaction presenting with acute respiratory distress and severe hypoxemia usually during or within 6 hours of transfusion in the absence of other causes of acute lung injury. TRALI is a syndrome clinically similar to acute respiratory distress syndrome (ARDS) but usually resolves within 96 hours. TRALI can be a life-threatening or fatal transfusion reaction.

Pathogenesis of TRALI: Exact pathogenesis is not fully understood. Two different hypotheses have been postulated.
1. **Immune TRALI**: It consists of an antibody-mediated, one-hit event. High-titer

Table 14.3: Allergic transfusion reactions.

	Mild allergic reactions (urticarial response)	Severe reactions (anaphylactoid or anaphylactic response)
Clinical signs and symptoms	Hives and itching develop within 20 minutes of transfusion	Sudden onset of severe wheezing, cough, dyspnea, bronchospasm, respiratory distress. No fever
Cause	Antibodies in the recipient against foreign plasma proteins or others like drugs and food consumed by donor	Recipient having IgA deficiency with IgG complement binding anti-IgA antibodies
Laboratory tests	Direct antiglobulin test (DAT) negative. No visible hemolysis	DAT negative, no visible hemolysis. Test for IgA antigen and anti-IgA
Complications	Nil	Shock. Loss of consciousness and death
Management	Transfusion to be stopped temporarily and antihistamines to be given	Stop transfusion, administer epinephrine and similar drugs, maintain open airways, and administer oxygen
Prevention	If the patient gives prior history of allergic reaction, give antihistamines before transfusion	Plasma-containing products from IgA-deficient donors

antibodies in the plasma of transfused blood component directed against the human leukocyte antigen (HLA) or human neutrophil antigens (HNA) react with recipient leukocytes. This produces aggregation of leukocytes in the pulmonary vasculature. The aggregates of leukocytes occlude the pulmonary circulation and release mediators that increase capillary permeability.
  - Leukocyte antibodies are most frequently found in the plasma of multiparous female donors and are not found in plasma of males unless they have been transfused.
  - Plasma containing components include whole blood, RBCs, platelets, cryoprecipitate, and fresh frozen plasma (FFP). **Transfusion of even as small as 15 mL of plasma can cause TRALI**.
  - Blood components containing large plasma volumes donated by alloimmunized donors have high risk of causing immune-mediated TRALI. Blood components with a large volume of plasma include plasma and platelets.
2. **Nonimmune TRALI**: It consists of a two-hit event. The risk depends on the patient's predisposition to this disorder.
  - **First hit (priming of patient's leukocytes)**: The trauma to lung or an infectious or inflammatory disease in the patient may result in priming of the patient's neutrophils. The proinflammatory priming event of the patient's endothelium primes the patient's neutrophils. This is a basic requirement for nonimmune TRALI. This priming can be triggered by physiological stressors such as sepsis, surgery, and massive transfusion.
  - **Second hit (activation of the primed neutrophils):** The transfused biologically active substances accumulated during storage or antileukocyte antibodies cause the activation of the primed neutrophils.

Both the immune and nonimmune TRALI lead to a final common pathway. This causes **damage to the endothelium** and leads to increased pulmonary capillary permeability. This, in turn, results in noncardiogenic **pulmonary edema**.

Signs and symptoms
TRALI is a clinical syndrome in which diagnosis depends on the assessment of clinical symptoms. It has many overlapping symptoms with transfusion-related sepsis, circulatory overload, and anaphylactic reactions.
- **Symptoms:** These include **dyspnea, hypoxemia, tachycardia**, nonproductive cough, fever, hypotension, and cyanosis. Fever (1 to 2°C increase), chills, and

hypotension, when present, are usually moderate and respond quickly to antipyretics and fluids.
- Characteristically, there are **no abnormal breath sounds**. A **chest X-ray** usually shows bilateral **pulmonary edema** in a generalized pattern (shows bilateral infiltrates) rather than only along the major vasculature, as seen in cardiac failure. Respiratory distress and pulmonary edema may develop during transfusion or within 6 hours.
- By definition, there are **no signs of cardiac failure**.

Risk factors: Patients with **hematologic malignancy, cardiac disease,** infection, surgery, and trauma have an increased risk for TRALI with a significant impact on morbidity and outcome. This may be because these patient groups receive the majority of platelet transfusions.

Mortality: This syndrome is the **leading cause of transfusion-associated mortality**, surpassing ABO incompatibility, and bacterial contamination. The mortality is about 20% and depends on the severity of the lung injury and the underlying clinical status of the patient.

Laboratory Investigations
- Suspected case of TRALI should be reported to the blood bank.
- The **serologic workup** of the recipient and the implicated donors for the presence of HLA/HNA antibodies should be done.

Prevention
- If HLA/HNA antibodies are detected in the donor causing TRALI, the leukocyte incompatibility between the donor and the recipient should be documented. Such a donor should be excluded from any further donations (permanent deferral).
- Collect plasma components, whole blood, and platelets from male donors, never-pregnant female donors, or females who have been tested since their last pregnancy and found to be not having HLA antibodies.

Box 14.8: Criteria for the diagnosis of TRALI.
- **Onset:** Within 6 hours of transfusion.
- **Oxygen saturation** of <90% on room air.
- **Chest X-ray:** Bilateral interstitial infiltrates.
- **Blood pressure:** Pulmonary artery occlusion pressure <18 mm Hg when measured or no evidence of left atrial hypertension.

(TRALI: transfusion-related acute lung injury)

Diagnosis: TRALI is a clinical diagnosis based on clinical **(Box 14.8)** and radiological parameters. It is characterized by:
- Noncardiogenic pulmonary edema.
- No increase in brain natriuretic peptide (BNP) from pre- to post-transfusion. But it is increased in circulatory overload.
- TRALI resolves within 48 to 96 hours from outset.

Differential diagnosis: These include circulatory overload, bacterial contamination, allergic reactions, acute respiratory distress syndrome (ARDS), pulmonary embolism, and pulmonary hemorrhage. Other causes of acute lung injury include aspiration, pneumonia, toxic inhalation, lung contusion, near drowning, severe sepsis, shock, multiple trauma, burn injury, acute pancreatitis, cardiopulmonary bypass, and drug overdose.
- Anaphylactic transfusion reactions: It is characterized by bronchospasm, laryngeal edema, severe hypotension, erythema, and urticaria. Fever and pulmonary edema are not found.
- TRALI may be difficult to differentiate from transfusion-associated circulatory overload (TACO). In TACO, pulmonary edema is cardiogenic and responds to diuretics. The patient with TRALI the pulmonary edema is noncardiogenic and does not respond to diuresis.
- Transfusion-related sepsis is characterized by high fever with hypotension and vascular collapse.

Treatment/Management
- Discontinue the transfusion.
- Managed with supporting therapy.
  - Respiratory support: Usually, oxygen is indicated. Severe TRALI may require mechanical ventilation.

- Circulatory support: Pressor agents to support blood pressure may be required.
- Corticosteroids have not been shown to improve the clinical outcome and hence are of little value.
- Blood bags from recently transfused units should be recovered.
- Consult the blood bank regarding the evaluation of TRALI.
- Diuresis is not indicated in the absence of signs of fluid overload.
- Salient features of transfusion-related acute lung injury are presented in Table 14.4.

Nonimmunological Acute Transfusion Reactions

Transfusion-associated Circulatory Overload

Transfusion-associated circulatory overload (TACO) is an acute, common, nonimmune, and preventable transfusion reaction (complication of transfusion). It presents as congestive heart failure during or shortly after transfusion.

CDC (Centers for Disease Control and Prevention) definition: TACO is defined as infusion volume that cannot be effectively processed by the recipient either due to high rate and/or volume of infusion or an underlying cardiac or pulmonary pathology.

Table 14.4: Summary of feature of transfusion-related acute lung injury.

Clinical signs and symptoms	Acute onset of fever (1 to 2°C rise), chills, rigors, hypoxia, dyspnea, cyanosis, nonproductive cough, new onset bilateral pulmonary edema, hypotension headache, vomiting
Cause	Immune or nonimmune
Laboratory tests	DAT-negative, no visible hemolysis, chest X-ray, WBC antibody screen in donor and recipient
Complications	Can be life-threatening and fatal
Management	Respiratory support
Prevention	Avoid plasma components from multiparous female having HLA antibodies

Risk factors: Volume overload should be anticipated in at-risk patients and should be prevented. Risk of developing TACO is observed in the following:
- **Preexisting disease:** Patients with **preexisting heart disease, diminished cardiac reserves, end stage renal disease, chronic anemia,** and those who are **very young or very old**, even with a small transfusion volume can produce TACO.
- **Rapid or massive transfusion** of blood.
- **Age:** Patients older than 70 years and infants.

Preventive measures
- **Slowing the transfusion rate:** In patients having risk of developing TACO, the transfusion rate should be slowed down. Rates of 2 to 4 mL/minute and 1 mL/kg of body weight per hour are recommended.
- **Extension of transfusion duration:** Usually in normal individuals, the transfusion should be completed within 4 hours. However, in patients with risk of TACO, if medically indicated, the duration of transfusion may be extended. If more than 6 hours is needed, however, alternative strategies should be considered. The blood component can be divided into smaller volumes and transfused over a longer period of time with adequate time between transfusions to allow for diuresis.
- **Splitting of unit using sterile technique:** To prevent additional donor exposures, a unit can be split using sterile technique and a portion retained in the blood bank for later transfusion.
- **Concentration of units:** It can be done by removal of plasma.
- **Use of diuretic:** A diuretic can be administered before or during the transfusion.
- **Packed RBC:** Transfusion in a patient susceptible to TACO should receive RBC units, not whole blood.

Signs and symptoms: It present with respiratory distress and hypoxemia. Signs and symptoms include dyspnea, cough, orthopnea, cyanosis, tachycardia, chest tightness, elevated blood pressure (hypertension), pulmonary edema, distention of jugular veins, elevated central venous pressure, pedal edema, headache, and elevated **pulmonary wedge pressure** during or after transfusion. TACO occurs when the patient's cardiovascular system's ability to handle additional workload is exceeded. It manifests as congestive heart failure.

TACO is also **associated with increased morbidity and mortality**.

Diagnosis: TACO does not have pathognomonic signs or symptoms. The chest radiography shows pulmonary edema, cardiomegaly, and distended pulmonary artery. Diagnosis of TACO on clinical and radiologic examination may be difficult. Elevation of brain natriuretic peptide can be helpful in making the diagnosis (refer below).

Differential diagnosis: It includes TRALI, allergic reactions, and causes of congestive failure not related to transfusion, such as valvular heart disease.

Laboratory assay
Assay of brain natriuretic peptide (BNP): BNP is a marker of congestive heart failure and its measurement may be used to aid the diagnosis of TACO. BNP is a peptide secreted from the ventricles in response to increased filling pressures. Increase in brain natriuretic peptide (BNP) from pre- to post-transfusion is observed in circulatory overload at a post-transfusion to pretransfusion BNP ratio of 1.5. A post-transfusion level equal or greater than 100 picograms per milliliter is taken as a cut-off point.

Treatment (Box 14.9)
Salient features of transfusion-associated circulatory overload are presented in Table 14.5.

Transfusion-associated Hypotension

Definition: Transfusion-associated hypotension (hypotensive transfusion reaction-HyTR) is defined as sudden and unexpected onset of clinically significant hypotension that occurs during transfusion of blood and blood components. It resolves quickly when the transfusion is discontinued.

Pathophysiology
The cause of transfusion-associated hypotension is not known definitively. However, it is most likely due to the release of bradykinin. Bradykinin is a vasoactive peptide produced via activation of kinin-kallikrein system

Box 14.9: Steps to be taken when TACO develops.

- As soon as symptoms suggest TACO or infusion of other fluids
- Stabilize the patient
- Contact physician and inform the blood bank
- Provide respiratory support: Place the patient in a sitting position, supplemental oxygen, ventilatory assistance
- Administer diuretics (if not contraindicated) to reduce intravascular volume
- Investigate to rule out other causes (e.g. hemolysis, sepsis, TRALI, etc.)

Table 14.5: Summary of transfusion-associated circulatory overload.

Clinical signs and symptoms	Acute respiratory distress (dyspnea, cough) Acute onset within 6 hours of transfusion Increased central venous pressure Left heart failure Positive fluid balance
Cause	Transfusion of large volumes of blood and fluids High flow-rates
Laboratory tests	Raised brain natriuretic peptide X-ray chest: Evidence of pulmonary edema Rule out TRALI
Complications	Acute pulmonary edema
Management	Respiratory support Diuretics (if not contraindicated) to reduce fluid volume
Prevention	Avoid infusion of large volumes of plasma Transfuse packed RBCs Transfuse blood at a slower rate

from its precursor called high-molecular weight kininogen. Factors which increase concentration of bradykinin in blood components include storage, filtration, and ACE activity in donors and recipients. Angiotensin converting enzyme (ACE) is the major enzyme that breaks down bradykinin in the circulation. ACE activity can be affected by ACE-inhibitors medication and cardiopulmonary bypass circuits (lung is the primary site of ACE activity). Hypotensive reactions are associated with red cell and platelet transfusions.

Diagnosis: The drop of blood pressure should be least 10 mm Hg in systolic or diastolic arterial blood pressure from the pretransfusion baseline. Usually, the systolic blood pressure (SBP) drops by >30 mm Hg or to <80 mm Hg in adults. Hypotension usually begins within first 15 minutes of transfusion. If hypotension persists beyond 30 minutes after discontinuation of the transfusion, it is not a transfusion-associated hypotension. Hence, other causes of hypotension should be considered.

Differential diagnosis: Hypotension may be observed in HyTR, anaphylaxis (associated with mucocutaneous allergic manifestations), septic transfusion (accompanied by fever), AHTR (associated with hemoglobinuria, pain, and fever), TRALI (associated with pulmonary insufficiency), or underlying disease or due to medication. All manifest within first minutes of transfusion, but there is absence of concomitant signs or symptoms of other transfusion reactions, such as fever, chills, dyspnea, urticaria, or flushing in HyTR. HyTR resolves quickly and promptly when the transfusion is discontinued when compared to other reactions associated with hypotension.

Treatment/Management
- If hypotension occurs, discontinue the transfusion and maintain intravenous access.
- Position the patient with head down and feet elevated (Trendelenburg position).
- Administer isotonic fluids.
- Pressor support is indicated only if the hypotension is severe and refractory to intravenous fluids.

Prevention
If a patient who experiences HyTR is on ACE-inhibitor, subsequent transfusion should be given slowly to prevent a recurrence of HyYR.

Transfusion-associated Sepsis

Transfusion-associated sepsis (TAS) is an **acute nonimmune transfusion reaction**. It presents with rise in **body temperatures usually 2°C or more above normal** and rigors. It can be associated with hypotension.

A serious and potentially fatal complication of transfusion is secondary to bacterial contamination and proliferation in donor units during storage. The transfusion of **even small quantity of blood contaminated with bacteria blood can be fatal** or cause serious morbidity.

Sources of bacterial contamination: The sources are mainly skin flora and, less frequently, gut flora associated with transient bacteremia in an asymptomatic donor.
- **Sources:**
  - **Clinical conditions predisposing to TAS:** Thrombocytopenia and pancytopenia in the patient/recipient.
  - **Colonized or infected central venous catheter**: It is important to know that a colonized or infected central venous catheter used for transfusion may be the source of the bacteria. These bacteria can cause the signs and symptoms of bacterial infection during transfusion.
  - Bacterial contamination of blood (Box 14.10).
- **Organism involved**: It depends on the type and storage of the blood component.

Box 14.10: Major sources of the bacterial contamination of blood in transfusion medicine.

- Donor has asymptomatic bacteremia at time of blood donation
- Rare bacterial infection which can survive in storage conditions
- Others: Defect (pinhole) in blood collection set, testing error, etc.

- **RBCs transfusions:** The contamination rate in association with red blood cell transfusions is less and there is lower risk for TAS. This is because at the required storage temperatures (1°C to 6°C) for the RBC component. Most bacteria that contaminate the donor unit are not able to survive and grow at 4°C and die after several days of storage. However, there are few organisms that can grow at 40°C. These include *Acinetobacter, Escherichia, Staphylococcus, Yersinia enterocolitica, Serratia liquefaciens,* and *Pseudomonas fluorescens. Listeria monocytogenes* is a Gram-positive bacterium that can thrive at cold temperatures and use iron for their growth.
- **Platelet concentrate transfusions:** Bacterially contaminated platelet concentrates are the most frequent component causing TAS. It is because their storage requirement is at room temperature. Platelet concentrate may contain Gram-positive cocci (e.g. *Staphylococcus* and *Streptococcus*), Gram-negative rods (e.g. *Acinetobacter, Klebsiella, Salmonella, Escherichia coli,* and *Serratia*), and Gram-positive rods (e.g. *Propionibacterium*). It was found that apheresis platelets have a lower incidence of septic reactions than pooled whole blood-derived platelets.

Pathophysiology

Bacterial endotoxins produced during the storage of blood products can cause a dramatic clinical picture on transfusion of the contaminated blood product. Transfusion recipients may rapidly develop shock rapidly. Fatalities of contaminated blood are more common after platelet transfusions.

Clinical presentation: The clinical presentation of a transfusion reaction is caused by transfusion of bacteria-contaminated blood components.
- **Time of presentation:** The symptoms usually develop dramatically (suddenly) and in most cases it occurs during the transfusion (shortly after the transfusion begins) or shortly after it. Presentation more than 1 day may rarely occur with contaminated platelet transfusions. Abrupt presentation may be similar to AHTR; milder cases may mimic a febrile nonhemolytic transfusion reaction (FNHTR).
- **Symptoms:** The number of organisms present in the transfused blood component may influence the clinical presentation and the clinical outcome. The clinical symptoms of bacterial contamination mimic AHTR. The most common symptoms are fever, chills, hypotension, headache, shock, muscular pain, nausea, vomiting, and diarrhea. Other symptoms include dyspnea, pain, and diarrhea. Development of high fever and hypotension during or shortly after transfusion is clues for transfusion of a contaminated unit.

Complications: Bacterial contamination of blood component may give rise to complication—shock, renal failure, DIC and death.

Mortality risks: The mortality rate is high in TAS and it depends on the type of component used, type and amount of the causative organism, and the clinical condition of the patient. Bacterial **endotoxins** generated during storage of blood component may contribute to TAS-related morbidity and mortality.
- **Risk factors for fatality:** These include contamination by Gram-negative rods, greater patient age, volume of component transfused, and storage time of platelet concentrate.

Laboratory Workup for the Diagnosis of TAS
- **Rule out hemolysis as the cause of reaction** (refer pages 304-5).
- **Inspect the returned blood component**
  - In **a red blood cell component**: For **color changes, presence of bubbles, hemolysis**
  - In a **platelet component**: For **absence of swirling, or presence of clumping**.

- **Gram stain and culture:**
  - A sample should be taken **from the remaining blood component** unit and perform **Gram stain and culture** of the implicated component. The sample must be obtained from the implicated container within the container and not a segment attached to the component.
  - Blood **cultures from the transfusion recipient** (patient) should also be collected. Blood should be drawn from a venous site different from the transfusion site.
  - Diagnosis of TAS: Key for the diagnosis of TAS is isolation of the same organism in both the implicated blood bag and the patient's blood. However, a positive blood culture from the patient without confirmation of the same organism in the transfused component is not sufficient for the diagnosis of TAS.

Differential diagnosis
- **AHTRs:** The abrupt onset and severity of signs and symptoms in TAS are similar to AHTRs.
- **FNHTRs:** Mild cases of TAS may resemble FNHTRs.

Key feature for diagnosis TAS is culture of the same organism from both the patient and the remainder of the component.

TAS prevention (Box 14.11)
- **Aseptic precautions:** Decreasing the risk of bacterial contamination **at the time of collection**.
- **Detecting contamination prior to transfusion:** Interventions to prevent the transfusion of a contaminated component are mainly done on platelet components. The risk of contamination at the time of collection in a single-donor platelet is lower than compared to prepooled and leukoreduced whole blood-derived platelets. This is due to the single venipuncture used in the collection of the former and the multiple venipunctures required with the latter. Visual checking of all donor units at the time of issue and any sample with visible discoloration, clots, cloudiness or hemolysis should not be issued for transfusion.

> **Box 14.11:** Interventions to prevent transfusion-associated sepsis.
>
> **Before blood donation**
> - Donor health check before donation
>
> **At the time of blood collection**
> - Proper phlebotomy technique: Scrub arm at and around the venipuncture site
> - Single arm collection technique
> - Use of closed sterile system of collection bags
>
> **Before storage**
> - Prestorage leukoreduction
> - Pathogen inactivation
> - Automated culture
>
> **At the time of transfusion**
> - Visual inspection
> - Biochemical markers
> - Microscopy/stains

Treatment/Management
- **Discontinue the transfusion immediately** upon suspecting a TAS. **Unit with its associated tubing should be removed**. Any other blood bags that have been recently transfused should be recovered.
- **Supportive treatment:** Supportive care of circulation and respiration should be initiated as required.
- **Initiating antibiotic therapy:** Usually, treatment must be initiated before the identification of the causative organism to prevent a fatal outcome. Initial antibiotic therapy should include broad-spectrum coverage such as a β-lactam and an aminoglycoside. Once the microbiologic stains or cultures indicate the causative organism, then adjust to more specific coverage based on the organism identified and its antimicrobial susceptibility. Blood cultures from the patient as well as the blood bag should be obtained.

Summary of acute transfusion reactions is presented in Table 14.6.

Table 14.6: Summary of acute transfusion reactions.

Type of acute transfusion reaction	Signs and symptoms	Lab findings and diagnosis	Treatment	Prevention
Immunologic				
Acute immune hemolytic transfusion reaction (AIHTR) due to red cell incompatibility	Fever/chills, Back pain, Hemoglobinemia, Hemoglobinuria, Hypotension, renal failure, oliguria, oozing from IV site, back pain, pain along infusion vein, shock, DIC	DAT positive, Plasma free hemoglobin (visual inspection) +, Further tests to detect hemolysis (decreased hemoglobin, increased LDH, increased bilirubin, decreased haptoglobin)	Stop transfusion, Maintain vascular access, Maintain blood pressure, Maintain renal blood flow, Treat DIC if present	Follow standard operating procedures for identification of the patient
Febrile nonhemolytic transfusion reaction (FNHTR) due to antibody to donor leukocytes, accumulated cytokines in bag	Fever/chills, rise in temperature (1°C), headache, nausea/vomiting, Tachycardia, Tachypnea, Increased blood pressure	DAT negative, Rule out hemolysis, Rule out bacterial contamination	Antipyretics (acetaminophen, no aspirin)	Prestorage leukoreduction of PRBC and platelets
Mild allergic reactions due to antibody to donor plasma proteins	Erythema/rash, Pruritus, urticaria, flushing	Clinical diagnosis, DAT not required	Temporary discontinue transfusion, Treat with antihistamines, If symptoms improve, restart transfusion	For repeated reactions, consider premedication with antihistamines
Severe allergic reactions and anaphylaxis usually idiopathic and rarely due to antibody to donor plasma proteins (most commonly anti-IgA)	Urticarial, erythema, anxiety angioedema respiratory distress/wheezing, Hypotension, Anaphylaxis	DAT negative, Anti-IgA (IgA deficiency workup when indicated)	Discontinue transfusion, Maintain vascular access, Treat with subcutaneous epinephrine, Maintain blood pressure, Provide respiratory support	For IgA absolute deficient Patients provide IgA deficient blood components
Transfusion-related acute lung injury (TRALI) due to WBC antibodies in donor (occasionally in recipient), other WBC-activating agents in components	Severe hypoxemia, respiratory failure, hypotension, fever, bilateral pulmonary edema, No evidence of left atrial hypertension	Chest X-ray: bilateral infiltrates, Donor test for HLA/HNA antibodies, Recipient test for HLA/HNA antigens, Rule out hemolysis (DAT, inspect for hemoglobinemia, repeat ABO)	Discontinue transfusion, Maintain vascular access, Supplemental oxygen, Mechanical ventilation	Use male only plasma, Exclude or screen female platelet donors

Contd...

Contd...

Type of acute transfusion reaction	Signs and symptoms	Lab findings and diagnosis	Treatment	Prevention
Nonimmunologic				
Acute nonimmune hemolytic transfusion reaction (ANIHTR) Due to physical or chemical destruction of blood (e.g. heating, freezing, hemolytic drug or solution added to blood)	Asymptomatic hemoglobinuria, hemoglobulinemia	DAT negative Rule out hemolysis (DAT, inspect for hemoglobinemia, repeat ABO) Test blood unit for hemolysis	Discontinue transfusion Maintain vascular access Maintain renal blood flow	Follow standard operating procedures for equipment operation
Transfusion-associated circulatory overload (TACO) due to volume overload	Dyspnea, orthophea, productive cough with pink, frothy sputum, tachycardia Severe hypoxemia Increased blood pressure Jugular vein distension Increased central venous pressure	Chest X-ray: pulmonary edema, cardiomegaly, distended pulmonary artery Rule out TRALI Brain natriuretic peptide (BNP)	Upright posture Supplemental oxygen Diuresis Phlebotomy	Slower transfusion rate Transfuse in smaller volumes
Transfusion-associated sepsis (TAS) due to bacterial contamination	Fever/chills Hypotension Shock	DAT negative Gram stain and culture of donor's blood component from bag Culture of patient's post-transfusion blood sample Rule out hemolysis (DAT, inspect for hemoglobinemia, repeat ABO)	Discontinue transfusion Maintain vascular access Consider initial broad-spectrum antibiotic coverage	Follow standard operating procedures for collection Implement bacterial detection intervention prior to transfusion

(DAT: direct antiglobulin test; DIC: diffuse intravascular coagulopathy; LDH: lactic dehydrogenase; PRBC: packed red blood cell)

DELAYED TRANSFUSION REACTIONS

Definition: Delayed transfusion reactions are defined as reactions in which signs and symptoms present after 24 hours of a transfusion. It has diverse etiology (Flowchart 14.3).

Delayed Immunological

Delayed Hemolytic Transfusion Reactions

Definition: Delayed hemolytic transfusion reactions (DHTRs) are defined as the detection of "new" red cell antibodies at least 24 hours after transfusion of the offending unit. DHTRs are also called delayed serologic/hemolytic transfusion reactions (DSHTRs).

It is an anamnestic response after transfusion with no signs of hemolysis. Acute

Flowchart 14.3: Etiology of delayed transfusion reactions.

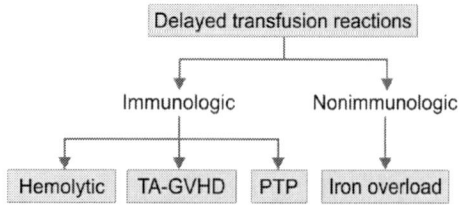

(PTP: post-transfusion purpura; TA-GVHD: transfusion associated graft-versus-host disease)

hemolytic transfusion reactions are usually associated with the transfusion of ABO incompatible red cells. In contrast, in delayed hemolytic transfusion reactions (DHTRs), the symptoms appear after 24 hours and are caused due to a secondary immune response. The recipient has been immunized (primary immune response) after red cell exposure from either a prior transfusion or pregnancy.

Normally, clinically significant antibodies are detected during pretransfusion testing. However, it may not be detected because of (i) the antibody levels below the detectable levels, (ii) missed in error, (iii) less sensitivity of the test and (iv) rarely an antibody to a low-frequency antigen which are not demonstrated on the screening cells.

Time of development: The time of diagnosis of a DHTR after receiving the transfusion is variable. Most patients develop DHTRs within the first 2 weeks after the transfusion. However, clinical DHTR may be recognized more than 6 weeks later.

Pathophysiology
Extravascular hemolysis is seen in delayed hemolytic transfusion reactions and is usually due to IgG antibodies (e.g. Rh, Kell, Duffy system).

Anamnestic response to a red cell antigen: Anamnestic response is an accentuated (rapid) antibody response following a secondary exposure to an antigen.
- **Primary immune response (alloimmunization)**: During **pregnancy or transfusion** (very rarely transplantation of a solid organ or hematopoietic progenitor cells), **exposure to non-ABO antigens** (that the individual is lacking) may stimulate the primary immune response. These non-ABO antigens associated with DHTRs include Kidd, Duffy, Kell, and MNS systems. Primary immune response in turn stimulates the **production of IgM antibodies** in the recipient, followed by **a switch to production of IgG antibody**. The primary immune response is usually asymptomatic and can be detected by immunohematology testing within weeks to months after transfusion. As the time passes (over months to years), these antibodies may diminish to undetectable levels (antibody titer too low to be detected) when repeat immunohematology testing is performed. These antibodies are weak to be detected during cross-match. This phenomenon of slow decrease of antibody titer after initial immune response is termed as "evanescence".
- **Secondary (anamnestic) immune response (refer page 9):** When the above-mentioned individuals are subsequently exposed (re-exposed) to incompatible red cells (by receiving the blood expressing non-ABO red cell antigens), they elicit a secondary immune response. This is called anamnestic response in which there is rapid production of IgG. This antibody can be detected between 2 days to 2 weeks after the re-exposure.

Almost all DHTRs are secondarily due to an anamnestic response to a red cell antigen to which the patient has previously made an antibody. The concentration of this antibody was too low to be detected in pretransfusion testing.

Rarely, a DHTR may be **due to primary alloimmunization to a red cell antigen.** This may occur during transfusion of incompatible blood during emergency or massive transfusion.

Hemolysis: The degree of accelerated red cell destruction depends on the characteristics of the responsible antibody. Thus, hemolysis depends on antibody specificity (usually antibodies directed against the Rh, Kidd, Duffy, and anti-Kell antigens), thermal activity range, and the ability to fix complement. Most frequently, the red cell destruction (hemolysis) is extravascular, but intravascular hemolysis may also occur. The hemolysis of DHTR is more protracted than AGTR and usually does not produce acute signs and symptoms of an AHTR.

Mononuclear phagocytes: Sensitized red blood cells (due to either immunoglobulin or complement) are removed from the circulation by the mononuclear phagocyte system. The macrophages in the spleen are the most active followed by the Kupffer cells of the liver.

Clinical presentation: Delayed hemolytic transfusion reactions (DHTR) are generally mild and may be overlooked. They tend to be much less severe than AHTRs.

- **Characteristic feature is development of fever and unexpected anemia** (unexplained or unexpected fall/drop in hemoglobin or hematocrit) days or weeks after transfusion of an RBC component.
- The patient returns to see the physician after a transfusion and complains of flu-like symptoms, with or without **jaundice**. Jaundice appears 5 days after transfusion. Hemoglobinuria is also observed. Other clinical features include chills, pain, or dyspnea. Renal failure and DIC are rare.
- DHTRs may be severe in chronically transfused patients such as patients with sickle cell disease. In patients with sickle cell disease, DHTRs may precipitate a sickle crisis.

First detectable signs of a delayed hemolytic reaction are given in Box 14.12.

Laboratory findings in DHTRs

Standard basic immunohematology testing off ABO/Rh, antibody screen, and when indicated antibody identification.

Immunohematology evaluation: These include **DAT** and, when indicated, **elution and antigen typing of the units recently transfused** and suspected to be implicated in the immune response.

- In a DHTR, antibodies may be found in the serum of patient/recipient on transfused red cells or both.

Box 14.12: First detectable signs of delayed hemolytic reaction.

- Inadequate increase in the level of hemoglobin following transfusion
- Rapid decrease of hemoglobin level back to pretransfusion levels
- Unexplained appearance of spherocytes in the peripheral blood smear

- Diagnosis of DHTRs should be done by routine antibody screening and antibody identification.
- DAT will be positive if transfused red cells are still present in the patient's circulation.
- If DAT is positive, an eluate may be required to demonstrate the presence of the implicated antibody.
- If samples from previous immunohematology testing are available, perform repeat testing.

Baseline and follow-up samples to assess ongoing hemolysis

- These include hemoglobin level (anemia), elevated lactate dehydrogenase (LDH), hyperbilirubinemia, low haptoglobin, leukocytosis, the presence of a new red cell antibody, and a positive reaction on a DAT.
- **Hyperbilirubinemia**: Estimate total and direct bilirubin. The degree of hyperbilirubinemia depends on the rate and amount of hemolysis, as well as on liver function. Usually, levels of unconjugated bilirubin are elevated during active hemolysis.
- **Low haptoglobin levels**: It does not necessarily indicate intravascular hemolysis, as they may also be seen with extravascular hemolysis.

Differential diagnosis

- **Blood contaminated with intracellular red cell parasite:** Fever and hemolysis may also develop after transfusion when the component has been contaminated with an intracellular red cell parasite (e.g. malaria, babesia).
- **Graft versus host disease and transfusion-transmitted viral disease (e.g. cytomegalovirus):** These are associated with fever without hemolysis.
- **Transplantation of a minor-ABO-incompatible organ**: It may cause hemolysis resulting from antibody production by donor passenger lymphocytes. For example, after transplantation of group O liver to a group A patient.

Prevention: If DHTR is caused by known antibody, it can be prevented by the transfusion of antigen-negative RBCs.

Treatment/Management
- DHTRs in general are mild and many patients tolerate it well. The patient may require only careful monitoring and to be followed carefully. Treatment, if necessary, should depend on the patient symptomatology. Provide supportive care when necessary.
- Usually, fluid loading and diuresis are not needed unless there is active intravascular hemolysis. Avoid transfusion till the causative antibody can be identified and antigen-negative units obtained.
- Correction of anemia if needed should be by transfusing antigen-negative RBCs.
- When antigen typing suggests a large burden of antigen-positive red cells and other laboratory results are consistent with ongoing hemolysis, a **red cell exchange transfusion** should be considered.
- The extravascular hemolysis in DHTRs is similar to autoimmune hemolytic anemia. Hence, a high-dose intravenous immunoglobulin (IVIG) infusion may be useful in the treatment of DHTRs also.
- Complications, such as renal failure or sickle crisis, should be treated as such. If there is suspicion of a sickle cell HTR syndrome, withhold further transfusions.

Differences between acute and delayed hemolytic transfusion reactions are presented in Table 14.7.

Table 14.7: Differences between acute and delayed hemolytic transfusion reactions.

Features	Acute hemolytic transfusion reactions	Delayed hemolytic transfusion reactions
Clinical signs and symptoms		
Development	Immediate or within 24 hours of transfusion	After 24 hours to 28 days after transfusion
Symptoms	Fever, chills, pain at the site of infusion, tachycardia, tachypnea, lower back pain	Fever, raised body temperature (increase >1°C or 2°F)
Signs	Hemoglobinemia, hemoglobinuria, hypotension	Unexplained decrease in hemoglobin or hematocrit level, jaundice, hemoglobinuria
Major complications	DIC, renal failure, shock, death	Anemia
Causes	ABO incompatibility Activation of complement	Anamnestic response to red cell antigen Alloantibody not demonstrable or missed during pretransfusion testing
Laboratory findings		
	Clerical check and visual inspection of post-transfusion blood sample. Repeat ABO grouping	Reduced hemoglobin and hematocrit
DAT	Positive or negative	Positive
Tests for hemolysis		
Plasma-free hemoglobin	Increased	Increased
Serum bilirubin	Increased	Increased
Serum haptoglobin	Decreased	Decreased
Hemoglobinuria	Present	Present
Management	Treat hypotension, DIC, maintain adequate renal blood flow	Identify causative antibody, transfuse antigen-negative blood
Prevention	Avoid clerical and misidentification errors and technical errors	Check patient's records for recent transfusion or pregnancy

Transfusion-associated Graft-versus-host Disease

Definition: Transfusion-associated graft-versus-host disease (TA-GVHD) is a delayed immune transfusion reaction due to an immunologic attack by viable donor T lymphocytes present in the transfused blood component against the transfusion recipient.

Pathophysiology

Transfusion-associated graft-versus-host disease (TA-GVHD) is a rare but highly lethal (90% mortality rate) complication of transfusion. This immune reaction is mediated by immunocompetent donor T lymphocytes in cellular blood components. After the transfusion of donor T lymphocytes to a recipient who is immunologically incompetent or closely HLA similar, the recipient/host immune system is unable to recognize donor T lymphocytes as foreign and cannot destroy the transfused donor T cells. The viable donor T lymphocytes proliferate, engraft, and recognize recipient/host as foreign. The donor T lymphocytes mount an immune response against the recipient/host tissues and reject the host tissue.

Requirements for development of GVHD:
Three conditions required for development of GVHD in a recipient/patient are:
1. Differences in the HLA antigen expression between the donor and recipient.
2. Presence of donor immunocompetent cells (T lymphocytes) in the transfused blood component.
3. The host/recipient incapable of rejecting the donor immunocompetent cells.

Primary Factors that Determine the Risk of Development of GVHD
- Degree of immunodeficiency in recipient
- Number of viable immunocompetent cells (T lymphocytes) in the transfusion. This in turn depends on the age of the blood component, leukocyte reduction status, and the irradiation status of the component. Fresher blood components contain more viable T lymphocytes.
- Degree of genetic diversity between the donor and recipient.

Risk factors for GVHD
- **Patients with marked cellular immunodeficiencies** (or immunocompromised) who are receiving blood products from donors that share similar HLA are at risk for TA-GVHD. These include congenital cellular immunodeficiencies (DiGeorge syndrome, severe combined immunodeficiency syndrome), immaturity of the immune system (intrauterine transfusions, very-low-birthweight infants), disease-associated immunodeficiencies (Hodgkin lymphoma, leukemia), and use of immunosuppressive drugs (hematopoietic progenitor cell transplantation or myeloablative chemotherapy). These patients should receive blood products that have been irradiated.
- **Patients with normal immunity** (intact immune system) may be at risk for TA-GVHD **if there is difference in HLA class I locus** (Fig. 14.7). TA-GVHD can occur when the patient is transfused with a cellular blood component from a donor homozygous for an HLA haplotype and the recipient is heterozygous but shares one haplotype with donor. In such settings, the recipient immune system does not recognize the homozygous HLA haplotype of the transfused donor lymphocytes as foreign and therefore will not eliminate them. In contrast, the transfused donor T lymphocytes are able to recognize the recipient nonshared haplotype as foreign and will mount an immune attack on the recipient (Fig. 14.7). This can occur in individuals receiving cellular blood components from close (first- or second-degree) blood relatives and patients receiving HLA matched or crossmatched platelets or granulocytes.

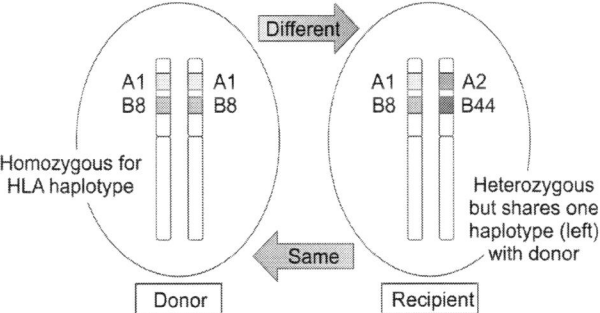

Fig. 14.7: Mechanism of TA-GVHD in an immunocompetent (normal immunity) patient. The triggering event involves the transfusion of a cellular blood component from a donor (graft) with a homozygous HLA haplotype (A1, B8) to a recipient (host) with a heterozygous HLA type (A1, B8 and A2, B44) of which one haplotype is shared with the haplotype with the donor (A1, B8). The recipient's T cells do not identify donor T cells as foreign but the grafted donor T cells recognize the recipient as foreign. In this illustration, the HLA haplotype shared is A1, B8. There is no foreign haplotype to be recognized by the recipient. However, the recognition of the foreign HLA haplotype (A2, B44) by the donor triggers an "unopposed" immune attack against the recipient.
(HLA = human leukocyte antigen; TA-GVHD = transfusion-associated graft-versus-host disease)

Clinical manifestation

Time of manifestation: TA-GVHD usually manifests 2 to 30 days (usually 10–12 days) after transfusion.

Characteristic findings: The presenting symptoms features include a **maculopapular** rash (usually pruritic, typically starting centrally and extending to the extremities), watery diarrhea (accompanied by bloody stools and abdominal pain), fever, nausea, elevated liver function tests, and pancytopenia (due to marrow failure). These symptoms occur following transfusion of a nonirradiated cellular blood component.

Diagnostic tests
- **Skin biopsy:** Superficial perivascular lymphocyte infiltrate, necrotic **keratinocytes**, and bullae formation.
- **Bone marrow examination:** Unlike the expected GVHD of allogeneic HPC (hematopoietic progenitor cell) transplantation, the bone marrow in TA-GVHD is of recipient type and is a target organ. Bone marrow is hypocellular or aplastic marrow (profound), with only the presence of macrophages.
- **Liver biopsy:** Degeneration and eosinophilic necrosis of small bile ducts, intense periportal inflammation, and lymphocytic infiltration.

Definitive diagnosis: It needs the identification of donor derived lymphocytes in the recipient circulation or tissues. However, the presence of donor-derived lymphocytes alone in the absence of clinical symptoms is not diagnostic for TA-GVHD.

Mortality: Transfusion-associated GVHD is a rare but potentially fatal complication of blood transfusion. It has high mortality and more than 90% die of infection within 1 to 3 weeks after appearance of first symptoms.

Treatment/Management
TA-GVHD is only rarely successfully treated. Hence, identifying the patients at risk and providing irradiated blood products are necessary. Irradiation eliminates the ability of leukocytes to replicate and mount an immune response. Treatment includes the following:
- Aggressive immunosuppressive treatments have been not successful.
- Stem cell transplantation may be the only curative option.

Prevention: Recognize the patient at risk of TA-GVHD and provide the interventions that prevent its occurrence.
- **Leukoreduction:** It does not reduce the risk of TA-GVHD.

- **Gamma irradiation**: TA-GVHD can be prevented by transfusing the irradiated blood/components in patients at risk. Exposing the cellular blood component to gamma irradiation reduces the number of viable lymphocytes and can prevent TA-GVHD. Box 14.13 lists the types of patients for whom irradiated blood components are indicated.

Salient features of transfusion-associated graft-versus-host disease are presented in Table 14.8.

Post-transfusion Purpura

Posttransfusion purpura (PTP) is a relatively uncommon, delayed immune complication of transfusion that occurs 5 to 12 days after transfusion of blood or blood products containing platelets. It presents with severe thrombocytopenia (with platelet counts below 10,000/μL) in the patient and frequently accompanied by generalized purpura, bleeding from mucous membranes, and the gastrointestinal and urinary tract.

Pathophysiology

The pathogenesis of PTP is related to the presence of platelet-specific antibodies in the patient. A patient may be previously exposed/sensitized to human platelet antigens by pregnancy or transfusion. PTP occurs when the same patient is re-exposed to the same antigen via a transfusion. PPT is characteristically more commonly associated with transfusion of RBCs or whole blood, expressing that human platelet antigen specificity and causing an anamnestic immune response. These platelet-specific antibodies formed may destroy not only transfused but also the autologous platelets. The most commonly (60%) involved antigen is the human platelet antigen (HPA)-1a and the corresponding antibody is HPA-1a. Antigen-negative individuals are at risk of developing PTP. PTP can also occur with transfusion of platelets or plasma. PTP is a self-limiting syndrome with the platelet count generally returns to normal within 2 weeks. However, in 13 to 16% of cases, mortality due to intracranial hemorrhage has been reported.

Diagnosis: It is confirmed by demonstrating the presence of antibodies in the patient's plasma against human platelet antigens and the absence of the implicated antigen specificity in the patient's platelets.

Differential diagnosis: It includes other causes of thrombocytopenia such as autoimmune thrombocytopenic purpura, heparin-induced

---

Box 14.13: Indications for transfusion of irradiation of cellular blood components for prevention of TA-GVHD.

Immunocompromised state (indicated by patient condition)
- **Absolute indications**
  - Congenital cellular immunodeficiency
  - Hematopoietic progenitor cell transplantation
  - Transfusions
    - Granulocyte transfusions
    - Intrauterine transfusions (IUTs)
    - Transfusion to neonates who have received IUT
    - Transfusions from biologic relatives
  - Hematologic malignancies or solid tumors (neuroblastoma, Hodgkin lymphoma)
  - Hodgkin lymphoma
  - Prematurity, low-birth weight infants (<1,200 g) or erythroblastosis fetalis in new borns
  - Fludarabine therapy
- **Probable indications**
  - HLA-matched platelet concentrates
  - High-dose chemotherapy, radiation therapy, and/or aggressive immunotherapy

Immunocompetent state (indicated by origin of blood component to be transfused)
- Directed donations from blood relatives (from family members or other related donors)
- HLA-matched platelets or granulocytes
- Crossmatched platelets or granulocytes
- Granulocyte components

Table 14.8: Summary of feature transfusion-associated graft-versus-host disease.

Clinical signs and symptoms	Occurs 3 to 30 days after transfusion. Presents with fever, erythematous maculopapular rash, diarrhea, abnormal liver function and pancytopenia
Cause	Donor immunocompetent T lymphocytes mounting an immune response against the recipient
Laboratory tests	HLA (human leukocyte antigen) typing to demonstrate disparity between donor T lymphocytes and recipient tissues
Complications	Marrow aplasia, hemorrhage, mortality about 90%
Management	No specific medical treatment
Prevention	Irradiation of blood products before transfusion in recipients at risk

thrombocytopenia, DIC, and drug-induced thrombocytopenia. Platelet serology may help in the diagnosis.

Treatment: Treatment includes plasmapheresis, exchange transfusion, and use of intravenous immunoglobulin (IVIG). The standard **treatment** is infusion of intravenous immunoglobulin, 0.5 to 1 grams per kilogram per day over a period of 2 to 10 days. The average response occurs within 4 days after initiating therapy.

Prevention: PTP usually does not recur with subsequent transfusions. However, patients with a known history of PTP should be given whenever possible, antigen-negative blood products (or autologous donations and directed from antigen-matched donors and family members) for subsequent transfusions.

Delated Nonimmunological Iron Overload (Transfusion Hemosiderosis)

Definition: Iron overload is a delayed, non-immune complication of transfusion. It presents with multiorgan (i.e. liver, heart, endocrine organs) damage secondary to excessive accumulation of iron.

Pathophysiology: Hemosiderosis is a condition characterized by the accumulation of excess iron in macrophages in various tissues. Iron overload, also called transfusion hemosiderosis, is a potential complication seen in patients with persistent hemolysis (e.g. thalassemia sickle cell disease) receiving long-term transfusions. Thalassemia is an inherited disorder causing anemia because of a defective production rate of either α or β globin chains of hemoglobin. Each unit of red blood cells contains about 200–250 mg of iron (250 mg/unit). Daily iron excretion is about 1 mg/day. There is no physiological mechanism in human beings to excrete excess iron. Persistence increase in iron lead occurs from transfusion (especially 10 to 15 units of red cell transfusions) and this leads to overload of iron (i.e. iron intake exceeds the daily loss). When the accumulated iron overload exceeds the capacity for safe storage, it accumulates in tissue and produce tissue damage. The excess iron gets deposited in reticuloendothelial cells of spleen, bone marrow, liver, heart, and endocrine glands. The excess iron accumulates in the liver, heart, spleen, pancreas, and endocrine organs. The resulting damage leads to heart failure, liver failure, diabetes, and hypothyroidism. Patients/recipients who are chronically transfused (who receive multiple transfusions over a period of few years) with red cell (e.g. thalassemia, sickle cell anemia, and other chronic anemia) have the greatest risk for developing iron overload, causing greater morbidity than the underlying anemia.

Prevention: The accumulation of toxic levels of iron stores can be prevented or reduced by use of iron chelators, therapeutic phlebotomy, or red cell exchange transfusion. The chelating agents (chelators) bind to iron in the tissues, helping its removal through the urine and feces. The chelating agents include: parenteral deferoxamine, oral deferiprone, and oral deferasirox.

Massive transfusions and its complications are discussed on pages 236-7.

Citrate Toxicity

The transfusion of large amount of citrated blood in a relatively short time can produce citrate toxicity for the patient receiving transfusion. Citrate is one of the components present in the formulation of the anticoagulants used in the blood collection. Citrate binds ionized calcium in the blood. Excess citrate may be toxic to patients receiving large volumes (e.g. massive transfusion) or in patients where citrate cannot be metabolized due to impaired liver function. Citrate toxicity occurs in preterm infants with severe hepatic or renal insufficiency who receive transfusion.

Management: Removal of the additive-containing plasma may be useful. Injections of calcium chloride or calcium gluconate may reduce the toxic effects if citrate.

Summary of delayed transfusion reactions is presented in Table 14.9.

SILENT TRANSFUSION-RELATED ADVERSE EVENTS

Some incidents or errors may occur with transfusions that need not be present with transfusion-associated symptoms. They are termed as *silent* adverse events. These events

Table 14.9: Summary of delayed transfusion reactions.

Type of delayed (>24 hours) transfusion reaction	Signs and symptoms	Lab findings and diagnosis	Treatment	Prevention
Immunologic				
Delayed hemolytic transfusion reaction (DHTR) Anamnestic immune response to red cell antigens	Flu-like symptoms Pallor (decreased hemoglobin) Mild jaundice	Antibody screen/ DAT + Reduced hemoglobin Increased total bilirubin	As needed transfuse antigen negative, AHG crossmatched compatible PRBC	Accurate record-keeping Obtain transfusion history Limit transfusions
Transfusion-associated graft-versus-host disease (TA-GVHD) Functioning donor lymphocytes transfused to immunosuppressed patient and mount attack on host tissues	Erythroderma, maculopapular rash, fever, anorexia, nausea, hepatitis, vomiting, diarrhea	Pancytopenia Identify donor engraftment Skin biopsy HLA typing	Immunosuppression	Gamma irradiation of cellular blood components for patients at risk (including components from related donors and HLA-selected components)
Post-transfusion purpura (PTP) due to recipient platelet antibodies (usually HPA-1a) destroy autologous platelets	Purpura, bleeding, fall in platelet count 8–10 days following transfusion	Thrombocytopenia Platelet antibody screen and identification— HPA antibodies	Intravenous immunoglobulin	Limit transfusions HPA-1a-negative platelets Plasmapheresis
Nonimmunologic				
Iron overload due to multiple transfusions in transfusion dependent patients (congenital anemias, aplastic anemia, etc.)	Multiorgan failure, cardiomyopathy, arrhythmias, hepatic (cirrhosis) and pancreatic (diabetes) failure	Iron studies-high serum ferritin levels Liver and cardiac iron concentration (MRI) Liver enzymes Endocrine function tests	Use of iron-chelating agents, e.g. deferoxamine	Prophylactic use of iron-chelating agents Red cell exchange

include transfusion sample collection errors, red blood cell alloimmunization, platelet alloimmunization, and transfusion over- or underdosing.

Sample Collection Errors

Transfusion sample collection errors can be divided into major collection errors and minor collection errors. These require appropriate intervention or corrective or preventive action.
- **Major collection errors**: In this, sample tubes are properly labeled containing all the required information and contain wrong blood sample in the tube drawn from the wrong patient. It can cause mistransfusion of incompatible blood.
- **Minor collection errors:** In this, samples are provided with missing required information.

Preventive measures for collection errors include improved patient identification mechanisms such as improved computer technology and barrier systems to prevent transfusion without precise recipient identification.

Red Blood Cell Alloimmunization

- **Risk of developing antibodies against the red cell antigens:** In patients who chronically transfused, the risk of developing antibodies against the red cell antigens (RBC alloimmunization) increases by 2% to 8%. In patients with sickle cell anemia, this risk is as high as 40%.
- **Factors influencing the rate of alloimmunization:** These include frequency of transfusion, antigenic differences, dose, recipient immune status, and immunogenicity of the donor HLA antigens.
- **Significance:** The presence of red cell antibodies
  - Makes it **difficult to allocate compatible, antigen-negative units**.
  - May **increase the risk of DHTR**.

Platelet Alloimmunization

- **Platelet transfusion refractoriness**: The most common immune cause of platelet transfusion refractoriness is the presence of antibodies against class I HLA antigens. These antibodies are formed after exposure to corresponding antigen expressed on contaminating WBCs in transfused blood components.
- **Development of antibodies against the HPA can also cause post-transfusion purpura**.

TRANSFUSION-RELATED ADVERSE EVENTS IN SPECIAL PATIENT SCENARIOS

A transfusion-related adverse reaction discussed earlier is usually based on recipients (mainly adults and older children) of allogeneic blood components. However, there are special patient populations and transfusion circumstances which need to be known. These include the following:
1. **Infusion of plasma derivatives:** Plasma derivatives include albumin and intravenous immunoglobulin (IVIg), and human-derived coagulation factor concentrates. Presently, common adverse events seen in association with the transfusion of plasma derivatives are nonviral transfusion reactions. These adverse events can be acute or delayed. Most of them are transient and have no clinical sequelae. However, rarely these plasma derivatives can produce life-threatening adverse reactions.
   - **Albumin infusion:** In patients on **ACE inhibitors** for the treatment of hypertension, **albumin infusion can produce hypotensive reactions** when used as the sole replacement fluid during plasmapheresis.
   - **IVIg infusion:** It can cause **numerous adverse effects** such as renal dysfunction, related to the use of sucrose

as a stabilizing agent; dose-related aseptic meningitis; positive direct antiglobulin test with or without hemolysis; anaphylaxis; TRALI; and thromboembolic events.
- **Infusion of human-derived coagulation factor concentrates**: It may be associated with allergic reactions and thrombosis.
2. **Therapeutic apheresis:** During therapeutic apheresis procedures using blood components as fluid replacement, transfusion reactions can occur, or inherent symptoms to the procedure may be aggravated. Adverse effects include perioral or acral **paresthesias**, seen when citrated plasma rather than albumin solution is used as the replacement fluid. Anaphylactoid reactions can develop with the use of albumin as the replacement fluid in patients receiving ACE inhibitors. The bacterial contamination of albumin solutions can also occur.
3. **Neonatal transfusions**
    - Transfusion adverse reactions in neonates may be difficult to recognize in the presence of other concomitant clinical factors.
    - **Acute immune-mediated transfusion reactions** are more commonly observed in adults and older children. They are **rarely seen in neonates** because of the immature underdeveloped immune system at birth.
    - **Metabolic complications**: Neonates have brittle physiological balance and may be more vulnerable to metabolic complications. Some symptoms may be caused by the anticoagulant or preservative solutions in the blood component. The metabolic complications in association with transfusion in neonates include hyperglycemia or hypoglycemia, hypocalcemia or hyperkalemia. They present with jitteriness, tremors, convulsions, **hypotonia,** lethargy, **apnea,** and **cyanosis.** Their treatment depends on their expected duration and the infant's underlying condition.
    - The neonatal lymphocytes cannot recognize foreign antigens. Hence, development of antibodies is extremely rare. If a rare acute immune-mediated transfusion reaction occurs, the reaction is due to the passively transfused antibodies. Some neonates may rarely develop graft-versus-host disease.
    - Infants are at a risk of developing TAS or mistransfusion in a similar fashion to the adult or older children population.
4. **Autologous blood transfusions:** The methods used to collect autologous blood are:
    - **Preoperative autologous donation** (PAD) in which planned collection and storage of patient's own blood until the time of surgery.
    - **Intraoperative hemodilution** (IOH) in which collection of a patient's own blood at the beginning of the surgery that is then returned to the patient at the end of surgery.
    - **Perioperative blood recovery** (POBR) in which the recovery of a patient's blood from the surgical field or postoperative drainage. This is washed and returned to the patient.

With the exception of transfusion-transmitted diseases, **autologous transfusions** may **be associated with all other adverse events associated with allogeneic transfusions** (FNHTR, TAS, TACO, mistransfusion, AHTR). These adverse events may be associated with increased morbidity and even death.

Prevention: Follow the same rules and regulations of allogeneic blood, as well as the manufacturer's instructions when utilizing perioperative blood recovery.

SUMMARY

- Transfusion reactions are classified according to time of development as acute transfusion reactions developing within (less than 24 hours and delayed transfusion reactions which occur after 24 hours). Both are further classified into immune or nonimmune.
- Acute transfusion reaction evaluation includes clerical check, examination for visual hemolysis, DAT, and patient ABO group confirmation.
- Acute transfusion reactions include acute hemolytic reactions, febrile nonhemolytic reactions, allergic reactions, transfusion-associated sepsis, TRALI, and TACO.
- Immune hemolysis develops when previously formed IgM (ABO) or IgG (non-ABO) antibodies in the recipient recognize the corresponding donor RBC antigen. It causes complement-mediated intravascular hemolysis.
- Nonimmune hemolysis may occur due to mechanical or chemical damage and present as an asymptomatic hemoglobinuria.
- Febrile nonhemolytic reactions occur when the recipient is exposed to the donor cytokines present in the WBC or plasma. It presents as an increase in body temperature of more than 1°C with or without chills.
- Allergic reactions can be mild (hives or itching) or severe (anaphylaxis).
- TRALI occurs when donor leukocyte antibodies react with the WBCs in the recipient's lung vasculature. It damages the endothelium and causes noncardiogenic pulmonary edema. Transfusion-associated sepsis may occur when bacteria are introduced to the patient via a contaminated blood product; it presents as increase in body temperature, rigors, and hypotension.
- TACO occurs when the patient's cardiovascular system is unable to handle the transfused volume. It leads to congestive heart failure.
- Delayed transfusion reactions include delayed serologic/hemolytic reactions, transfusion-associated graft-versus-host disease, post-transfusion purpura, and iron overload.
- Delayed serologic/hemolytic reactions manifest secondary to an anamnestic or primary immune response directed to red cell antibodies.
- Transfusion-associated graft-versus-host disease develops when the donor T lymphocytes attack and destroy the recipient immune system, causing pancytopenia and death. It is prevented by using irradiated blood components for transfusion to patient at risk.
- Post-transfusion purpura manifest as a severe thrombocytopenia. Anti-HPA-1a is the most common implicated antibody.
- Iron overload occurs due to long-term accumulation of iron in the body tissues from multiple RBC transfusions. This causes organ damage especially liver, heart, spleen and endocrine organs.

SELF-ASSESSMENT EXERCISE

Long essay on:
- Discuss the diagnosis, management and prevention of mismatched blood transfusion
- Discuss in detail about complications of blood transfusion and their preventive measures

Write short essays/notes on:
- Immune-mediated (immunological) transfusion reactions
- Describe the complications of blood transfusion
- TRALI (Transfusion-Related Acute Lung Injury)
- Enumerate the transfusion reactions
- Problems in blood transfusion
- Hazards of blood transfusion
- Discuss in brief hemolytic transfusion reactions
- Nonhematological blood transfusion reactions
- Discuss blood transfusion reactions
- Graft versus host disease in blood transfusion
- Transfusion associated GVHD
- Post transfusion reactions

CHAPTER 15

Investigations in a Case of Transfusion Reaction

CHAPTER OUTLINE

☞ Investigation (work up) of suspected adverse transfusion reactions

INTRODUCTION

It is mandatory to check all the identifying information and document before the transfusion of any blood component. Before starting the transfusion, it is also necessary to record vital signs (includes body temperature, blood pressure, pulse, and respiration rate) of the recipient. After the initiation of transfusion, the concerned medical personnel should remain with the patient for the first few minutes of the infusion to detect any signs and symptoms of acute hemolysis, anaphylaxis, or bacterial contamination. After the first 15 minute period, the patient should be observed and the vital signs should be recorded. Clinical personnel should periodically continue to observe the patient throughout the transfusion and 4-6 hours after completion. Any acute transfusion reactions (e.g. febrile reactions or acute lung injury) should be detected immediately. The diagnosis of an acute transfusion reaction may be challenging. This is because of the following reasons:
- Signs and symptoms are not specific for each type of reaction
- All possible signs and symptoms may not be observed with every reaction
- Different types of reactions can occur simultaneously. This should always be considered when the patient presents with atypical findings.
- Similar signs and symptoms may be observed in different reactions (e.g. bacterial sepsis, allergic, and anaphylactic reactions can all present with cutaneous symptoms).

Because of above reasons, it is important to completely follow-up and perform investigation on every reported transfusion reaction. When investigating a transfusion reaction, both the clinical evaluation and the laboratory work-up are important to correctly diagnose the cause/etiology of the transfusion reaction. Differential diagnoses based on primary presenting symptom are presented in Table 15.1.

INVESTIGATION (WORK-UP) OF SUSPECTED ADVERSE TRANSFUSION REACTIONS

It is necessary to understand the typical clinical presentation for each type of reaction (discussed in detail in Chapter 14) so that a differential diagnosis can be done. It is very essential to *stop the transfusion* if the patient's symptoms and signs suggest a possibility of transfusion reaction because the initial presentation of acute HTR may be subtle or may not present with the classic symptoms of back pain and feelings of impending doom. Immediately report/notify all (except mild

Table 15.1: Differential diagnoses based on primary presenting symptom.

Symptom	Possible reaction type	
	Immunological	*Nonimmunological*
Fever	Acute hemolytic transfusion reaction* Febrile, nonhemolytic*	Transfusion-associated sepsis (TAS) *
Hemolysis	Acute hemolytic* Delayed hemolytic	Nonimmune hemolysis*
Dyspnea	Transfusion-related acute lung injury (TRALI)* Anaphylaxis/anaphylactoid*	Transfusion-associated circulatory overload (TACO)*
Rash	Anaphylaxis/anaphylactoid* Minor allergic* Transfusion-associated graft versus host disease (TA-GVHD)	
Hypotension	TRALI* Acute hemolytic* Anaphylaxis/anaphylactoid*	
Cytopenia	TA-GVHD Post-transfusion purpura (PTP)	

*Indicates reactions are acute.

allergic/hypersensitivity) acute transfusion reactions to the blood centre/bank which has supplied the blood or blood component.

Clinical Findings That May Suggest Immediate Transfusion Reaction

Recognition of a transfusion reaction: Clinical signs and symptoms of a transfusion reaction are listed in Box 15.1. It may be associated with more than one type of reaction. Early recognition and evaluation are very important for the best outcome.

- Fever
  - **Fever is common** in most types of reactions. However, it is **not observed in allergic transfusion reactions or with**

> **Box 15.1:** Clinical signs that suggests a transfusion reaction.
>
> - Fever >1°C increase or >38°C, chills and rigors
> - Hypotension or hypertension
> - *Respiratory*: Wheezing, coughing, dyspnea, cyanosis
> - *Cutaneous*: Urticaria, rash, flushing, edema
> - *Pain*: Abdominal, chest, flank or back, infusion site
> - Nausea or vomiting
> - *Renal*: Oliguria or anuria
> - Jaundice or hemoglobinuria
> - Abnormal bleeding

  anaphylaxis. Thus, fever can be useful to help to differentiate between severe hypotension associated with fever (e.g. bacterial contamination, acute hemolysis or TRALI) and hypotension without fever (e.g. anaphylactic shock).
  - **Increases in temperature of at least 1°C and/or chills**: These may suggest HTR, transfusion-associated circulatory overload (TACO), **bacterial contamination**, or febrile nonhemolytic transfusion reactions (FNHTRs).
- **Hypotensive changes and tachycardia**: They may occur with HTRs, TACO, anaphylaxis, bacterial contamination, or air embolus.
- **Hypertensive changes**: They may occur with TACO, but may also be seen with transfusion-related acute lung injury (TRALI).
- **Respiratory symptoms:** These include coughing, shortness of breath, pain or difficulty with breathing, wheezing, and respiratory failure. They are not specific and may occur with HTR, acute lung injury (ALI) including transfusion-associated ALI, *circulatory overload* from any cause, anaphylaxis, bacterial contamination, air embolus, or hypothermia. If there is

respiratory distress, a stat chest radiograph should be obtained. Sudden, bilateral pulmonary edema is found in both transfusions associated ALI and circulatory overload.
- **Hives and itching**: These are usually found in an allergic or urticarial reaction.
- **Pain and anxiety**: Abdominal, chest, flank or back pain, pain at the infusion site. Pain and anxiety can occur with HTRs, any type of *febrile reaction*, and citrate reactions.
- **Renal failure (oliguria/anuria)**, jaundice, **hemoglobinuria, and hematuria**: They can occur with both immune and nonimmune HTRs.
- Nausea/vomiting/abnormal bleeding.

Understanding the Clinical Presentation and Differential Diagnosis

Following clinical clues can help in the differential diagnosis.

Patient History:
- **Reason for the patient's admission and current diagnosis**: It may give some clue to the type of reaction. For example, if the patient is transfused for anemia and also in congestive heart failure, **TACO** could be the cause of the reaction.
- **Previous history of transfusion or pregnant**: They can lead to alloimmunization to red cell and leukocyte antigens, and they are known to be associated with certain types of reactions (**acute hemolytic, FNHTR**).
- **Recent blood components transfused**: If plasma containing products have recently been transfused, the reaction could be due to passive infusion of antibody or soluble allergens that may now be reacting with the product being transfused.
- **Previous history of reactions during transfusion**: Some patients are prone to develop recurrent FNHTR and/or allergic reactions when transfused.
- **IgA-deficient patient**: Some patients with IgA deficiency develop anti-IgA antibodies. When they are transfused with IgA containing blood component, it may cause anaphylactic transfusion reactions.

Medications:
- Determine whether the patient is receiving or has received medication. Examples, pyrogenic agents such as amphotericin or monoclonal antibodies can cause fever; ACE inhibitors have been associated with hypotensive reactions, etc.

Type of Blood Component Being Transfused:
- **Component with significant volumes of plasma**: Transfusion of plasma is associated with reactions such as allergic, anaphylactic, TRALI, and acute hemolysis caused by passive antibody incompatibility with the patient's red cells.
- **Component with significant number of red cells**: If more than 50 mL of red cells are present in the component, acute hemolysis is likely to be the possible cause of the adverse reaction.
- **Storage temperature of component**: Platelets stored at room temperature have a greater risk of bacterial contamination. Blood products stored at colder temperatures can be contaminated with bacteria.
- **Leukocyte or nonleukocyte reduced component**: Nonleukocyte-reduced blood components (especially platelets) have a higher risk of FNHTR. Prevention of FNHTR to platelets is highly effective when prestorage leukocyte reduction is performed whereas poststorage leukocyte reduction has only limited effectiveness. However, both post and prestorage leukocyte reduction are effective in preventing most FNHTR to red cells.

Volume of Component Transfused:
- Some types of reactions are **dose dependent**. Such reactions are likely to occur toward the end of the transfusion after most of the component has been given. These reactions include **allergic reactions, FNHTR, and TRALI**.
- **Anaphylactic reactions** can develop even with a **small amount of component** transfused (1–10 mL).

- The symptoms of **acute hemolytic reactions usually need at least 50–100 mL of red cells** to be transfused.

Record the Information

Once there is suspicion of reactions, **stop the transfusion immediately** and record the following on the patient's case sheet/file:
- **Type of transfusion reaction** with presenting signs and symptoms.
- **Start and stop time of the transfusion** (including the length of time after the start of transfusion that the reaction occurred).
- **Approximate amount/volume and type of component transfused**.
- Record the pre-, 15 minute, and post-transfusion vital signs.
- Ensure that the patient's medical needs are addressed.

Management

Using all the information discussed above, the clinician must take a decision whether to stop the transfusion temporarily or discontinue the transfusion. Stopping and investigating every transfusion reaction is the safest for the patient. But this decision should be dependent on other morbidities such as bleeding or respiratory/cardiovascular morbidity which may necessitate transfusion essential. Hence, clinical judgment also should depend on the balance between risk and benefit.

Initial Steps (Actions to be Taken) in Management of Acute Transfusion Reaction (Box 15.2)

Box 15.2: Initial steps to follow if there is suspicion of adverse reaction.

- **Prompt recognizing of an adverse transfusion reaction**
- **Stop the transfusion**
- **Keep IV open with saline:** Maintain an intravenous line (for administration with blood) with normal saline
- **Notify immediately** to the blood centre/bank and the patient's physician
- **Monitor/record vital signs**
- **Evaluate the patient** by attending physician to determine clinical intervention and potential medical management

- **Prompt recognizing of an adverse transfusion reaction** (e.g. hemolytic reaction) is crucial and becomes a high priority. In the event of an acute hemolytic transfusion reaction (AHTR), the key interventions for limiting damage for all types of acute hemolytic transfusion reactions are:
  – **Stop the transfusion immediately**. The severity of some reactions is dose dependent. For example, the severe morbidity and mortality with acute hemolysis is usually proportional to the volume of component transfused—immediately stop (discontinue) transfusion.
  – **Keep the IV line open with saline** (or other appropriate IV solution). Replace the giving set. Maintain the intravenous line/access open with saline and use it for supportive therapy. This will be used in case decision is taken to continue the transfusion or the patient requires other IV therapy. Insert a urinary catheter and monitor the urine output.
  – **Supportive therapy**: Depends on the patient's clinical symptoms.
  – **Inform the patient's physician** and notify to the blood centre/bank when there is any suspicion of the adverse reaction. All suspected transfusion reactions should be reported promptly to the blood centre/bank. The laboratory evaluation should be started.

Steps to be Followed When the Transfusion is Discontinued (Box 15.3)

These include:
- **Check for clerical errors**: Perform a clerical verification/check for any errors in identification. The first step is a prompt

Box 15.3: Steps to be followed when the transfusion is discontinued.

- Perform clerical check for any errors
- Visual check for hemolysis at bedside
- Collect post-transfusion sample:
  ○ Post-transfusion blood sample
  ○ Post-transfusion urine sample
- Return of the blood bag to blood centre/bank

review/recheck of clerical information to confirm proper reidentification of patient and transfused blood component/product.
- **Perform a bedside clerical check** to ensure that the name/labels on the blood component, on the patient records, and requisition match the patient's identification.
- **Check of the blood labels for any identification errors.** The identity of the patient and the unit or units of blood component should be reconfirmed for any errors relating to identification. All records should be double checked.
- **Check the identity of the patient/ donor/sample correctly** and all relevant papers.
- **If such misidentification/discrepancy/error is identified during clerical verification,** take immediate necessary steps to determine whether another patient (e.g. with a similar name) is involved and other patient may be at a risk for receiving incompatible blood. To prevent adverse transfusion reaction in other patients take immediate action. **Inform the blood centre/bank immediately.** The source of the error is evaluated to determine where the system failed.
- **Visual check for hemolysis or icterus at bedside: If hemolysis is suspected,** look carefully at the remaining **postreaction** (post-transfusion) blood component **for any evidence of hemolysis or particulate matter.** Also (if available in the laboratory) **examine the patient's pre-reaction** (pre-transfusion) **plasma** from EDTA sample for any evidence hemolysis. Compare postreaction with the pre-transfusion sample. In case of hemolytic reaction, the red cells immediately release free hemoglobin or increased bilirubin into the plasma during intravascular hemolysis. Pink or red discoloration (Figs. 15.1A and B) of postreaction plasma indicates the presence of free hemoglobin due to destruction of red cell (hemolysis).

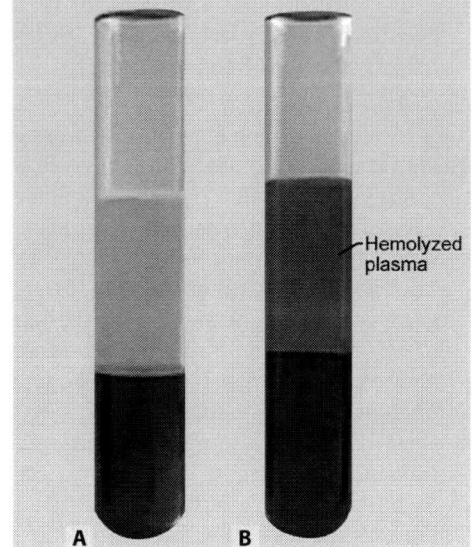

Figs. 15.1A and B: (A) Normal plasma; (B) Hemolyzed plasma.

- On inspection, if the postreaction blood sample appears hemolyzed, request a second sample to verify that the hemolysis is not secondary to a difficult blood draw.
- Yellow or brown discoloration of postreaction plasma drawn 3–8 hours after transfusion indicates the presence of increased bilirubin. The bilirubin is formed due to the degradation of free hemoglobin to bilirubin. Bilirubin levels usually peak at 5–7 hours after a hemolytic event.
- **Draw the post-transfusion reaction blood and urine samples:** If signs and symptoms suggest a possibility of acute hemolytic transfusion reaction (AHTR), anaphylaxis, TRALI, transfusion-induced sepsis, or other serious complications, collect the draw the **following samples from the patient and send it to the blood centre/ bank** for evaluation with a completely filled transfusion reaction form and all the specimens labeled properly.
  - **A post-transfusion blood sample** [tests to be done includes direct antiglobulin

test (DAT), repeat ABO and Rh grouping and cross matching, serum bilirubin].
- **A post-transfusion urine sample:** If possible, the first voided post-transfusion reaction urine sample is also collected for evaluation [tests to be done includes occult blood, methemoglobin, and microscopy for red blood cells (RBCs)]
- **A pre-transfusion blood sample** if available.
- **Return of the blood bag to blood centre/bank:** If the blood has been discontinued, return the blood bag with any remaining blood component and the infusion tubing intact to the blood centre/bank with the **transfusion/administration set and attached intravenous solutions.** Label this specimen properly and also send all related forms and labels (tests to be done in donor's remaining sample includes repeat ABO and Rh grouping, antibody screening, and cross matching).
- If the presenting clinical signs and symptoms are indicative of **urticarial or circulatory overload, there is no need to evaluate any post-transfusion reaction blood and urine sample.**

Initial Standard Laboratory Investigation of a Suspected Transfusion Reaction

Actions to be taken in the laboratory
- Perform **clerical check** of the component bag, label, and patient sample as mentioned above. When a transfusion reaction is reported to the blood centre/bank, always perform a clerical check to verify that the paperwork is accurate and that the correct component was issued for transfusion.
- **Visual check for hemolysis in the blood centre/bank:** It is done in both pre-transfusion and post-transfusion sample. Compare the color of plasma of patient's pre- and post-transfusion samples (pink/red/yellow-brown).
  - **Centrifuge the post-transfusion** and **pre-transfusion sample** of the patient's blood and **observe the plasma for any visual evidence of hemolysis.**
  - **If hemolysis** (i.e. presence of free hemoglobin in blood) has been established only **in the post-transfusion sample, the case is considered as hemolytic transfusion reaction.** Hemolysis is not visible if <50 mg/dL of hemoglobin (approximately 10 mL of red cells in an adult) is present.
  - Check of the blood bag, tubing, and segments also for hemolysis. Color of plasma on centrifuged sample for evidence of free hemoglobin or bilirubin can be done also colorimetrically.

Laboratory investigation
The transfusion laboratory will perform relevant investigations. To rule out hemolysis from the differential diagnosis, the screening tests should be performed as listed in Box 15.4.
- **Confirmation of post-transfusion ABO-Rh:**
  - **Repeat** (regroup) **ABO group determination** and Rh typing on the patient's **post-transfusion** blood **sample.**
  - **Regroup and retype the original donor pilot blood sample**, the original patient's cross-match sample, the blood in the blood bottle or tubing.
- **Direct antiglobulin test (DAT) on post-transfusion blood sample:** Perform DAT on EDTA **samples** taken from the patient and if positive, also on the most recent *pre-transfusion sample.*

Box 15.4: Initial standard laboratory investigation of a suspected transfusion reaction.

- Perform clerical check of the component bag, label, and patient sample
- Visual check for hemolysis* in the blood centre/bank: If hemolysis is established only in the post-transfusion sample, it indicates hemolytic transfusion reaction
- Laboratory investigation:
  ○ Confirmation of post-transfusion ABO-Rh
  ○ Post-transfusion direct antiglobulin test (DAT)

*Serum hemoglobin also may be present in nonimmune hemolysis, red cell fragility syndromes, hemoglobinopathies, severe burns, polyagglutination, or infusion of hemoglobin-based oxygen-carrying solutions.

- Post-transfusion serum hemoglobin (qualitative) may also be performed.

Blood centre/bank policy for retaining the blood sample and record:
- *Patient's original cross-match specimen:* Should be preserved for at least 48 hours after dispatching the blood or its products.
- *Donor's pilot tube/bottle:* Preserved for 48 hours after complete serological work-up.
- All the blood centre/bank records that are related to transfusion reactions, clinically significant antibodies or special transfusion requirements.

If the **clerical check indicated above does not indicate any problem** and the **screening tests are negative**, **acute hemolysis** as the cause of the reaction can **usually be eliminated.**

Further Work-up of a Suspected Immune Hemolytic Reaction

The hemoglobin (visual hemolysis) and antiglobulin tests are useful for screening purposes. If immune hemolytic reaction is suspected further testing/investigation are necessary (Box 15.5).

All prereaction testing is to be repeated using the postreaction specimen.

These tests include antibody screen, crossmatching, and any antigen typing of the units crossmatched.
- **If any of the repeated tests with the postreaction sample** show a **positive result**, then repeat tests with the prereaction sample.
- **Perform DAT:** Perform DAT on both prereaction and postreaction sample of the patient. DAT demonstrates sensitization of patient's red cells by immune antibodies (IgG) or by complement (C3d).
  - **If the postreaction DAT is positive:** It is positive when **alloantibody-coated transfused** donor **red cells** are present in recipient. In other words, a positive DAT usually indicates the presence of recipient antibodies on the surface of donor red cells. However, if all the donor cells are already destroyed, the test may be negative. This may occur if the patient's blood sample is drawn several hours after suspected reaction. DAT may also be positive because of the effects of drugs, autoimmune disease, or autoantibodies.
  - **If postreaction DAT is positive,** then **perform DAT on a stored prereaction sample.** If **DAT performed in the postreaction sample shows a "new" or stronger positivity than the prereaction sample** then further workup should be done with the postreaction sample. This may suggest the presence of incompatible transfused RBCs. If transfused incompatible RBCs are present in the circulation, DAT may give "mixed-field" appearance when the DAT is read microscopically.
  - If the **both post-transfusion and prereaction sample shows DAT positivity, then the DAT is not valid** for the purpose of **detecting, or excluding,** the presence of **alloantibody-coated transfused cells** and further testing is required.
  - **Further work-up:** These consist of complete serological work-up as listed in Box 15.6. This includes repeating the DAT with IgG and C3d reagents and performing an eluate. Incompatible RBCs may absorb sufficient quantities of antibody to make them undetectable in plasma, resulting in a negative antibody screen.
  - **If the prereaction DAT** shows a **stronger positivity when compared with the postreaction sample:** Then perform further DAT work-up with the prereaction sample.

Box 15.5: Conditions where further work-up is needed in transfusion reaction.
- If either of the **visual hemolysis or DAT is positive** or
- If the evaluations such as clerical and **ABO and Rh typing indicate a possible hemolytic reaction** or
- If the **patient's symptoms are severe** and **consistent with** a clinical suspicion of **hemolytic reaction**

- **Repeat the compatibility test of patient's serum** (prereaction and postreaction) **against donor red cells** from bag or the segment of the tube attached to the blood bag by using most sensitive technique, i.e. indirect antiglobulin test.
- **Check the donor plasma against patient's red cells by indirect antiglobulin test** technique to exclude any antibodies in the donor's plasma.
- **Tests to assess ongoing hemolysis**: Tests on baseline and follow-up samples in the patient also should be performed to know whether hemolysis is continuing or came to halt. These tests include free plasma hemoglobin, hemoglobin; lactate dehydrogenase (LDH); total and direct bilirubin; and haptoglobin, free urine hemoglobin, hemosiderin in urine.

Laboratory findings in acute hemolytic transfusion reactions (AHTRs) are presented in Box 15.6.

Box 15.6: Laboratory findings in acute hemolytic transfusion reactions (AHTRs).
- Hemoglobinemia
- Hemoglobinuria
- Elevated lactate dehydrogenase
- Hyperbilirubinemia
- Low haptoglobin
- *If renal injury develops:* Elevated blood urea nitrogen and creatinine
- *Direct antiglobulin test (DAT):* It may be positive with a mixed-field pattern if transfused incompatible red cells are present in the circulation. A negative DAT does not rule out immune hemolysis
- *Red cell antibody identification studies:* It may or may not be positive. It depends on the specificity of the antibody involved and the amount of antibody in the serum

Note:
- **Common cause of a false-positive test for free hemoglobin**: Drawing a blood sample through an indwelling catheter using inappropriate technique.

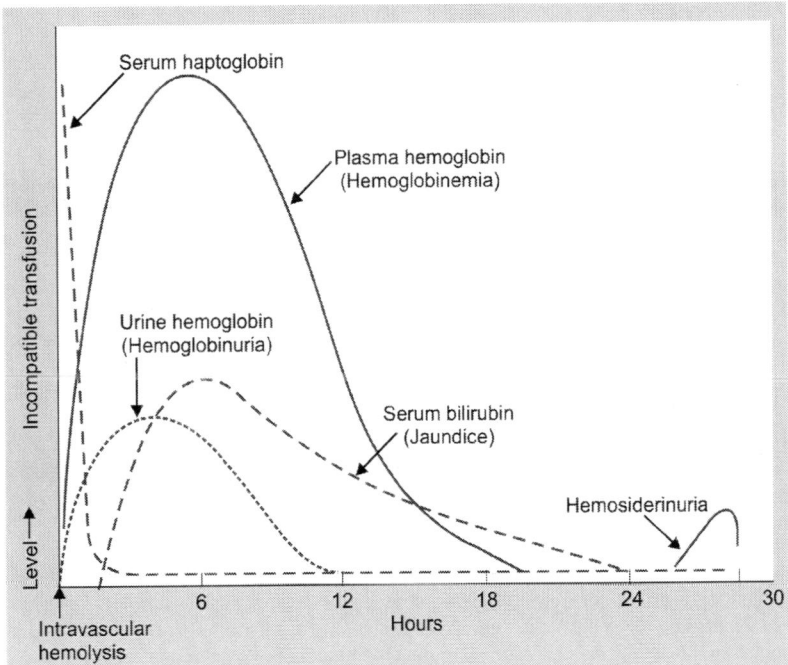

Fig. 15.2: Relationship of the changes in serum levels and time frames in acute intravascular hemolytic transfusion reaction (not to scale). Within a few hours of an acute hemolysis, free hemoglobin is cleared from plasma by forming complex with haptoglobin. It leads to fall in the serum haptoglobin falls to undetectable levels. If there is no further hemolysis, the serum haptoglobin level recovers. The presence of hemosiderin in the urine (hemosiderinuria) indicates prior hemolysis.

- **Cause of false-negative test for free hemoglobin:** Too much time has been allowed to elapse before obtaining the postreaction specimen.

Relationship of the changes in serum levels and time frames in acute intravascular hemolytic transfusion reaction are depicted in Figure 15.2.

Sample collected following a mismatched blood transfusion and the tests performed is presented in Table 15.2.

Complete serological work-up in hemolytic reaction is presented in Box 15.7.

Interpretation of results

1. **Pyrogenic/allergic reaction:** If the clerical errors are ruled out there was **no evidence of hemolysis in the blood** and **no free hemoglobin in the urine**, the patient, the hemolytic reaction is ruled out. It may be due to pyrogenic/allergic reaction.
2. **Hemolytic transfusion reaction:** It shows **evidence of hemolysis in the blood** and **hemolysis in the urine** (hemoglobinuria).
3. **Error in the crossmatching:**
   - If the **recrossmatching shows incompatibility** (both pretransfusion and post-transfusion), then it indicates that there was an **error in first crossmatch**.
   - If the **recrossmatch with the original patient specimen is compatible, but the crossmatch with the new patient specimen is incompatible**, the mistake is due to **mistaken identification of the patient.** This might be either when the first sample for crossmatch was done, or at **the time of giving the transfusion.**

Table 15.2: Sample collected following a mismatched blood transfusion and the tests performed.

Donor sample	Post-transfusion blood sample	Post-transfusion urine sample
Blood group and Rh typing	DAT	Occult blood
Crossmatching	Repeat grouping and cross matching	Methemoglobin
Antibody screening	Serum bilirubin	Microscopy: RBC

Box 15.7: Complete serological work-up in hemolytic reaction.

- **Repeating the compatibility** (crossmatch) **testing** on both **the pre- and post-transfusion patient samples** with donor blood
- **Performing an antibody screen** on the post-transfusion sample; antibody identification panels on pre- and postreaction samples, enhanced antibody screening method: PEG, extended incubation, gel, enzymes. Incompatible red blood cells (RBCs) may absorb sufficient quantities of antibody to make them undetectable in plasma, resulting in a negative antibody screen
- **Red cell eluate on pre-and postreaction samples**: To elute the antibody from the patient's RBCs (even if the DAT is negative)
- **Specific tests to assess ongoing hemolysis**: Tests on baseline and follow-up samples in the patient also should be performed to know whether hemolysis is continuing or came to halt. These tests include the following:
  - **Quantitative** free plasma hemoglobin, total and direct bilirubin (performed within 5–12 hours after the reaction), **lactate dehydrogenase** (LDH), **haptoglobin,** and methemalbumin
  - **Urine hemoglobin and hemosiderin** in urine: Evaluate the first post-transfusion urine **sample** (after 5–6 hours) **for products of hemolysis.** The products of hemoglobin (**hemoglobinuria**) or **bilirubin** can be detected by using dipsticks. Centrifuge the urine to see if the red color stays in the supernatant (hemoglobinuria) or goes down with the sediment (hematuria). Perform Prussian blue reaction (Perl's test) on urine sediment for hemosiderin
- **To establish the cause of hemolysis:**
  - **Gram stain and bacterial culture of blood bags**: If bacterial contamination is suspected, a Gram stain and bacterial culture from both the returned blood bag or tubing and patient should be performed

- If the **saline crossmatches are compatible** but the **Coombs' crossmatches are incompatible** then it may be due to an **immune antibody incompatibility**—the **most common** being the **Rh incompatibility**.

Optional investigations that may be useful in hemolytic reaction:
- Investigation of transfusion technique and blood storage conditions
- Enhanced crossmatches: PEG, enzymes
- Minor crossmatches of implicated units
- Hemoglobin electrophoresis
- Serum BUN and creatinine
- Peripheral blood smear
- Serial hemoglobin, hematocrit, and platelet count
- Blood coagulation studies (PT, fibrinogen, FDP)
- DAT on donor units
- Serum bilirubin in pre- and post-transfusion samples
- *Methemalbumin* in pre- and post-transfusion samples

Basic work-up and testing in the evaluation of an acute transfusion reaction is summarized in Flowchart 15.1.

Secondary testing in the evaluation of an acute transfusion reaction is summarized in Flowchart 15.2.

Laboratory tests in suspected delayed hemolytic transfusion reactions are presented in Flowchart 15.3.

Treatment

The work-up and treatment of a transfusion reaction must be predicated on the clinical picture/response of the patient, especially in

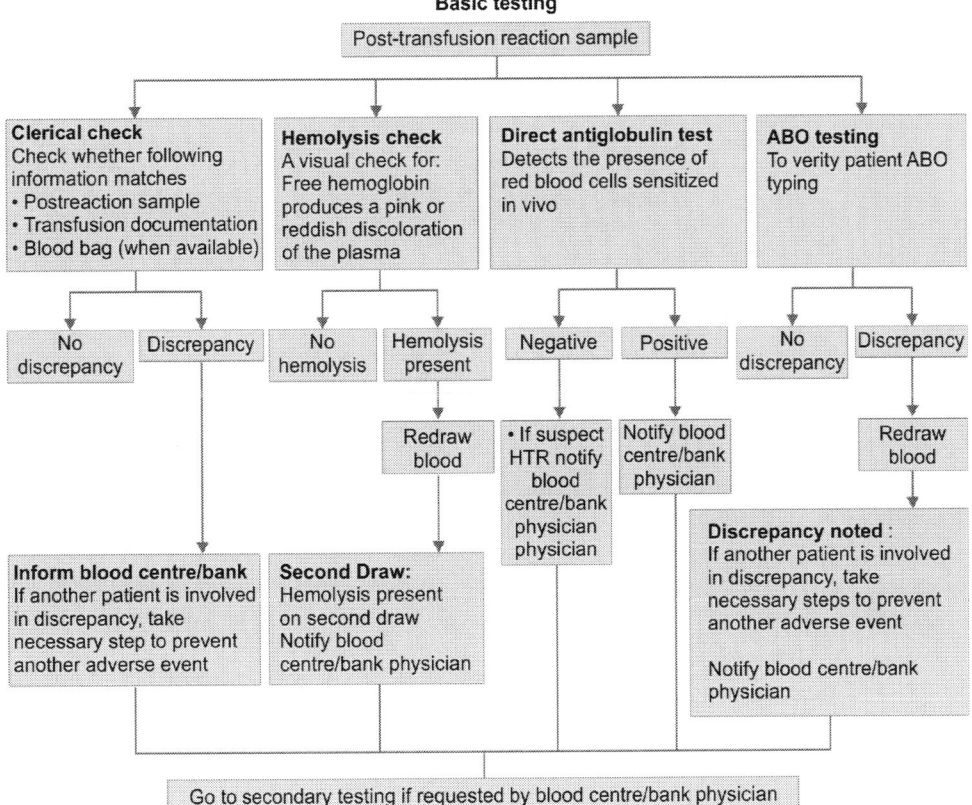

Flowchart 15.1: Basic work-up and testing in the evaluation of an acute transfusion reaction.

Flowchart 15.2: Secondary testing in the evaluation of an acute transfusion reaction. If basic test suggests hemolysis, further testing is necessary to investigate the cause of hemolysis as shown below.

```
                    Post-transfusion and pre-transfusion reaction sample
                                          │
                                    Basic testing
                          ┌───────────────┴───────────────┐
                      Hemolysis                       No hemolysis
```

Hemolysis branch:

- Check for hemolysis on prereaction sample
  - Hemolysis present: Hemolysis can be caused by nonimmune mechanisms
  - No hemolysis: Postreaction sample repeat: ABO grouping, Antibody screen, Crossmatches, Antigen typing of units → If any of the above are positive repeat testing on prereaction sample
- DAT on prereaction sample
  - Positive or negative:
    - Postreaction sample repeat: ABO and Rh typing, Antibody screen, Crossmatches, Antigen typing of units (Any positives, repeat testing on prereaction sample)
    - DAT–positive on post-pre-reaction samples: Perform DAT with IgG C3d, and eluate on sample with stronger reactivity
    - Baseline and follow-up testing:
      - Plasma hemoglobin
      - Hemoglobin
      - LDH
      - Total and direct bilirubin
      - Haptoglobin
      - Urine hemoglobin
- Repeat ABO testing on prereaction sample
  - Check of clerical errors
  - If another patient is involved in discrepancy, take necessary steps to prevent another adverse event

No hemolysis branch:

- TAS: Culture and gram stain of blood component blood culture-recipient
- ALTR:
  - IgA levels
  - Anti-IgA
- TRALI:
  - Chest X-ray
  - HLA and HNA antibody screen in donor
- TACO:
  - Chest x-ray
  - BNP

(ALTR: allergic transfusion reaction; BNP: brain natriuretic peptide; C3d: complement fragment 3d; DAT: direct antiglobulin test; HLA: human leukocyte antigens; HNA: human neutrophil antigens; IgG: immunoglobulin G; LDH: lactic dehydrogenase; TACO: transfusion-associated circulatory overload; TAS: transfusion-associated sepsis; TRALI: transfusion-related acute lung injury)

atypical cases. Consult appropriate medical specialists early in the course.

Minimal symptoms: If patients have minimal symptoms, they may be managed by careful observation.

Severe reactions: Needs vigorous intervention which may be lifesaving. The severity of AHTRs directly depends on the volume of incompatible blood transfused. The essential steps of treatment are:

- **First step:** Early recognition of AHTR, **discontinuation of the transfusion**, and prevention of the transfusion of additional incompatible units.
- **Cardiovascular support:** Maintaining adequate blood pressure. If there is hypotension, fluid resuscitation and

Flowchart 15.3: Laboratory tests in suspected delayed hemolytic transfusion reactions (DHTR). It may consist of one or more of the basic and secondary tests performed during the evaluation of an acute immune hemolytic transfusion reaction.

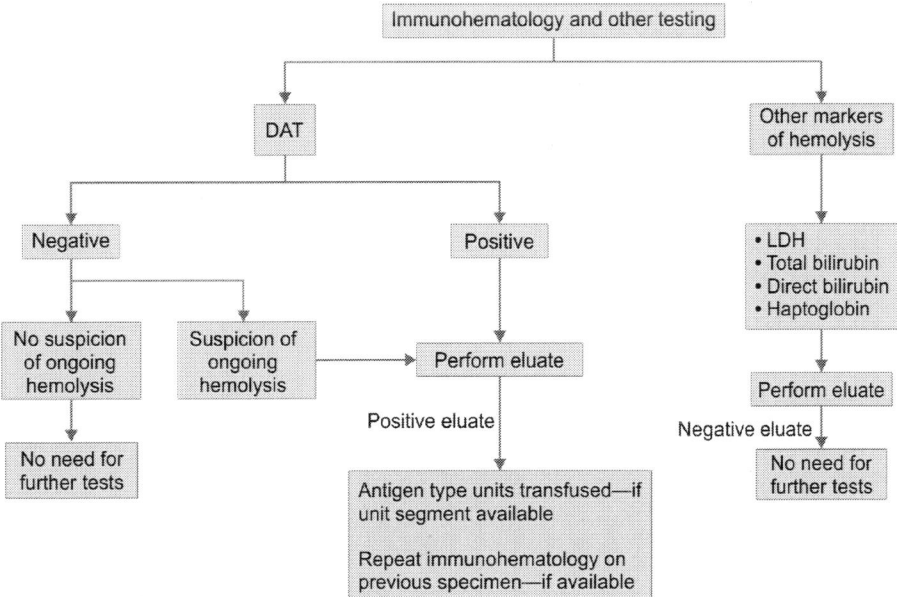

(DAT: direct antiglobulin test; LDH: lactic dehydrogenase)

pressor support may be needed. Avoid fluid overload, especially in patients with impaired cardiac or renal function.
- **Prevention of renal failure:** Renal impairment/failure should be prevented by early treatments of hypotension and disseminated intravascular coagulation (DIC). Urine output should carefully be monitored. Maintenance of urine output with intravenous fluids and diuretics, mannitol or furosemide, early in the course of the reaction. Hydration with normal saline and 5% dextrose (1:1 ratio) and sodium bicarbonate to maintain the urine pH above 7.0 should be given.
- **Disseminated intravascular coagulation:** Rare but is extremely difficult to treat.
- **Red cell exchange:** The load/volume of incompatible transfused donor red cells in the recipient circulation dictates the severity of the symptoms and course of AHTRs. Further, transfusion of red cells should be avoided until the cause of the reaction has been established. However, for symptomatic patients with a strongly reacting DAT, a red cell exchange transfusion with antigen negative blood may be used once the implicated antibody specificity has been identified. If possible, group O RBCs lacking other known clinically significant antigens to which the patient currently has an antibody should be obtained.
- **Exchange transfusion:** The focus of attention in most AHTRs is on red cells. However, care should be taken to avoid the transfusion of plasma or platelets that may aggravate hemolysis. This is especially so when ABO incompatibility is a possible cause. If the hemolytic process

> **Box 15.8:** Differential diagnosis of hemolytic transfusion reaction.
>
> - Alloantibody-induced hemolysis
> - Autoimmune hemolytic anemia
> - Cold hemagglutinin disease
> - Nonimmune hemolysis:
>   - Incompatible fluids
>   - Improper storage
>   - Small needles
>   - High hematocrit
>   - Improper deglycerolization
>   - Bacterial contamination
>   - Mechanical thrombectomy
> - Hemolytic anemia
>   - G6PD deficiency
>   - Congenital spherocytic anemia
>   - Hemoglobinopathies
>   - Sickle cell disease
> - Drug induced hemolysis
> - Microangiopathic hemolytic anemias (TTP, HUS, HELLP syndrome)
> - Bleeding
> - Artificial heart valve dysfunction
> - Paroxysmal nocturnal hemoglobinuria
> - Polyagglutination
> - Infections (e.g. *Clostridium perfringens*, Malaria, Babesiosis)

(TTP: thrombotic thrombocytopenic purpura; HUS: hemolytic uremic syndrome; HELLP: hemolysis, elevated liver enzymes, low platelet count)

is well tolerated, it is not appropriate to expose a patient to the added risk for infectious disease. The decision to perform an exchange transfusion depends on the clinical response of the patient to initial treatments. With ABO incompatibility, an exchange transfusion may greatly reduce the chance of morbidity or death.

- **Serologic tests**: The clinical judgment should be exercised depending on the results obtained from serologic tests performed up to this point.

Differential diagnosis of hemolytic transfusion reaction is given in Box 15.8.

Special Laboratory Investigations for Selected Reactions

These may be needed for investigation of some nonhemolytic transfusion reactions such as anaphylaxis, sepsis or TRALI. They are discussed in their respective sections. If **TRALI is suspected**, examine chest radiographs and medical records. Test the blood samples collected in acid citrate dextrose tubes for human leukocyte antigen (HLA) and HNA testing.

Summary of transfusion reactions, their clinical features, and relevant investigations are summarized in Table 15.3 and summary of steps for transfusion reaction is presented in Flowchart 15.4.

Table 15.3: Summary of transfusion reactions, their clinical features and relevant investigations.

Type of suspected transfusion reaction	Clinical features	Action needed and diagnostic tests required
Immune-mediated hemolytic transfusion reaction		
Acute hemolytic	Chills, fever, hypotension, hemoglobinuria, renal failure, oozing from intravenous sites, petechia (disseminated intravascular coagulation), back pain, pain along infusion vein	• Clerical check • Direct antiglobulin test (DAT) • Visual inspection of plasma for hemolysis • Repeat patient's ABO on pre- and post-transfusion sample • Further tests depending on the possible cause of hemolysis
Delayed hemolytic	Fever, anemia, new positive antibody screening test, jaundice	• Antibody screen • DAT • Tests for evidence of hemolysis (e.g. bilirubin, plasma hemoglobin, lactate dehydrogenase, urine hemosiderin)
Nonimmune-mediated hemolytic transfusion reaction		
Nonimmune hemolysis	Hemoglobinuria, hemoglobinemia	Rule out immune-mediated hemolysis (DAT, repeat patient ABO)
Nonhemolytic transfusion reaction		
Immunological		
Febrile, nonhemolytic	Fever, chills/rigors, headache, vomiting	Rule out hemolysis (DAT, hemoglobinemia, repeat patient ABO) Rule out bacterial contamination (culture of component and patient's blood culture)
Allergic/urticarial	Urticaria, pruritis	Rule out hemolysis (DAT, hemoglobinemia, repeat patient ABO)
Anaphylactic/anaphylactoid	Urticaria, hypotension, respiratory distress, wheezing	Rule out hemolysis (DAT, hemoglobinemia, repeat patient ABO) IgA quantitation and anti-IgA screen
Transfusion-related acute lung injury (TRALI)	Hypoxemia, respiratory failure, hypotension, fever, bilateral pulmonary edema	• Rule out hemolysis (DAT, hemoglobinemia, repeat patient ABO) • Rule out cardiogenic pulmonary edema (brain natriuretic peptide level) • Chest X-ray • Human leukocyte antigen (HLA) antibody screen in donor and recipient
Transfusion-associated graft versus host disease (TA-GVHD)	Erythroderma, maculopapular rash, anorexia, nausea, vomiting, diarrhea, hepatitis, pancytopenia, fever	• Skin biopsy • HLA typing
Post-transfusion purpura (PTP)	• Purpura and bleeding • Thrombocytopenia 5–12 days after transfusion	Platelet antibody screen and identification
Nonimmunological		
Transfusion-associated circulatory overload (TACO)	Dyspnea, orthopnea, cough, tachycardia, hypertension	Rule in cardiogenic pulmonary edema (brain natriuretic peptide level) Chest X-ray
Hemosiderosis	Diabetes, cirrhosis, cardiomyopathy	• Serum ferritin level • Liver enzyme levels

Flowchart 15.4: Summary of steps for transfusion reaction.

```
                    Transfusion reaction
                            │
                            ▼
                     Severity of
                    signs/symptoms
                    ┌───────┼────────┐
                    ▼       ▼        ▼
                  Mild   Moderate  Severe
```

Mild:
Decide depending on
- Patient's reaction history
- Co-mortoid clinical factors
- Amount of the product transfused
- Product type: Leukocyte-reduced/pre- or post-storage
- Product age if non-leukocyte-reduced platelets

Options
- Temporarily stop the transfusion, treat symptoms, resume transfusion when symptoms subside and monitor closely
- Slow the rate of infusion, treat symptoms, monitor closely

Moderate: Whether the transfusion be stopped and investigated — No → (Options above); Yes → Immediately stop the transfusion

Severe:
- Immediately stop the transfusion
- Provide supportive measures
- Perform bedside clerical check and notify blood centre/bank
- Return the remainder of the product to the blood centre/bank for further investigations:
  - Confirmation of bacterial contamination (gram's stain, cultures)
  - Screen for hemolysis (caused by passive antibody infusion or transfusion of incompatible red cells)
  - Tests for IgA deficiency TRALI and/or TACO (beta-natriuretic) peptide [BNP])

Complete transfusion reaction form and send to the blood bank

SUMMARY

- Initial investigation in a suspected case of transfusion reactions should include clerical checks and the following tests on a post-transfusion blood sample namely: visual check for hemolysis, direct antiglobulin test (DAT), and ABO group
- Positive DAT indicates immune-mediated hemolysis
- New antibody screen test positivity or additional identified antibody suggests a delayed hemolytic transfusion reaction
- Other useful tests that indicate hemolysis include urinalysis, serum bilirubin, or lactate dehydrogenase levels, hemoglobinuria, increased bilirubin, and/or increased lactate dehydrogenase
- Bilateral pulmonary infiltrates on chest X-ray support a diagnosis of transfusion-related acute lung injury
- IgA deficiency and presence of anti-IgA supports a diagnosis of anaphylactoid reaction
- Skin or liver biopsy shows characteristic changes in graft versus host disease

SELF-ASSESSMENT EXERCISE

Write Long essay/short notes on:
- Describe blood groups and discuss transfusion reactions and complications
- Discuss adverse reactions to blood transfusion. What are the laboratory test that may be done in investigating a case of transfusion reaction?
- Discuss the protocol for investigations of mismatched blood transfusion
- Describe the laboratory investigations in blood transfusion reactions
- Write down complications of blood transfusion and investigation of transfusion reactions
- Laboratory investigation and management of acute transfusion reaction
- Discuss (Give an account of) blood transfusion reactions and their investigations in brief
- Investigations in a mismatched blood transfusion
- Investigations in a blood transfusion reaction
- Laboratory diagnosis of mismatched blood transfusion
- Transfusion reaction—causes and diagnosis
- Investigation of hemolytic transfusion reaction

CHAPTER 16

Transfusion-Transmitted Diseases

☙ CHAPTER OUTLINE

☞ Transfusion-transmitted diseases
☞ Screening blood donors for transfusion-transmitted infections
☞ Prion disease
☞ Safety measures in laboratory during testing for HIV and hepatitis
☞ Detection of malaria in blood donors

■ INTRODUCTION

Blood is a lifesaving resource and blood components should be tested so that it makes them extremely safe and reduces the risk to minimum of the likelihood of a transfusion-transmitted disease (TTD). TTD is the infectious complications of blood transfusion. A variety of infectious agents including bacteria, viruses, parasites (Table 16.1), and prion pathogens can get effectively transmitted through blood transfusions. If they are not detected in the testing process, it can cause harm and even death.

▎TRANSFUSION-TRANSMITTED DISEASES

Human Immunodeficiency Virus and Acquired Immunodeficiency Syndrome

Acquired immunodeficiency syndrome (AIDS) is caused by the retrovirus **human**

Table 16.1: Transfusion-transmitted infectious (TTI) agents.

Viral	Bacterial	Parasitic
Common		
• Human immunodeficiency virus (HIV) • Hepatitis B virus (HBV) • Hepatitis C virus (HCV)	*Treponema pallidum* (syphilis) is not common nowadays	*Plasmodium* species (malaria)
Other less common TTIs		
• Epstein-Barr virus (EBV) • Cytomegalovirus (CMV) • Human T lymphotrophic virus-1 (HTLV-1) • Human T lymphotrophic virus-2 (HTLV-2) • West Nile virus • Parvovirus B19 (B19) • Dengue virus (few cases reported)	Brucella	• *Babesia* species • *Toxoplasma gondii* • *Trypanosome cruzi* (Chaga's disease) • *Leishmania* species
Others: Prion		

immunodeficiency virus (HIV). AIDS is a clinical condition characterized by severe involvement of the patient's immune system. This leads to a sharp decline in CD4 lymphocytes and results in pronounced acquired immunodeficiency in humans. This, in turn, predisposes to increased host susceptible to any infection.

Route of Transmission

Transmission of HIV occurs when there is an exchange of blood or body fluids containing the virus or virus-infected cells. The **three major routes** of transmission are:

1. **Sexual transmission:** It is the **main route of infection** in more than 75% of cases of HIV.
   - **Homosexual or bisexual men** or **heterosexual contacts:** It may be male-to-male or male-to-female or female-to-male transmission.
   - **HIV is present in genital fluids** such as vaginal secretions and cervical cells (in women) and semen (in men).
   - Risk of sexual transmission of HIV is increased when there is coexisting sexually transmitted diseases, especially those associated with genital ulceration (e.g. syphilis, chancroid, and herpes).
     - **Viral transmission** can occur in two ways: **Direct inoculation of virus or infected cells into the blood vessels** at the site of breach caused by trauma, and
     - **By uptake into the mucosal dendritic cells** (DCs).
2. **Parenteral transmission:** Three groups of individuals are at risk.
   i. **Intravenous drug abusers:** Transmission occurs by **sharing of needles and syringes contaminated** with HIV-containing blood.
   ii. **Hemophiliacs:** Mainly those who received large amounts of factor VIII and factor IX concentrate before 1985. Now increasing use of recombinant clotting factors has eliminated this mode of transmission.
   iii. **Transfusion of blood or blood components:** Recipients of blood transfusion of **HIV-infected whole blood or components** (e.g. platelets, plasma) were one of the modes of transmission. Screening of donor blood and plasma for antibody to HIV has reduced the risk of this mode of transmission. Because recently infected individual may be antibody-negative (seronegative), there is a small risk of acquiring AIDS through transfusion of blood. Organs from HIV-infected donors can also transmit AIDS.
3. **Perinatal transmission (mother-to-infant transmission):**
   - **Major mode of transmission of AIDS in children.**
   - Transmission of infection can occur by **three routes**:
     i. **In utero:** It is transmitted by transplacental spread.
     ii. **Perinatal spread:** During normal vaginal delivery or child birth (intrapartum) **through an infected birth canal** and in the immediate period (peripartum).
     iii. **After birth:** It is transmitted by ingestion of breast milk or from the genital secretions.

Transmission of HIV infection to health care workers: There is an extremely small risk of transmission to healthcare professional, after accidental needle-stick injury or exposure of nonintact skin to infected blood.

Etiology

Properties of HIV

AIDS is caused by HIV, which is a **nontransforming human retrovirus** belonging to the lentivirus family. Retroviruses are **RNA viruses having an enzyme called reverse transcriptase**, which **prepares a DNA copy of the RNA genome of the virus in host cell**. It belongs to the lentivirus subfamily of retroviridae. Human is the only host.

Genetic forms: HIV occurs in two genetically different but related main forms, **HIV-1 and HIV-2**.
- **HIV-1** is most common in the United States, Europe and Central Africa. The most

common cause of AIDS in India is HIV-1 group M subtype C.
- **HIV-2 is common** in West Africa and confined to western and southern India.

Structure of HIV (Fig. 16.1)
- HIV-1 is **spherical enveloped** virus which is about 90–120 nm in diameter.
- It consists of electron-dense, cone-shaped core surrounded by nucleocapsid cell which is covered by lipoprotein envelope.
A. **Viral core:** It contains:
  1. **Major capsid protein p24:** This viral antigen and the antibodies against this are **used for the diagnosis of HIV infection** in enzyme-linked immunosorbent assay (**ELISA**).
  2. **Nucleocapsid protein p7/p9** (not shown in Figure 16.1).
  3. **Two identical copies of single-stranded RNA genome.**
  4. **Three viral enzymes: (1) protease, (2) reverse transcriptase** (RNA-dependent DNA polymerase) and **(3) integrase.** When the virus infects a cell, viral RNA is not translated, instead **transcribed by reverse transcriptase into DNA.** The **DNA form of the retroviral genome** is called a **provirus** which can be **integrated into the chromosome of host cell.**
B. **Nucleocapsid:** The **viral core is surrounded by a matrix protein p24 and p17**, which **lies underneath the lipid envelope** of the virion.
C. **Lipid envelope:** The virus contains a lipoprotein envelope, which **consists of lipid derived from the host cell and two viral glycoproteins.** These glycoproteins are: (**1**) **gp120,** project as knob-like spikes on the surface and (**2**) **gp41,** anchoring transmembrane pedicle. **These glycoproteins are essential for HIV infection of cells.**

Serological Profile Following HIV Infection

The patterns of serological markers following HIV infection are shown in Figure 16.2.

Window period: Following infection, the interval of varying length (usually 4–6 weeks) between infection and the before development of any demonstrable circulating markers of infecting virus (HIV antigen or anti-HIV antibody) is known as the "window period/phase." Screening test for HIV detects anti-HIV (HIV antibody). During window period, the individual is infectious but the screening tests are negative for anti-HIV (HIV-1/HIV-2 antibodies). Thus, in spite of testing for

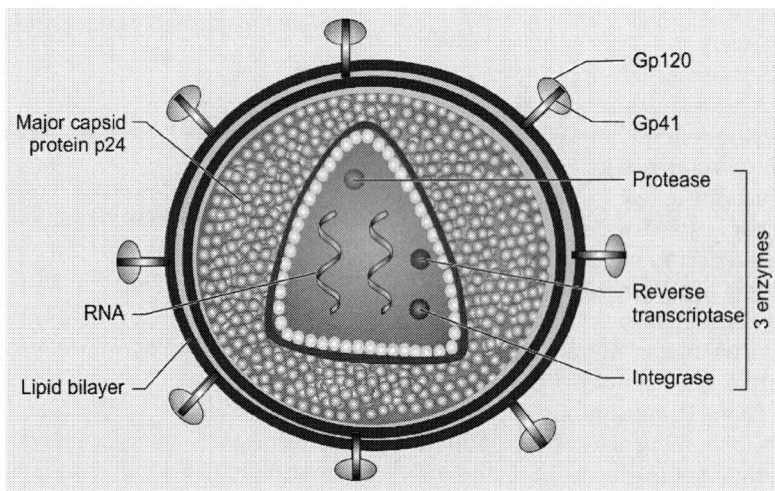

Fig. 16.1: Diagrammatic representation of structure of the human immune deficiency virus (HIV)-1 virion. The viral particle is covered by a lipid bilayer derived from the host cell and studded with viral glycoproteins gp41 and gp120.

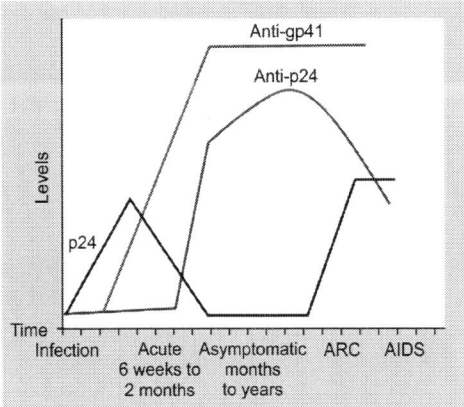

Fig. 16.2: Serologic markers in HIV infection.
(ARC: AIDS-related complex; AIDS: acquired immunodeficiency syndrome)

anti-HIV, transmission of the virus could still occur from blood donated during the window period. The blood donation during this window period may be potentially infectious. Antibodies are detectable at about 22 days after infection.

- **HIV antigen testing:** During window period, the virus is present and HIV antigen (p24 antigen) may be detected (as early as 30 days following infection) by an ELISA (using sandwich antibody-antigen antibody) in some individuals prior to their becoming HIV antibody positive. Hence, HIV antigen testing will not be helpful during window period. It is generally used to detect evidence of HIV infection during late window period when antibody assays are negative.
- **Nucleic acid amplification (NAT) testing (refer Chapter 17):** During window period, before the appearance of anti-HIV, HIV-RNA in infected individuals' blood may be detected by nucleic acid-based assays such as the polymerase chain reaction (PCR) for plasma HIV RNA (reverse transcriptase polymerase chain reaction—RT-PCR) or HIV DNA (in peripheral blood mononuclear cells) and the branched-chain DNA (bDNA) assay. HIV RNA in plasma of infected individuals can be detected 6 to 10 days (during early window period) after infection. It is generally used to detect evidence of HIV infection period when both antigen and antibody assays are negative. Unfortunately, even NAT cannot detect all infectious units of blood and so a very small number of cases of transfusion-transmitted HIV still can occur.
- **HIV isolation (culture):** HIV can be cultured in T4 lymphocytes. However, it is a laborious and expensive process. Hence, it is not used to diagnose HIV infection.

Following an initial window period (during which no markers can be detected), viral RNA is the first marker to appear. Following this viral capsid antigen appears and finally anti-HIV antibodies appear. The diagnosis of HIV infection is most commonly confirmed by demonstrating antibody to the virus or its components. Development of antibodies does not result in eradication of the virus but it indicates previous infection and probable present infectivity. Once present, in most of the cases, anti-HIV persists until the individual becomes symptomatic. Thus, the test for HIV-1 antibody is used to detect infectious donated blood.

- **HIV-1 antibody tests:** The HIV-1 antibody **detection** (anti-HIV gp120-gp41) test is an excellent and the most widely used test using an enzyme-linked assay. However, the test **becomes positive only after** an average **45 days following infection**. The specificity and sensitivity of the HIV antibody test is excellent. However, the predictive value of a positive HIV antibody test in blood donors is low because of the low prevalence of HIV infection in that population.

Laboratory tests to detect HIV infection are summarized in Box 16.1. Flowchart 16.1 shows test and decision to be taken in patients suspected for HIV infection.

Hepatitis B Virus

Structure of HBV

- Hepatitis B virus (HBV): It is a **hepatotropic DNA virus** belonging to the family hepadnaviridae.

Box 16.1: Laboratory tests to detect HIV infection.

To detect antibodies
- Screening tests are highly sensitive but may lack specificity. Hence, the reactive samples in screening should be confirmed by highly specific confirmatory tests.
  - Enzyme-linked immunosorbent assays (ELISA)—particle agglutination
  - Specialized rapid tests
- Confirmatory or supplementary test
  - Western blot detects antibodies to specific HIV proteins
  - Immunofluorescence (IF)
  - Radioimmunoassay (RIA)

To detect antigens
- Isolation of virus
- ELISA (capture ELISA assay)
- Nucleic acid amplification (NAT) testing: Polymerase chain reaction (PCR)

- **HBV virion**: It is spherical and **double-layered**.
- **Dane particle**: It is the complete viral particle/virion.

Genome of HB

It consists of partially double-stranded circular DNA and has four genes (Fig. 16.3).
- **HBsAg (S gene)**: HBsAg, hepatitis B surface antigen is a product of S gene, which is **secreted into the blood in large amounts**. HBsAg is **immunogenic**.
- **HBcAg (C gene)**: The **C** gene produces two antigenically different products: Hepatitis B core antigen:
  - **HBcAg:** It remains intracellular within the hepatocytes and do not circulate in

Flowchart 16.1: Test and decision for human immunodeficiency virus, types 1 and 2 (anti-HIV-1, -2) of blood donors. If enzyme immunoassay (EIA) testing is nonreactive, nucleic acid amplification testing must also be nonreactive before release of a donation.

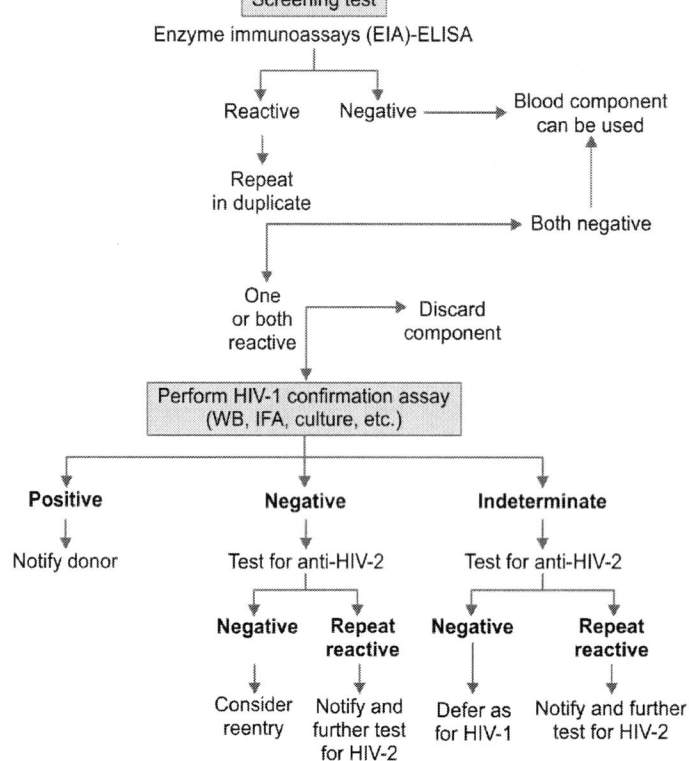

(IFA: immunofluorescence assay; WB: western blot; ELISA: enzyme-linked immunosorbent assay)

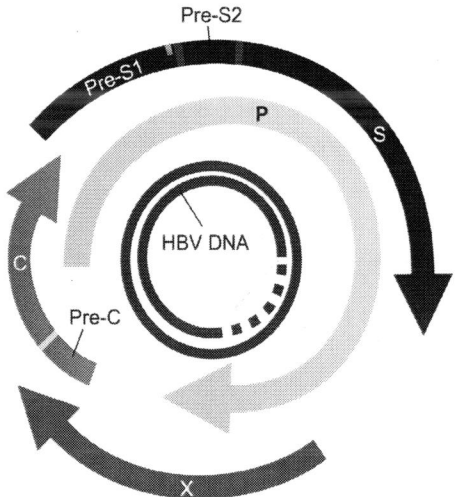

Fig. 16.3: Diagrammatic representation of various genes and respective encoded proteins in HBV. HBV-DNA encodes four proteins, namely, (1) DNA polymerase required for viral replication (P), (2) surface protein (S), (3) core protein (C), and (4) X protein.

the serum. Hence, it is not detectable in the serum of patients.
- **HBeAg:** It is secreted into serum and is a surrogate (substitute) marker for high levels of viral replication. It is essential for the establishment of persistent infection.
- **HBV polymerase (P gene): A polymerase (Pol)** is a product of P gene and DNA polymerase enzyme is **needed for virus replication.**
- **HBxAg (X gene): HBx protein** is **necessary for virus infectivity** and has been implicated in the pathogenesis of liver cancer in HBV infection.

Source of infection: Human suffering from **hepatitis or carrier** is the only source of infection.

Mode of Transmission

- **Vertical/congenital transmission:** From mother [who is carrier for HBV (90% HBeAg+, 30% HBeAg–)] to child may occur in utero, **during parturition, or soon after birth.**
- **Horizontal transmission:** It is the **dominant mode** of transmission.
- **Parenteral:**
  - **By percutaneous and mucous membrane:** Exposure to infectious body fluids, through minor cuts/abrasions in the skin or mucous membranes. HBV can survive for long periods on household articles, e.g. toys, toothbrushes, and may transmit the infection.
  - **Intravenous route:** Through transfusion of unscreened infected blood or blood products. This mode of spread is rare now, because of routine screening of all blood donors for HBV and HBC. Other modes include intravenous drug abuse with sharing of needles and syringes, tattooists or acupuncturists.
- **Close personal contact:** Unprotected heterosexual or homosexual intercourse. The virus can be found in semen and saliva.

Incubation period: It ranges from **4 to 26 weeks**.

Sequence of Serological Markers for HBV Hepatitis (Fig. 16.4)

The natural course of the disease can be followed by serum markers (Figs. 16.4A and B).
HBsAg: It is the **first virologic marker**, which appears in serum before the onset of symptoms. It peaks during the disease and becomes undetectable within 3–6 months. HBsAg is also named Australia antigen, because of its first detection in Australian aborigine.
- **Significance: Present in the serum in both acute and chronic hepatitis B; indicates an infectious state. Loss of HBsAg** plus the development of anti-HBs **denotes recovery**.

Anti-HBs: It is antibody to HBsAg and **detectable in serum after the disappearance of HBsAg**.
- **Significance:** Anti-HBs is a **protective antibody** and present in the serum in the recovery phase and in immunity (i.e. vaccination) and **may persist for life providing protection.** This is the basis for current vaccination using noninfectious HBsAg.

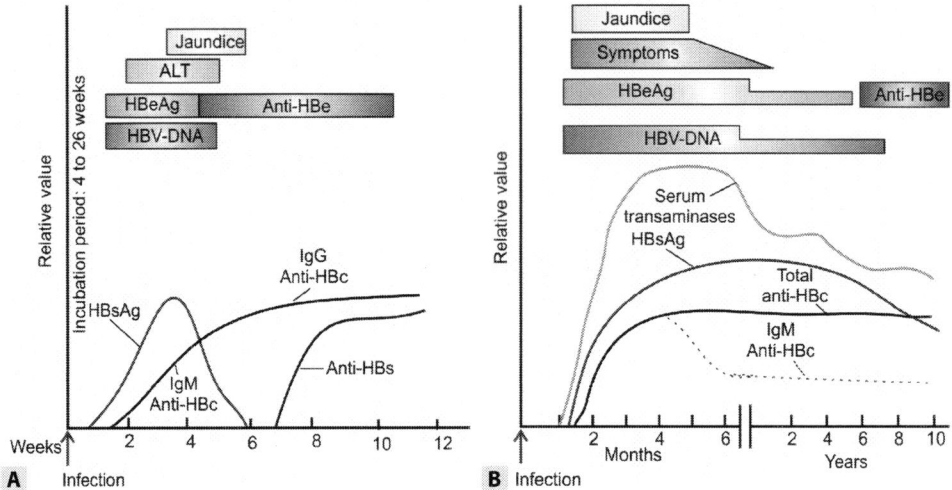

Figs. 16.4A and B: Sequence of serologic markers in hepatitis caused by hepatitis B virus. (A) Acute hepatitis with resolution; (B) Chronic hepatitis caused by HBV.

HBeAg and DNA polymerase: They appear in serum soon after HBsAg.
- **Significance:** Usually not helpful in the diagnosis of hepatitis B, but may be **valuable in assessing prognosis**. They **indicate active viral replication**.

HBeAg or HBV-DNA: Their persistence 6 weeks after the onset of symptoms indicates infectivity and probably develops chronic hepatitis B. Their absence is a favorable serologic finding and if associated with appearance of anti-HBe antibodies indicates low infectivity.

Anti-HBe is present in the serum in the recovery phase.

Anti-HBc: HBcAg **is not found in the serum**. But its antibody, IgM anti-HBc appears in serum a week or two after the appearance of HBsAg. After about 6 months, the IgM anti-HBc antibody is replaced by IgG anti-HBc.
- **Significance:** IgM anti-HBc is the **earliest antibody marker** seen in the serum, long before anti-HBe or anti-HBs.

IgM anti-HBc indicates recent infection (first 6 months).

IgG anti-HBc indicates remote infection (beyond 6 months). IgG anti-HBc remains lifelong in the serum and its presence **indicates previous infection with HBV** even when all the other viral markers are not detectable.

HBV-DNA: It is the first marker to appear and can be detected by polymerase chain reaction (PCR) testing before HBsAg reaches detectable levels. PCR is helpful in confirming the diagnosis.

Interpretation of HBV serology is presented in Table 16.2.

The screening of donated blood for the presence of HBsAg is now routinely done and has considerably reduced the occurrence of post-transfusion hepatitis B.

Laboratory Diagnosis of HBV Infection

- HBsAg assay-enzyme immunoassay (EIA/ELISA), chromatographic immunoassay (CIA), and HBsAg neutralization test
- IgM anti-HBcAg assay-ELISA
- Total (IgG+IgM) anti-HBcAg assay-ELISA
- Anti-HBeAg assay-ELISA
- HBV-DNA in blood by PCR.

Hepatitis C Virus

HCV is a **small, enveloped (contains specific proteins), single-stranded RNA virus**. It is a member of the *Flaviviridae* family. It is the major cause of liver disease.

Mode of spread: It mainly spreads by the **parenteral route** as a blood-borne infection. It may also spread by **sexual contact**. The

Table 16.2: Summary of serological findings in HBV.

Antigens		Antibodies			Interpretation
HBsAg	HBeAg	Anti-HBc	Anti-HBs	Anti-HBe	
+	+	IgM	–	–	**Acute hepatitis B**, highly infectious
+	+	IgG	–	–	**Chronic infection** or carrier state, **high infectivity**
+	–	IgG	–	+/–	**Chronic infection** or carrier state, **low infectivity**
–	–	–	+	–	**Immunity** following HBV vaccine

major route of infection in children is vertical perinatal transmission from the mother.

Incubation period: 2–26 weeks (mean 6–12 weeks).

Laboratory Diagnosis of HCV Infection (Fig. 16.5)

- HCV antigen assay by ELISA
- Anti-HCV by ELSIA: The antibodies are generally detectable after 10 weeks of infection. This is the most widely used screening method.
- HCV RNA RT-PCR is also available.

Syphilis

Introduction: Spirochetes are Gram-negative, slender corkscrew-shaped bacteria covered in a membrane called an outer sheath, which may mask its antigens from the host immune response.

Syphilis (lues) is a **chronic, sexually transmitted** disease **caused by spirochete *Treponema pallidum*.** Untreated syphilis manifests by three distinct clinical stages, namely—*primary, secondary,* and *tertiary syphilis*.

Mode of Transmission

- **Sexual contact:** It is the usual mode of spread.
- **Transplacental transmission:** From mother with active disease to the fetus (during pregnancy) → congenital syphilis.
- **Blood transfusion.**
- **Direct contact:** With the open lesion is rare mode of transmission.

Laboratory Diagnosis of Syphilis

Serological Tests

Serological tests form the **mainstay of laboratory diagnosis.** Serologic tests for

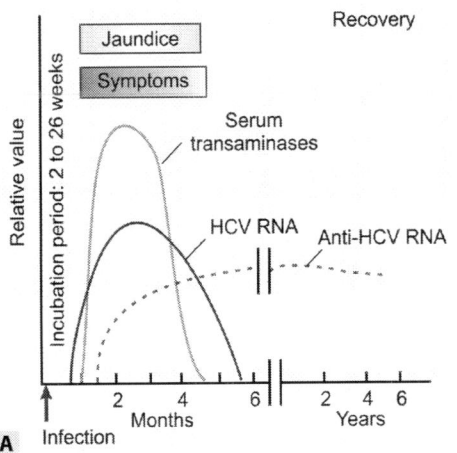 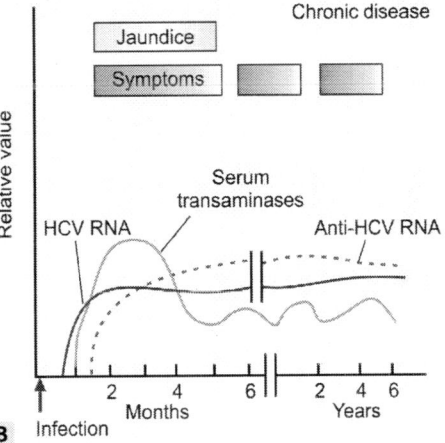

Figs. 16.5A and B: (A) Sequence of serologic markers for acute hepatitis caused by HCV; (B) Sequence of serologic markers for chronic hepatitis caused by HCV.

syphilis measure the presence of **two types of antibodies**, namely—**treponemal** (specific/confirmatory tests) and **nontreponemal** (nonspecific/screening tests).

Nontreponemal (reaginic tests) antibody-screening tests

Nontreponemal (regain) antibodies are **often known as *reagin* antibodies** and are produced in infected patients against components of mammalian cells. Syphilis infection causes breakdown of human tissue and releases fatty substances. The fatty substances combine with *T. pallidum* protein to form an antigen. The antigen in turn leads to formation of nonspecific and specific *T. pallidum* antibodies in the serum of infected patients. These nontreponemal antibodies are called reagin antibodies. Reagin is a mixture of highly purified cardiolipin, lecithin, and cholesterol present in both host tissues and *T. pallidum*. Reagin circulates in the blood and is a **fairly sensitive marker of recent/active syphilis infection**, though it is **not particularly specific.**

These nontreponemal (regain) tests detect regain antibody. These antibodies are detected by the **two most widely used nontreponemal serologic tests**, namely, the (i) **Venereal Disease Research Laboratory** (VDRL) and (ii) **rapid plasma reagin** (RPR) tests. **VDRL/RPR test is the choice for screening blood** for *T. pallidum*. Each of these tests is a flocculation (or agglutination is a type of precipitation reaction) test, in which soluble antigen particles are coalesced to form larger particles. These large particles are visible as clumps when they are aggregated in the presence of antibody. The **VDRL is used as a quantitative test** and usually performed on serum.

Venereal disease research laboratory (VDRL) test

This is a nontreponemal (reaginic tests) antibody-screening test.

Aim: VDRL is a slide flocculation test used for screening patients for infection with *T. pallidum*.

Principle: Patients infected with *T. pallidum* produce nonspecific antibodies. These antibodies can react with the cardiolipin test antigen. Cardiolipin is a lipid antigen extracted from beef heart and it contains cardiolipin, lecithin and cholesterol.

Significance

- The VDRL test is usually **positive within 1 to 2 weeks** after the appearance of the primary lesion (primary chancre).
- The test is reactive in late phase primary syphilis and highly reactive in secondary syphilis. The results will slowly decrease and become less reactive in late or tertiary syphilis.
- VDRL test is also useful in the diagnosis of congenital syphilis.
- Maternal antibodies can cross the placenta and a positive VDRL immediately following birth may be due to the presence of maternal antibodies. The RPR antigen consists of cardiolipin, lecithin, and cholesterol. Hence, a quantitative titer at birth followed by a second titer approximately 1 month following birth is needed to know whether the infant is having congenital syphilis. No increase in titer will rule out the possibility of congenital syphilis.

Specimen: Patient serum or CSF samples. The serum must be inactivated before the test by heating at 56°C for 30 minutes. This inactivates serum proteins such as complement present in the serum. CSF samples should not be heated prior to testing.

Method

1. Take 50 µL of patient sample, a positive reactive, and a negative nonreactive control into separate circles on the test card.
2. Place 20 µL of reagent next to the sample and stir each. Make sure to completely cover the circle on the test card. Use a separate stirrer for each sample to avoid contamination.
3. Place the test card on a rotator or shaker at 180 rpm for 4 minutes.

Interpretation
- **Strongly reactive**: Presence of large visible clumps.
- **Weakly reactive**: Appearance of small clumps.
- **Nonreactive:** Appear as a diffuse, evenly turbid reaction.

Limitations
1. Read the results immediately to avoid drying of sample and the appearance of clumping due to evaporation.
2. **Biologic false positives (BFP)** are discussed below.

Quality control
Run a reactive and nonreactive control in each assay.

Rapid plasma reagin (RPR) card test and automated reagin test (ART)
This is another nontreponemal (reaginic tests) antibody-screening test.

Aim: It is a **presumptive serologic screening test** for syphilis.

Principle: The test depends on the presence of a nonspecific antilipid antibody, namely, reagin, found in the serum of patients infected with *T. pallidum*. The nonspecific (reagin) antibody combines with the test antigen and forms flocculation. The flocculation incorporates charcoal particles in the antigen preparation on a white test card and makes it visible.

Specimen
Patient serum or plasma is tested at room temperature, 20 to 25°C.

Method
1. Take 50 µL of patient serum or plasma, positive, and negative controls into three separate circles on the test card.
2. Gently mix the RPR-carbon (charcoal) reagent before applying to each circle.
3. Add exactly one drop (20 µL) of reagent to each sample.
4. Carefully mix the specimen and reagent with a stirrer. Spread each sample over the entire surface of the circle. Use a clean stirrer for each sample.
5. Keep the test card on a mechanical rotator or shaker at 80 to 100 rpm for 8 minutes.
6. Read the results prior to drying.

Interpretation
- **Reactive:** Presence of small to large clumps.
- **Weak positive:** May show fine granulation or partial clumping.
- **Nonreactive:** No clumping or very slight roughness.

Limitations
1. Room temperature affects the slide flocculation tests. Hence, all test reagents and specimens should be warmed to room temperature before testing.
2. Results must be read within 8 minutes. Otherwise it may lead to drying and the appearance of false-positive results.
3. Samples should not be hemolyzed, lipemic, or contain a high concentration of bilirubin. Their presence may interfere with test results.

Quality control
- Positive controls should demonstrate readily visible flocculation.
- Negative controls will appear uniformly turbid.

Biologic false-positives (BFP) VDRL/RPR tests
Though reaginic antibodies are almost always produced in patients with syphilis, they are found in other physiologic or pathologic conditions.

Physiological
Increasing age, pregnancy, menstruation, trauma, and recent immunization (vaccination).

Pathological
- **Other infectious diseases:** These include lepromatous leprosy, tuberculosis, chancroid, leptospirosis, malaria, rickettsial disease, trypanosomiasis, lymphogranuloma venereum (LGV), measles, chickenpox, hepatitis, and infectious mononucleosis.
- **Noninfectious conditions**: These include drug addiction, hypergammaglobulinemia of any cause and immunologic disorders such as autoimmune disorders, including

rheumatoid disease and systemic lupus erythematosus.

Specific Treponemal Tests— Confirmatory

Treponemal antibodies are produced against antigens of the organisms themselves. Specific treponemal or confirmatory serological tests include **fluorescent treponemal antibody-absorbance (FTA-ABS)** test, *T. pallidum* **indirect hemagglutination** (TPHA), microhemagglutination assay (MHA-TP), automated enzyme immunoassays (EIAs), and particle gel immunoassay (PaGIA). Once positive; these tests are of limited use because these tests tend to positive throughout the patient's life. The confirmatory tests can be done using live or killed *Treponema pallidum* or using its extract.

Tests using live T. pallidum
- *Treponema pallidum* **immobilization (TPI):** In this test, the test serum is incubated with suspension of live *T. pallidum* and complement. They are maintained anaerobically. If the test serum contains antibodies, the treponemes will be immobilized (i.e. rendered nonmotile). Test is considered positive if more than 50% of treponema is immobilized when examined under dark ground illumination. Once, TPI was considered the **gold standard** in syphilis serology. However, because of its complexity, TPI test has now been replaced by others such as FTA-ABS and TPHA which are quite as specific and much simpler.

Test using killed T. pallidum
- **Fluorescent treponemal antibody (FTA) test:** It is an indirect immunofluorescence test. Nicholas strain of *T. pallidum* is smeared on slide (which can be stored in deep freeze for several months). Patient's serum is allowed to act on smear. This is treated with antihuman gamma globulin fluorescence conjugate. Excess of unfixed conjugate is washed off. The slide is examined under ultraviolet microscope. If the test is positive, treponema is seen as fluorescent objects.

Test using T. pallidum extract
T. pallidum **hemagglutination assay (TPHA):** This assay is an indirect hemagglutination assay that uses sensitized (sensitized with a sonicated extract of *T. pallidum* as antigen) red blood cells that aggregate when exposed to positive patient serum (containing antibody).

Advantages: The following advantages have made TPHA as a standard confirmatory test.
- TPHA is just as specific and almost as sensitive (except in the primary stage of syphilis) as FTA-ABS (discussed below).
- Much simpler technique and more economical.
- No special equipment is needed.
- Kits (Fig. 16.6) are available commercially.
- Have good quality control.

Microhemagglutination assay for T. pallidum (MHA-TP): It is a passive hemagglutination assay of sensitized erythrocytes that are tested against the patient's serum. The procedure in microhemagglutination test (MHA-TP) can be automated.

Fluorescent treponemal antibody-absorbance (FTA-ABS) test: It is the indirect immunofluorescent and is the modification of the FTA test. In this test, the test serum (patient's serum) is first allowed to react with

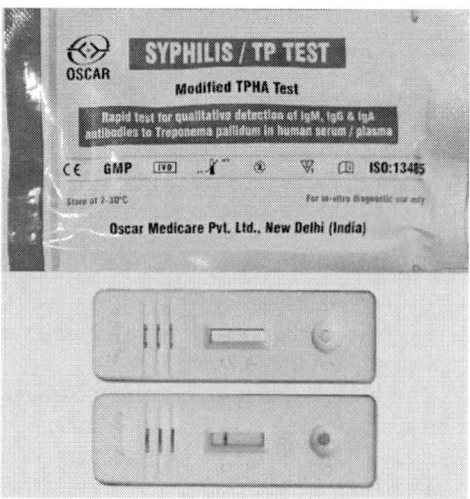

Fig. 16.6: *T. pallidum* hemagglutination assay (TPHA). The lowest figure shows a colored band indicating the test as positive. The middle one is a card before performing test.

treponemes fixed to slides and then reacted with antihuman globulin antibody labeled with fluorescent dyes (fluorescein-conjugated antihuman antibody reagent). If antibodies to the treponeme are present in the test sera, the fluorescently labeled antihuman globulin antibody will bind to the *Treponema* on the slide. The result is highly visible with a fluorescence microscope. Before starting the test proper, first the test sera are preabsorbed with extract of Reiter's treponema which is non-*T. pallidum* treponemal antigens (sorbent, to remove group-specific reactive antibody), hence the term absorbance. This absorbance reduces the nonspecific cross-reactivity. FTA-ABS is as specific as the TPI test. However, it can perform only in suitably equipped laboratories; it is not available for routine testing and is presently used as a standard reference test. This test is usually performed following a positive VDRL or RPR screening test.

Enzyme immunoassays (EIA)
It is a rapid agglutination test that uses latex particles coated with three immunodominant proteins of *T. pallidum* as antigens, obtained by recombinant technology. It is claimed to be as specific as TPHA, and more sensitive.

Particle gel immunoassay (PaGIA) test
It uses gel immunoassay technology (an established method in blood group serology). The assay contains recombinant antigens for the detection of *T. pallidum* antibodies in the patient's serum or plasma. The results can be obtained within 15 minutes.

T. pallidum particle agglutination (TP-PA) test
TP-PA tests utilize gelatin particles sensitized with *T. pallidum* subsp. *pallidum* antigens. The test is performed in a microdilution well. Serum of patient is diluted in a microtiter plate and sensitized gelatin particles are added. The presence of specific antibody causes the gelatin particles to agglutinate and form a flat mat across the bottom of the microdilution well.

SCREENING BLOOD DONORS FOR TRANSFUSION-TRANSMITTED INFECTIONS

Donor Testing
Once a donor passes the medical screen and donor questionnaire, the serologic tests should be performed for the transfusion-transmitted disease (TTD). Routine screening of donor's blood in India is presented in Table 16.3. Performing these tests can make blood transfusion safer than ever before.

Apart from the transfusion-transmitted diseases listed in Table 16.1, many other organisms may also be transmitted by transfusion. However, tests for these organisms are not routinely performed in the blood screening process. These include other viruses such as Epstein-Barr virus (EBV), cytomegalovirus (CMV), parvovirus B19 (B19), bacteria (presently is the leading cause of death from transfusion), parasites such as *Babesia microti* and *Trypanosoma cruzi*, malaria, and prion diseases.

Table 16.3: Routine serological tests and screening methods used for testing donor blood in India.

Transfusion-transmitted diseases	Required serological tests	Screening method
Human immunodeficiency virus (HIV)	Antibodies to human immunodeficiency virus (anti-HIV 1/2 RNA) and p24 antigen	ELISA, particulate agglutination, simple rapid assays
Hepatitis B virus	Hepatitis B surface antigen (HBsAg), antibody to hepatitis B core antigen (anti-HBc)	ELISA, simple rapid assays
Hepatitis C virus	Antibody to hepatitis C virus (anti-HCV), HCV RNA	ELISA, simple rapid assays
Syphilis	Nonspecific antibody: serological tests for syphilis (STS)	VDRL or RPR
Malaria	Trophozoite/gametocyte	Microscopy or QBC

Presently performed test methods are extremely sensitive. Hence, confirmatory tests are used only to detect false-positives. These tests depend on the disease to be confirmed and include polymerase chain reaction (PCR), Western blot (WB), radioimmunoprecipitation assay (RIPA), and recombinant immunoblot assay (RIBA).

It is important to select a safe donor to provide a safer donation. The safest donors are regular, voluntary, and nonremunerated. Blood for donation should be screened for TTDs.

Test samples: Most of the assays use either serum or plasma. The instructions with the assay must be followed strictly.

Terminology

The terminologies used in classifying the results of the assays are mentioned in Table 16.4.

Principles of Screening Assays or HIV HBV and HCV

Enzyme Immunoassays

Enzyme immunoassay (EIA) is an alternative method to immunofluorescent assays. EIA exists in many forms and procedures can used to **detect either antigen or antibody or hapten** in clinical samples. EIA **procedure can be automated** to test large numbers of samples. The term enzyme immunoassay includes all assays based on the measurement of enzyme-labeled antigen, antibody. In immunofluorescent assays, an antibody is labeled with a fluorochrome. In EIA, **enzyme molecules are conjugated to specific antibodies** and thus **preserve the activities of both enzymatic and antigen-binding**. Furthermore, the antibody binding sites remain free to react with their specific antigen. Advantages of enzyme immunoassays are presented in Box 16.2.

Solid-phase immunoassay: Most commercially available EIAs used for detection of infectious agents require physical separation of the specific antigens from nonspecific complexes found in clinical samples. For detection of antigen by ELISA in the clinical specimen, this separation is achieved through firmly binding the antibody specific for an antigen of interest to a solid phase or matrix to the walls of a plastic microtiter well or the outside of a spherical plastic or metal bead or some other solid matrix. Such systems are called **solid-phase immunosorbent assays (SPIAs)**. It is named **immunosorbent** because this technique uses a solid support such as a plastic microtiter plate that can *adsorb* (bind to its surface) the reactants. The absorbing material is specific for one of the components of the reaction: the antigen or antibody. The solid-phase support is an inert surface to which reagent Ag or Ab is attached. A variety of solid matrix platforms are commercially

Table 16.4: The terminologies used in classifying the results of the assays.

Terminology	Meaning
Positive/negative	These terms are used when a confirmatory test is done
Reactive/nonreactive	These terms are used when a screening test is done
Equivocal/indeterminate	It is a WHO terminology that is used for a result that cannot be classified as clearly positive or negative (usually around the cut-off value) is equivocal

Box 16.2: Advantages of enzyme immunoassays.

- Commercial enzyme immunoassay (EIA) kits are available for a large number of infectious agents.
- Enzyme itself is not changed during activity. Enzyme can catalyze the reaction of many substrate molecules, greatly amplifying the reaction and enhancing detection.
- EIA tests can be automated and thus allowing more tests to be performed in shorter times.
- Enzyme-conjugated antibodies are stable and can be stored for a relatively long time.
- Colored end products allow direct observation of the reaction or automated spectrophotometric reading. Automation makes the interpretation of test results objective rather than subjective.

available. These include individual wells of polystyrene microtiter trays spheric plastic beads, or magnetic beads. The solid matrix allows for separation or washing, of the sample and reagent to decrease nonspecific binding or background activity. ELISA is usually done using 96-well microtiter plates suitable for automation. Enzyme immunoassays or more specifically, solid-phase EIAs [enzyme-linked immunosorbent assay (ELISA)] are the most popular and widely used types of immunoassay in use today.

Enzyme-linked immunosorbent assay

Enzyme-linked immunosorbent assay (ELISA) is simplest and most commonly used "enzyme immunoassay" test. In this technique, immobilized antigen/antibody captures corresponding specific antibody/antibody present in the test sample. In radio-immunoassay (RIA), a radioactive anti-antibody is used. In ELISA, to generate a signal, an enzyme-linked indicator (either antibody or antigen) is used to visualize antigen-antibody reactions. During reaction, it generates either color (chromatogenic reaction) or photons (chemiluminescent reaction). Because antibody/antigen has an enzyme attached to them, the term *enzyme-linked* is used. The most commonly used antigen detection assays are based on the use of immobilized antibody. ELISA is much more sensitive than fluid-phase agglutination or SPRCA assays (refer pages 17-9). ELISA assay is an important diagnostic tool for hepatitis Bs (surface) and hepatitis Be (early) antigens and HIV p24 protein, all indicators of early, active, acute infection. However, false positives can occur and a verification test (such as a Western blot) may be necessary. Advantages of ELISA procedures are listed in Box 16.3.

Enzyme-linked antiglobulin test: ELISA usually uses purified or recombinant antigens or antibodies, depending on the analyte to be detected. However, intact RBCs can be sued to screen for RBC antibodies. This test is termed enzyme-linked antiglobulin test.

Applications/uses of ELISA (Box 16.4): ELISA can detect antigen, hapten or antibody. Most

---

Box 16.3: Advantages of ELISA procedures.

- ELISA assays are popular because they require little interpretive skill to read
- Results tend to be clearly positive or clearly negative
- Many ELISA tests are available for clinical use in the form of commercially prepared kits
- Procedures are often highly automated. The results read by a scanner and printed out by computer
- Some ELISA tests are also available for use by the public (e.g. pregnancy test)

Box 16.4: Applications of ELISA.

Tests used to screen the blood donors: To protect recipients of blood products from infection
- HIV detection: HIV antibodies can be detected within 6 weeks of infection
- Infectious diseases: Hepatitis, EBY, cytomegalovirus IgM/IgG, dengue IgG, influenza, TORCH panel, etc
- Syphilis IgG/IgM

Other tests
- *H. pylori* IgG and antigen detection
- Detection of rotavirus in fecal specimens and enterotoxin of *E. coli* in feces
- Food toxins, e.g. chloramphenicol, streptomycin, penicillin, aflatoxins, etc.
- Food adulterants, e.g. *E. coli*, *Campylobacter* and *Salmonella* antigens
- Mycobacterial antibody detection in tuberculosis
- Human allergen-specific IgE and IgA ELISA

ELISA systems are used for the detection of antibody against antigen/infectious agents.

ELISA plays a major role in the diagnosis of many diseases (Box 16.4). Enzyme immunoassays are commonly and popularly used for the serologic diagnosis of infectious diseases.

Interpretation of the test: It is based on comparison of the results to a cut-off value. If a specimen is reactive, the test should be repeated in duplicate on the same specimen.

Main Types of ELISA

Three main types of ELISA are commonly used in blood screening, namely, (i) indirect ELISA, (ii) competitive ELISA and (iii) sandwich ELISA. They can be used to detect antibody or antigen, depending on the specific design format of the assay. A microtiter plate with numerous shallow wells (96-well microtiter plates are popular) is used in these procedures. The advantages of these microtiter plates are that are large number of tests can be performed and the serum volume required is small.

Indirect ELISA

The indirect ELISA is the simplest form of EIA. It is used to detect any microbe-specific antibodies in a patient's sera (test sample) rather than an antigen. The detection of antibody by indirect ELISA is used, for example, to screen blood for specific antibodies (anti-HIV antibody to HIV).

Procedure (Fig. 16.7): Usually, it is performed using microtiter plate well. In this immunoassay, an immobilized antigen (either purified or recombinant) is bound to the surface of the wells of the microtiter plate. These plates are provided by the manufacturer, ready coated and standardized for use.

- It uses purified inactivated viral antigen (e.g. HIV antigen) that is adsorbed on to the surface of a microassay plate well.
- The serum test sample is then added to the microtiter wells and incubated at 37°C for 30 minutes. (The period of time at the correct temperature varies according to the manufacturer's instructions.) If antibody is present in the specimen, stable antigen–antibody complexes form when the sample is added to the matrix.
- Unbound antibodies are removed by thoroughly washing the microassay plate well. The commonly used wash fluid is phosphate buffered saline. The wash process removes the excess sample from the well without dislodging and removing any bound, specific antibody.
- After washing, a secondary antibody (serves as a reporter, e.g. anti-IgG) complexes to an enzyme, i.e. anti-antibody–enzyme complex is added to the well. It is incubated for 30 minutes. The enzymes often used are alkaline phosphatase or horseradish peroxidase. This enzyme-bound antibody will bind to the Fc portion of the patient's antibody. If the serum contains antibodies against the virus (e.g. anti-HIV antibody), it will form a stable complex (i.e. antigen-antibody complex) with the antigen (e.g. HIV) on the plate. The enzyme catalyzes a reaction and produces a visible (colored) end product while attached to the antibodies. The intensity/amount of color development is directly proportional to the amount/concentration of antibody present. This end product can be quantified spectrophotometrically.

Inference

- **Positive result:** If the patient's serum contains antibodies, the viral antigen in the well has attached to each other and will remain in the well. The product in such a

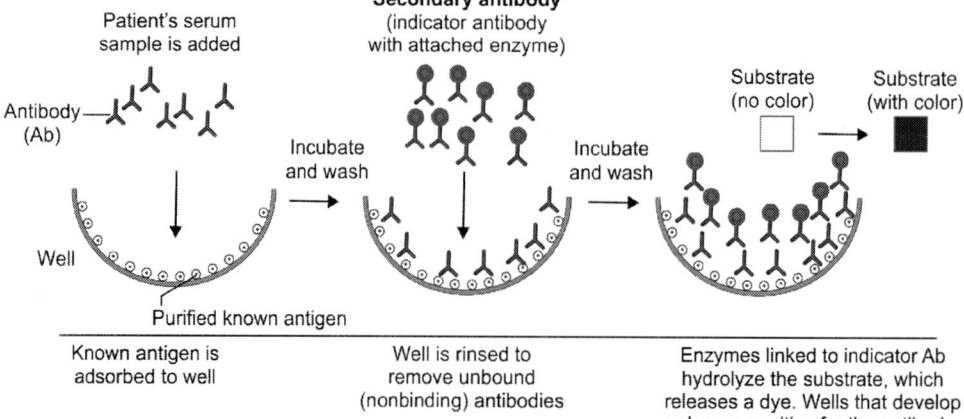

Fig. 16.7: Different steps in indirect ELISA.

case will be a colored substance. Thus, the color change in the well indicates a positive result/test.
- **Negative result**: If the patient's serum did not contain the correct antibody, there will be no enzyme to produce a colored product.
- Always run positive and negative controls along with test sera.

Sandwich ELISA

Sandwich ELISA is a highly specific type of EIA. This can be used for screening either antigen such as HBsAg and HIV antigen or antibody in the patient sample. It can detect and quantify a specific soluble antigen. Specific antibody (or antigen) in the test sample is bound to immobilized specific antigen (or antibody) and then detected by enzyme-labeled specific antigen (or antibody).

Principle: The **antigen is sandwiched between two layers of antibodies** (i.e. capture and detection antibodies). The basic principle of the sandwich ELISA is that the specific antigen binds to immobilized antibody present on the microtiter plate wells and the presence of the antigens is then detected using conjugate (an enzyme HRP) labeled specific secondary antibody.

Described below is the procedure for the detection of antigen in the test sample.

Procedure (Fig. 16.8): This assay uses two different antibodies (capture antibody and reporter antibody) which are usually monoclonal antibodies (MoAbs). Each antibody binds separate epitopes (When an antibody binds to a protein, it does not bind to the entire full-length antigen. Instead, it binds to a segment of that antigen known as an epitope.) on the same target antigen in the sera of patients without cross-interference. Suitable positive and negative controls should also be run.

- **Microtiter plate wells** are first **coated with** one **specific monoclonal antibody** (which is called the "capture" antibody).
- When performing an ELISA to detect an antigen, a clinical/**test sample** (serum) is **added to the microplate wells** (solid matrix). The wells are incubated for the defined time and at the correct temperature. During this time if the test sample (serum) contains specific antigen of interest, it will bind to the capture antibody bound to the surface of the microplate well (solid matrix) and will form a stable complex.
- At the end of the incubation period, the **microplate wells are washed to remove unbound antigens** in the test sample (serum).
- Next, a **second MoAb** (called reporter antibody) specific for the antigen but recognizes epitopes different from those bound by the first antibody is added. The second antibody is **attached (linked/conjugated) to a reporter enzyme** (horseradish peroxidase or alkaline phosphatase). The microplate wells are incubated for the defined time and at the correct temperature. Because this antibody

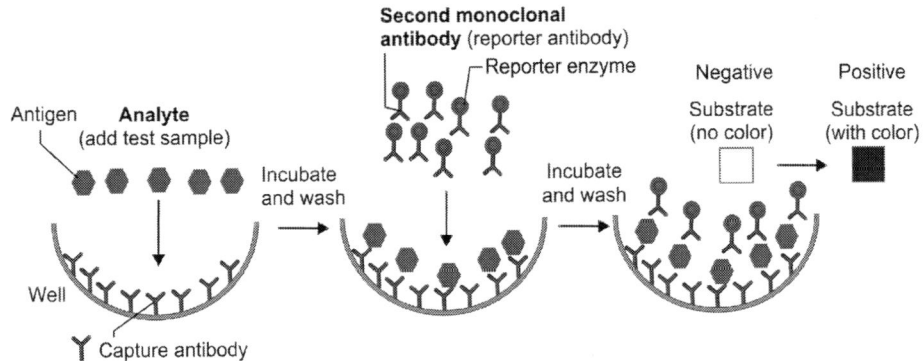

Fig. 16.8: Sandwich ELISA technique.

is specific for the target antigen (in the specimen/serum of patient), the reporter antibody binds to the well only if the antigen is already bound via the capture antibody. If the target antigen is present, it binds the second antibody, forming a sandwich with antigen in the middle (sandwich" of antibody/antigen/enzyme-linked antibody).
- The microplate wells are washed to remove the unbound labeled antibody antibodies. After washing, the enzyme substrate is added, the intensity of the color produced being proportional to the amount of bound antigen.

Inference
- **Positive:** If antibody with enzyme has been bound to the target antigen, the enzyme attached to the second antibody converts the enzyme substrate to produce a detectable colored product. An ELISA reader provides quantitative (intensity of color produced) color recordings which are directly proportional to the quantity of antigen present in the test sample.
- **Negative:** If the sample does not contain antigen, there is no significant color change.

Competitive ELISA

Competitive ELISA begins similar to indirect ELISA with the target/specific antigen already bound (immobilized) to the wells of microplate. But this is a slightly more complex assay.

Principle: In this assay, **specific antibody** that may be present **in a test sample** (unknown antibody) **competes with enzyme labeled specific antibody (known antibody)** with each other for binding sites for a fixed amount of **immobilized specific antigen on the wells** of microplate. Competitive ELISA yields an inverse curve, where higher values of antibody in the samples/standards yield a lower amount of color change. It is normally used for hapten (refer page 3) detection. Though competitive ELISAs are more difficult to optimize than sandwich ELISAs, competitive ELISAs do not require two separate antibodies against different epitopes on the target antigen.

Procedure
For detection of antigen in the test specimen:
- The target/specific antigen (known standard antigen) is bound (immobilized) to the wells of microplate.
- The test sample (serum) is preincubated with solution-phase antibody, and this mixture is added to the well.

Inference
- **If no antigen is present in the test sample** specimen, then **reagent antibodies bind freely to the solid-phase antigen on the wells of microplate**.
- If **antigen** (unknown antigen in sample) **is present in the test sample specimen**, the antigen binds to the reagent antibodies **preventing them from binding to the solid-phase antigen** on the wells of microplate.
- As the amount of soluble antigen in the test sample specimen increases, the amount of reagent antibody free to bind to the solid-phase antigen on the wells of microplate decreases. Thus, the competitive ELISA yields an inverse curve. The signal generated is **inversely related to the amount of soluble antigen in the** test sample **specimen**. A higher signal (higher values of antigen in the test specimen) is generated if the antigen level in the sample is low or absent.

Competitive ELISA can also be used for the detection of antibody. Schematic representation of competitive ELISA is presented in Figure 16.9.

Technical problems with ELISAs
- False negative can occur due to the presence of inhibitors of enzymes in the test samples.
- False positive can occur due to nonspecific enzyme activity in the test samples.
- **Hook effect:** Falsely low signals can be seen if the amount of antigen exceeds the amount of antibody. This phenomenon is termed hook effect. This can be readily overcome by diluting the antigen.

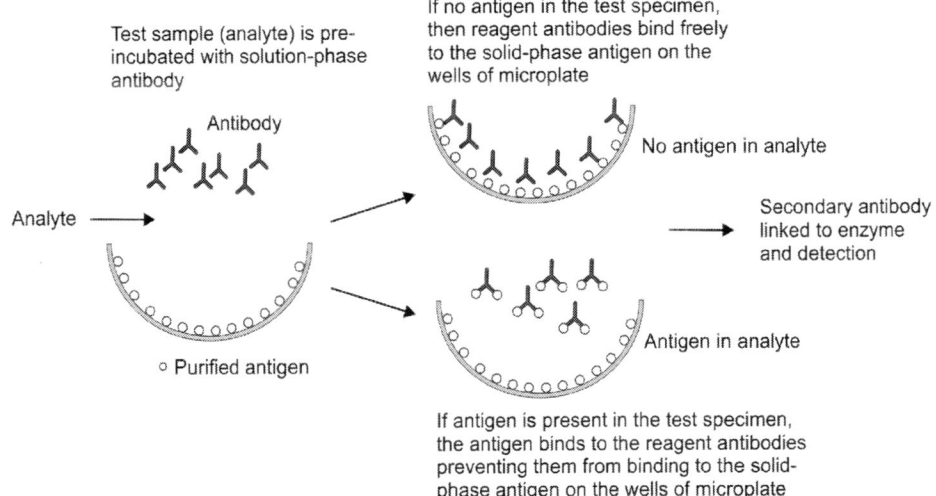

Fig. 16.9: Schematic representation of competitive ELISA.

- In patients exposed to mice or mouse-based biological drugs may develop human mouse antibodies (HAMAs) that crosslink the capture antibody and/or detection antibody in sandwich ELISAs. This may give rise to very high signals.

Membrane-bound SPIA: The flow-through and large surface area characteristics of nitrocellulose, nylon and other membranes have been made use to increase the speed and sensitivity of ELISA reactions. An absorbent material below the membrane draws the liquid reactants through the membrane. This helps to separate nonreacted components from the antigen–antibody complexes bound to the membrane and also simplifies the washing steps.

Capture ELISA is more specific and on this antibody is captured by antihuman immunoglobulin onto a solid phase. Capture ELISA specific for IgM antibody is also available. Immunometric assays are highly sensitive and specific.

Rapid tests

There are several variations of the ELISA technique which provide simple diagnostic tests. A number of 'rapid tests' have been introduced for this purpose. These include cassette ELISA, immunochromatographic tests (ICT), coated particle agglutination, immunoperoxidase, and cardor dipstick tests. Some of them can be used both in clinical laboratory and at the bedside as singly-use disposable devices. Tests using blood from finger-prick, dried blood on filter paper, saliva, and urine have also been developed. They give results in minutes rather than hours and, in most cases, with good sensitivity. Assays of this format are available which detect antibody (e.g. anti-HIV, anti-HCV) and antigen (e.g. HBsAg).

Cylinder or cassette ELISA: It is a simple modification of ELISA. Advantages of cylinder or cassette ELISA are listed in Box 16.5.

Dot Blot Assay: It is an **example of cassette ELISA and is used for the detection of HIV type 1 and 2 antibodies.**

Box 16.5: Advantages of cylinder or cassette ELISA.

- Useful for testing one or a few samples of sera at a time
- Each specimen is tested in a separate disposable cassette
- Test is rapid (10–15 minutes)
- No need for microplate washers or readers
- Result is read visually
- In-built positive and negative controls are usually provided for validation of the test procedure

- **Procedure:**
  - Specific type 1 and 2 **antigens are immobilized** at separate **fixed sites on the nitrocellulose membrane in the cassette**.
  - Test **serum is added on the membrane and allowed to filter into absorbent material placed below it in the cassette base. Antibody, if present in the serum, will bind to** the appropriate **antigen**.
  - **Washing is done** to remove the unbound antibody. Then an **enzyme labeled anti-human immunoglobulin antibody is added**.
  - Additional washing is done to remove the unbound conjugate. A substrate yielding a colored product is added.
- **Result:**
  - **Positive result: If the test serum contains a specific antibody against the antigens immobilized at separate fixed spots on the nitrocellulose membrane in the cassette,** it binds to the antigen. Result is considered positive if a colored spot develops at the site of the antigen and antibody binding.
  - Human immunoglobulin immobilized at a spot on the membrane acts as a control for the test procedure, as shown by the development of color at the site.

Particle Agglutination Assays

Principle: Particle agglutination assays detect the presence of specific antibody or antigen in a test sample through the agglutination of particles (e.g. gelatin, latex, microbeads) coated with the complementary specific antigen or antibody, respectively.

Advantages and disadvantages of particle agglutination assays are shown in Table 16.5.

Basic test procedure
- The particles are added to the diluted sample and are incubated, usually at room temperature (18–25°C). The incubation period varies considerably, but is usually between 0.5 and 2.5 hours.
- During the incubation period, the particles are agglutinated by any antibody present in the sample. The agglutination is similar to that observed with red cells and blood group antibodies.
- At the end of the incubation period, the test can be read. Particle agglutination assays are generally read by eye and the results are recorded as either positive or negative.

Table 16.5: Advantages and disadvantages of particle agglutination assays.

Advantages	Disadvantages
No need for expensive equipment	Subjective error can occur when the reaction is weak
Test procedure is simple. They do not have a lot of different stages and do not need wash equipment	False positive reaction may occur due to antibodies in patient's sample reacting against carrier particles
Result can be read visually	At times prozone reaction can occur

Settle method: This method is most commonly recommended by the manufactures.
- **Reactive result:** It appears as an even mat of agglutinated particles across the bottom of the well.
- **Nonreactive result:** It appears as a button or ring of unagglutinated particles that have settled in the center of the well.

Confirmatory Test for HIV: Western Blot

ELISA tests even though highly sensitive are prone to false positive results when the antigen used to coat the well is not pure (e.g. cell lysates of viruses grown in tissue culture). This will lead to cross-reactivity with other components in the antigen preparation.

It is very essential that the confirmatory test must be highly specific. This should help in confirming the diagnosis when the samples are reactive in screening assay. Sometimes the confirmatory tests may also produce indeterminate results which need further testing to resolve. The most common confirmatory test is western blot (WB).

Western Blot or Immunoblot/Immunoelectroblot

Serologic test methods for detecting antibody such as IFA assays and enzyme immunoassays

(EIAs) provide excellent sensitivity and specificity in most clinical applications. However, their ability to resolve the complex antibody response occurring during infection by most infectious agents is limited. This is because most antigens used in these assays are crude microbial and viral extracts and a positive result may be due to an antibody response to one or too many antigens. The EIA test can be designed to detect antibody to a number of individual antigens. But this needs expensive and labor-intensive process of purifying antigens and running multiple EIAs. As an alternative, the Western blotting technique is used which combines the sensitivity of enzyme immunoassay (EIA) with much greater specificity.

In some individuals, EIA may produce nonspecific reactions. Hence, it is necessary to perform a confirmation test on all repeatedly reactive tests. The test most commonly used is the western blot. This procedure involves immunoelectrophoresis and immunoblot technology.

Western blotting is often simply called *immunoblotting*. In **western blot, proteins or antigen mixtures** are first separated by high-resolution protein electrophoresis, using polyacrylamide gels. These separated proteins are transferred to a membrane to serve as the solid phase for probing within an antibody-containing patient sample. Western blot can be used to identify a specific protein in a mixture. When this specific protein is an antibody, the technique is valuable in diagnosing disease. Western blotting is extensively used to confirm antibodies to human immunodeficiency virus type 1 (HIV-1) in patients whose sera have been repeatedly reactive in EIA tests. Thus, western blot test is considered to be the definitive/confirmatory test for the serodiagnosis of HIV infection. Western blot test detects the antibodies to various components of HIV antigens. Western blot tests are available for HIV-1 and HIV-2.

Western blot technique allows for characterization of multiple antibodies to an infectious agent. It is a highly specific and sensitive method to identify or verify the presence of microbial-specific antigens or antibodies in a patient sample. The technique is a combination of three separate procedures:

1. **Separation of ligand–antigen** (microbial or viral antigens or protein) mixture from a bacterial cell or virus components via electrical charge in a polyacrylamide gel electrophoresis. This results in distribution/separation of antigens/proteins throughout the gel.
2. The antigens separated by electrophoresis are **transferred or blotted on solid support nitrocellulose membrane** strips (special protein-binding sheet/filter called blotted membrane or blotter).
3. **Enzyme immunoassay (or radioimmunoassay)** to detect antibody in test sera against the various ligand fraction bands. The filter is incubated with a patient's serum (containing antibody). The antibody in the serum that is specific for the antigen/protein of interest, called the *primary antibody*. During incubation, if the test serum contains antibodies to the microbe, they will bind to the antigens on the nitrocellulose strip/filter paper. Since the patient's antibodies are not "labeled", the binding is not visible. To make antibodies bound to the antigens visible, a second enzyme-linked antibody (designed to combine with the Fc portion of human antibody as the antigen) is applied to the filter paper. The second antibody is called secondary *antibody that is specific for the primary antibody*. This will turn a colorless substrate into a colored product. The principle of detection of antibody is the same as that of ELISA except that the colored end product is insoluble. After incubation, sites of specific antigen-antibody binding will appear as a pattern of bands. These bands can be compared with known positive and negative controls.

If a definite pattern does not exist (bands are missing), the bands which do not meet the criteria for positive results are considered indeterminate. It is usually recommended that such a sample be retested in several weeks (after 3–6 months). If the blood sample is found reactive (positive), it should be destroyed by incineration.

PRION DISEASE

Creutzfeldt-Jakob Disease

Creutzfeldt-Jakob disease (CJD) is one of the transmissible spongiform encephalopathies (TSE). These are rare diseases characterized by fatal neurodegeneration and produce sponge-like lesions in the brain. A definitive diagnosis can be done only by a post-mortem biopsy of the brain and testing cerebrospinal fluid for the Tau protein and protein 14.3.3, which may be done before death. However, a preliminary diagnosis can be made depending on the neurological signs and symptoms and disease progression. TSE can affect humans as well as animals (sheep, goats, cattle, cats, minks, deer, and elk).

Types of humans CJD: These include sporadic, inherited, and iatrogenic CJD and are considered as the classic CJD.

- **Sporadic CJD** is the most common (85–90%) form. It usually occurs in late middle age (average age of 60 years).
- **Inherited CJD** form due to a gene mutation is responsible for 5% to 10% of cases.
- **Iatrogenic CJD** acquired through contaminated neurosurgical equipment, cornea or dura mater transplants or human-derived pituitary growth hormones (no longer allowed). It constitutes less than 5% of cases.

A variant form of CJD (vCJD) affecting younger individuals was identified in 1996 and epidemiological evidence this to bovine spongiform encephalopathy, probably due to eating contaminated beef.

Causative agent: All TSEs are believed to be a "prion". Prion is a self-replicating protein and does not contain nucleic acid. It is formed when the confirmation of the normal cell surface glycoprotein, the prion protein, is changed to an abnormal form.

Features of prion: Prion is abnormal forms that accumulate in the brain. After its involvement, the brain tissue becomes highly infectious. It is resistant to inactivation by heat, radiation, and formalin.

Incubation period: In humans, it ranges from 4 to 20 years or longer in some cases.

Involvement of blood: CJD does not involve blood. In **vCJD**, prion particles have been found in lymphoreticular tissues, including the tonsils, spleen, and lymph nodes. Because blood is intimately involved with the lymphoreticular system, there is possibility of patients with vCJD to **transmit the prion to recipients of blood or blood products.**

Diagnosis: Currently, there is no reliable diagnostic test to detect asymptomatic patients. Therefore, **deferral of donors should be done to prevent transmission.**

Prognosis: All cases of CJD are fatal. Death usually occurs within 1 year of the onset of symptoms.

SAFETY MEASURES IN LABORATORY DURING TESTING FOR HIV AND HEPATITIS

- **Specimens** should be treated as infectious and universal safety precautions to be taken for all blood samples.
- **Laboratory personnel**
  - Must wear disposable gloves while handling specimens. Also wear laboratory coats to ensure that the clothes are kept free from infectious agents.
  - If there are any cuts or scratches on hands, they must be covered and protected.
  - Mouth pipetting is forbidden.
  - Hands should be properly washed before leaving laboratory.
- **Laboratory equipments and materials**
  - The working table, equipments in laboratory, etc. should be cleaned everyday with disinfectants before and after work.
  - Any spills must be immediately decontaminated with one of disinfectants listed in Table 16.6.
  - All the glassware used in the lab should be properly autoclaved.
- **Disposal of materials**: All the disposable materials used in the laboratory must be properly decontaminated before disposal either by autoclaving or incineration (as per biological waste management).

Table 16.6: Main disinfectants used in laboratory.

Type of disinfectant	Concentration and dilution
Sodium hypochlorite (0.5% available chlorine)	10%
Calcium hypochlorite (70% available chlorine)	7.0 g/L
Ethyl alcohol (ethanol)	70%
Isopropyl alcohol	70%
Methylated spirit (denatured alcohol)	70%
Hydrogen peroxide	6%
Glutaraldehyde	2%
Povidone iodine (PVI)	2.5%

Main disinfectants used in laboratory are listed in Table 16.6.

New testing methodologies: Nucleic acid testing (NAT) is the next step in further reduction of the window period in HIV infection (Discussed in detail in Chapter 17). NAT is very sensitive and specific and involves detection of the viral protein itself.

Pathogen inactivation: The safety of the blood can be improved with screening of donors and testing of the blood product. However, pathogen inactivation methods may be useful to eliminate or reduce the risks due to serologic window periods and possibly the newly emerging pathogens that can be transmitted by blood transfusion.

DETECTION OF MALARIA IN BLOOD DONORS

Microscopic Examination of Peripheral Blood Smears (Thick and Thin Smears)

Examination of blood film is considered as the gold standard for diagnosis of suspected cases of malaria. However, it is not suitable for screening large number of blood donors. This is because it is difficult to find parasites in the blood film in short time especially the density of parasites is less than 100 per microliter of blood.

Macroscopic Tests

1. **Tests for malarial antibody:** Malarial antibody can be detected either by direct fluorescent antibody (IFA) test or by ELISA. This serological screening test is appropriate only for nonendemic areas. It is not ideal for malaria endemic areas (e.g. India) because there are likely chances of many blood donors showing positive reaction and many donors will be rejected if these tests are used.
2. **Malaria antigen test (Fig. 16.10):** Detection of malaria antigen is the method of choice for detection of malaria in blood donors. Sensitive tests using monoclonal antibodies for detecting malarial antigens are available.
   Principle: This test is based on the chromatographic immunoassay principle. It is a one-stage, simple, economical, and reliable technique. The test is claimed to be nearly as sensitive and specific as EIA tests.
   – The test system is a small cassette containing a membrane precoated with antibody colloidal gold dye conjugate on the test region. The antibodies used are monoclonal anti-LDH antibody (which is nonspecific for all *Plasmodium* species) and/or histidine rich protein 2 (HRP-2 is specific for *P. falciparum*). The control band contains captured immunoglobulin which is anti-IgG.

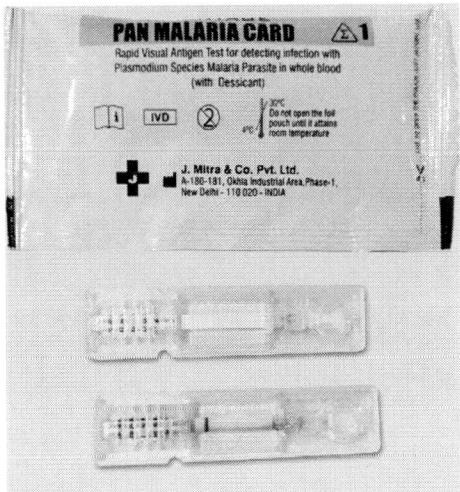

Fig. 16.10: Malaria antigen test. The lowest figure shows colored band indicating the positive test. The middle figure shows card before the test.

Procedure: The membrane is exposed at three windows on the cassette. During the test, the blood/serum is dropped into the first window and allowed to react with colloidal gold conjugate precoated with monoclonal anti-LDH antibody and/or histidine rich protein 2 antibody. The mixture moves/travels up chromatographically due to capillary action.

Interpretation

- **Positive reaction:** If the blood/serum contains malarial antigens, a colored band will be formed at the second window (test site/region). This is band is due to the formation of an antigen–antibody conjugate complex and indicates that the reaction is positive. A colored positive band at LDH region indicates infection with any *Plasmodium* species whereas if colored bands are seen on both test regions (LDH and HRP-s), it indicates infection by *P. falciparum*.
- **Negative reaction:** Absence of a colored band at the test site indicates a negative reaction.
- **Control:** Simultaneously, a colored band should appear in every case at the third window. This control band serves as a procedural in-built control. In the absence of color band at control, the test is considered invalid.

3. **Other tests**
   - Nucleic acid and immunofluorescence for detection of plasmodia within the RBCs.
   - Gel diffusion, counter immunoelectrophoresis, radioimmune assay, and enzyme immunoassay for malaria antigens in body fluids.
   - Hemagglutination tests, indirect immunofluorescence, enzyme immunoassay (EIA), immunochromatography, and western blot for antiplasmodial antibodies in the serum.

SUMMARY

- The most important step in transfusion medicine is to ensure that transfused blood will not transmit a pathogenic virus to the donor from the donor blood component.
- Four categories of pathogens within the blood supply are viruses, prions, bacteria, and parasites.
- HIV and HTLV are retroviruses and HIV is the causative agent of AIDS.
- HIV can be transmitted by transfusion. Diagnosis of HIV-1 and HIV-2 infection depends on the demonstration of antibodies to both envelope and core proteins. HIV-positive persons with less than 200 CD4+ T cells per μL are considered to have AIDS in the absence of symptoms.
- The window period for HIV can be shortened by using the polymerase chain reaction (PCR). PCR detects HIV infection before tests for antigen or antibody are positive.
- The hepatitis viruses HBV and HCV can be transmitted through transfusion.
- The first serological marker that appears with HBV infection is HBsAg, followed by HBeAg and IgM anti-HBc within the first few weeks of exposure.
- Majority (60–70%) of HCV infections are asymptomatic. NAT testing for HCV has reduced the window period to 10 to 30 days.
- Transfusion transmission of the prion disease classic CJD has not been reported so far. However, contaminated human growth hormone and transplant material have caused transmission of CJD.
- Routine donor testing includes tests for HBV, HCV, HIV I and II, syphilis and malaria.
- Parasitic infections associated with transfusion include babesiosis, Chagas disease, trypanosomiasis, malaria, leishmaniasis, and toxoplasmosis.

SELF-ASSESSMENT EXERCISE

Write short essays/notes on:
- Transfusion-transmitted diseases
- Infectious complications of blood transfusion
- Prion and blood transfusion
- Enumerate transfusion transmitted diseases and relevance of donor screening test
- Diseases transmitted through blood transfusion
- Transfusion Transmitted Infections (TTI)
- Write short note on transfusion transmitted infection
- Advances in TTI testing
- Prion diseases and blood safety

CHAPTER 17

Nucleic Acid Amplification Test in Blood Banking

CHAPTER OUTLINE
- Nucleic acid amplification test
- Polymerase chain reaction (PCR and RT PCR)
- Transcription-based amplification

INTRODUCTION

Routinely blood banks perform screening test on a sample of blood from each donor using for presence of any infectious agents. This screening test is very important because most blood components (e.g. red cells, platelets, plasma, and cryoprecipitate) are infused to the recipient without sterilization, pasteurization, or other methods to inactivate infectious agents. If the screening test does not detect any infectious agents present in donor's blood at the time of donation, the infectious age can be transmitted to the recipient. Blood components are prepared from blood so that more than one patient can benefit from a single donation. If components are prepared from a single unit of blood collected from a donor in the window period of infection; transfusion of the various components may transmit the infections up to four recipients of blood-derived products.

Mandatory Screening Tests

The five tests that are mandatory as per Food and Drug Administration (FDA) for the donated blood units are HBsAg, HIV Ab, HCV Ab, VDRL and malarial parasites.

The conventional tests require the presence of pathogen, antibodies or antigens to produce a positive test.

Conventional Serological Tests for Infectious Agents

Conventional serological screening tests are used to detect antibody or antigen by using enzyme immunoabsorbent assays (EIAs) or chemiluminescent immunoassay (CLIA). If the screening test is nonreactive, the test result is considered as negative, i.e. there is no evidence of infection. If the test is reactive during initial testing, the test should be repeated in duplicate (refer Flowchart 16.1). If both the repeat results are nonreactive, the blood is considered as nonreactive (i.e. there is no evidence of infection), and the unit may be used for transfusion. If one or both of the repeat tests are reactive (i.e. repeatedly reactive), this unit should not be used for allogenic transfusion.

Enzyme Immunoassay

Current screening testing methods used in blood bank for detection of viral infection in blood are based on the principle of EIA (refer pages 359-64). EIA screening tests are used for detection of antigens (HBsAg, HIV p24 antigen) and antibodies (anti-HIV-1/2, anti-HBc, and anti-HCV) in donor blood.
- **Not useful during window period**: EIA-based blood tests detect not the causative virus but detect either virus-induced antibodies or viral antigens. The production

of detectable amount of antibodies by the body after a viral infection takes some time. The period from the time of exposure to infection to the time that produces detectable level of antibodies (that can be detected by a laboratory test) is called the "seroconversion window" or "window period". The greatest threat to the safety of blood transfusion is blood collected from "seronegative" donors during "window period" of initial infection. Samples obtained during window period have low viral load. Hence, detection of very low viral load samples requires highly sensitive assays.

- **Hepatitis B:** Current screening techniques detect markers such as core antibodies or surface antigens in hepatitis B. However, these markers do not appear up to eight weeks after an infection. Thus, HBV infection has a higher residual risk of transmission by transfusion than HCV or HIV. The window period in HBV infection is the real issue in the transfusion.
- **High rate of false positives:** EIA screening tests have a very high rate of false positives. This will result in perfectly healthy donors being labeled as "positive."

Chemiluminescence (CL)

It is the emission of light by molecules in an excited state with a limited amount of emitted heat (luminescence) from a chemical reaction. In chemiluminescence, an excited electron state is produced by a chemical reaction (most often an oxidation) of the luminescent compound. When the electrons move from this "excited" or more energetic state back to their more natural "relaxed" state, they release energy in the form of light. The emitted light is read with a luminometer or may be captured on photographic film. Chemiluminescence is the most sensitive technique for immunoassays, because even low levels of light emission can be detected. Also there are only few naturally occurring molecules which can emit light under the conditions used for chemiluminescence, leading to very low backgrounds. Most chemiluminescent reagent compounds are acridinium esters and derivatives of isoluminol; both can be excited by sodium hydroxide and hydrogen peroxide. These reagents are stable and relatively nontoxic. Chemiluminescent labels can be attached to an antigen or an antibody, depending on the assay format. The light from the label is emitted in the form of a flash lasting for 1 to 5 seconds. The highest intensity is used for the measurement. The photomultiplier tube is used to detect emitted light. Advantages of chemiluminescence are (i) they are stable, (ii) relatively nontoxic, (iii) very sensitive, (iv) reagent use is less than ELISA and (v) the reactions are quick (less turnaround time).

Application of Molecular Genetics to Blood Banking

Serological tests for HIV HCV, and HBV cannot detect the transmission of these diseases while donor is (i) in preseroconversion window period, (ii) infected with immunovariant viruses and (iii) a nonseroconverting chronic carrier. One of the important contributions of recent advances to biological science is the procedures based on the detection or analysis of DNA and RNA. This molecular technology is used in blood banking and transplantation and is used for HLA typing, red cell typing, viral marker testing, and determination of engraftment in hematopoietic progenitor cell (HPC) transplantation.

NUCLEIC ACID AMPLIFICATION TEST

Nucleic acid testing (NAT) or nucleic acid amplification test (NAAT) is a general term used for molecular-based methods of screening for infectious agents. A nucleic acid test (NAT) is a method useful to detect a particular genetic material (nucleic acid) of virus or bacteria which acts as a pathogen in blood, tissue, urine, etc. The NAT differs from these conventional tests in that it detects genetic materials rather than antigens or antibodies. The nucleic acid may be deoxyribonucleic acid (DNA) or ribonucleic acid (RNA) in donation samples. Use of nucleic acid testing (NAT) into the blood screening process has added an extra layer of safety against transmission of transfused viral infections. NAT was first introduced in 1999 for screening of HIV and HCV RNA.

All molecular procedures involve the direct manipulation and analysis of nucleic acid sequences rather than the analysis of gene products. Because nucleic acids are common to all living entities, most can be used for the diagnosis of viral, fungal, parasitic or bacterial infections. This technique needs the extraction of nucleic acid from donor plasma followed by amplification to detect the viral genetic sequences. A specific RNA/DNA segment of the virus is targeted and amplified *in vitro*. The amplification step helps in the detection of virus even present at low levels in the original sample and increases the amount of specific target to a level that can be easily detected. If the test shows a specific nucleic acid, it indicates the presence of the virus and blood donation is likely to be infectious. Fully automated systems are now available for donor viral nucleic acid testing. They use multiplex assay platforms that can detect HIV RNA, HCV RNA, and HBV DNA in a single reaction chamber. ID-NAT is an individual donation (ID) screening for nucleic acid test (NAT). MP-NAT is a minipool (MP) screening for nucleic acid test (NAT).

The RNA viruses routinely tested using NAT technology are HIV and HCV, and DNA virus HBV. Polymerase chain reaction (PCR) testing and transcription-mediated amplification are two examples of testing procedures using NAT.

Advantages (Box 17.1)

When an individual gets infected by a pathogen (virus or bacteria), the pathogen can be present in the blood/tissue. During this period, the diagnosis can be made by culture to identify the pathogen. Some time is needed for the appearance of antigens and antibodies in the bloodstream/tissue, etc. Hence, the detection of antigens/antibodies requires some time after the infection with the pathogen. If the pathogen cannot be cultured or identified by other

> **Box 17.1:** Benefits and advantages of nucleic acid testing (NAT).
>
> - Detects very low numbers/levels of RNA or DNA of the pathogens (e.g. HIV, HBV, HCV) in the bloodstream before the appearance of antibodies
> - Higher level of specificity and sensitivity than serologic laboratory assays
> - NAT is also useful in detecting mutants, emerging pathogens, occult cases, and false negatives from serology
> - Detects infection earlier than conventional methods thereby narrowing the window period
> - Provides additional safety to blood supply in transfusion medicine

conventional tests/methods to detect antigens/antibodies, NAT is useful sensitive test in such situation (i.e. before seroconversion). NAT is a direct test that identifies/detects pieces of the infectious agent's genetic material (DNA or RNA) and allows an early diagnosis of an infectious disease. The amount of a certain genetic material (e.g. viral RNA or DNA) is usually very small in donated blood during window period. So, NAT includes an amplification step of the genetic material (even when present at low level). NAT significantly reduces the "seronegative window period" or the time between the exposure to pathogen and the appearance of antibodies (or when antibodies may be below detectable levels). In transfusion medicine, it allows for earlier detection of the infection and thus reduces the possibility of transmission by transfusion. NAT technique has approximately reduced the "window period" for detection of HIV from 15 days to 9 days, for HCV, it is reduced from 59 days to 7.4 days, and for HBV, from 67 days to 38 days. Usual time sequences of the appearance of various markers in infection are depicted in Figure 17.1.

In contrast to conventional serologic testing, if an individual specimen is reactive on NAT screen for HIV, HCV, or HBV, the corresponding blood unit should be discarded. There is no need to repeat NAT.

Applications of NAT (Box 17.2)

After extraction of nucleic acid, it needs to be amplified followed by detection of viral

Manual of Transfusion Medicine

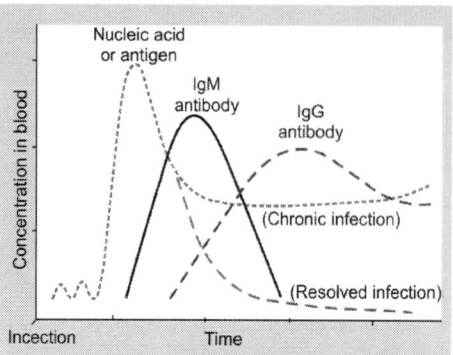

Fig. 17.1: Time sequences of the appearance of various markers in infection.

Box 17.2: Applications of NAT (nucleic acid testing).

- Transfusion medicine
- Detection of hepatitis C, HIV and HBV virus
- Other diagnostic applications
- Diagnosis of gonococcal and other *Neisseria* infections
- Diagnosis of urogenital *C. trachomatis* infections
- Detection of *Mycobacterium tuberculosis*

(HBV: hepatitis B virus; HIV: human Immunodeficiency Virus)

genetic sequence (in case of viral infections). Presently, fully automated NAT systems are available. These use multiple/triplex assays and they simultaneously detect HIV RNA, HCV RNA, and HBV DNA in one reaction chamber.

Techniques of Nucleic Acid Testing

These tests detect nucleic acid of either DNA or RNA of the pathogen in donor's/patient's blood sample. The various steps for many molecular pathological tests follow a similar scheme are shown in Figure 17.2.

Extraction of nucleic acid: NAT requires extraction of nucleic acid from a donor plasma or serum.

Amplification: DNA cloning is the term used for making multiple identical copies (clones) of a DNA sequence of interest, the target DNA. The increase in copy number is called amplification. There are several ways of amplification of nucleic acid as listed in Box 17.3. All nucleic acid amplification methods and detection technologies detect the

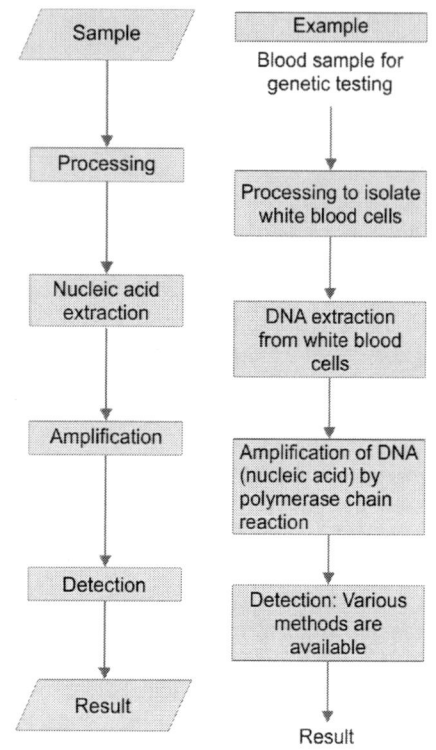

Fig. 17.2: Different steps in nucleic acid amplification test.

Box 17.3: Various techniques of nucleic acid amplification.

- Polymerase chain reaction (PCR)
- Strand displacement assay (SDA)
- Branched DNA (bDNA)
- Transcription mediated assay/amplification (TMA).
- Nucleic acid sequence-based amplification (NASBA).

presence of infectious agents in donor blood by amplifying the nucleic acid sequences specific to the pathogenic microorganism. It has a much higher level of sensitivity and specificity than routine EIA test.

POLYMERASE CHAIN REACTION (PCR AND RT PCR)

It is a powerful, rapid, highly sensitive, simple, molecular biology technique used for *in vitro* (laboratory) to amplify pieces of DNA (nucleic acid) of specific interest. PCR process was first developed in 1984 by Karry Mullis (Nobel Prize, 1993). The polymerase chain reaction (PCR) is a laboratory (*in vitro*) method/**technique for** synthesis (**generating**) **large quantities** of a specific DNA (nucleic acid) sequence. By PCR, large amounts (thousand to **millions of times**) of a specific segment of DNA can be quickly synthesized/**replicated** from a small/minute amount of **genetic material** within a few hours. The **starting genetic material could be a single molecule of rRNA, mRNA of DNA.** In contrast, cloning of DNA needs week to months. Thus, PCR allows rapid and reliable detection of genetic markers of infectious diseases, cancer and genetic disorders. The amplified products obtained by PCR are then analyzed by other methods (refer page 375). One requirement of PCR is that there should be some knowledge of the DNA sequence of the gene that is to be amplified.

Principle of PCR

PCR involves *in vitro* enzymatic amplification of a DNA sequence/fragment (defined target genomic sequence of interest). Identifying of a target sequence is done by using specific oligodeoxynucleotide primers and the amplification to produce millions of copies (amplicons) of the target DNA sequence from template molecule is performed using a DNA polymerase. The amplification products produced during each cycle act as a new template for the successive rounds of amplification.

Steps in PCR (Fig. 17.3)

The **PCR is a cyclical process** and each cycle consists of **three steps.** These are (i) **denaturation of the DNA duplex, (ii) renaturation** and (iii) **synthesis which** are repeated again and again to produce multiple copies of target DNA. The different components of the PCR reaction are mentioned in Table 17.1.

1. **Denaturation of the DNA duplex:** The double-stranded DNA of interest is denatured to separate it into two individual DNA strands (i.e. single-stranded DNA). Double-stranded DNA can be denatured/disrupted by heat or high pH.

2. **Renaturation or primer annealing:** Annealing of primers select the area of the DNA for amplification. The single-stranded

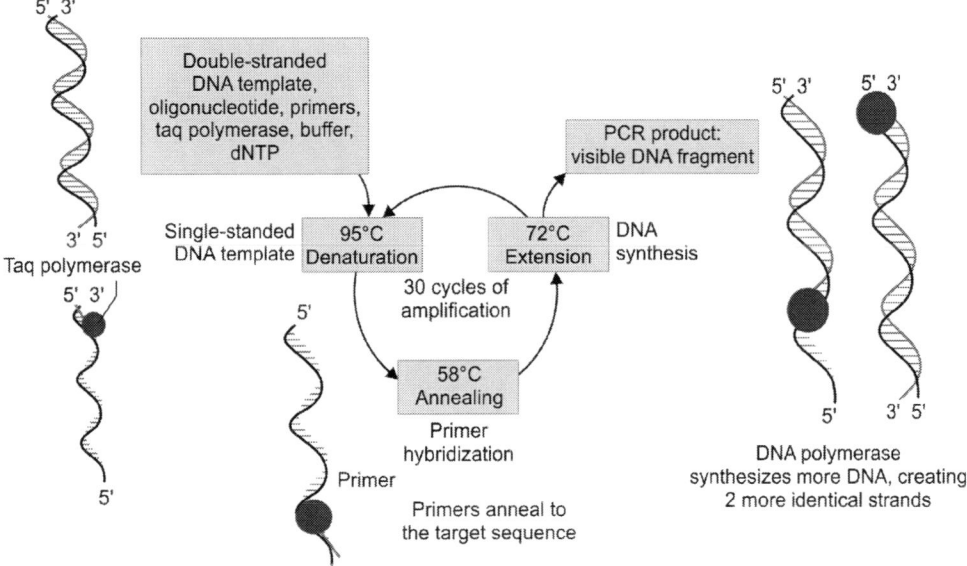

Fig. 17.3: Three steps and typical temperatures for each step in a single PCR cycle. One cycle of PCR amplification is shown. Each cycle consists of three steps: (1) template denaturation, (2) primer annealing, and (3) primer extension. Each step usually occurs over 15–30 seconds and can vary depending on the instrument.

Table 17.1: Components of the polymerase chain reaction (PCR) reaction.

Component	Description
Target DNA	DNA that contains the region of the DNA fragment to be amplified
Taq polymerase	Thermostable enzyme. It catalyzes the replication of template DNA into copies
Primers	Short pieces of single-stranded DNA which are complementary to the opposite strands that flank the target DNA. They amplify the DNA sequence and provide the initiation site on each DNA
Nucleotides	dNTPs (deoxynucleotide triphosphates) are the building blocks for the newly synthesized DNA
$MgCl_2$ and buffer	Maintains proper pH and divalent cations required for the functioning of the enzyme

DNA serves as a template for synthesis of a complementary strand. During the annealing step, oligodeoxynucleotide primers recognize and hybridize (hydrogen bond) to the target sequence contained in the single-stranded template. The primers are synthetic oligonucleotides (21 to 25 nucleotides in length) that are complementary to the 5' region of the single stranded DNA. Each single-stranded DNA template strand is then cooled to permit the primers to anneal to the target DNA in a sequence-specific manner (annealing). These DNA templates hybridize with a primer (renaturation) by replicating enzymes, DNA polymerases.

3. **Primer extension (replication):** In this step, DNA polymerase synthesizes a new DNA strand by extending the 3' ends of the primers. The primer-template duplex in the presence of deoxynucleotide triphosphates (dNTP) and enzyme DNA polymerase (after which the method is named) synthesizes a new copy (complimentary sequence) of the designated DNA sequence. Replication result in a million-fold copies of a specific area of DNA.

PCR system used to amplify segments of DNA are depicted in Figures 17.4A and B.

At the end of each PCR cycle, there is theoretically doubling of the PCR products.

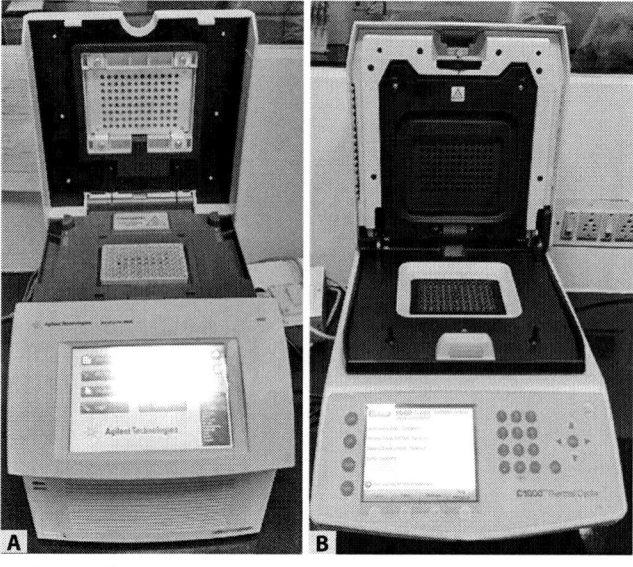

Figs. 17.4A and B: Inside view of PCR system (DNA amplifier) used to amplify segments of DNA via the polymerase chain reaction (PCR): (A) Thermocycler/thermal cycler (qualitative); (B) Thermocycler (quantitative/real time PCR).

Thus, after number of PCR cycles, the target sequence can be amplified two-fold. Each cycle of PCR takes about 3–5 minutes. Amplified product is known as an amplicon.

The whole procedure of PCR is performed in a programmable thermal cycler. This cycler precisely controls the temperature at which the steps occur, the duration of the reaction at the different temperatures, and the number of cycles.

Analysis/Detection of PCR Products

Various methods for analysis of PCR products are available. The method of choice depends on the type of information that is required. **Electrophoretic separation and ethidium bromide staining is the usual method employed**. These include:
- **Agarose gel electrophoresis:** It is most commonly used and it effectively separates DNA products over a wide range of sizes (100 bp to 0.25 kbp).
- **Polyacrylamide gel electrophoresis:** It is the method of choice when greater resolution or separation power is needed, such as in the analysis of very small PCR products (100 bp). DNA products are easily visualized by ultraviolet illumination after ethidium bromide staining.

Reverse-transcriptase Polymerase Chain Reaction

- Original PCR is a technique used for amplification of DNA. Reverse-transcriptase PCR (RT-PCR) was developed if the template of interest is ribonucleic acid (RNA).
- This technique uses an enzyme, namely, reverse transcriptase that works like DNA polymerase but uses RNA as a template and makes RNA/DNA complex. Then replaces the RNA with DNA. The resulting strand is referred to as cDNA or complementary DNA. After the cDNA strand is made from the RNA template, the remaining cycles can be carried out with DNA polymerases, using standard PCR protocols.
- RT-PCR basically consists of four-steps: (1) RNA isolation, (2) reverse transcription, (3) PCR amplification and (4) PCR product analysis.

Branched DNA

Branched DNA (bDNA) detection is a sensitive signal amplification technique. Branched DNA is used most often to quantify viral nucleic acids from clinical specimens. The technique is available for quantification of RNA from hepatitis C virus and HIV and quantification of DNA from hepatitis B virus. It is a solid-phase, sandwich hybridization assay in which multiple target-specific probes (sets of synthetic oligonucleotide probes) are used. These multiple target-specific probes capture the target nucleic acid on to the surface of a solid support mechanism, such as a microtiter well/tray.

Steps (Fig. 17.5)

Capture probes: A branched DNA assay begins with a solid-phase microtiter well. The well is covered with small, single-stranded DNA molecules called capture probe DNA molecules (**capture probes microwell**).

Capture extender (capture probes solution): Next capture extender is added. Each capture extender has two domains; one that hybridizes to the capture probe and one that "hangs out" in the air. The capture extender has two purposes: (i) it creates more available surface area for target DNA molecules to bind and (ii) it allows the assay to be easily adapted to detect a variety of target DNA molecules.

Adding the test sample: The test sample is then added to the microtiter well. The capture probe along with capture extender binds to the target molecules in the sample.

Target probe: Next second set of target-specific probes is added. The target probes binds to a different region of the target nucleic acid in the sample than the capture probes.

Target/label extender: Then a second extender, namely, target/label extender is

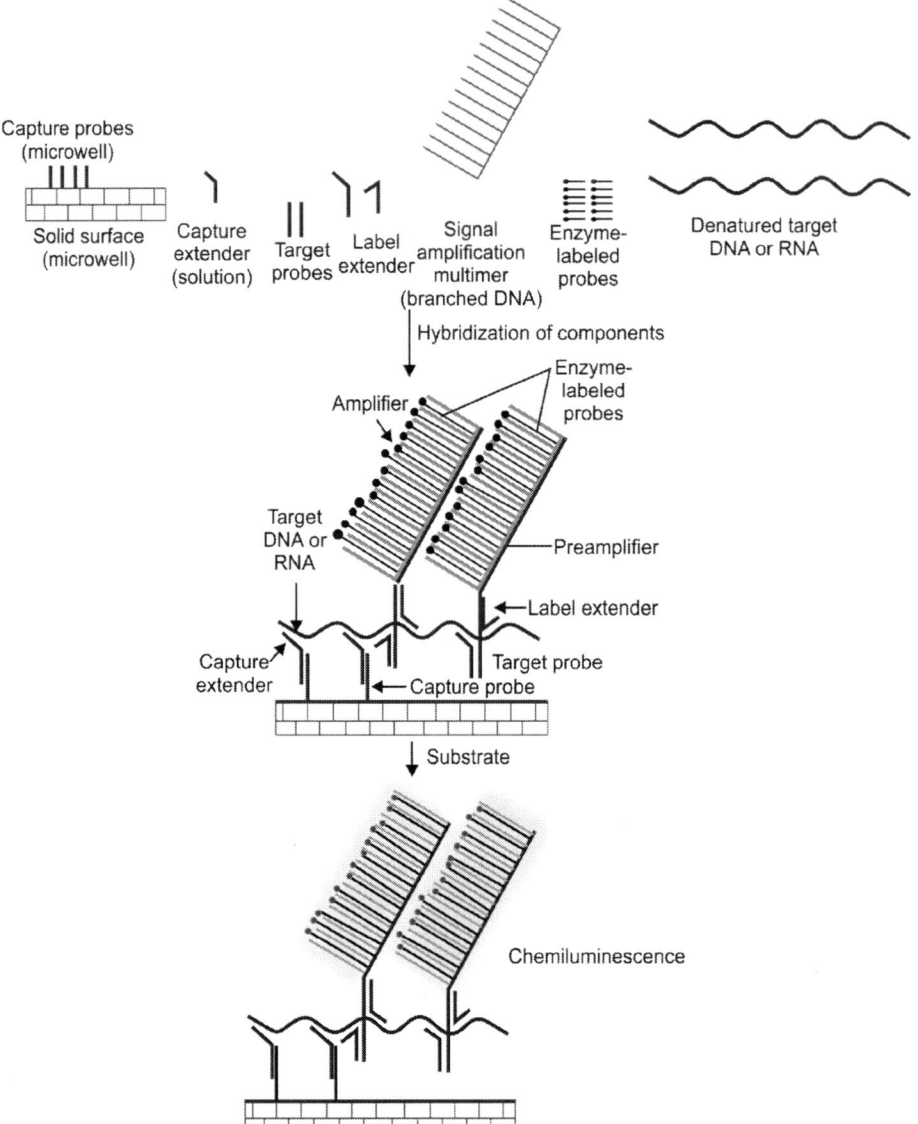

Fig. 17.5: Different steps involved in branched DNA (bDNA).

added. This label extender has two domains (similar to the first capture extender): one that hybridizes to the target and other to a pre-amplified molecule.

Preamplifier molecule: Preamplifier molecules/probes have two domains. First, it binds to the second set of target probes and label extender and second, it binds up to eight bDNA amplifiers.

Amplifier molecule: The amplifier molecule/probe is the key in this technique. The amplifier molecule is a DNA molecule (set of oligonucleotide chain) with 15 identical branches. The amplifier probes are then added which bind to the preamplifier probes. This forms a branched DNA structure. Finally, probes labeled with alkaline phosphatase (AP) are added. Each branch of the amplifier binds/hybridizes to three alkaline-phosphatase (AP)-labeled probes. At this stage, signal amplification takes place.

Detection: Next step is detection of the bound labeled (e.g. alkaline-phosphatase-labeled) probes. It is done by incubating the complex with an enzyme-triggerable substrate, dioxetane, and chemiluminescence results. The light emitted is collected by an analyzer, measured in a luminometer, and reported as light units. The signal generated is directly proportional to the amount/quantity of target nucleic acid present in the test sample. This is determined from an external standard curve.

Various steps are summarized as follows: Base → capture probe → capture extender → target → target probe → label extender → pre-amplifier → amplifier.

Background signals: It may be produced due to nonspecific hybridization of any of the amplification probes and nontarget nucleic acids. In third-generation bDNA assays, increased target-specific amplification without any increase in background was achieved by incorporating the nonnatural bases isocytidine (isoC) and isoguanosine (isoG) in the amplification probes. This also greatly enhances the detection limits. IsoC and isoG bases pair with each other but not with any of the four naturally occurring bases of genetic material.

Uses: Branched-DNA (bDNA) technology is used for the detection and quantitation of pathogens such as HIV-1 RNA, HBV, DNA, and hepatitis C virus (HCV) RNA.

TRANSCRIPTION-BASED AMPLIFICATION

Transcription is the process by which the information in a strand of DNA is copied into a new molecule of messenger RNA (mRNA). Transcription-based amplification converts RNA into DNA and then use the DNA as a template for transcription of multiple copies of RNA. These methods include: **(i) transcription-mediated amplification (TMA) and (ii) nucleic acid sequence-based amplification (NASBA)**. Both TMA and NASBA are isothermal (operates at a single temperature) nucleic acid amplification techniques and do not require any thermal cycler. Both are essentially similar to retroviral replication *in vitro*. They convert RNA into DNA and then use the DNA as a template for transcription of multiple copies of RNA.

Process: The process begins with release of an RNA target. Since RNA is single-stranded in most cases, there is no need for thermal denaturation (required only when double stranded) of the template before amplification. Then a sequence-specific DNA primer is added which binds to the RNA target. Reverse transcriptase then extends the primer and produces a DNA-RNA heteroduplex. The 5' end of the sequence specific primer contains the promoter for a T7 bacteriophage polymerase. This synthesizes a DNA strand complementary to the initial RNA target.

- **Transcription-mediated amplification (TMA)**: It uses two enzymes, namely, reverse transcriptase and T7 RNA polymerase. In TMA, **the degradation of the initial RNA template is caused by the reverse transcriptase enzyme itself**. The degradation occurs as it synthesizes its complementary DNA.
- **Nucleic acid sequence-based amplification (NASBA):** It uses three enzymes, namely, reverse transcriptase, RNAseH, and T7 RNA polymerase. In NASBA, the **degradation of the initial RNA template is caused by** a separate enzyme called **RNAseH**. RNAseH selectively cuts off the RNA portion from the DNA-RNA heteroduplex but it cannot degrade RNA alone.

Advantages of TMA and NASBA: They have distinct advantages over other RNA amplification techniques.
- **No need of initial denaturation** for the amplification. This will prevent denaturation of dsDNA sequences and DNA cannot bind to primers. Hence, NASBA and TMA eliminate the problem of DNA contamination giving rise to falsely elevated RNA.
- **No need for sophisticated thermocyclers**: These methods are isothermal processes

and occur at a single temperature. Hence, there is no need for thermocyclers because of the whole process.
- **Prevent cross-contamination of amplicon in the laboratory:** This technique can be combined with molecular beacons or other sequence-specific probes. These can be added directly to the amplification mixture and create a closed-tube system. This will prevent cross-contamination amplicon in the laboratory.

Uses: NASBA and TMA have a wide variety of clinical qualitative and quantitative applications especially in infectious diseases such as detection of *Neisseria gonorrhoeae, Chlamydia trachomatis, Trichomonas vaginalis,* and human papilloma virus (HPV). They are also used for **viral load tests in HIV-1 and HCV.**

SUMMARY

- Nucleic acid testing (NAT) or nucleic acid amplification test (NAAT) is a molecular-based method of screening for infectious agents.
- It helps in identifying very low levels of virus even during window period.
- In this method, first nucleic acid is extracted from the donor's serum, followed by its implication either by polymerase chain reaction or transcription-based amplification.

SELF-ASSESSMENT EXERCISE

Write short essays/notes on:
- NAT in blood banking
- Merits of NAT over serological methods.
- Nucleic acid technology in blood donor screening
- What is the role of NAT in transfusion medicine?

CHAPTER 18

Hemolytic Disease of Newborn

CHAPTER OUTLINE

- Etiopathogenesis of HDFN
- Rh (D) hemolytic disease of the fetus and newborn
- Antenatal management of Rh immunization
- Postnatal management of infant
- Prevention of Rh (D) HDFN
- ABO hemolytic disease of fetus and newborn
- Alloantibodies causing hemolytic disease of the fetus and newborn other than anti-D

INTRODUCTION

Definition: Hemolytic disease of the fetus and newborn (HDFN) also known as erythroblastosis fetalis is the destruction of the red blood cells (RBCs) of a fetus (in utero) and/or neonate (after delivery) by red cell IgG antibodies produced by the mother.

Salient Features of HDFN

Premature destruction of the fetal red blood cells: Maternal IgG antibodies that are directed against fetal antigens, cross the placenta, sensitize fetal red cells, and shorten red cell survival. The destruction of fetal red cells by maternal IgG antibodies leads to hyperbilirubinemia. It is commonly also known as **hemolytic disease of the newborn** (HDN).

Range of HDFN clinical presentation: This premature red cell destruction results in disease that can range from a clinically unaffected newborn (mild anemia) with a positive direct antiglobulin test (DAT) result to severe anemia and occasionally death of fetus in utero.

Conditions that cause antibody production: The mother can be stimulated to form the antibodies by **previous pregnancy, transfusion or transplantation** and sometimes during the second and third trimester of pregnancy.

Types of antibody: Most of the HDFN were caused by antibodies in the mother directed against the **Rh antigen D**, or **Rh (D)**. However, the incidence of HDFN caused by anti-D has decreased with the introduction of **Rh-immune globulin** (RhIG). Other causes of HDFN are listed in Box 18.1.

Classification of HDFN

Hemolytic disease of the fetus and newborn is classified into three categories depending on antibody specificity: Rh (D), ABO, and other antibodies (Box 18.1).

Role of Transfusion Service in HDFN

It plays an important role in the **prediction, diagnosis, treatment**, and **prevention** of this potentially life-threatening disease. Depending on the period which the test is done to prevent or predict HDFN, following terms are used:

- **Prenatal** (time period before birth), **antenatal** (time period before birth), **and antepartum** (period between conception and onset of labor with reference to the mother): These are the terms used to refer the testing done before delivery.

Box 18.1: Classification of hemolytic disease of the fetus and newborn (HDFN) based on the specificity of IgG antibodies.

- Rh (D) hemolytic disease of fetus and newborn caused by:
  o Anti-D alone
  o Other Rh antibodies: Anti-D in combination with anti-c, anti-E, anti-C, or anti-e
- ABO hemolytic disease of fetus and newborn caused by anti-A, anti-B in group O woman
- Antibodies against antigens in other blood group systems. For example, anti-K, anti-k, anti-Fy^a, anti-Jk^a, anti-Jk^b, anti-N, anti-S, anti-s).

- **Neonatal testing:** This refers to testing done in the newborn up to 28 days after delivery.
- **Perinatal period** extends from 28 weeks of gestation to 28 days after delivery

ETIOPATHOGENESIS OF HDFN

Role of placenta during pregnancy includes:
- Placenta functions as the site of **exchange for oxygen, nutrient, and waste material**.
- Placenta also **acts as a barrier between maternal and fetal circulations**. During pregnancy, the placental barrier limits the entry of the number of fetal red cells into the maternal circulation and thereby reduces the chances of antibody production.

Protection by ABO incompatibility: ABO incompatibility between mother and fetus can also provide additional protection against immunization. In such situations, the maternal antibodies (anti-A or anti-B) cause intravascular hemolysis of ABO incompatible fetal red cells. This destruction of fetal RBCs reduces exposure to fetal red cells carrying foreign antigens to the mother.

HDFN results from blood group incompatibility between mother and fetus. In HDFN, the destruction of the RBCs of a fetus is caused by antibodies produced by the mother.

Sequence of events during delivery: At the time of delivery, the placenta gets separated from the mother's uterus. At this period, a significant number of fetal red cells escape into the maternal circulation due to **Fetomaternal hemorrhage** (FMH)]. If there is incompatibility (ABO or Rh) between mother and fetus, fetal red cells escaped into mother can stimulate the production of antibody by mother's immune system.

Antigenic Exposure during Gestation and at Delivery

Variable numbers of incompatible fetal RBCs may enter the maternal circulation during gestation or delivery. If the fetal red cells carry antigens that are different from the mother (paternal antigens), then they can stimulate an active immune response in the mother. This results in the production of IgG antibodies in the mother.
- **During gestation:** Immunization can result from fetal red cell exposure during gestation and can be caused by **fetomaternal hemorrhage**.
  – Minor **fetomaternal hemorrhage** (FMH) spontaneously occurs in many women during gestation. During gestation, transplacental hemorrhage of fetal RBCs into the maternal circulation can occur in up to 7% of women.
  – Fetomaternal hemorrhage **can also occur during trauma to the abdomen**, placenta previa, abruptio placentae, ectopic pregnancy, interventions such as amniocentesis, fetal blood sampling or cordocentesis (procedure that punctures the umbilical vein at the point of placental insertion and aspirates a sample of fetal blood), chorionic villus sampling and intrauterine manipulations, or spontaneous or induced abortion.
- **During delivery:** Fetomaternal hemorrhage occurs in more than 50% when the placenta separates from the uterus.

Alloimmunization in the mother: After the entry of incompatible fetal red cells (with antigen) into the maternal circulation, the maternal immune system forms red cell antibody and is called causes alloimmunization. Alloimmunization can also result from transfusion of incompatible red cells. This causes formation of IgG antibodies.

Consequences during Subsequent Pregnancies in Mother

During subsequent pregnancies, IgG antibodies formed during alloimmunization in the maternal circulation cross the placental barrier by an active transport mechanism. Only the immunoglobulin G (IgG) type antibodies can be actively transported across the placenta whereas other immunoglobulin classes (e.g. IgA and IgM) are not transported. Normally, most IgG antibodies are directed against bacterial, fungal, and viral antigens. Hence, the transfer of these IgG antibodies from the mother to the fetus is beneficial (but not IgG antibodies against RBCs). IgM antibodies are not implicated in HDFN as they do not cross the placenta. D antigen is the most important cause. As little as 0.1 mL to 1 mL of D-positive red cells can stimulate production of alloantibody.

Consequences during Pregnancy (i.e. before Delivery) (Fig.18.1A).

- **Hemolysis:** Maternal IgG antibodies that have crossed the placenta, bind to the corresponding antigens present on the fetal red cells. In HDFN, the antigens on the fetal RBCs are inherited from the father. These IgG antibody coated fetal red cells are removed from the circulation by the macrophages (fetal monocyte-macrophage system) of the fetal spleen and liver. This results in **immune destruction of fetal red cells** (hemolysis) in the fetal spleen and liver. The rate of RBC destruction depends on antibody titer and specificity and on the number of antigenic sites on the fetal RBCs.
- **Hyperbilirubinemia:** Large amount of **hemoglobin is liberated** from the hemolyzed fetal red cells. It is metabolized to unconjugated bilirubin and form complexes with albumin in the blood. The **unconjugated bilirubin** (bound to albumin) **is transported across the placenta** to the mother. In the mother, unconjugated **bilirubin is converted to conjugated bilirubin by** glucuronyl transferase in **the maternal liver** and becomes water soluble and harmless. The conjugated bilirubin is excreted by the mother into the GI tract. This prevents marked increase in total plasma bilirubin level in the fetal circulation and amniotic fluid even with severe hemolysis. Hence, they do not produce any clinical disease in the fetus.
- **Anemia:** As fetal red cell destruction (hemolysis) continues, **the fetus becomes increasingly anemic.**
- **Accelerated erythropoiesis:** The fetal liver and spleen increases (accelerates) erythropoiesis (increased production of red cells) in an effort to compensate for the anemia due to red cell destruction. This caused enlargement of liver and spleen (hepatosplenomegaly) and both show increase in the hematopoietic tissues. The increased erythropoiesis releases immature red cells (**erythroblasts**—nucleated cells) into the fetal circulation. The term *erythroblastosis fetalis* was used to describe this finding of erythroblasts in a fetus.
- **Hydrops fetalis:** The clinical severity of HDFN can range from serologic abnormalities detected in an asymptomatic to infant intrauterine death. In severe cases, severe anemia due to hemolysis and hypoproteinemia due to decreased hepatic production of plasma proteins (decreased albumin synthesis and decreased colloid osmotic pressure) lead to the development of high-output cardiac failure (secondary to severe anemia). This will result in generalized edema, effusions (fluid accumulation in fetal pleural cavities), and ascites (fluid accumulation in fetal peritoneum). These features are

characteristics of condition called **hydrops fetalis** (edema in the fetus). The cardiac failure is the greatest threat to the fetus. Anemia can also lead to tissue hypoxia and death in utero (stillbirth).

Consequences after Delivery (Fig. 18.1B).

- **Hemolysis after birth**: After delivery, the newborn infant faces a different challenge. The destruction of RBC continues even after the delivery of such an infant if alive. It can continue till there is presence of maternal antibody in the circulation of newborn infant. After the delivery of child, there is no additional entry of maternal antibody through the placenta into the infant's circulation. Hence, there is decreased rate of destruction of fetal RBC after birth. However, IgG is distributed both extravascularly and intravascularly and has a half-life of 25 days. This leads to continuation of antibody binding and hemolysis of RBCs for several days to weeks after delivery.
- **Hyperbilirubinemia**: In utero, unconjugated bilirubin is conjugated in the maternal liver and excreted by the mother without any damage to fetus. Red cell destruction continues in the newborn releases unconjugated bilirubin. The unconjugated bilirubin binds to albumin and transported to infant's liver. After birth, the infant becomes dependent on its own hepatic glucuronyl transferase (the liver enzyme needed to convert unconjugated bilirubin to conjugated bilirubin) for conjugation of bilirubin. The glucuronyl transferase enzyme is poorly developed at birth. The newborn infant's liver cannot conjugate efficiently (especially in premature infants), the unconjugated bilirubin produced by RBC destruction.

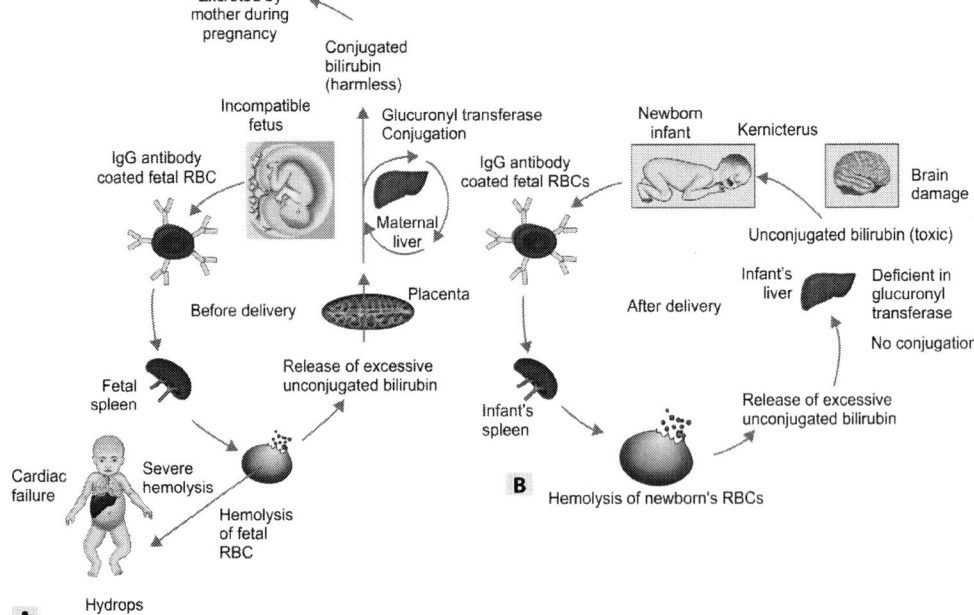

Figs. 18.1A and B: Metabolism of bilirubin in hemolytic disease of fetus and newborn: (A) Before delivery, the bilirubin released from the breakdown of sensitized red cells in the fetal spleen is safely metabolized by the maternal liver; (B) After delivery, the newborn's liver cannot produce glucuronyl transferase and therefore not able to convert toxic unconjugated bilirubin to harmless, water soluble and excretable conjugated form. This leads to excessive collection of unconjugated bilirubin in tissues and causes brain damage.

- **Kernicterus:** When the levels of unconjugated bilirubin increase to a level that exceeds the binding capacity of the albumin, unconjugated bilirubin binds to tissues and results in jaundice. When there is moderate to severe hemolysis, the unconjugated bilirubin may reach about more than 18 to 20 mg/dL, it is toxic to central nervous system. If not treated, this toxic level can cross through CSF because of poorly formed blood–brain barrier (BBB) and reach to the infant's brain. In the brain, it may bind with tissues of the central nervous system (CNS) and cause permanent damage to parts of the brain (**kernicterus**). This results in deafness, mental retardation, or death.

Basic factors required for the development of HDFN

Three important factors are needed for the development of HDFN. These are as follows:
- **IgG type of antibody (Fig. 18.2):** The red cell antibody produced by the mother must be of the IgG types. Only IgG type is capable of crossing the placental barrier. This active transport across the placenta depends on the fragment, crystallizable, or Fc portion of the immunoglobulin molecule. IgM antibodies (e.g. anti-Lea, anti-Leb, anti-M, anti-N, and anti-P1) do not cause HDFN.

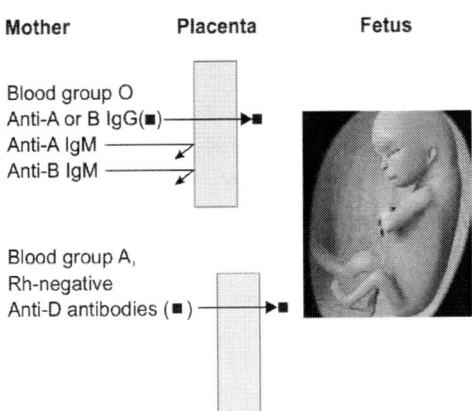

Fig. 18.2: IgG antibodies can cross placenta whereas IgM antibodies cannot cross placenta.

- **Fetus must possess an antigen that is lacking in the mother:** The gene for the antigen in the fetus for HDFN is inherited from the father. If the father is homozygous for the gene, all his children inherit the gene and have a risk for HDFN. If the father is heterozygous, only 50% of the children may inherit the gene and are at risk.
- **Fetal antigen must be well developed at birth:** Some blood group antigens (e.g. Lewis, P1, and I) are not well developed at birth. Antibodies to these antigens cannot cause HDFN because the antigen is not available to bind with the maternal antibody.

Rh (D) HEMOLYTIC DISEASE OF THE FETUS AND NEWBORN

Definition: Hemolysis of Rh-D antigen positive fetal RBCs caused by IgG Rh D antibodies acquired through the placenta from a sensitized RhD-negative mother.
- The antigen that most frequently cause alloimmunization is D antigen of the Rh blood group system. The anti-D IgG antibodies are the main cause of severe HDFN. D antigen is a potent immunogen. HDFN develops if father is Rh-positive (D+), mother is Rh-negative (D-) and fetus is Rh-positive (D+). Isoimmunization of Rh (D) negative mother may occur due to Rh (D) positive pregnancy or transfusion of Rh-positive blood.
- First pregnancy (first-born) Rh-positive infant of a Rh-negative mother is usually not affected by Rh(D) HDFN because the mother has not yet been immunized.

Mechanism of Immunization of Rh-negative Mother (Figs. 18.3A to D and Flowchart 18.1)

Antigenic exposure during gestation and at delivery: Variable numbers of fetal RBCs may enter the maternal circulation during gestation or delivery (refer earlier under pathogenesis).

In most cases, D-negative mothers become alloimmunized or sensitized at delivery in the first pregnancy with a D-positive baby.

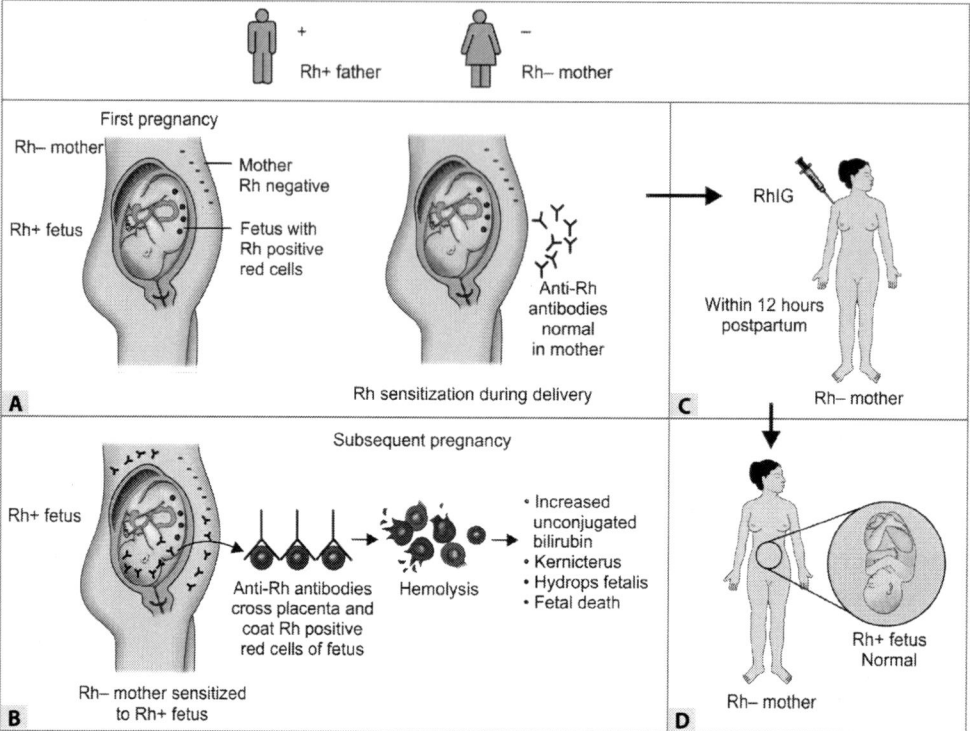

Figs. 18.3A to D: Pathogenesis of fetal Rh hemolytic disease of the newborn caused by Rh incompatibility: (A) During the first pregnancy involving an Rh (D) negative mother and Rh (D) positive fetus, fetal red cells will circulate in mother after delivery or rarely during pregnancy; (B) If mother is not given RhIG, mother can mount an immune response to the fetal red cells and form anti-D. In the subsequent pregnancy with Rh (D) incompatibility, the maternal IgG antibodies cross the placenta and enter fetal circulation. Rh (D) positive fetal red cells will become sensitized and destroyed by the maternal anti-D; (C) If within 12 hours of delivery RhIG is given to the mother, there will not be sensitization in the mother; (D) The subsequent pregnancy in a mother who has been given RhIG will be normal.

It is very rare to demonstrate HDFN in the first pregnancy.

Immunization of Rh-negative mother: If the fetal red cells are Rh-positive because of inheritance of D antigen from the father, the fetal D+ red cells released either during gestation or delivery enters the circulation of Rh-negative mother. It usually occurs in the last trimester and during delivery. The production of anti-D by mother occurs weeks later. In most of the cases, the volume of fetomaternal hemorrhage is small. However, hemorrhage as little as 1 mL of fetal RBCs can immunize the mother. The D antigens stimulate the production of anti-D in the mother and the mother becomes immunized to D antigen. Immunization can also result from transfusion of incompatible Rh-positive red cells to Rh-negative mother.

Consequences: After production of anti-D by the mother, subsequent D-positive fetuses are affected to varying degrees.

- **Mild affection:** In mild cases, the maternal anti-D binds to fetal D-positive red cells and causes a positive direct antiglobulin test (DAT). The signs of red cell destruction are minimal.
- **Moderate affection:** These infants develop jaundice with raised bilirubin levels during the first few days of life.
- **Severe affection:** These D-positive infants, show rapid red cell destruction, anemia in utero. They develop jaundice within hours of delivery. Exchange transfusion may be

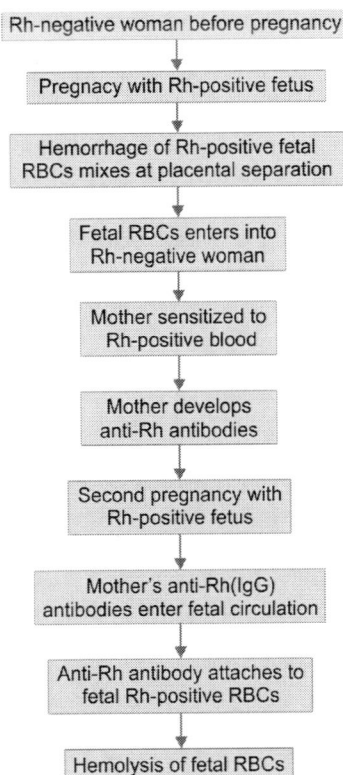

Flowchart 18.1: Sequence of events in erythroblastosis fetalis.

antigens of paternal origin present on the Rh-positive red cells of fetus (and absent from the maternal cells).

Consequences during subsequent pregnancies in mother are discussed in detail on page 381.

Factors affecting immunization and severity of HDFN: Factors affecting the production of Rh antibodies and severity of HDFN include host factors, immunoglobulin class, antibody specificity, and influence of the ABO group.

1. **Amount of fetomaternal hemorrhage:** A small amount of fetal RBCs may enter the maternal circulation in the 3rd trimester, but this quantity is not sufficient to cause antibody production in the mother.
   - **First pregnancy:** During normal delivery, transplacental hemorrhage is not uncommon. At this time, about 1 mL to 10 mL or more fetal blood can enter the mother's circulation. The entry of these Rh (D) positive fetal RBCs into the circulation of Rh-negative mother can stimulate the production of anti-Rh (D) in about 5–9% of the Rh-negative mothers. This anti-D are found in the maternal circulation within 6 months of delivery and about 7–12% of these mothers becomes sensitized. But they may not show demonstrable levels of antibodies till they come across secondary antigen stimulus during subsequent pregnancy.
   - **Subsequent pregnancy:** During the next pregnancy with a Rh (D) positive fetus, the small numbers of D positive fetal red cells can enter the maternal circulation in the 3rd trimester (from about 24th week of gestation). They cause a secondary immune response in the sensitized mother. This results in either sensitized mother to produce antibody or cause rapid increase in the titer of existing anti-D. Since anti-D is IgG, it can cross the placenta into fetal circulation. It combines with Rh (D) positive fetal red cells and causes hemolysis.

required to reduce bilirubin levels and to prevent development of kernicterus after delivery.

Prevention of immunization of Rh-negative mother: Anti-D formation in mother can be prevented with anti-D immunization immediately after birth. The introduction of Rh immune globulin (RhIG) in 1968 has reduced the incidence of Rh HDFN. Rh immune globulin (RhIG) is a human-source gamma globulin consisting of high-titered anti-D. It is used in preventing alloimmunization to the D antigen in Rh-negative mother.

Effect of the maternal antibody on the fetus and its consequences: Once the Rh-negative mother is immunized, all her subsequent offsprings who inherit the D antigen will be affected. In the next pregnancy (if baby is Rh+) the maternal IgG anti-D (alloantibody) crosses the placenta and binds to (coats) the specific

2. **Host factors:** The ability of individuals to produce antibodies in response to antigenic exposure varies.
   - *Parity:* Usually the first pregnancy is not affected by HDFN and in about 70% of cases, it develops in 2nd and 3rd pregnancy.
3. **Zygosity of father:** If father is heterozygous for the implicated antibody, there is 50% possibility of child being affected by Rh-HDFN. If father is homozygous for the implicated antibody, there is 100% possibility of child being affected by Rh-HDFN.
4. **Immunoglobulin class/type:** The severity of the HDFN depends on immunoglobulin class and subclass of the maternal antibody. Of the different classes of immunoglobulin (i.e. IgG, IgM, IgA, IgE, and IgD), only IgG (all subclasses of IgG) can cross the placenta. The active transport of IgG across the placenta begins in the second trimester and continues till birth. Of the four subclasses of IgG antibody, the more efficient hemolysis of RBC is caused by IgG_1 and IgG_3 rather than IgG_2 and IgG_4.
5. **Antibody specificity:**
   - **D antigen:** Of all the RBC antigens, D is the most antigenic and is the most important cause of HDFN. Hence, if transfusion is needed to Rh-negative females during childbearing period, it is essential to transfuse only Rh-negative blood.
   - **Other antigens:** Other antigens in the Rh system, namely C, E, and c, are also potent immunogens (although less than D) and can cause HDFN. Of the non-Rh system antibodies, anti-Kell can cause clinically significant HDFN. **Kell antigens** are found on immature erythroid cells in the bone marrow. Hence, in HDFN due to anti-Kell, there is not only destruction of circulating RBCs but also the precursors producing severe anemia.
6. **Effect/influence of ABO incompatibility between mother and fetus:** If the mother is ABO incompatible with the fetus (major incompatibility), there is **decreased incidence of Rh immunization**. Thus, ABO incompatibility likely to protect against Rh immunization. This may be due to the destruction of Rh (D) positive fetal red cells immediately as they enter the maternal circulation by maternal ABO alloantibodies (anti-A and anti-B). This occurs before they can sensitize the mother.
   - **History of blood transfusion:** It is very important to avoid transfusing Rh-positive blood/components to Rh-negative females of childbearing age. This is because anti-D stimulated by transfusion can cause severe HDFN even in the first pregnancy with a D positive fetus. Rh antigen load is much greater in transfusion. The immunization in Rh-negative women is greater with transfusion than previous Rh-positive pregnancy.
7. **Medical termination of pregnancy (MTP) or miscarriage:** These can also immunize Rh-negative mother.

Diagnosis and Management

Serologic Testing of the Mother (Prenatal/Antenatal Evaluation of Rh-HDFN)

Purpose: Prenatal or antepartum testing has two purposes:
1. To identify D-negative women with a high risk of delivering a baby with Rh HDFN and who require RhIG.
2. To identify women with antibodies capable of causing HDFN. This helps to assess the risk to the fetus.

Serologic and clinical tests of mother should be carried out at appropriate times during the pregnancy. Usually investigation should be started at about 12th week (first trimester) of pregnancy or the first prenatal / antenatal visit.

Recommended investigations (Table 18.1): These include performing the ABO and D phenotyping and antibody screen. These can accurately determine the level of antibody in the maternal circulation, the potential

Table 18.1: Prenatal testing to identify women at risk of hemolytic disease of the fetus and newborn.

Time period of performing test	Nature of investigation
Initial visit	• ABO grouping and Rh typing • Antibody screen for IgG antibodies • If antibody screen is positive, identify the antibody and antibody titration for IgG antibodies
Follow-up visits (if IgG antibody was identified during initial visit)	• To exclude other clinically antibodies—select reagent cell panel • Perform antibody titration at an interval of 2–4 weeks

26–28 weeks gestation	• Confirm Rh typing
	• Repeat antibody screening:
	  – Before starting Rh immune globulin (RhIG) in Rh-negative mother
	  – In third trimester if mother was previously transfused or gives history of unexpected antibodies

of the antibody to cause HDFN, and the severity of RBC destruction during gestation. Thus, they will help to estimate degree of involvement for proper management. If clinical and serologic data indicate that the fetus is becoming severely anemic, interventions (e.g. intrauterine transfusion) can be used to treat the anemia and prevent the development of severe disease.

Assessment of Rh-HDFN

A. Detailed history:
1. **Obstetric history**: A detailed obstetric history of previous pregnancies and their outcomes should be obtained. These include bad obstetric history (hydrops fetalis, stillbirth or HDFN, etc.) or earlier Rh immunization. Previous severe disease and poor outcome predict similar findings in the present pregnancy. If a woman who gives a history of HDFN secondary to anti-D, a subsequent D-positive fetus has a more chance of being affected. If there is a history of a previously affected infant, it will be useful in predicting the prognosis for future pregnancies.
2. **History of prior blood transfusion**: If Rh-negative women are transfused with Rh-positive blood, it may immunize the women.

B. Investigations:
1. **ABO and Rh grouping:** The prenatal specimen must be typed for ABO and Rh including D^u grouping.
2. **Antibody screening**: On the first antenatal visit, sera of both Rh (D) positive and Rh (D) negative women should be screened for red cell antibodies. This is because some IgG antibodies (e.g. Kell, Duffy, Kidd, Ss) can also cause HDFN and may be seen in Rh (D) positive women. The antibody screening method must be able to detect clinically significant IgG alloantibodies that are reactive at 37°C and in the antiglobulin phase. On the first visit, screening for IgG antibody(ies) should be done with at least two separate "O" group screening cells covering all common blood group antigens (preferably homozygous), should be used. They should be tested by indirect antiglobulin test, using polyspecific antiglobulin serum and by two stage enzyme technique (greater sensitivity). For tube testing, an antibody-enhancing medium [e.g. polyethylene glycol (PeG) or low-ionic strength solution (LISS)] can increase sensitivity of the assay. If the antibody screen is nonreactive, it is advisable to repeat the test before giving RhIG therapy in Rh-negative prenatal patients and in the third trimester if the patient has been transfused or has a history of unexpected antibodies.
3. **If antibody(ies) is/are found at any stage then following should be performed:**
   i. **Antibody titration**: The **antibody titration** determines the relative

concentration of all antibodies capable of crossing the placenta and causing HDFN. In this test, the patient serum or plasma is serially diluted and tested against appropriate RBCs to determine the highest dilution at which a reaction occurs. The method must include the indirect antiglobulin phase using anti-IgG reagent. The result is expressed as either the reciprocal of the titration endpoint or as a titer score. Antibody titration should be performed in the first trimester, served as baseline and this specimen should be frozen for future testing. Severity of the disease is usually but not always correlated with the titer of the antibody titer and titer should be repeated every month. Only a difference of more than 2 dilutions, or a score change of more than 10 (16 is considered the critical titer), is considered a significant change in titer. A titer of 1:32 or above and a rising titer at repeated testing is important. A titer repeatedly at 32 or above is an indication for color Doppler imaging to assess middle cerebral artery peak systolic velocity (MCA-PSV) after 16 weeks' gestation. It is an indication for amniocentesis. When the titer is below 32, it should be repeated at 4-week intervals, beginning at 16–20 weeks' gestation and then every 2–4 weeks during the third trimester. Follow-up should be done when the titer is more than 8. Antibody titer alone cannot predict severity of HDFN. Though antibody titters are useful in assessing the extent of intrauterine fetal anemia during the first affected pregnancy, antibody titers are less predictive in subsequent pregnancies.

ii. Identify the antibody(ies) with 8–10 cell panel (refer pages 198, 199).

iii. Perform Rh phenotype to confirm the implicated antibody.

4. **Paternal phenotype and genotype: Father's probable Rh genotype**—specimen of the father's blood should be obtained and the father's RBCs are tested with anti-D, C, E, c, and e to determine Rh phenotype.

5. **Fetal DNA testing:** If the mother has anti-D and the father is likely to be heterozygous for the D antigen, D typing the fetus can be done using polymerase chain reaction to amplify DNA obtained from amniocentesis or chorionic villous sampling. It can be performed as early as 10–12 weeks' gestation. During the second trimester, the fetal genotyping may be determined by testing plasma of the mother. Testing can be done for the genes coding c, e, C, E, K, Fya, Fyb, Jk^a, Jk^b, M, and others.

6. **Antibody-dependent cell-mediated cytotoxicity (ADCC) test**: There is correlation between ADCC and severity of HDFN. A high ADCC indicates serious HDFN.

7. **Color Doppler middle cerebral artery peak systolic velocity:** Further diagnosis and treatment are started at about 16–20 weeks' gestation. Earlier intervention is needed for patients with a history of a severely affected fetus or early fetal death. The fetal **middle cerebral artery peak systolic velocity** (MCA-PSV) can be measured using color Doppler ultrasonography. Color Doppler indicates the direction of blood flow, using red for arterial flow and blue for venous flow. The middle cerebral artery is used because of its easy accessibility. MCA-PSV is noninvasive procedure which can reliably predict anemia in the fetus and does not produce any adverse effects for the fetus. The peak systolic (arterial) velocity is plotted on a standardized graph to determine the critical point for cordocentesis.

8. **Cordocentesis (percutaneous umbilical blood sampling):** It is a procedure in which clinicians obtain a

sample of fetal blood using advanced sonography. The umbilical vein is visualized at the level of the cord insertion into the placenta by using high-resolution ultrasound with color Doppler enhancement of blood flow. A sample of the fetal blood is obtained by inserting a spinal needle into the umbilical vein. The fetal blood sample can be tested for hemoglobin, hematocrit, bilirubin, blood type, direct antiglobulin test (DAT), and antigen phenotype, and genotype.

9. **Amniocentesis**: Amniotic fluid is normally almost colorless and in a fetus with severe hemolysis it appears bright yellow due to the presence of bilirubin.

    Procedure: Amniocentesis is usually performed between 28th weeks and 32nd weeks of gestation. Amniotic fluid is obtained by USG-guided amniocentesis by inserting needle through abdominal wall into the uterine cavity.

    Indications for amniocentesis: (a) Titer of maternal IgG by IAT is 1:32 or above or a rising titer on repeated testing by about 28 weeks of gestation, (b) previous obstetric history of stillbirth, hydrops fetalis or neonatal death in Rh (D) negative mothers.

    Significance: The amniotic fluid obtained by amniocentesis is tested for bilirubin by spectrophotometry. The concentration of bilirubin pigment in amniotic fluid indicates the extent of fetal hemolysis and helps in predicting the degree of hemolytic process in pregnancy and severity of HDFN. High values indicate severe and often life-threatening hemolysis (fetal hemoglobin less than 8 g/dL) and needs urgent intervention. Based on amniotic fluid analysis, three options exist: (i) allow the pregnancy to continue to term, (ii) perform intrauterine transfusion or (iii) induce early labor.

    Precautions:
    - The first amniocentesis is usually not performed before 26th weeks of gestation because the fetus is too small size for any kind of intervention.
    - It should not be done without a clear indication because of complications such as infection and enhancement of maternal immunization.
    - Amniotic fluid obtained should be protected from light which oxidizes bilirubin and gives low value.
    - Sample should not be contaminated with meconium or fetal and maternal blood. They increase the optical density and gives wrong reading.

10. **Fetal maturity**: Maturity of fetal lungs and thereby the ability of the fetus to survive after early delivery, can be predicted by estimation of lecithin/sphingomyelin (L/S) ratio in amniotic fluid. L/S ratio of less than 2.0/1.0 indicates that the lung is immature and may need intrauterine transfusion. The fetal conditions can also be evaluated by ultrasound scanning and replaced amniography.

    - **Fetal genotyping**: Molecular typing can be done on fetal DNA on maternal plasma during the second trimester. Fetal genotyping for blood groups, particularly the D antigen, can help in predicting the risk of HDFN. It can avoid amniocentesis or cordocentesis if the fetus lacks the antigen for the maternal antibody.

Investigation (Serologic Testing) of Newborn Infant (Box 18.2)

Investigation of cord blood sample from a Rh-negative mother is important for the confirmation of HDFN and its management.

Umbilical cord is divided after delivery and blood sample is obtained from the maternal side of the umbilical cord, by inserting a needle attached to a syringe into the umbilical vein.

> **Box 18.2:** Investigations performed in newborn in HDFN.
>
> - ABO grouping
> - Rh typing including D^u
> - Direct antiglobulin test (DAT)
> - *Elution:* Screening and identification of antibody in cord's serum (is necessary)
> - Estimation of hemoglobin in cord blood
> - Cord blood bilirubin level
> - *Hematological parameters on cord blood:* It shows increased number of nucleated red cells and reticulocyte count, but it is not specific for HDFN

(HDFN: hemolytic disease of fetus and newborn)

1. **One blood sample is taken in an EDTA** (1 mg EDTA in 1 mL) anticoagulant. It is used for ABO and Rh grouping, antiglobulin test and for measuring hemoglobin value.
2. **Second blood sample is taken in a dry plain tube.** The serum is separated and is used for estimation of bilirubin and screening antibody.

- **ABO grouping:** In newborn infants, ABO antigens are not fully developed. Hence, newborns may show weaker reactions than older children and adults. ABO grouping on newborn is based on cell grouping only. This is because infants do not have their own isoagglutinins/alloantibodies and alloantibodies in the cord blood are those of the mother (maternal origin). So reverse grouping cannot be used to confirm the ABO group. Before performing cell grouping, red cells should be washed 4–5 times to avoid false positive results due to contamination with Wharton's jelly present in the umbilical cord.
- **Rh typing:** Rarely, the infant's RBCs can be heavily coated with anti-D IgG antibodies derived from mother. This causes difficulty in Rh grouping and may give a false-negative Rh type, or false positive what has been called *blocked Rh*.
- **Causes of false Rh (D) positive:**
  - Red cells contaminated with Wharton jelly.
  - Rh (D) negative cells heavily coated with antibody(ies) other than anti-Rh (D).

  Problem can be solved by:
  - Using red cells washed 4–5 times in saline
  - Gentle elution of antibody and repeating Rh typing. An eluate from these RBCs will reveal anti-D, and typing of the eluted RBCs will show correct reaction with anti-D.

  Causes of false negative or weak positive result:
  This can occur with saline anti-D when the newborn is Rh-positive and the red cells are fully coated with maternal anti-D that no sites are available to react with the reagent serum. In such situation, baby's red blood cells give a strong positive DAT. The maternal anti-D can be removed from these cells by heat elution.

- **Direct Antiglobulin Test** (DAT)
  Direct antiglobulin test with anti-IgG reagent is the most important serologic test for diagnosing HDFN. DAT is strongly positive if HDN is due to anti-D and is negative in HDN due to ABO. Positive DAT test indicates that the anti-D antibody is coating the infant's RBCs. However, the strength of the reaction does not correlate with the severity of the HDFN. A positive DAT may also be found in infants without clinical or other laboratory evidence of hemolysis (e.g. mother received RhIG).

- **Elution**
  The maternal Rh antibody may or may not be found in the infant's serum. It is not necessary to routinely eluate all infants with a positive DAT result. Elution is also not needed in known cases of HDFN and postnatal ABO incompatibility, because results of eluate do not change therapy. The preparation of an eluate of cord red blood cells may be helpful to identify antibody when the cause of HDFN is not known.
  - **Cord hemoglobin value:** Normal level of cord blood Hb is 18.6–19.6 g/dL. The cord hemoglobin values correlates well with the severity of HDFN and serves as a guide to assess the severity of HDFN (Table 18.2).
  - **Cord blood bilirubin:** Normal cord blood bilirubin value is 0.7–3.1 mg/dL. Cord bilirubin level also is correlated with

Table 18.2: Cord Hb values and severity of HDN.

Hb level (g/dL)	Severity of HDN
Above 14	Unaffected
11–14	Mild to moderate
8–11	Moderate to server
Below 8	Severe

(Hb: hemoglobin; HDN: hemolytic disease of newborn)

severity of HDFN but its correlation is less close than cord hemoglobin. However, when Hb value is within normal limits, cord bilirubin level is valuable to assess the severity of the disease. It is unusual to have a cord bilirubin above 4 mg/dL and if present, suggests a very severe disease. The bilirubin levels reach peak levels usually by the third or fourth day of life.

Antenatal Management of Rh Immunization

Antenatal management depends upon the levels of anti-D in the fetus, the results of amniocentesis and past obstetric history. If the obstetrician is convinced that the fetus might not survive a full-term pregnancy, the following steps can be taken.

Intrauterine Transfusion

Indications for intervention in the form of intrauterine transfusion is needed when one or more of conditions listed in the Box 18.3 are present.

Goal: To maintain fetal hemoglobin above 10 g/dL.

Procedure: Intrauterine transfusion is done by accessing the fetal umbilical vein (cordocentesis) under USG guidance and injecting donor RBCs directly into the vein. Packed RBCs of group O Rh (D) negative, less than 5 days old, leukocyte depleted, irradiated and preferably compatible with mother's blood is given. The first intrauterine transfusion is done after about 24–26 weeks of gestation and it is repeated every 2–4 weeks till delivery. The first intrauterine transfusion is rarely performed after 36 weeks' gestation. Intrauterine transfusion probably suppresses the RBC production by the bone marrow of fetus. After birth, the infant may need additional RBC transfusion during the first few weeks.

Complications: Cordocentesis, intrauterine transfusion, and amniocentesis procedures carry several risks. These include infection, premature labor, and trauma to the placenta. These procedures may cause fetomaternal hemorrhage which may increase the antigenic challenge resulting in increased antibody titers in the mother.

Plasmapheresis

Intensive plasmapheresis can reduce antibody level in the mother's serum, thus increase the chance of survival of fetus. About 200-600 mL plasma can be exchanged every week, beginning at 10-20 weeks of pregnancy till the baby is delivered at 34-35 weeks gestation. The replacement fluid given is 4-5% human albumin and small supplement of FFP from Rh (D) negative donors to maintain normal IgG levels, coagulation factors, etc.

Premature Induction of Labor

The decision to induce premature labor depends on analysis of amniotic fluid, previous obstetric history, antibody titers, and fetal maturity on ultrasound examination. Those pregnancies having high risk of HDFN can be terminated after 34 weeks of gestation. This will lower the incidence of stillbirth and will reduce the severity of HDN in live born infants.

Intravenous Immune Globulin

Mechanism of action: The IVIG competes with the mother's antibodies for the FC receptors on the macrophages in the infant's spleen, thereby reducing the amount of hemolysis.

Box 18.3: Indications for intrauterine transfusion.

- MCA-PSV indicates anemia
- Fetal hydrops identified on ultrasound examination
- Cordocentesis blood sample shows hemoglobin level less than 10 g/dL
- Amniotic fluid Delta OD 450 nm results are high

(MCA-PSV: middle cerebral artery peak systolic velocity)

Intravenous immune globulin (IVIG) infusion can be used both antenatally and postnatally.

Antenatal: Intravenous immune globulin (IVIG) infusion can be used to stabilize anti-D titers and best results are observed if started before 28 weeks of gestation and when fetus is not hydropic.

Postnatal: Intravenous immune globulin (IVIG) can also be used to treat hyperbilirubinemia of the newborn caused by HDFN.

Postnatal Management of Infant

About 40% of newborns are born with DCT/DAT positive. They are usually asymptomatic and require no treatment. Rest of them, if not treated may die within few hours due to cardiac failure or may develop severe jaundice and develop kernicterus at any stage after birth.

Phototherapy to Reduce Serum Bilirubin Concentration

After delivery, the neonate can become deeply jaundiced (hyperbilirubinemia due to raised unconjugated bilirubin). Phototherapy is exposure of newborn infants to fluorescent light. On exposure to light in the region of 460–490 nm, unconjugated bilirubin gets converted to the nontoxic pigment isomer, biliverdin, and lowers serum bilirubin concentration. These isomers are less lipophilic and less toxic to the brain. Relatively high doses of phototherapy are given to neonates by using two banks of lights to surround the infant's body. Phototherapy, when applied early enough and with sufficient intensity, is usually sufficient for infants with mild-to-moderate hemolysis or history of intrauterine transfusion. This can avoid the need for exchange transfusion in many infants. Recently, the efficacy of phototherapy has been improved by use of a fiberoptic blanket that delivers phototherapy to the anterior and posterior surfaces of the infant simultaneously. This device almost doubles the reduction in serum bilirubin concentration in low-birthweight infants with hyperbilirubinemia.

For details about intravenous immune globulin (refer page 391).

Blood Transfusion

- Infants with mild HDN (less than a week old) with only anemia are treated by transfusion with red cell concentrate to correct the anemia.
- Moderate to severe HDN require exchange transfusion.

Exchange transfusion

Newborn transfusions: Exchange transfusion is the use of whole blood or equivalent, to replace the neonate's circulating blood. The bilirubin level in the newborn can be successfully reduced by phototherapy and the use of IVIG and have markedly reduced the need for exchange transfusion. Less than 50% of the cases of HDFN are caused by anti-D, so the majority is generally less severe and does not need exchange transfusion.

The newborn may receive small aliquot transfusions to correct anemia. In newborn treated by small aliquot or exchange transfusions, the suppression of erythropoiesis may cause anemia to occur immediately after the neonatal period.

Exchange transfusions in **newborn** mainly remove the high levels of unconjugated bilirubin and thereby prevent kernicterus. The requirement of exchange transfusions is more likely in premature newborns than in full-term infants. This is because the liver of premature infants has less capability to conjugate the raised unconjugated bilirubin into conjugate bilirubin. Advantages of exchange transfusion are listed in Box 18.4 which help in interrupting the production of bilirubin due to hemolysis.

Criteria for exchange transfusion: It depends on: (a) hemoglobin level in the cord blood, (b) bilirubin level, and (c) birth-weight. Bilirubin estimation should be done at every 4–8 hours intervals. Criteria for exchange transfusion are as follows:
- **Before birth:** (i) cord blood hemoglobin below 12 g/dL and (ii) serum bilirubin above 5 mg/dL.

Hemolytic Disease of Newborn

> **Box 18.4:** Advantages of exchange transfusion in HDFN.
>
> - Lowers the serum bilirubin level and to prevent kernicterus
> - Removes antibody-coated fetal red cells (sensitized RBCs) and replaces them with antigen-negative cells
> - Corrects anemia without expanding blood volume
> - Removes/reduces the level of circulating maternal antibody
> - Replaces incompatible RBCs with compatible RBCs with adequate oxygen carrying capacity and thereby treating fetal anemia.

(HDFN: hemolytic disease of fetus and newborn)

- *After birth:* (i) capillary blood hemoglobin below 12 g/dL and falling in first 24 hours, and (ii) serum bilirubin above 20 mg/dL in first 48 hours.

Selection of Blood for Intrauterine and Neonatal Transfusion

- **Blood should be as fresh as possible. Traditionally, blood units less than 5 days from collection** from the donor are selected. This will ensure long survival of red cells in infant and to avoid high level of plasma potassium in the transfused blood. Special circumstances, such as mother's blood with high-incidence antibodies are involved, older blood units can be safe and effective for the newborn when infused slowly.
- If **baby's ABO group is same as mothers**, then Rh (D) negative blood of same ABO group should be used.
- If **baby's ABO group is not compatible with mothers**, then O Rh (D) negative blood, free from hemolysins anti-A and anti-B should be used. The RBCs must be antigen negative for the mother's respective antibodies.
- **Rh-negative units are used for fetuses and neonates whose blood types are unknown or are Rh-negative.**
- If **exchange transfusion is repeated**, then the **subsequent blood should be of the same ABO and Rh type as that transfused first time.**
- **In ABO HDN** the red cells used must be **group O cells**.
- Group O RBCs for intrauterine and neonatal transfusions is used in most of the centers treating HDFN.
- Donors should be usually **cytomegalovirus (CMV)-negative**.
- Blood transfused to the fetus and premature infant, and blood for exchange transfusion should be **irradiated to prevent graft-versus-host disease**.
- **Blood should not contain hemoglobin S**. This is because the decreased oxygen tension which may occur early in the neonatal period may cause hemoglobin S trait blood to sickle.
- If the antibody in the mother is reactive against a high frequency antigen and no compatible blood is available then the following options can be considered:
  - Test the mother's siblings or other close relatives for compatible blood. Blood from relatives should be irradiated.
  - Collect a unit of blood from mother. Separate the red cells and resuspend it in AB plasma to the desired hematocrit.
  - If clinical situation is urgent, exchange transfuse with incompatible donor blood. The exchange will reduce the bilirubin load, the most heavily antibody-coated cells and the number of unbound antibody molecules. Because without transfusion the infant may die.

Selection of ABO Group blood for exchange transfusion in Rh-HDN is mentioned in Table 18.3.

Table 18.3: ABO Group blood selection for exchange transfusion in Rh-HDN.

Infant's blood group	Mother's blood group	Blood selected for exchange transfusion
A	A, AB	A or O
	O, B	O
B	B, AB	B or O
	O, A	O
O	A, O, B	O
AB	A	A or B
	B	B or O
	AB	AB, A, B or O

Volume and Hematocrit of Blood for Exchange Transfusion

Volume of blood for exchange transfusion: It should be equal of twice the infants blood volume (blood volume of a full-term infant is about 85 mL/kg).

Hematocrit
- For intrauterine transfusion, the hematocrit level of the RBCs should be greater than 70% because of the small volume transfused and the need to correct severe anemia.
- Hematocrit of the transfused blood should be maintained at about 50–55%. This is achieved by using partially concentrated red cells.
- For the rare exchange transfusions, one practice is to prepare RBCs from whole blood units and then replace the plasma with group AB plasma to reduce the amount of blood group antibodies transfused. This procedure is not necessary if both the neonate and the mother are the same ABO group.

Compatibility Testing for Exchange Transfusion

- If ABO group of mothers and infant are compatible, then use serum from mother for cross matching.
- If ABO group of mother and infant are not compatible, or if mother's group is not known, then use infant's serum for cross matching.
- The blood to be transfused should be cross matched against mother's serum by IAT and enzyme method.

■ PREVENTION OF Rh (D) HDFN

Rh Immune Globulin (RhIG)

Principle: Active immunization induced by RBC antigen can be prevented by the concurrent administration of the corresponding RBC antibody. This principle is used to prevent immunization to D antigen by using high-titered RhIG.

Risk of sensitization: Fetal and maternal blood can get mixed during pregnancy and delivery. If the mother is Rh-negative and carries a Rh-positive fetus, the mother has up to a 16% possibility of being stimulated to form anti-D. As little as 1 mL of fetal RBCs can elicit an immune response.
- **Before delivery**: The risk of sensitization is 1.5–1.9% in susceptible women. This indicates that a significant amount of fetal RBCs can enter the maternal circulation during pregnancy.
- **At delivery**: The greatest risk of immunization to Rh is at delivery.

Mechanism of Action of RhIG

RhIG is an antibody administered to the Rh-negative mother during pregnancy and after delivery. This RhIG attaches to the fetal Rh-positive RBCs in the maternal circulation. The antibody-coated RBCs are removed by the macrophages in the maternal spleen. The mechanism of action of RhIG is not certain. Probably it interferes with B-cell priming to make anti-D.

Indications

The clinical indications for administering RhIG to the mother during pregnancy and after delivery. Box 18.5 lists indications for RhIG administration.

Box 18.5: Indications for RhIG.

Antenatal
- Amniocentesis
- Chorionic villus sampling
- Abdominal trauma
- Greater than 40 weeks' gestation

Postpartum
- Delivered a Rh (D) positive baby and has not developed anti-D in the serum
- Undergone abortion (spontaneous and induced) or medical termination of pregnancy
- Ectopic pregnancy
- Have had antepartum hemorrhage

Transfusion
Accidental or inadvertent transfusion

(RhIG: Rh immune globulin)

Antenatal

There is a known risk of Rh immunization during pregnancy. Hence, RhIG should be administered to the mother early in the third trimester, or at about 28 weeks' gestation. It may produce a positive DAT result in the newborn.

Postpartum

Nonimmunized Rh-negative mother should receive RhIG soon after delivery of a Rh-positive infant. If the Rh type of the infant is not known (e.g. if the infant is stillborn), RhIG should also be administered. A full dose of RhIG (about 300 µg) is sufficient to counteract the immunizing effects of 15 mL of D positive red cells or 30 mL of fetal whole blood. It is given intramuscularly within 72 hours after delivery to Rh (D) negative woman. But even after the elapse of more than 72 hours, still RhIG should be given, as it may be effective and is not contraindicated.

Massive fetomaternal hemorrhage: Massive fetomaternal hemorrhage of more than 30 mL of whole blood can occur in less than 1% of deliveries. A full dose of RhIG (about 300 µg) is not sufficient for immunization in such cases and they need adequate RhIG. To prevent undertreatment of these cases various methods to screen large fetomaternal hemorrhage are available.

a. **Microscopic weak D**: Look for D-positive RBCs in the mother's D-negative blood by examining microscopically the antiglobulin phase of the test for D (microscopic weak D test). Mixed-field reactivity indicates significant admixture of D positive red cells.

b. **Rosette technique (Fig. 18.4):** It demonstrates small number of D positive fetal red cells in a D negative maternal red cells. A maternal blood sample is obtained within 1 hour of delivery. The blood is incubated with anti-D reagent of human origin. During incubation, anti-D molecules in the reagent bind to D-positive fetal red cells in the suspension. The suspension is washed thoroughly, and indicator D positive red cells are then added, which react with antibody bound to the surface of already present D positive fetal red cells. They form visible agglutinates (rosettes) around these D-positive fetal cells. The blood suspension is placed on a slide and examined microscopically for the appearance and number of rosettes. A positive and negative controls should be simultaneously run to ensure valid test results. A positive test indicates significant fetomaternal hemorrhage (FMH) and suggests the need for more than one dose of RhIG. The rosette test detects a bleed of only 10 mL and therefore rosette assay should be used as a screening test only. For the rosette test to be valid, the fetal cells must be D-positive and the mother must be D-negative. A false-positive result may be found if the mother is weak D-positive and a false-negative result may be found if the fetus is positive for weak D.

c. **Kleihauer–Betke acid-elution test:** If rosette test is positive, quantitation of the hemorrhage must be done by Kleihauer-Betke or by flow cytometry. Kleihauer-Betke test is used to quantitate the amount of fetal red cells in maternal circulation.

Principle: Kleihauer–Betke test depends on principle that fetal hemoglobin resist acid-elution compared to adult hemoglobin.

Method: A maternal blood smear is prepared, treated with acid and then stained with counterstain. Fetal red cells contain fetal hemoglobin (HbF) is resistant to acid and will remain pink. The maternal red cells are not acid resistant and will appear as ghosts (Fig. 18.5). After 2,000 red cells are counted and the percentage of fetal cells in maternal circulation is determined. The volume of fetal hemorrhage is calculated using the formula mentioned below.

$$\text{Volume of fetomaternal hemorrhage} = \frac{\text{Number of fetal cells} \times \text{Maternal blood volume}}{\text{Number of maternal cells}}$$

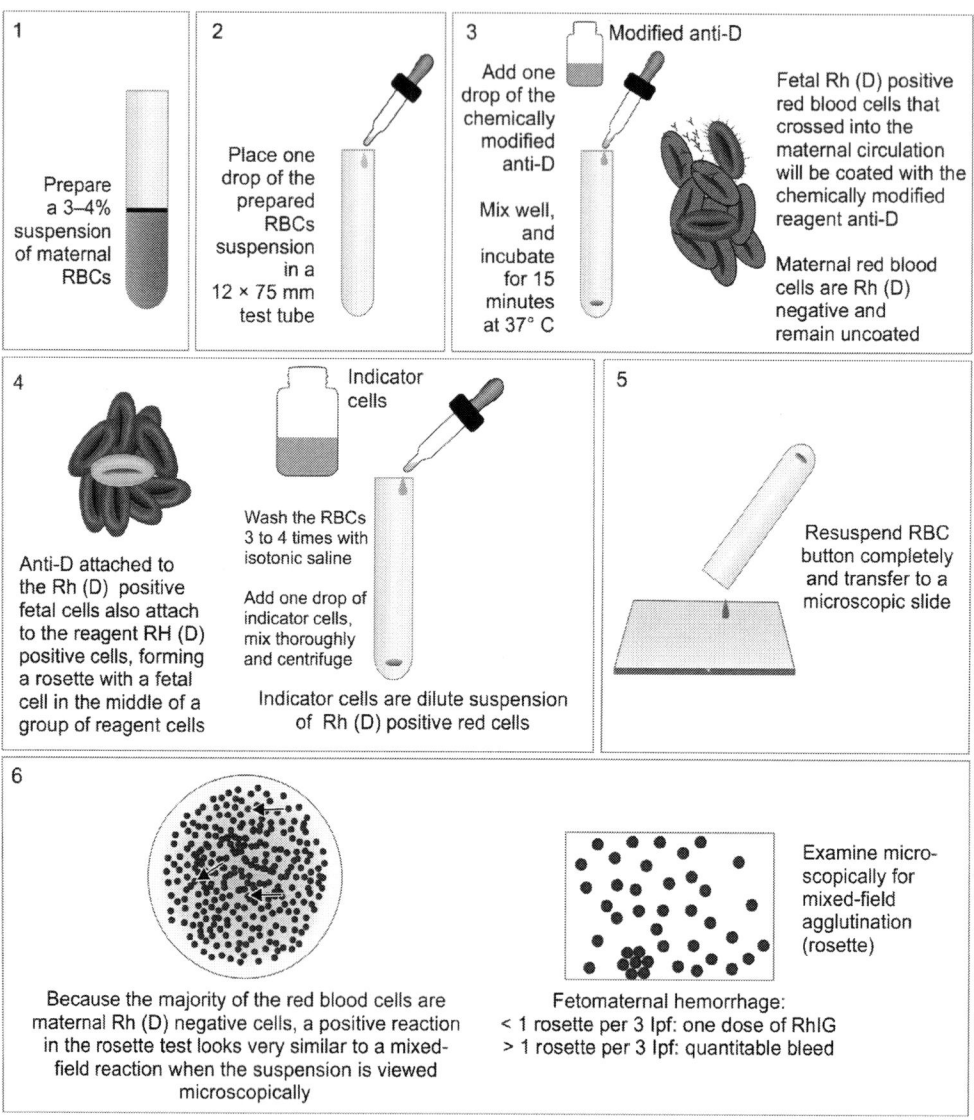

Fig. 18.4: Various steps in rosette test for detection of fetomaternal hemorrhage.
(RhIG: Rh immune globulin; lpf: low power field)

As mentioned earlier, 300 µg (one vial) of RhIG is sufficient to protect against fetomaternal hemorrhage (FMH) of 30 mL D positive fetal blood. The number of doses of RhIG is determined by dividing the calculated volume (as mentioned in formula above) of fetomaternal hemorrhage by 30. This will determine the number of required vials of RhIG (each vial has 300 µg). For example:

- If Kleihauer–Betke test results show 1.3% (percentage of fetal cells in maternal circulation)

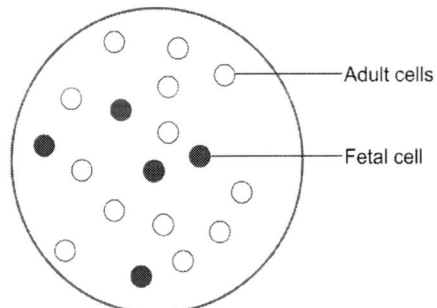

Fig 18.5: Acid elution test for determination of hemoglobin F. Blood smear is prepared from maternal blood. It is treated with acid and then stained with counterstain. Fetal hemoglobin resists acid elution and remains intact. Thus, the fetal red cells appear dark pink. The adult red cells lose the hemoglobin and do not take up the stain. Thus, the adult cells appear as pale ghost cells.

- Volume of blood in a pregnant woman of 50 kg = 50 × 100 mL = 5,000 mL
- Therefore the volume of fetomaternal hemorrhage = $\frac{1.3 \times 5000}{100}$ = 65 mL
- The dose of RhIG needed = 65/30 = 2.2 doses
Alternatively a simpler method to calculate the dose is to multiply the percentage fetal red cell by 50. This gives the volume of fetomaternal hemorrhage in milliliters. Because the Kleihauer–Betke is an estimate, one vial is added to the calculated answer.

Prevention of undertreatment:
- If the number to the right of the decimal point is less than 5, it should be rounded to the number and one dose should be added. For example, if it is 2.2, give 3 doses.
- If the number to the right of the decimal point is more than 5, it should be rounded to the next number and one dose should be added. For example, if it is 2.8, give 4 doses.

Note: More than 5 doses of RhIG should not be injected at one time intramuscularly. If more quantities are required, injections can be spaced over a 72-hour period.

RhIG is available both for intramuscular (IM) and intravenous (IV) injections. The intramuscular form must be given intramuscularly only, but IV form can also be given intramuscularly. However, the intramuscular preparations must not be given as IV injections, because it can cause severe anaphylactic reactions. RhIG also contains IgA and may be contraindicated in patients with anti-IgA and IgA deficiency who have had anaphylactic reactions to blood products.

Other Considerations of RhIG

- **Active versus passive immunization:** Once an individual has been actively immunized and has formed anti-D, there is no benefit of giving RhIG. However, it is necessary to distinguish women who have been passively immunized by antenatal administration of RhIG from those who have been actively immunized by exposure to Rh-positive RBCs.
- **If infant is D-negative:** RhIG is not indicated for the mother if the infant is D-negative.
- **If fetus D status cannot be determined:** Usually, the Rh type of fetuses in abortions, stillbirths, and ectopic pregnancies cannot be determined. Hence, RhIG should be administered in these situations.
- **Not for newborn infant:** RhIG must not be given to the newborn infant.
- **No risk of transmission of the viral diseases:** Such as hepatitis A and B and HIV with the administration of RhIG.

ABO HEMOLYTIC DISEASE OF FETUS AND NEWBORN (HDFN)

ABO incompatibility between the mother and newborn infant can cause HDFN. As the incidence of HDFN caused by Rh (D) has decreased, ABO incompatibility has become the most common cause of HDFN. ABO-incompatible between mother and infant are observed one in every five pregnancies. Most of them are subclinical and do not necessitate treatment.

ABO HDFN occurs in group A or group B infants born to group O mothers. It is caused by IgG anti-A, anti-B or isolated IgG anti-A or anti-B in the mother's circulation. These IgG antibodies can cross the placenta and attach to the ABO-incompatible antigens of the fetal RBCs. These antibodies occur without a history of previous exposure to human red cells. ABO HDFN can occur in any pregnancy including the first. However, destruction of fetal RBCs (hemolysis) leading to severe anemia is very rare and the infant is rarely symptomatic at birth. More commonly, it manifests as mild hyperbilirubinemia (elevated bilirubin) and jaundice developing within 12–48 hours of birth. The hyperbilirubinemia can be treated with phototherapy. Severe cases requiring exchange transfusion are extremely rare. Comparison of ABO versus Rh HDFN is presented in Table 18.4.

Table 18.4: Comparison of hemolytic disease of the fetus and newborn (HDFN) due to incompatibility of ABO versus Rh.

Features	HDFN due to ABO incompatibility	HDFN due to Rh incompatibility
Incidence	Uncommon	Common
Blood group association	Mother must be group O, and the fetus must be group A or B	Mother can be any blood group
Rh association	ABO HDN is protective against Rh sensitization with the exception of an O Rh-positive baby	The mother must be Rh-negative, and the fetus must be Rh positive
First pregnancy affected	Yes	Rare
Clinical findings		
• Jaundice	Mild to moderate	Moderate to severe
• Edema	Absent	Mild to severe
Serological findings		
Direct antiglobulin test on cord blood	Negative or weakly positive	Strongly positive
Indirect antiglobulin test on cord blood	Usually positive	Positive
Disease predicted by titters	No	Yes
Type of IgG antibody	Anti-A, anti-B, anti-A, B	Anti-D
Bilirubin level at birth	Normal range or mildly elevated, peaks at 24–48 hours after birth	Moderate to severely raised
Hematology results		
Anemia at birth	Mild to no anemia	Frequent, moderate to severe
Reticulocyte count	Mild increase	Greatly increased
Morphology	Spherocytes in the peripheral blood	Macrocytes, hypochromic
Nucleated RBCs (red blood cells)	Mild increase	Marked increase
Usefulness of phototherapy	Yes	Yes
Exchange transfusion requirement	Rare	Uncommon
Intrauterine transfusion requirement	None	Sometimes
Serious consequences (stillbirth, hydrops fetalis, and kernicterus)	Very rare	Rare but may occur

Factors Affecting Incidence and Severity

ABO antibodies are found in the plasma of all individuals whose RBCs lack the corresponding antigen. These antibodies are produced due to environmental stimulus.

Can affect first pregnancy: The occurrence and severity of the disease is not related to the previous history of transfusions or pregnancies in mother. Thus, ABO HDFN can occur in the first pregnancy and in any, but not necessarily all, subsequent pregnancies. Affection of the first pregnancy is because of the presence of naturally occurring ABO antibodies. It has been found that administration of tetanus toxoid and helminth parasite infection during pregnancy can produce high-titered IgG ABO antibodies and severe HDFN.

ABO blood groups affected: ABO HDFN occurs most commonly in fetus or infants with group A or B of mothers with group O. Group O individuals have higher titers of IgG ABO antibodies compared with other ABO groups.

Causes of Mild Course of ABO HDFN

The possible cause for the mild red cell destruction in spite of presence high levels of maternal antibody are the following:

- **Presence of A or B substances/antigens in the fetal and infant tissues and secretions**: They can bind or **neutralize the** ABO antibodies **(anti-A and anti-B) of the mother.** This reduces the amount of ABO antibody available to destroy fetal red cells.
- **Poor development of ABO antigens on fetal** or infant **RBCs**: ABO antigens are not fully developed till after the first year of life.
- Reduced number of A and B antigen sites on fetal or infant red blood cells.

Diagnostic Criteria for HDFN due to ABO Incompatibility

- **Exclude the presence of antibodies to other blood group antigens**. This is done by checking the mother's serum with panel of reagent RBCs.
- **A or B infants of group O mothers:** ABO antibodies are more frequently found as high-titered IgG antibodies in group O individuals than in group A or B individuals. Hence, ABO HDFN is almost always limited to **A or B infants of group O mothers** with potent anti-A, B.
- Anti-A and anti-B titre higher than 1:128 and presence of hemolysins in the mother may further support the diagnosis.
- Direct antiglobulin test is often negative or occasionally weakly positive.
- **Hematological findings:** Microspherocytes and increased RBC fragility in the jaundiced infant are characteristic of ABO HDFN, but not of Rh HDFN. The bilirubin peak is seen later, at 1–3 days.

Severity of the disease: It is independent of the presence of a positive DAT or demonstrable anti-A, anti-B, or anti-A, B in the eluate of the infant's RBCs.

Consequences: The serious consequences of Rh and other blood groups causing HDFN are stillbirth, hydrops fetalis, and kernicterus. These are extremely are in ABO HDFN.

Investigation in ABO HDFN

Prenatal Screening in the Mother

- ABO grouping and Rh typing
- Estimation of IgG anti-A and anti-B in the mother's serum. Titer above 32 is considered significant.
- Antibody-dependent cell-mediated cytotoxicity (ADCC) test: Using mother's serum correlates with severity of ABO HDFN.

However, ABO HDFN is diagnosed best after birth.

Postnatal Diagnosis—Tests in the Infant

Collection of blood: It is recommended to collect cord blood samples from all delivered infants. The sample should be collected by venipuncture to avoid contamination with maternal blood and Wharton's jelly (the material surrounding the blood vessels). Use anticoagulant for storage.

Tests: No single serologic test is diagnostic for ABO HDFN. When a newborn develops jaundice within 12-48 hours after birth, the causes of jaundice should be investigated and ABO HDFN is only one of them.
- **Direct antiglobulin test (DAT):** Performed on the cord or neonatal RBCs and is the most important diagnostic test.
  - DAT result are positive in all cases of ABO HDFN that need transfusion therapy
  - DAT result can be positive in the newborn infant even when there are no signs and symptoms of clinical anemia. These infants may have compensated anemia or the RBCs are not destroyed by the reticuloendothelial system.
  - If DAT result is negative, the eluate of the cord RBCs always reveals ABO antibodies.
- **ABO grouping and Rh typing**
- **Serum bilirubin:** Moderately increased. It can be controlled by phototherapy but very often may need exchange transfusion.
- **Hematological parameters:**
  - Reticulocytosis 5%
  - Increased osmotic fragility
  - Spherocytes in peripheral blood smear.

Management of ABO HDFN

It is very rare to have severe anemia and therapy is usually required to control hyperbilirubinemia.
- For slowly rising bilirubin levels—phototherapy (treatment with ultraviolet light rays) is usually enough.
- Rapidly increasing bilirubin levels—IVIG or exchange transfusion with group O RBCs may be required.

1. **Phototherapy:** Discussed on page 394.
2. **Blood transfusion:** Infants having mild ABO HDFN with only anemia may be transfused with red cell concentrate. The blood should be not more than 5 days old.
3. **Exchange transfusion:** It may be needed when bilirubin level exceeds 20 mg/dL. The whole group O blood of infant's Rh type is used for exchange transfusion. The blood should have low titer of anti-A and anti-B and should also be free from hemolysins. When O group blood is transfused to an infant with group A, B, or AB, it is necessary to used red cell concentrate. It is better to use packed cells resuspended in one-third volume of fresh AB plasma (or A plasma or B plasma as appropriate). The volume and hematocrit of the blood used for exchange transfusion is same as that for Rh HDFN mentioned on page 394.

ALLOANTIBODIES CAUSING HEMOLYTIC DISEASE OF THE FETUS AND NEWBORN OTHER THAN ANTI-D

Any IgG antibody can produce HDFN if the fetal red cells have the antigen and the antigen is well developed at birth. After anti-D, anti-c, and anti-K are the next most common antibodies to cause HDFN. Less commonly other antibodies such as anti-E, anti-k, anti-Kp^a, anti-Kp^b, anti-Js^a, anti-Js^b, anti-Jk^a, anti-Fy^a, anti-Fy^b, anti-S, anti-s, and anti-U can cause HDFN. Antibodies to low-frequency antigens (e.g. Js^a, Kp^a), may not be detected by the antibody screening or panel cells. If there is evidence of HDFN, testing paternal red cells with the mother's serum may show a positive reaction not detected with reagent red cells.

SUMMARY

- HDFN occurs when the fetal red cells, carrying antigens inherited from the father, stimulate the mother to produce IgG antibodies. Maternal IgG antibodies cross the placenta and destroy fetal red cells.
- HDFN is characterized by the destruction of the RBCs of the fetus and neonate by IgG antibodies produced by the mother. Only antibodies of the IgG type can be transported across the placenta.
- HDFN can be caused by ABO, Rh, or other IgG antibodies.
- HDFN caused by anti-D is the most severe form of HDFN. It occurs in D-negative women with anti-D who deliver D-positive infants. In Rh HDFN, the Rh-positive infant of first pregnancy of Rh-negative mother is not affected. This is because the mother has not yet been immunized. The Rh-negative mother is sensitized usually during delivery, but can also be immunized during pregnancy. During sensitization, the fetal cells carrying the Rh antigen immunize the Rh-negative mother and stimulate production of anti-D.
- ABO HDFN is the most common type of HDFN and occurs most commonly in group O mothers who deliver group A or B babies. In ABO HDFN, the first infant as well as subsequent pregnancies may be affected.
- Red cell destruction (hemolysis) in utero and the splenic removal of the IgG-coated RBCs causes anemia. There is excessive erythropoiesis and liberation of erythroblasts/immature RBCs into the circulation of fetus. Erythroblastosis fetalis is characterized by the presence of immature RBCs or erythroblasts in the fetal circulation. If anemia is severe, it can proceed to heart failure and possibly death.
- Bilirubin released from hemoysis in the fetus is removed by the mother's circulation before birth.
- Red cell destruction (hemolysis) after delivery increase bilirubin level in infant, causing jaundice. Before the newborn's liver becomes fully functional, the bilirubin can cross the blood–brain barrier and damage to the CNS (kernicterus).
- Prenatal serologic tests for obstetric patients to predict, prevent, or monitor HDFN include an ABO, Rh, and antibody screen on the mother during the first trimester of pregnancy.
- Titration of the maternal antibody helps in deciding when to perform diagnostic and invasive procedures.
- D-negative mothers should receive prenatal RhIG. RhIG administered to the Rh-negative mother within 72 hours following delivery prevents active immunization by the Rh (D) antigen on fetal cells. RhIG attaches to fetal Rh-positive RBCs in maternal circulation, blocking immunization and subsequent production of anti-D.
- After delivery, HDFN is monitored, prevented, and treated by cord blood testing, A cord blood workup includes tests for ABO and Rh as well as DAT.
- RhIG dosage is determined by the fetal screen (rosette) and Kleihauer–Betke test performed on the mother.
- A Kleihauer–Betke test or flow cytometry is used to quantitate the number of fetal Rh-positive cells in the mother's circulation which are the result of a fetomaternal hemorrhage.
- Depending on the severity of HDFN, treatment can begin in utero or after delivery.
- After delivery, exchange transfusion is used to correct anemia, remove sensitized red cells, and reduce levels of maternal antibody and bilirubin.
- Blood used for exchange and intrauterine transfusion should be less than 7 days old, irradiated, CMV negative and negative for the antigen corresponding to the maternal antibody.

SELF-ASSESSMENT EXERCISE

Long essay on:
- Discuss Rh incompatibility, its diagnosis and management.

Write short essays/notes on:
- Write about fetal hydrops.
- Hemolytic disease of fetus and newborn.
- Exchange transfusion.
- What are the tests done using the cord blood in a setting of Rh incompatibility?
- What are the tests done in investigating a case of Rh incompatibility?

CHAPTER 19

Transfusion Therapy in Selected Patients and Blood Substitutes

CHAPTER OUTLINE

- Transfusion therapy in selected patients
- Autologous transfusion
- Alternatives to transfusion
- Blood substitutes
- Plasma substitutes

INTRODUCTION

Transfusion therapy provides patients with the correct component for many types of diseases and conditions. In this chapter, few selected clinical conditions that commonly require transfusion support are briefly discussed. Transfusion of blood component can provide support for many patients with unique hematologic disorders. Few patients (e.g. sickle cell disease patients) need this support throughout their life. For others, it may be an urgent requirement for surgery or following trauma.

TRANSFUSION THERAPY IN SELECTED PATIENTS

Cardiac Surgery

When performing cardiopulmonary bypass surgery, the patient's blood is circulated through an oxygenating pump outside the patient's body.

Risk factors for bleeding during cardiac surgery (Box 19.1): Extracorporeal circulation of blood causes a reduction in number as well as function of platelets. Because of hemodilution and the use of cell salvage instrument, there is also decrease in coagulation factors. Other risk factors that affect hemostasis during cardiac surgery include hypothermia, transfusion of shed blood, thrombin-mediated activation, and residual heparin. Hence, these risk factors increase the need for component support both perioperative and postoperative period. The demand of blood and its components varies with each patient.

Heparin effect in cardiac surgery: During and after cardiac surgery, heparin prolongs the activated partial thromboplastin time.

The thrombin time confirms heparin excess and this **heparin excess can be treated with a protamine sulfate** rather than fresh frozen plasma (FFP). **Indications for FFP are usually only factor deficiency or massive transfusion from severe bleeding during cardiac surgery**. The effects of preoperative warfarin therapy also contribute to postoperative blood loss

Box 19.1: Risk factors for bleeding during cardiac surgery.

- Time of oxygenating pump
- Age of patient
- Previous history of cardiac surgery
- Type of present cardiac surgery: Valve replacement, coronary artery bypass graft (CABG)
- Preoperative medications: Aspirin and anticoagulant
- Effect of heparin
- Hypothermia (reduces platelet function)

and thereby increase the requirement of transfusion.

Neonatal and Pediatric Transfusion

Unique Aspects of Neonatal Physiology

There are three unique aspects of neonatal physiology namely: Fetal red blood cells (RBCs), erythropoietin (EPO) response, and immunologic status.

Fetal red blood cells
The fetal RBC differs from adult RBC in many ways.
- Fetal RBC is **larger** and **contains mainly hemoglobin F** (HbF; about 70% at term). Premature infants have a higher percentage of HbF, which may be as high as 97% in very premature children, than full-term infants.
- Fetal RBC has a shorter lifespan of 90 days when compared to 120 days in adult.
- **HbF has a higher affinity** or capacity **to bind oxygen**.
- At birth, a full-term infant has a hemoglobin level between 14.0 and 20.0 mg/dL (140–200 g/L). Since much of the increase in hemoglobin occurs during the last weeks of gestation, infants born prematurely can be expected to have lower hemoglobin levels.
- HbF interacts poorly with 2,3-diphosphoglycerate (2,3-DPG). Hence, there is decreased delivery of oxygen to the tissues of the premature neonate, especially if the amount of hemoglobin is also low.

Erythropoietin response
- After birth, all newborns show a decline in the amount of circulating RBCs which is called the physiologic anemia of infancy.
- Erythropoietin is a growth factor that stimulates the proliferation and differentiation of stem cells into RBC precursors in the bone marrow. This increases the production of RBC and releases more RBCs into the blood.
- **Site of production: In the fetus**, erythropoietin is produced **mainly in the liver** whereas in the adults, erythropoietin is produced mainly in the kidneys. The switch in production of erythropoietin from the liver to the kidney starts during fetal life, but a complete transition occurs when the infant is several months old. The liver is less responsive to tissue hypoxia/anemia than kidney.
- In the full-term infant, levels of hemoglobin gradually decrease during the first 1–2 months of age and then begin to increase. Usually, the infants can tolerate this change without difficulty and require no treatment. In a premature infant, who are already born with a lower hemoglobin level, there will be even more dramatic decrease in hemoglobin levels following birth. This **"anemia of prematurity"** may be **due to low erythropoietin** levels, a suboptimal erythropoietin response, decreased iron stores, decreased survival of RBCs, and high levels of HbF. This anemia may be further aggravated when repeated phlebotomies are performed to obtain blood samples for testing of the sick infant.

Immunologic status
The immune system is **not fully developed at birth**. This involves both humoral and cellular immunity. The newborns are at increased risk for a variety of infections. Though the infant can produce some IgM in response to antigens, sufficient levels of IgG are not produced till the infant attains first year of age. Most of the infant's circulating IgG is derived from the mother via placental transfer, while the infant's IgA comes from breast milk.

Transfusion Issues Unique to Neonates (Box 19.2)

Transfusion issues in neonates and pediatric patients are significantly different from transfusion issues for adults. This is because of the small size, hemoglobin changes, and erythropoietin response in early infancy. Neonates usually receive RBC transfusions than other adult patients. Because of the unique physiology of the neonatal period it is necessary to have some differences in

> **Box 19.2:** Transfusion issues unique to neonates.
>
> - Shifting from fetal to adult hemoglobin causing physiologic anemia of infancy
> - Iatrogenic blood loss (blood collection for laboratory tests)
> - Decreased response of erythropoietin
> - Low tolerance of hypothermia
> - Decreased ability to metabolize citrate and potassium
> - Decreased ability to restore 2,3-Diphosphoglycerate (2,3-DPG) in older blood units
> - Greater risk of cytomegalovirus infection due to immature immune system

the approach in infants compared to older children or adults.

Shift from fetal to adult hemoglobin: Fetal red cells contain HbF. HbF has a higher affinity or capacity to bind oxygen. During the intrauterine period, the HbF increases oxygen transfer from maternal red cells to fetal red cells. There is gradual switch from fetal to adult hemoglobin which starts at about 32 weeks' gestation. This is responsible for higher level of fetal hemoglobin in preterm infants than infants born at term. The change from fetal to adult hemoglobin occurs during the first few weeks of life, and this process is responsible for a condition called physiologic anemia of infancy. In a full-term infant of normal birth weight, this change from fetal to adult hemoglobin is well tolerated. However, treatment may be necessary in an infant born prematurely with low birth weight.

Neonates receive RBC transfusions because of anemia of prematurity, hemolytic disease of the newborn (HDN), or iatrogenic blood loss. The unique physiology of the neonatal period and the relative fragility of the developing brain vasculature necessitate some differences from the approach to older children or adults.

Iatrogenic blood loss: Apart from the shift in hemoglobin (fetal to adult), the need for frequent laboratory tests contributes to the transfusion requirement in neonates and pediatric patients. Blood loss caused by treatment (e.g. collection of blood samples for laboratory testing) is called as iatrogenic blood loss and is the most common indication of transfusion in a preterm infant with low birth weight. Newborns do not compensate for hypovolemia.

Decreased response to erythropoietin: In adults, erythropoietin is released from the kidneys in response to low levels of oxygen (hypoxia). In an infant, erythropoietin is produced in the liver and less responsive to low levels of oxygen. This lower level of response of erythropoietin to low oxygen levels (hypoxia) protects the infant from producing excess number of red cells (polycythemia) during fetal life. This is responsible for low level of response to anemia in the immature infant which is not a desirable effect.

Low tolerance to hypothermia: It is also different from an adult's response. In a neonate, the metabolic rate, hypoglycemia, and acidosis can produce temporary cessation of breathing, or apnea. Apnea can lead to hypoxia, hypotension, and cardiac arrest. This is the reason for using a monitored blood warmer to administer RBCs, especially for exchange transfusions.

Decreased ability to metabolize citrate and potassium: In newborns, the ability to metabolize citrate and potassium is more difficult due to the immature nature of liver and kidneys during neonatal period. This is the basis of using washed or fresh red cells in newborns. The potassium increases when blood is irradiated and hence, it is recommended to wash irradiated RBCs.

Decreased ability to restore 2,3-DPG: The level of 2,3-diphosphoglycerate (2,3-DPG) decreases during storage of blood. So, transfusion of fresh blood will maximize the level of 2,3-diphosphoglycerate (2,3-DPG) in newborns because of their limited ability to compensate for hypoxia.

Cytomegalovirus (CMV) infection: Premature and low birth weight infants are at greater risk for CMV infection and graft-versus host disease.

Transfusion issues unique to the infants are summarized in Box 19.2.

Red Blood Cell Transfusions in Infants less than 4 Months of Age

When transfusion is needed in infants, the neonate's physiology must be considered.

Following are the general features to be considered before transfusion in neonates.

- **Indications for RBC transfusion:** In neonates, RBC transfusion is indicated for any infant with signs or symptoms of **anemia** (anemia of prematurity), **HDN, or preterm infants to replace iatrogenic blood loss**. It may be necessary in neonates, with hemoglobin value less than 13 g/dL during the first 24 hours of life and in an ill neonate with loss of about 10% blood volume.
- **Volume:** RBC transfusions in infants are usually given frequently in **small volumes** prepared from (pediatric) multiple-pack systems. The pediatric units for infants are prepared by dividing a full unit of RBCs into sterile portions. **RBC transfusion of 10–15 mL/kg is administered slowly over a period of 2–4 hours**. Usually it will increase the Hb by 2–3 g/dL Most infants tolerate transfusion of RBCs stored until outdate, without adverse effects. When a large volume transfusion (e.g. exchange transfusion or cardiac surgery) is needed, it is indicated to transfuse fresh RBCs (usually <10 days old).
- **Compatibility testing: Red cell antibodies are not formed** in infants **during the first 4 months** of life, therefore no crossmatching is needed. The testing required consists of a forward ABO and Rh type on RBCs either from the cord or a heel prick sample. However, if maternal red cell alloantibody is detected in infant's plasma or serum, it is necessary to transfuse antigen-negative blood. Antibodies detected in the newborn are maternal in origin. At 4–6 months of age, infants begin to produce their own ABO antibodies and are capable of producing antibodies, if immunologically sensitized by transfusion of RBC.
- **Antibody screening:** It can be done on the serum or plasma of either the mother or the neonate.
  - **If this initial antibody screen is negative**, there is no need to crossmatch the donor RBCs
  - **If the antibody screen is positive** due to a clinically significant antibody, **compatibility testing should be performed** with the neonate or mother's serum or plasma, or with an eluate prepared from the infant's RBCs.
- **Blood group selection for transfusion:** During the first 4 months of age, RBC units chosen for transfusion should be **ABO identical, or ABO compatible with the mother as well as with the neonate**. For example, for the neonate with group A and the mother of group O, the RBC units should be group O. For this reason, many transfuse group O RBCs to all neonates, rather than ABO type-specific blood. The selected **blood unit should be D-negative or the same as the infant's D type**. Before issuing nongroup O RBCs, it is necessary to test the infant's plasma or serum to detect passively acquired maternal anti-A or anti-B and also an antiglobulin phase test.
- **Risk of CMV:** In preterm infants of less than 1,200 g weight who are born to seronegative mothers or to mothers whose CMV status is unknown, there is a risk of transfusion-transmitted CMV. This can be prevented by transfusing irradiated CMV antibody negative blood to neonates. If leukocyte reduced component is used, leukocyte reduction should be done using highly efficient leukocyte removal filters. This is because CMV resides within the white blood cell.

Transfusion of Other Blood Components

Sometimes, neonates and babies may require a transfusion of a blood product other than RBCs. These components include platelets, granulocytes, and components necessary to restore hemostasis.

Platelets

Indication for platelet transfusion is thrombocytopenia or qualitative defects in platelet function. Adults may tolerate a platelet count as low as 10,000/µL (10×10^9/L), but newborns often cannot. This is especially in case of premature infants who are at higher risk of intraventricular hemorrhage (IVH) due to the immaturity of the brain. In neonates, generally **a minimum platelet count of 50,000/µL (50×10^9/L) is necessary to maintain hemostasis.** However, the sick premature infant may require a platelet count as high as 100,000/µL (100×10^9/L) to prevent bleeding. Whenever possible, the platelets selected for transfusion should be leukocyte reduced and ABO compatible with the infant. Similarly, whenever possible, Rho(D) negative infants should be transfused with Rho(D) negative platelets. Dosage is calculated depending on body weight; 5-10 mL of platelets/kg of the baby's body weight should increase the platelet count by 40,000-50,000/µL ($50-100 \times 10^9$/L). As with RBC units, when appropriate irradiated and/or CMV reduced-risk platelets may be used.

Granulocytes

Granulocyte transfusions are very rarely required. However, they are transfused more frequently in the neonates and pediatrics patients than in adults.

Indication: Granulocyte transfusion is reserved only for those with **severe neutropenia**, an absolute neutrophil count <500/µL, (<0.50 $\times 10^9$/L) and a **bacterial or fungal infection not responding to standard antimicrobial therapy** for at least 24-48 hours. In addition, there must be a reasonable chance of marrow recovery.

Granulocytes collection: For newborns, granulocytes should be collected **from CMV-seronegative donors and must be irradiated** before transfusion **to prevent transfusion-associated graft versus host disease** (TA-GVHD) by any donor lymphocytes present.

Dose: The determination of dose of granulocytes required is difficult to determine, but generally the children who are given higher doses have a better response. For an infant, a recommended dose is $1 \times 10^9 - 2 \times 10^9$ PMN/kg. This dose is generally repeated for five daily transfusions. The granulocytes have short lifespan and should be given as fresh as possible and not later than 24 hours after collection. In a critically-ill infant, it is often transfused immediately after collection and before the completion of test for infectious disease.

Crossmatching: In a granulocyte concentrate, there will also be RBCs. Hence, it is **necessary** to perform a crossmatch.

Transfusion to enhance hemostasis

Newborns have lower levels of some coagulation factors at birth.
- **Fresh frozen plasma** is usually transfusion **to prevent bleeding when multiple** (such as the vitamin K-dependent) **factors are required.** FFP transfusion is mainly used for bleeding due to either an acquired deficiency of coagulation factors such as disseminated intravascular coagulation (DIC) or a congenital factor deficiency for which no specific factor concentrates are available. FFP should be ABO compatible with the infant. The usual dose is 10-15 mL/kg of body weight and this will raise factor levels by 15-20%.
- **Cryoprecipitate** contains fibrinogen, factor VIII, factor XIII, and von Willebrand factor (vWF). In newborns (as in adults), it is transfused mainly **for treating hypofibrinogenemia.** Cryoprecipitate should be ABO compatible with the infant. A dose of 1-2 units/10 kg of body weight will raise the fibrinogen level by 60-100 mg/dL.

Exchange transfusion of the neonate for hyperbilirubinemia is usually indicated when the total bilirubin level is more than 25 mg/dL. Exchange transfusion is discussed in page 392 of Chapter 18.

Guidelines for neonatal transfusion are summarized in Box 19.3.

> **Box 19.3:** Guidelines for neonatal transfusion.
>
> **RBC transfusion**
> - Hct <20% with symptomatic anemia
> - Hct <30% with supplemental O_2
> - Hct <35% with supplemental O_2
> - Hct <45% with cyanotic congenital heart disease or extracorporeal oxygenation
>
> **Platelet transfusion**
> - Platelet count <30,000/µL in term infant with platelet production failure
> - Platelet count <50,000/µL in stable premature infant
> - Platelet count <100,000/µL in unstable premature infant
>
> **Plasma transfusion**
> - Coagulation factor deficiency, unavailability of factor concentrates, and bleeding or prior to surgery
> - Disseminated intravascular coagulation (DIC)

Transplantation

The transfusion service provides support for transplantation of organs and hematopoietic progenitor cells (HPCs).

Solid Organ Transplantation

Transfusion support required varies because of the nature of the transplant organ. Usually, transplantation of kidney, liver, heart, and lung are performed. The **donor organs are usually ABO compatible** and except for kidney transplants, human leukocyte antigen (HLA) matching is often not needed. ABO compatibility is very important for the success of vascularized grafts, such as livers, kidneys, and hearts. **Generally, leukoreduced blood products are transfused to the recipients of solid organ transplant** to diminish HLA alloimmunization. However, it is not necessary to transfuse irradiation blood products. Since, TA-GVHD in solid organ transplant is very unusual, it is not necessary to use irradiated blood products. CMV reactivation occurs following transplantation, so CMV-reduced risk products should be used.

Liver transplantation: It requires a complicated surgery because of its vascular natures and can be associated with massive hemorrhage. Liver synthesizes clotting factors and is involved in clearance of coagulation inhibitors. Hence, **hemostatic problems are major complications of liver transplant**. The pre-existing liver disease also contributes to the excessive bleeding during the surgical procedure. Historically, significant blood loss during liver transplantation has been treated with large autologous transfusions of RBCs, FFP, platelets, and cryoprecipitate. The metabolic and coagulation abnormalities were treated with drugs along with the blood products. Improvements in operative techniques and use of drugs that minimize loss of blood have minimized the requirement of transfusion.

Heart and heart lung transplants: In cardiopulmonary bypass, hemostasis can be affected secondary to hypothermia, use of heparin, priming fluid used for the bypass instrument, and duration of surgery. These patients should be transfused with leukocyte-reduced components to prevent sensitization and complications caused by HLA antibodies.

Renal transplant: In kidney transplant, cyclosporine is used for immunosuppression and reduced the need of transfusion. Use of erythropoietin has also reduced the need for transfusion in patients with kidney disease. Leukocyte-reduced blood products have reduced the alloimmunization to HLA antigens in renal transplant. It is difficult to obtain compatible kidney when a potential kidney transplant recipient develops HLA antibodies.

Hematopoietic Progenitor Cell Transplantation

Hematopoietic progenitor cells can be obtained from bone marrow, peripheral blood, and cord blood. HPC is discussed in detail in chapter 24.

Transfusion support for HPC transplants
Before transplantation: Transfusion support is given before transplantation and consists of transfusing leukocyte-reduced blood products to avoid HLA alloimmunization, CMV infection, and febrile reactions.

After transplantation: Patients usually need extensive platelet and RBC support for about 2 weeks. If the ABO types of the transplant recipient and donor are not matched, careful monitoring is required, and additional RBC support may be needed if hemolysis develops.

Patients receiving transplants undergo immunosuppression and have the serious risk of graft versus host disease (GVHD) (refer Chapter 24). After transplant, only irradiated blood products should be transfused. However, the progenitor cell product must never be irradiated because this will prevent engraftment. Another complication due to immunosuppression is CMV infection, which can be avoided with leukocyte-reduced or seronegative blood products. **The progenitor cell product should never be administered through a leukocyte reduction filter.**

HLA compatibility is very important for successful engraftment of myelosuppressed patients with HPCs. However, ABO compatibility is not essential. In these HPC transplants, the early committed and uncommitted cells do not possess A, B, and H antigens (ABH antigens). Hemolysis can develop after a minor ABO-incompatible transplant (e.g. group "O" HPC donor to group "A" recipient). After transplant of ABO mismatched grafts, the components transfused must be compatible with the blood type of both the donor and the recipient.

Oncology

A patient with cancer may undergo chemotherapy or radiation treatment. They require many blood products. Chemotherapeutic agents are used with the purpose to target cancer cells. At the same time, they also affect epithelial cells of the gastrointestinal tract and germinal epithelium of the hair follicles. In the bone marrow, they reduce differentiation of hematopoietic cells into megakaryocytes, erythrocytes, and leukocytes. As treatment with chemotherapy progresses, there will be decrease in platelet, leukocyte, hemoglobin, and hematocrit levels. The most common complications are bleeding, anemia, and infection. To determine component therapy required depends on laboratory findings and clinical conditions associated with bleeding and anemia. Commonly, irradiated blood products are transfused after intensive chemotherapy and radiation therapy. In some patients, multiple platelet transfusions may cause refractoriness or the inability to achieve desired therapeutic results. If the cause of refractoriness is alloantibodies to HLA antigens, it may necessary to transfuse HLA-matched platelets. Nowadays, colony-stimulating factors are more widely used to prevent the risks of infection and bleeding associated with chemotherapy.

Chronic Renal Disease

Patients undergoing dialysis for renal conditions may develop many hematologic complications that require transfusion of usually RBC component. Severe uremia may lead to alteration in the shape of red cell. This altered shape may result in hemolytic anemia. The dialysis process also causes as breaking of the red cells and can contribute to hemolysis. Patients with chronic renal disease do not produce sufficient levels of erythropoietin because of the nonfunctioning kidney. This will also reduce the erythrocyte production and contribute to anemia.

Factors contributing to anemia in patients with chronic renal disease are summarized in Table 19.1.

Careful monitoring of hemoglobin and hematocrit levels is necessary along with clinical symptoms to determine the need of transfusion therapy. The use of recombinant erythropoietin has significantly reduced the need for transfusion. However, in acute anemia

Table 19.1: Factors contributing to anemia in chronic renal disease.

Contributing factors	Effect
Uremia	Alters red blood cells (RBC) shape and causes their premature destruction
Dialysis procedure	Breaking of RBCs
Low erythropoietin level	Decreased production of RBC

there is need for RBC transfusions. To reduce the need for an additional venipuncture, transfusions are usually given while the patient is on dialysis equipment. Leukocyte-poor RBCs are the preferable to prevent the development of HLA antibodies, which may cause difficulty in finding a compatible kidney for transplantation in future.

Hemolytic Uremic Syndrome and Thrombotic Thrombocytopenic Purpura

Hemolytic uremic syndrome (HUS) and thrombotic thrombocytopenic purpura (TTP) have many overlaps in their clinical symptoms. These clinical symptoms are as follows:
- Microangiopathic hemolytic anemia
- Thrombocytopenia
- Renal dysfunction
- Central nervous system involvement

In both HUS and TTP, damage to the vessel endothelium is activated and there is consumption of platelets and coagulation proteins. This causes formation of microthrombi in the kidney.
- Thrombotic thrombocytopenic purpura is caused due to a deficiency or antibody to a protease (ADAMTS13) that cleaves vWF. **Therapeutic plasma exchange** removes the inhibitor and large-molecular-weight multimers and simultaneously replaces the deficient protease (ADAMTS13) enzyme.
- Hemolytic uremic syndrome usually seen in young children below 1 year of age. It usually follows a severe viral infection, bacterial gastroenteritis, or treatment with certain cytotoxic drugs. **Therapeutic plasma exchange** is a supportive treatment for HUS due to an autoantibody to factor H or complement factor deficiencies.

Anemias Requiring Transfusion Support

Sickle Cell Anemia

Hemoglobinopathy is a genetic (inherited) disorder of hemoglobin (the oxygen-carrying protein of the RBCs). Sickle cell disease contains hemoglobin S and is one of hemoglobinopathy. This is due to a structural variance in the β-chain of the hemoglobin molecule in which there is substitution of an amino acid valine at the sixth position by glutamic acid. This molecular change alters the solubility of the hemoglobin molecule. At low oxygen (hypoxia), hemoglobin S polymerizes causing the characteristic sickling of the cell. These sickled cells can block the microvasculature and are responsible for "sickle cell crisis," characterized by endothelial damage, thrombosis, and pain. The red cells with hemoglobin S have a decreased lifespan and cause hemolytic anemia. Serious complications of sickle cell disease are stroke, acute chest syndrome, and multiorgan failure.

Hematopoietic stem cell transplantation has the ability to cure sickle cell disease and is recommended in patients with the most severe complications.

Hemoglobin and hematocrit values are usually reduced in sickle cell disease before they become symptomatic.

Indications for transfusion in sickle cell disease are summarized in Box 19.4.

Transfusion

Indications for **transfusing RBCs** to patients with sickle cell disease have two purposes: (i) to increase hemoglobin and thereby increase oxygen-carrying capacity and (ii) to dilute RBCs containing HbS with healthy donor RBCs. Patient with sickle cell disease need RBC transfusion throughout most of their life time. This is responsible for high chances of alloantibody production. To avoid this, these patients should be transfused with phenotypically matched (C, E, and K) antigens

---

Box 19.4: Indications for transfusion in sickle cell disease (SCD).

Acute anemia due to:
- Bleeding
- Increased hemolysis
- Infection
- Sequestration of cells in the spleen and liver

To prevent:
- Stroke: To reduce sickling which blocks blood vessels
- Recurrent pain episodes due to sickling in joints

early in the treatment by transfusion. Once the patients develop a red cell antibody, extend the matching of additional antigens to Fy, Jk, and S to reduce the chance of developing life-threatening delayed hemolytic transfusion reactions.

RBC transfusions: Clinical symptoms associated with pulmonary or cardiac insufficiency require RBC transfusions. The RBCs in sickle cell disease can be transfused either as a simple transfusion or as part of a RBC exchange.

Red cell exchange: In patients with severe pain and crisis, automated RBC exchange (therapeutic red cell exchange) may be needed. In a RBC exchange, the transfusion of donor cells is infused and there is removal of patient cells with HbS.

Iron overload: Repeated transfusions can produce iron overload. Each unit of RBCs contains about 250 mg of iron. Normally, an average of 1 mg of iron can be excreted daily. Iron overload can be treated with using oral iron chelators. They bind to iron in the body and remove it. Red cell exchange therapy is another method to avoid iron overload.

Thalassemia

Thalassemia is an inherited syndrome caused by a deficiency in hemoglobin α-chain or β-chain production. It causes anemias ranging from mild to severe.
- α-thalassemia is characterized by reduced or absence of synthesis of α-chain production and total absence of α-chain synthesis is fatal in utero.
- β-thalassemia is characterized by reduced or absence synthesis of the β-chain and is classified as thalassemia major, intermedia, and minor.

In thalassemia, hemolysis leads to anemia. To compensate anemia, hematopoietic tissue proliferates and results in bone deformities (due to excessive medullary hematopoiesis) and enlargement liver and spleen (due to excessive extramedullary hematopoiesis).

Transfusion in children with thalassemia suppresses ineffective erythropoiesis and prevents early complications.

To determine whether transfusion is required, it is necessary to monitor hemoglobin and hematocrit values. The transfusion needed may be:
- RBC transfusion
- Leukocyte-reduced red cells are preferred

Similar to sickle cell disease, thalassemia patients need multiple transfusions. Hence, iron chelation must accompany blood transfusions to prevent the iron overload.

Immune Hemolytic Anemias

Immune hemolytic anemias are characterized by decreased survival of the RBCs because of antibody coating the red cell membrane. This sensitization causes premature removal of red cell from the circulation compared to normal removal by 120 days. These disorders can be produced due to several mechanisms.
- **Autoimmune hemolytic anemia:** In this type, the antibody reacts with a self-antigen on the red cell. These RBCs are removed by the spleen and causes anemia. Based on serologic tests, these anemias can be further divided into those due to cold or warm autoantibodies.
- **Drug-induced hemolytic anemia:** In these hemolytic anemias, either the drug is adsorbed directly onto the red cell membrane or the drug-antibody combination becomes adsorbed onto the red cell. Some drugs can also induce the production of an autoantibody.
- **Alloimmune hemolytic anemia:** This anemia occurs when RBC destruction by alloantibodies produced against transfused RBCs or against fetal cells in hemolytic disease of the fetus and newborn.

Hemostatic Disorders

Hemostatic disorders may be due to:
- A decrease or absence of production of one or more of the coagulation proteins.
- Normal production of an abnormal structure resulting in a nonfunctioning protein.

von Willebrand disease: vWF is required for platelets to adhere to endothelium and also for factor VIII for correct functioning and maintenance of adequate levels. Quantitative or qualitative abnormalities of vWF can cause bleeding.

Hemophilia A (factor VIII deficiency) and hemophilia B (factor IX deficiency)

Clinically coagulation factor deficiencies present with prolonged bleeding, bleeding into joints, and subcutaneous bleeds.

Treatment:
- **Most of the hemostatic disorders** are treated with factor concentrates or desmopressin (DDAVP). 1-deamino-8-d-arginine vasopressin (DDAVP) stimulates the release of preformed factor VII and vWF from cellular stores. It is used for treating type 1 von Willebrand disease.
- **Hemophilia:** Replacement of factor VIII or factor IX is used for the management of patients with severe hemophilia. It can be administered before a medical procedure, in response to a bleed, or as long-term prophylaxis to prevent bleeding episodes.
- **Disadvantages of coagulation factor concentrate:** Their administration can lead to the development of antibodies, or inhibitors to one or more of the factors. This, in turn, can lead to further bleeding episodes.
- **Cryoprecipitated antihemophilic factor (AHF):** It is used only in urgent situations when the preferred concentrate is not available.

Disseminated intravascular coagulation:
It is an acquired hemostasis disorder characterized by inappropriate activation of coagulation cascade. This leads to formation of microthrombi which consume platelets and fibrinogen. It may occur in several conditions (e.g. during surgery, massive blood loss, amniotic fluid embolism, snake or insect bite). Strands of fibrin trap platelets. Patients with DIC can spontaneously bleed or form a thrombus.

Management:
- Identify and treat or remove the cause of DIC. Immediate and appropriate determination and treatment or removal of the underlying condition/cause is essential to prevent tissue ischemia and shock.
- Maintain blood volume and also stabilize the patient.
- Maintain hemostatic functions: If PT and aPTT are prolonged

Therapeutic apheresis is discussed in Chapter 13.

Massive transfusion is discussed on pages 236-8 of Chapter 11.

AUTOLOGOUS BLOOD DONATION AND TRANSFUSION

Autologous transfusion is transfusion to a patient of their own blood.
- Advantages of autologous blood transfusion are given in Box 19.5.
- Disadvantages of autologous blood transfusion are given in Box 19.6.
- Contraindications for autologous blood transfusion are given in Box 19.7.

The patient must not suffer from a disease that would put them at risk from this procedure. They may not be able to tolerate phlebotomy.

Preliminary Steps
1. **Identification of patient-donor:** It is important.
2. **Consent:** A written consent should be obtained from patient-donor after explaining the procedure. If the patient

---

Box 19.5: Advantages of autologous blood transfusion.

- Prevents
  - Transfusion transmitted diseases. Compared to allogeneic, it prevents the transmission of blood-borne pathogens
  - Red cell alloimmunization: It may be useful in patients having antibodies to very common RBC antigens and where compatible allogeneic components are not available
  - Some adverse transfusion reactions (e.g. hemolytic, febrile allergic reactions)
- Provides
  - Compatible blood for patients with alloantibodies and rare blood groups
  - Reassurance to patients concerned about blood risks
- Supplements the blood supply

Box 19.6: Disadvantages of autologous blood transfusion.

- Does not affect
  - Risk of bacterial contamination
  - Risk of ABO incompatibility error
- More expensive/costly than allogeneic blood
- Results in wastage of blood, if not transfused
- Increases prevalence of adverse reactions to autologous donation
- Patients are prone to develop perioperative anemia

Box 19.7: Contraindications for autologous blood transfusion.

- Evidence of infection and risk of bacteremia. Bacterial contamination is the most serious consequence of autologous transfusion
- Cardiovascular contraindications
  - Scheduled surgery to correct aortic stenosis
  - Unstable angina
  - Severe left main coronary artery disease
  - Recent (within 6 months of donations) myocardial infarction or cerebrovascular accident
  - Patients with significant cardiac or pulmonary disease
  - Cyanotic heart disease
- Uncontrolled hypertension
- Active seizure disorder
- Hemoglobin concentration: Should not be significantly anemic (Hb level not less than 11.0 g/dL)

is a minor, parents or guardian must give consent.

3. **Request from patient's physician:** Requires a written request from patient's physician indicating the requirement and/or the advantage.
4. **Age:** No minimum or maximum age limits. Each case has to be evaluated individually. The lower age limit is determined by the capacity of the child to understand and cooperate.
5. **Volume of blood to be collected:** It depends on age and weight of patient. Volume should not exceed 10.5 mL/kg of the donor's body weight.
6. **Examination:** Medical interview and examination should be structured to the special needs of donor patients. Any contraindication (Box 19.7) to autologous transfusion should be ruled out.
7. **Serologic testing:** ABO and Rh typing must be determined on all units. Antibody screening and crossmatch are optional if only autologous units are ordered for transfusion. Screening for blood transmissible disease is required for the first unit collected from the donor in a 30-day period.
8. **Labeling:** The unit should be clearly marked for "**autologous use only**" and carry the statement autologous donor. Units should be clearly labeled with name and age of patient-donor, identification number, name of collection center, name of hospital, date of collection and expiry, ABO and Rh group, and signature of patient-donor.

Pre-transfusion Testing

The patient's blood sample should be tested for ABO and Rh grouping. It is optional to test for unexpected antibodies and crossmatching. The blood unit must be retested to confirm the ABO and Rh group using a sample obtained from segment of tubing attached to bag.

Criteria for unused autologous blood for homologous use are given in Box 19.8.

Types of Autologous Transfusion

Types of autologous transfusion are given in Box 19.9.

Box 19.8: Criteria for using unused autologous blood for homologous use.

- If the patient-donor does not need the blood, same can be given to another patient if donor gives a consent to use it for other patients
- If all standard criteria for donor selection for homologous transfusion are met for autologous blood
- If the blood unit is tested for VDRL, HBsAg, HIV, and malarial parasite (MP) as per standards required for homologous blood transfusion

Note: Blood collected intraoperatively should not be used for other patients.

> **Box 19.9:** Types of autologous transfusion.
> - Preoperative collection
> - Perioperative blood collection
>   - Acute normovolemic hemodilution (ANH)
>   - Intraoperative blood collection
>   - Postoperative collection

Preoperative Collection

In this procedure, the blood is drawn and stored prior to anticipated need. Patients suitable for preoperative collection are stable patients scheduled for surgical procedures in which blood transfusion is likely.

Collection schedule: Usually, a weekly schedule is used. Two or three units of blood may be collected several weeks before surgery by autologous donation. There should be sufficient interval from donation to surgery. The last collection should be done not before 72 hours of the scheduled surgery and preferably be longer. This period helps for recovery of a substantial portion of the collected red cell mass and for adequate volume repletion. During this period, iron supplementation may be needed. Erythropoietin stimulation can be used as an adjunct to autologous donation. It is to be noted that there is no indication for single unit autologous transfusion in an adult.

Indications: Preoperative autologous collections are most beneficial for patients undergoing:
- Major orthopedic procedures
- Vascular surgery, cardiac or thoracic surgery
- Radical prostatectomy.

Perioperative Blood Collection

- **Acute normovolemic hemodilution (ANH):** In this type, blood is collected before start of surgery. In order to maintain the circulatory blood volume, it is replaced simultaneously with colloid or crystalloid solution. Hematocrit is allowed to come down to 25–30%. The blood collected is reinfused either during or after surgery. The blood units are reinfused in the reverse order of collection. Thus, the first unit collected and therefore, the last unit transfused has the highest hematocrit and concentration of coagulation factors and platelets.
  Indications: It is useful in cardiac surgery because:
  - Due to hemodilution there is reduced loss of red cells. This is because the whole blood shed during surgery is having a low hematocrit.
  - The blood collected by ANH is stored at room temperature and is returned to the patient within 8 hours of collection. Thus, there is little deterioration of platelets or coagulation factors and results in preservation of hemostasis.
- **Intraoperative collection:** In this type, bloodshed from the surgical field is recovered by circulatory devices. The shed blood is processed by machines called shell savers and then infused/transfused into the same patient.
  Indications: This type of autologous transfusion is useful in:
  - Cardiovascular surgery
  - Ruptured
    - Spleen or liver
    - Ectopic pregnancy
    - Aneurysm
  - Traumatic penetrating injuries
  Contraindications:
  - When procoagulant materials (e.g. topical collagen) are applied to surgical field, it may result in systemic activation of coagulation.
  - Malignancy
  - Contamination of blood with fecal matter, urine or bile, etc.
- **Postoperative collection**: In this type, blood is collected from drainage devices and reinfused to the patient with or without processing. Postoperative shed blood may be collected into sterile canisters and reinfused after passing through microaggregate filter. Postoperatively recovered blood is dilute, partially hemolyzed and may contain high concentrations of

cytokines. Hence, a maximum of 1,400 mL of unprocessed blood can be reinfused within 6 hours of initiating collection.

ALTERNATIVES TO TRANSFUSION

Introduction

Blood is a limited resource and transfusion is associated with risks of transfusion-transmitted diseases and adverse reactions. For this reason, research is going on to substitute blood products with an alternatively safer, more effective, and more readily available products. Developing a safe blood substitute has been a goal of medical researchers for decades. These were found to be necessary after observing the urgent need of large amount of blood needed during the traumas of World Wars, as well as more recent wars in Asia and the Middle East. Apart from this, the recognition of blood-borne infections, especially hepatitis B and C, and HIV also further added the need of blood substitute. The long search for a goal of "artificial blood" has still not been achieved.

Functions of Blood

Before identifying the blood substitute, we should know the basic functions of blood (Box 19.10).

Various alternatives to blood transfusion are presented in Box 19.11.

Blood Substitutes or Artificial Blood

Considerable effort has been made to develop blood substitutes or artificial blood. The usual term "blood substitute" is a misnomer because most substitutes carry and transfer oxygen, just one of the many functions (refer Box 19.10) of transfused blood. Most commonly,

Box 19.10: Functions of blood.
- To maintain intravascular volume
- To deliver oxygen to tissues
- To provide coagulation factors
- To transport metabolic waste products
- To provide some defense mechanisms

Box 19.11: Various alternatives to blood transfusion.
- Hemoglobin or red cell substitutes (artificial blood)
  - Perfluorocarbon (PFC) emulsions/perfluorochemical emulsions
  - Hemoglobin-based oxygen carriers (cell free hemoglobin solutions (HBOCs)
  - New formulations by chemical modification of the molecule (e.g. liposome-encapsulated hemoglobin [LEH])
- Platelets substitutes
- Ex vivo generation of blood cells
- Hematopoietic growth factors
  - Erythropoietin (EPO)
  - Colony-stimulating factors (CSFs)
  - 1-deamino-8-D-arginine vasopressin (DDAVP)
- Factor concentrate
- Plasma substitutes
  - Crystalloid solutions
  - Colloid solutions

these products are small molecules which are capable of carrying out only delivery of oxygen efficiently. Hence, they are **better termed as hemoglobin or red cell substitutes** (RCS) than the original term *blood substitutes*. Recently, the terms **oxygen therapeutics** and **artificial oxygen carriers** have been used. They were originally developed to be used in trauma situations such as accidents, combat, and surgery. However, despite years of research, RBC substitutes are still not in routine use today.

Need of blood substitutes: There is shortage in blood and it is being an increasing problem that has worsened over recent years. Blood substitutes can alleviate shortages of donated blood. They are needed:
- To maintain a constant supply of safe alternative and prevent shortages.
- To overcome complex procedures of blood collection and processing.
- To eliminate the need for refrigeration, limited shelf-life, compatibility, immunogenicity, and transmission of infectious agents.

Potential benefits of artificial oxygen carriers are given in Box 19.12.

Features required for the ideal RCS are given in Box 19.13.

Box 19.12: Potential benefits of artificial oxygen carriers.

- Abundant supply
- Readily available for use (e.g. remote locations)
- Stock can be maintained for emergencies
- No need for blood grouping/typing or crossmatching
- Available for immediate infusion
- Could be stored at room temperature for a long period (long shelf-life of 1–3 years)
- Free of blood-borne pathogens and transmission of disease
- Free of toxicity
- Provides full oxygen capacity immediately
- Can deliver oxygen to tissue that is inaccessible to RBCs
- Less expensive than units of blood

Box 19.13: Features required for the ideal red cell substitute.

- Should uptake adequate oxygen in the lungs and deliver adequate oxygen to the tissues
- Nontoxic without any undesirable effects (if any)
- Need no compatibility testing or crossmatching
- Remain stable at room temperature during prolonged storage and readily available for use
- Long shelf-life and easy to store
- Long circulation time and should persist in the circulation of the recipient
- Should be easily reconstituted
- Should be cheap
- Rapidly excreted without causing harm
- Lower the risk of transfusion-transmitted infection or blood donation
- Easily sterilizable
- Free of any side effects

Types of Hemoglobin or Red Cell Substitutes

Situation that needs RCS: It is needed in situation where blood/RBCs are not immediately available. For example, trauma outside of the hospital, including in the military setting. It may also be useful when there is acute, unanticipated blood loss in surgery, and moderate blood loss during and after surgery, especially when there is shortage of blood for patients who are difficult to transfuse. In such situations, time is critical and immediate stabilization of a trauma victim in the first hour after the insult (the "golden hour") leads to the maximal survival rate. Valuable time can be lost in crossmatching blood and during this time acellular oxygen-carrying resuscitation fluid is the best solution during this golden hour.

Potential **hemoglobin or** RCS fall into three general classes.

1. **Perfluorocarbon (PFC) emulsions/ Perfluorochemical emulsions:** Perfluorochemicals are synthetic liquids, chemically inert, hydrophobic molecules with an almost unlimited ability to dissolve gases including oxygen (is highly soluble i.e. 20 times more than water). They also have the capacity to transport carbon dioxide. They are excreted unchanged through the lungs. Because these molecules are structurally similar to hydrocarbons, in which all the hydrogen atoms have been replaced with fluorine. Thus, they have carbon backbone with fluorine substitutions and they are not water soluble. Hence, they must be emulsified with surfactants before they are suitable for intravenous use. This emulsification process is a complicated process and their preparation and storage is a difficult. They were proved to be unsuitable in controlled clinical trials. Hence, no clinical studies with these compounds are conducted.
Advantages of PFCs are given in Box 19.14. Disadvantages of PFCs are given in Box 19.15.
2. **Hemoglobin-based oxygen carriers (cell free hemoglobin solutions):** Immense efforts have been made to develop a safe and effective synthetic oxygen-carrying solution with the functionality of packed RBCs and without the significant limitations associated with blood (i.e. immune suppression, loss of efficacy with storage, and risk of viral contaminants).

> **Box 19.14:** Advantage of perfluorocarbons (PFCs).
>
> - High respiratory gas solubility: Dissolves large volumes of both oxygen and carbon dioxide
> - Synthesized from nonbiological sources. Hence, adequate supply, and least chance for disease transmission
> - Highly stable and no need for chemical modification (unlike hemoglobin-based substitutes). Requires only simple storage.
> - No biochemical reaction in the body, and can be excreted from the body via the lungs
> - Easily sterilizable
> - Low cost

> **Box 19.15:** Disadvantage of perfluorocarbons (PFCs).
>
> - Does not mix with water and blood plasma. Hence, before administration, it must be prepared as emulsions. Do not last long in the blood
> - Needs high oxygen levels. To dissolve adequate quantities of oxygen into PFCs, the patients' needs to breathe 70–100% oxygen through a mask during surgery
> - Flu-like symptoms may occur in some

This has resulted in the development of modified hemoglobin solutions, commonly called hemoglobin based oxygen carriers (HBOCs). It is well known that 98% of blood oxygen is carried by nature's oxygen transport protein called hemoglobin. Hence, cell-free hemoglobin with similar characteristics can be used as RCS. This can be used in place of blood or packed RBCs. However, the hemoglobin tetramer is stabilized while inside the red cell membrane, whereas when present outside the red cell, hemoglobin is vulnerable to oxidative inactivation. The oxygen affinity of hemoglobin in solution is much higher than that of intracellular hemoglobin.

Sources and preparation: Hemoglobin-based oxygen carriers (HBOCs) are prepared by using either human, animal or recombinant DNA-produced hemoglobin. Hemoglobin can be prepared in solution by lysis of red cells and the cellular debris of remaining red cell stroma is removed by washing. Then it is pasteurized, filtered and passed over chromatographic columns to ensure purity. The tetramer is then chemically modified by various methods to provide molecules of different size, molecular weight, oxygen affinity, viscosity, and oncotic activity. The stroma free hemoglobin is nonantigenic. However, this has two short comings: (i) it has a short intravascular lifespan and (ii) a low P50 (the point at which 50% is saturated). These two disadvantages can be overcome by modifying the structure of the hemoglobin molecule (crosslinking or polymerization) or binding hemoglobin to other molecules. Potential difficulties with hemoglobin-based oxygen carriers are given in Box 19.16.

Applications: HBOCs have two different roles namely correction of anemia, and resuscitation of hypovolemic blood loss.

- **Immediate restoration of oxygen delivery:** Though HBOC cannot replace allogeneic blood (or red cell transfusions), a safe HBOC would help in stabilization of hemodynamic status or immediate restoration of oxygen delivery (e.g. in trauma, or urgent replacement when there is massive blood loss) till the blood is available. This will be without any transmission of infectious agent or transfusion reaction.
- **During surgery:** It may be used for a resuscitation solution or as an oxygen-carrying adjuvant in hemodiluted patients undergoing surgery. HBOCs also have long shelf lives and can be used when blood is

> **Box 19.16:** Potential difficulties with hemoglobin-based oxygen carriers.
>
> - Should be stored in an oxygen-free environment
> - Hemoglobin in solution gradually oxidizes to methemoglobin
> - Rapid clearance of the hemoglobin
> - Has hypertensive (both systemic and pulmonary) effects and produces bradycardia in the recipients
> - Changes the oxygen dissociation curve
> - Produces hemoglobin metabolites
> - Immunogenic
> - Can produce bacterial sepsis
> - Nephrotoxicity (renal toxicity)
> - Poor oxygen delivery to tissues

in short supply or fully tested blood often unavailable especially for the developing world. These situations and inexpensive RCS may save hundreds of thousands of lives. Due to the short half-life of these substitutes, they cannot be used for long-term red cell replacement (e.g. in chronic anemic).

- **Military or civilians:** Since blood typing and crossmatching is not needed, the substitutes might be carried in emergency situations or used by the military or civilians in situations where access to blood is limited.
- **Other uses:** In organ perfusion and preservation, prior to transplantation and improving oxygen delivery to tissues having an impaired blood supply.

New formulations

The problems of cell free hemoglobin (Hb) can be overcome by new formulation. They improve the oxygen delivery of Hb and its stability in the bloodstream. This is achieved by chemically-modifying the molecule by: (i) conjugation, (ii) cross-linking, (iii) polymerization, and (iv) encapsulation.

- **Conjugation:** The surface of hemoglobin is "decorated" (surface-decorated or conjugated hemoglobins) by adding molecules such as polyethylene glycol (PEG), pyridoxylated hemoglobin polyoxyethylene (PHP) or polyethylene glycol-modified human hemoglobin. This changes the oxygen-binding properties of the hemoglobin and helps prevent it from damaging the kidney.
- **Cross-linking:** Chemical modifications join the components of hemoglobin together, preventing it from falling apart.
- **Polymerization:** Chemical cross-links are created between different hemoglobin molecules. This results in holding hemoglobin molecules together and preventing them from falling apart.
- **Encapsulation:** In liposome-encapsulated hemoglobin (LEH), the hemoglobin molecules are encapsulated in liposomes/lipid membrane which can contain high concentrations of hemoglobin. This discourages it from falling apart and prolongs its intravascular circulation. However, success of liposomal hemoglobin is not clear. Advantages of LEH are listed in Box 19.17.

Platelet Substitutes

Lyophilized synthetic platelets: These are microspheres of human albumin coated with human fibrinogen.

Ex Vivo Generation of Blood Cells

The human blood cells can be produced in laboratory from the hematopoietic progenitors present in peripheral blood and from umbilical cord blood. Considerable progress has been made in the production of therapeutic quantities of mature human erythrocytes.

Major hurdles in ex vivo generation of RBCs include:
1. Induction of a substantial proliferation of primitive progenitors
2. Triggering of differentiation of progenitors into a pure cell lineage
3. Complete terminal maturation into functional (enucleated) cells.

It is possible to generate erythroid cells from human embryonic stem cells (hESC) and induced pluripotent stem (iPS) cells.

Hematopoietic Growth Factors

Hematopoietic growth factors are glycoproteins, which stimulate the bone marrow to produce erythrocytes, platelets, and leukocytes. They are used for patients with chronic anemia and various conditions causing low blood cell counts. They are also useful for patients undergoing chronic

---

Box 19.17: Advantages of liposome-encapsulated hemoglobin (LEH).

- Circulation time is longer
- Vasoactivity is less
- Diffusion of oxygen is closer to that of RBCs
- Metabolized by the reticuloendothelial system (RES) of the liver and spleen in a similar to RBCs

transfusions and renal dialysis and patients undergoing chemotherapy.

Groups: Hematopoietic growth factors are divided into four functional groups.
1. Lineage specific: Granulocyte colony-stimulating factor (G-CSF), erythropoietin, thrombopoietin (TPO)
2. Multilineage factors: *Interleukin-3* (IL-3), granulocyte-macrophage colony stimulating *factor* (GM-CSF)
3. Stem cell factors (Steel factors)
4. Accessory or synergistic factors: IL-1, IL-6, IL-11

List of factors which can be used as an alternative to transfusion along with their potential uses are presented in Table 19.2.

Factor Concentrate (Table 19.3)

Essential components or factors involved in the coagulation cascade include factor VIII, factor IX, and antithrombin concentrate. These factor concentrates are blood derivatives formulated to replace factor deficiencies as well as overcome the effects of inhibitors. The use of heat and detergent treatment of these factors has **reduced the risk of transmitting**

Table 19.2: Alternatives to transfusion and their potential uses.

Factor	Names	Uses
Erythropoietin (EPO)	EPO rHuEPO (human recombinant erythropoietin. This is prepared by recombinant technology)	• Chronic renal failure • Preoperative for cardiac surgery • Cancer patients with active myelosuppressive therapy
Colony-stimulating factors (CSFs)	• Granulocyte CSF • Granulocyte-macrophage CSF • Recombinant interleukin-11	• To decrease infection in patients on chemotherapy • Congenital agranulocytosis • Acute leukemia • Myelodysplastic syndrome • Aplastic anemia in children • Bone marrow transplant • Cancer patients with thrombocytopenia
1-deamino-8-D-arginine vasopressin (DDAVP)	Desmopressin (Promotes hemostasis by release of von Willebrand factor [vWF])	For hemophilia A, von Willebrand disease, and some platelet function disorders

Table 19.3: Factor concentrates as alternatives to transfusion.

Blood derivative	General information/preparation	Indications
Factor VIIa (FVIIa)	Recombinant (rFVIIa)	Bleeding in patients with an inhibitor to factor VIII or factor IX and congenital factor VII deficiency
Factor VIII (FVIII)	Produced by recombinant (rFVIII) or fractionation of pooled human plasma antihemophilic factor (AHF)	• Hemophilia A • von Willebrand disease
Factor IX	Produced by recombinant and plasma-derived sources	Hemophilia B
Prothrombin complex concentrate	Crude preparations of factor IX (contains other vitamin K-dependent factors)	• Deficiency of factor II, IX, and X • Overdose of warfarin
Antithrombin concentrate	Inhibitor of coagulation; prepared from pooled plasma	Hereditary deficiency of antithrombin
Protein C concentrate	Inhibitor of coagulation	Congenital deficiency of protein C

viruses. Presently, recombinant technology is used for formulating these blood derivatives. Only disadvantage being they are substantially **more expensive.** The factor concentrates are **sterile, stable, and lyophilized.** These properties make administration of these factor concentrates more convenient than administration of blood components.

■ PLASMA SUBSTITUTES

Plasma substitutes provide colloid osmotic pressure (i.e. colloid) or expand the plasma volume (crystalloids). They are also known as **volume expanders.** Various types of volume expanders are listed along with their use in Table 19.4. These products are usually dispensed by the pharmacy rather than the blood bank. They are used with or in place of blood for hypovolemia. Volume expanders as alternatives to transfusion include crystalloid and colloid solutions.

Crystalloid Solutions

Replacement type crystalloid solutions are used to correct body fluid deficits. They expand the plasma volume temporarily.

Crystalloid (salt) intravenous solution/ fluids contain small molecular weight solutes that can be either ionic (e.g. sodium [Na^+], chloride [Cl^-]) or non-ionic (e.g. glucose, mannitol). They are used to replace blood volume either during surgery or to treat traumatic blood loss. These fluids enter both the plasma and interstitial fluid compartment without shifting the osmotic balance. Because of this, infusion of large volume of these fluids is needed to expand the intravascular plasma volume. In most patients where the volume of blood lost is small, its administration does not produce any untoward incident. However, in patients with extensive blood loss, they should be judiciously administered to avoid flooding of the extravascular space, particularly in pulmonary edema. The characteristics of crystalloid fluids must be understood if important complications are to be avoided. Crystalloid fluids are **inexpensive compared with blood products and artificial colloids**.

- Replacement crystalloids are isotonic with respect to sodium concentration.
- **Common crystalloids** include 0.9% saline (0.9% sodium chloride solutions), Hartmann's solution, Ringer's lactated, acetated ringer's, 5% dextrose in water, 5% dextrose in 0.45% saline, 2.5% dextrose in saline, plasmalyte A, 3% saline and 7.5% saline.

Colloid Solutions

Colloid solutions (Table 19.4) can also be used to replace blood. Colloid solutions include solutions containing larger molecular weight solutes such as albumin or hetastarch. These include:
1. Dextrans: They consist of mixtures of polysaccharide molecules of different molecular weight (e.g. Dextran 40 and Dextran 70).
2. Hydroxyethyl starch (HES) 450
3. Others: Gelatin plasma protein fraction, albumin

The advantages and disadvantages of crystalloid and colloids solutions are presented in Table 19.5.

Transfusion support in selected patients is summarized in Table 19.6.

Table 19.4: Volume expanders as alternatives to transfusion.

Type	Examples	Use
Crystalloids	• Normal saline • Ringer's lactate • 5% dextrose in 0.45% saline	Shock due to hemorrhage and burns
Colloids	Hydroxyethyl starch (HES)	
	Dextran	Prolonged expansion of extravascular volume
	Plasma protein fraction (PPF)—5%	
	Albumin (25% or 5%)	

Table 19.5: Advantages and disadvantages of crystalloids and colloids.

Advantages	Disadvantages
Crystalloids	
• Readily available • Cheap • Nonimmunogenic • Do not transmit diseases • Do not inhibit synthesis of albumin • Storage and administration are easy	Plasma has oncotic pressure whereas crystalloids lack oncotic pressure and do not provide oncotic pressure
Colloids	

• Readily available
• Do not transmit diseases
• Provide oncotic pressure
• Storage and administration easy
	• Short half-life in circulation
	• Mild immunogenic
	• May interfere with:
	  – Blood grouping and crossmatching
	  – Hemostasis
	• May delay replacement of albumin

Table 19.6: Summary of transfusion support.

Disease or condition	Problem/risk faced	Required transfusion therapy
Massive transfusion	Risk of hypovolemic shock	Crystalloids, colloids, plasma, RBCs
Cardiac surgery	Heparin, hypothermia, platelet destruction	RBCs, platelets, plasma
Premature infant and neonate	Iatrogenic loss of blood, hemoglobin F, low erythropoietin response	Leukocyte-reduced, CMV antibody negative irradiated RBCs <7 days old
Liver transplant	Reduced levels of vitamin K-dependent factors, bleeding	RBCs, FFP, platelets, cryoprecipitated AHF
Progenitor cell transplant	Immunosuppression, irradiation of bone marrow	Irradiated and leukocyte-reduced platelets and RBCs
Oncology	Chemotherapy and irradiation reduce production of red cell and platelet	Leukocyte-reduced platelets and RBCs, colony-stimulating factors
Chronic renal disease	Absence of erythropoietin production, red cell damage due to dialysis and uremia	Erythropoietin, leukocyte-reduced RBCs
TTP and HUS	Consumption of platelet and coagulation factors	Therapeutic apheresis, FFP, and RBCs
Sickle cell anemia	Chronic hemolysis due to sickling of red blood cells	Phenotypically matched RBCs to prevent production of alloantibody
Hemostatic disorders	Factor deficiencies: von Willebrand disease, hemophilia A and B	Factor derivatives specific for deficient factor

(AHF: antihemophilic factor; CMV: cytomegalovirus; FFP: fresh frozen plasma; HUS: hemolytic uremic syndrome; RBC: red blood cell; TTP: thrombotic thrombocytopenic purpura)

SUMMARY

- Transfusion of blood component can provide support for many patients with unique hematologic disorders. Targeted blood component therapy can minimize blood exposure and the subsequent risks of adverse transfusion complications.
- Platelet function defects and some degree of reduction in number of platelets (thrombocytopenia) occur frequently after cardiac bypass surgery.
- The newborn has an immature immune system and most antibodies for the first 4 months of life are derived from the mother. The mechanisms underlying the anemia of prematurity include phlebotomy blood losses for laboratory testing and deficiency of plasma erythropoietin due to insufficient production.
- Newborns are very sensitive to volume changes and low platelet counts. It is advisable to transfuse fresh group O red blood cell units that are CMV-risk-reduced and irradiated to decrease the risk of CMV infections or transfusion-associated graft versus host disease (TA-GVHD) in immune-suppressed newborns.
- Transfusion support required for transplantation varies depending on of the nature of the transplant organ.
- Therapeutic plasma exchange will be helpful in TTP and HUS.
- Transfusion support is required for many patients with hematological disorders
- Sickle cell disease is inherited disorder characterized by HbS (hemoglobin S) and is associated with hemolytic anemia. It requires multiple blood transfusions.
- Regular blood transfusions should be started from an early age in severe β-thalassemia syndromes on the basis of symptoms rather than a particular Hb level or genotype.
- Blood transfused to both sickle cell disease and thalassemia should be fully matched for Rh and Kell blood groups, with more extensive phenotypic matching for those already alloimmunized.
- Most of the hemostatic disorders are treated with factor concentrates or desmopressin (DDAVP). Replacement of Factor VIII or Factor IX is used for the management of patients with severe hemophilia.
- Disseminated intravascular coagulation, where there is bleeding associated with severe thrombocytopenia, platelet transfusions should be given in addition to coagulation factor replacement.
- Autologous transfusion is transfusion to a patient of their own blood.
- Considerable effort has been made to develop blood substitutes or artificial blood.
- Hematopoietic growth factors stimulate the bone marrow and are used for patients with chronic anemia and various conditions causing low blood cell count.
- Plasma substitutes provide colloid osmotic pressure (i.e. colloid) or expand the plasma volume (crystalloids).

SELF-ASSESSMENT EXERCISE

Write short essays/notes on:
- Problems in pediatric blood transfusions
- Autologous blood transfusion
- Discuss blood cell substitutes
- Newer blood cell substitutes
- Red cell substitutes
- Describe the advantages and disadvantages of blood substitutes
- Benefits and hazards of autologous blood transfusion
- Give an account of pediatric transfusion
- Artificial substitute for red cell
- Discuss blood substitutes and its uses
- What are the alternatives to whole blood transfusion.

CHAPTER 20

Automation and Recent Advances in Blood Bank

CHAPTER OUTLINE

- Automation in immunohematology
- Automated testing in transfusion medicine
- Recent advances in blood banking
- Virtual blood bank
- Recent advances in therapy
- Safe blood transfusion
- Protocols in blood bank

AUTOMATION IN IMMUNOHEMATOLOGY

In the last 10–20 years important changes have taken place in the blood transfusion laboratory which makes transfusion laboratory practice safer. These changes include new technologies, the replacement of some manual systems by semi or fully automated systems and the use of information technology (IT) systems. Automation is defined as the use of various control systems for operating equipment or processes requiring no, minimal or reduced human intervention. Advances in test technologies and robotics have provided new opportunities for automation to meet the requirements of medium-sized blood banks and hospital transfusion services. Automation in blood banks is being adopted by more and more blood centers.

Automation: It is the process in which an analytical instrument performs many tests with only minimal involvement of analysts/persons. It has following features:
- Steps in a procedure are mechanized.
- Gel technology and solid phase red cell adherence assays (SPRCAs) can be performed on automated platforms.
- Automation makes it easier to do things the right way and more difficult to do the wrong things.

Advantages of automation: Automation improves quality of testing by:
- Reduces human errors in patient identification. Human errors in sample identification are often responsible for a significant cause of near miss events and transfusion reactions due to mismatched blood transfusion.
- Reduces human errors while performing tests and subjective variations during interpretation of results.
- Prevents transcription errors during documentation of results.
- Improves objectivity, reproducibility, and storage and retrieval/archiving of results of immunohematology tests.
- Improves traceability of all variables during testing including, samples, reagents, and operating staff.
- Reduces manual input and therefore need less manpower.
- Provides quality patient care with lesser turnaround time.

Forces/Factors Driving the Change to Automation

Although automation is used for many years within the clinical laboratory, its use in the blood bank has received significant attention only more recently. Apart from the availability

Automation and Recent Advances in Blood Bank

Box 20.1: Factors that drive for change to automation in blood bank.

- Pressures to operate more efficiently and round the clock
- Reduce manual errors due to fatigue/erroneous sample identification
- Reduced turnaround time (TAT)
- Increased productivity: Higher volume of tests to be carried out. More number of analysis and methods can be adopted in one system
- Opportunity to reduce the operating costs through reduction of laboratory expenses in labor, reagents and supplies, and biohazardous waste disposal
- Increased quality: Standardization of testing and technology
- Compliance with increased regulations: Quality assurance
- Shortage of skilled technologists
- Reduction in staff positions
- Reduce the cost of maintenance

of new technology for automated systems, many other factors have been responsible for use of automation in the blood bank. These factors have been listed in Box 20.1.

Disadvantages: Automation needs:
- Significant financial investment
- Infrastructure remodeling and increased floor space
- Highly technical personnel
- Personnel team building.

Use of Automation in Various Stages in Laboratory Investigations

Preanalytical Stages in Laboratory

Automation in sample delivery:
- Blood drawers or runners/courier facility
- Pneumatic tube delivery system
- Conveyers or track system
- Mobile robots

Automation in sample processing: It has three phases:
1. **Precentrifugation:** All measurements can be completed within 45 minutes
2. **Centrifugations:** Blood (plasma/serum)
3. **Postcentrifugation.**

Preanalytical modules:
- Labeling: Barcode label system
- Sorting: Stopper color, size, tests ordered, and instrument design requirements
- Decapping
- Aliquoting
- Recapping
- Storage/retrieval
- Automated identification methods.

Barcode label system:
- A barcode consists of a series of vertical bars and spaces arranged in various combinations to represent different characters.
- Different barcode systems are available. Each system follows different rules governing the representation of the characters (e.g. CODABAR system uses ABC symbols).
- By combining the numbers, letters and other characters, a series of barcodes can be built up. Barcoded labels are nowadays used commonly on blood groups, donation numbers, blood components, reagents, and patient samples.
- An eye readable number or description is included with the machine-readable code.
- Device which will interpret barcodes pass a beam of light across the code making use of two levels of optical reflectance (it is the measure of the proportion of light striking a surface which is reflected off it) visually the black bars and white spaces.
- Barcode labeling system has resulted in safer transfer of information, free from the transcription errors associated with manual methods.

Analytical Stage

In this stage, automation can be used for following tasks:
- Sample identification
- Centrifugation and volume determination
- Decapping and aliquoting
- Sorting
- Sample introduction and transport to cuvette or dilution cap
- Addition of reagent
- Mixing of sample and reagent
- Incubation
- Detection
- Calculation
- Read out and result reporting.

Postanalytical Stage

- Electrical signal generated by detector analyzers is analyzed by microprocessor/computers and converted into digital signal.
- Chemistry analyzer computers display graphical information as calibration curves, flags.
- Data processing: It includes data acquisition and calculation.
- Monitoring and display in the form of charts and curves.
- Performing statistics on patient and control value, and displayed as flags.

Automation is more secure over manual testing and may help in performing abbreviated pretransfusion testing (e.g. stopping duplicate D typing or reverse ABO grouping in the presence of a valid historical group).

Total laboratory automation: The automation can be used for all aspects of compatibility testing and is safer than manual techniques. Automation brings several or all of the tests of compatibility testing into a single-platform process. In total laboratory automation, integration of several instruments, processing specimen management, transportation systems, analyzers, digital interpretation, and dispatch of results are done in an automated manner.

Blood Bank Information Systems (BBIS)

Analyzer computers have capacity to link the laboratory to information system. Laboratory information management systems (LIMS) store patient details and results of laboratory tests. This is useful for timely and accurate access of the important information. In blood bank, BBIS system is used.

Blood bank information systems are computer systems that have been **developed specifically to assist the blood bank professionals in management of the patients, donor and blood component information.** BBIS consists of hardware, software, and users.

Advantages: It helps to assess trends and decide future policies by accessing the statistical information. It also helps to correlate the laboratory data with donor records and help to trace the donor records following transfusion reactions.

Characteristics of an Ideal Instrument for the Blood Bank

An "ideal" instrument should possess a proven track record with the ability to automate sampling, testing, and data handling.

Important criteria in the automation of sample handling are listed in Box 20.2.

Important criteria in the automation of testing should have some basic criteria (Box 20.3).

Important criteria in the automation of data handling are listed in Box 20.4.

Box 20.2: Important criteria in the automation of sample handling.

- Detection of any clot in the specimen
- Detection of liquid
- Barcode reading of specimen labels
- Positive identification link between sample tube and test results
- Closed-tube sampling of whole blood to reduce the risk of infectious disease
- Automated sampling of RBCs and plasma with precision and negligible carryover
- Acceptance of multiple sample tube

Box 20.3: Important criteria in the automation of testing.

- Automatic reagent dispensing and reagent recognition
- Precision pipetting
- Simultaneous multiple analyses
- Extensive testing menu
- Automated reader for reactions
- No need for excessive preventive maintenance

Box 20.4: Important criteria in the automation of data handling.

- Flexible software
- Laboratory information system (LIS) interface capabilities
- Automatic update of patient files in the LIS
- Automatic comparison of current and previous test results to flag discrepancies, if any

Selection of Automation to Meet Laboratory Needs

When we consider switching from manual to automated testing, it is important first to identify the appropriate need and assess the automation needed for the blood bank. It is necessary to assess the: i) vendor, ii) base technology, and iii) instrument.

AUTOMATED TESTING IN TRANSFUSION MEDICINE

Automated testing systems available at present are available for: **i) solid-phase, ii) gel technology and iii) microtiter plates**. These systems can perform ABO and Rh phenotyping, antibody selection and identification, and crossmatching. They are discussed in detail on pages 78-83.

Hemagglutination Assays

Uses of hemagglutination assays are outlined in Box 20.5.

Hemagglutination assays are performed in microplates and use the same principle as tube agglutination but in a smaller medium. Barcoded patient samples, reagents, and microtiter plates used in this technique. Barcode system helps in ensuring positive identification and system verification. In this technique, the sample and reagent are pipetted first. The plate is then automatically centrifuged and read by the camera reader present in the instrument.

Box 20.5: Uses of hemagglutination assays in blood bank.
Used for testing the following: • ABO and D antigen phenotype • Antigen typing • Immediate-spin crossmatch

Agglutination indicates a positive reaction and is seen as a button of agglutinated cells, whereas a negative reaction does not show any red cell button (Fig. 20.1). Grading and interpretations of the results are performed by the instrument and is displayed on the computer monitor. It is the responsibility of the operator to verify the reactions and interpretations before releasing results.

Immediate-spin crossmatch: This can also be performed by automated solid-phase hemagglutination methods. It has the advantage where the barcode technology enhances patient and donor sample identification and verification. If online with the hospital information system, previous test results can also be checked for ABO/Rh and antibody history results. This technology is helpful especially when performing the computer (electronic) crossmatch.

RECENT ADVANCES IN BLOOD BANKING

Transfusion medicine is a technology-based discipline undergoing continuous change. The recent rapid technological changes include changes related to blood collection and component processing, and cellular therapies. Recent advances in blood component production include automation, standardization, and a focus on quality and safety products.

New Technologies in Blood Banking (Box 20.6)

These new technologies are also available as user-friendly semi-automated and fully automated equipment for immunohematology tests. The new technologies in blood transfusion are next-generation advances. Cost is the

Sample ID	Interpretation	Flags	Control	Anti-A	Anti-B	Anti-D	A1 Cells	B Cells
XYZ	O Pos		0	0	0	3+	4+	3+

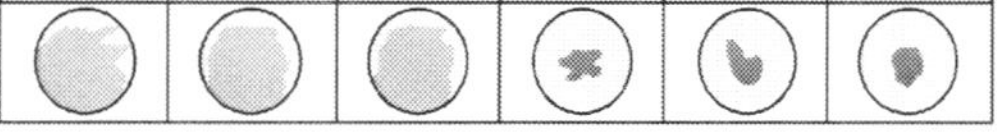

Fig. 20.1: Interpretation of an ABO/Rh phenotype using hemagglutination test. The development of agglutination indicates a positive reaction, whereas in negative reaction there is no agglutination. In this test, the blood group is O, D-positive.

Box 20.6: New technologies in blood banking.

- Immunohematological progress
- Grouping and crossmatching
  - Column agglutination technology (CAT) for immunohematology
    - Gel technology
    - Glass bead technology
  - Solid-phase red cell adherence assays
  - Erythrocytes magnetized technology
- Pathogen reduction (PR) technology
- Apheresis
- Automation
- Peripheral blood stem cell and cord blood banking
- IT system
- Transport system using drone
- Alternatives to transfusion
- Molecular techniques (refer Table 20.1)
  - Red cell (blood group) genotyping using allele specific primers
  - PCRs for Duffy, Kell, Kidd, MN, ABO, fetal RhD typing, and HLA typing

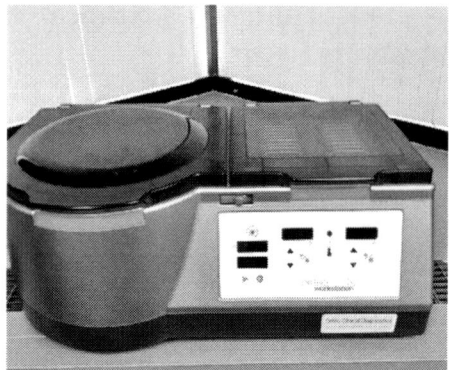

Fig. 20.2: Semiautomated immunohematology (IH) analyzer for column agglutination technology.
Courtesy: Ortho-Clinical Diagnostics, Raritan, New Jersey 08869, United States of America.

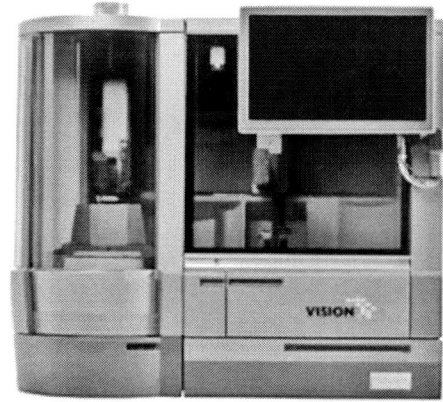

Fig. 20.3: Fully automated immunohematology (IH) analyzer for column agglutination technology. They are used for blood grouping, crossmatching, antiglobulin tests and antibody screening.
Courtesy: Ortho-Clinical Diagnostics, Raritan, New Jersey 08869, United States of America.

greatest barrier for their implementation and all the advances need highly skilled personnel.

Grouping Antibody Screening and Crossmatching

Various methods for ABO blood grouping are discussed in detail on pages 71-5. The conventional test tube technique has been replaced by newer techniques such as CAT, solid phase red cell adherence assay (SPRCA), and erythrocyte-magnetized technique. These new technologies are adaptable to automation and semi and fully automated equipment for immunohematology tests in the blood bank are presently available in the market.

Column agglutination technologies (CAT) systems

Gel card/microtyping system: This is discussed in detail on pages 78-82.

Glass bead technology (Figs. 20.2 and 20.3)

Glass bead technology of CAT is similar to gel technology, however instead of gel, glass microbeads are used.

Principle

- It is performed in a microcolumn prefilled with glass microbeads suspended in antihuman globulin serum, any diagnostic reagent or neutral isotonic solution.
- Detection of sensitized red blood cells (RBCs) is based on the sieving effect of glass microbeads similar to gel in gel technique.
- RBCs and serum are incubated at the upper part of a column over the glass microbeads suspension. These microbeads are calibrated.
- After centrifugation, positive reaction sensitized RBCs form agglutination and the unsensitized RBCs sediment at the bottom (negative reaction).

Advantages
- More objective, consistent, and reproducible interpretation of results.
- Minimum incubation time of 10 minutes for antibody screening or crossmatching.
- Centrifugation time is only 5 minutes.
- In anti-human globulin (AHG) test, no need to wash RBCs or to use sensitized RBCs for confirmation.
- No need to shake tube or resuspension of cell button which may lead to variation in reading and grading the agglutination.
- Provision of centrifuge calibrated to spin at optimal speed for fixed and correct length of time reduces error during this phase.

Disadvantages
- Expensive
- Special centrifuge is required to accommodate glass microbeads cassettes
- Special incubators to incubate the glass microbeads cassettes
- Need pipettes to dispense 10 µL, 40 µL, 50 µL.

Erythro-magnetic technology

Erythrocyte-magnetized technology (EMT) is a relatively recent technology for ABO grouping Rh/K phenotyping and antibody detection. EMT is a great innovation in the field of blood banking and has brought out short comings and improved the quality of testing and the reproducibility of results. Tests can be performed manually on a fully-automated system. This method does not require centrifugation steps and in this, magnetic RBCs and a magnetic plate are used.

Principle
In this technology, hemagglutination method is used in combination with a magnetic field.
- This technique is based on the magnetization of RBCs. Paramagnetic particles are adsorbed on to the surface of RBCs in a microplate well. Once antibodies in plasma/antisera react with antigens on RBCs in a microplate well, a magnetic force is applied at the bottom of the microplate using a magnetic plate.
- This magnetic force causes magnetization (magnetic force replaces the centrifugation) of RBCs and the magnetized RBCs migrate (pulled towards bottom) and form a pellet at the bottom of the well. In this method, the magnetization of RBCs avoids the need for centrifugation and washing steps.

Bromelin is used to enhance hemagglutination. Bromelin is a proteolytic enzyme that induces a marked decrease in the electronegative charge on the surface of RBCs. This enables RBC agglutination by normally non-agglutination antibodies in saline medium.

Technique
Forward grouping
- The test RBCs are suspended in a solution of iron chloride and bromelin.
- Then the RBC suspension is dispensed into the microplate well precoated with antisera.
- It is followed by gentle shaking and incubation for 10 minutes.
- Microplate is put on a magnetic plate. The magnetized RBCs gather at the bottom of the plate.
- After shaking, free RBCs are resuspended.
- On shaking (after the above step) the free RBCs are resuspended, whereas agglutinated RBCs form a button at the bottom of the well.

Reverse grouping
The premagnetized RBCs are mixed with test plasma in the microplate wells followed by the same steps as above.

Interpretation
- **Positive reaction:** Presence of agglutinate.
- **Negative reaction:** Absence of agglutinate.

Uses
- For **blood grouping and Rh/K phenotyping**, the microplate contains monoclonal IgM antibodies.
- The wells of the microplate can be used to perform antibody screening and crossmatching.
  - **For antibody screening**: EMT can detect only IgG antibodies. The wells

of microplate are coated with murine monoclonal anti-human globulin: anti-IgG.
- **For crossmatching**: The wells of microplate are coated with anti-IgG + anti-IgM.

Advantages

- **Quality:** Clear-cut reactions produces an unequivocal result
- **Comfort:** Centrifugation step is not required during the analytical process
- **Sensitivity:** Comparable to other existing techniques (e.g. gel technology).

Disadvantages

- Stages in the procedure to be carried out in succession without interruption
- Only qualified personnel should use the reagents
- Reactions should be read at the latest within 2 minutes of the last shaking.

Automated testing is also available for transfusion-transmitted infections (Fig. 20.4).

Pathogen Reduction Technology

New technologies include pathogen reduction (PR) technology, photochemical treatment of plasma and platelets, etc. PR technology is utilized to inactivate viruses, bacteria, and lymphocytes in platelet and plasma products. This has reduced the hazard of bacterial contamination occurring during platelet transfusions. Emerging and new infectious agents, such as chikungunya, dengue and *Anaplasma phagocytophilum*, will also be likely inactivated. PR will reduce the need for infectious disease tests thereby eliminating cost, longer platelet shelf-life.

Various methods of transfusion-transmitted diseases (TTD) testing:
- Enzyme-linked immunosorbent assay (ELISA)
- Chemiluminescent microparticle immunoassay (CMIA)
- Nucleic acid amplification testing (NAT)
- Automation in TTD testing.

Other New Technologies in Blood Banking

- Apheresis (refer Chapter 13)
- Automation
- Peripheral blood stem cell and cord blood banking (refer pages 521-4 of Chapter 24).

IT system
One of the requirements is sophisticated IT systems which link blood donors and patients, blood centers, and hospitals.

Transport of specimens
The barrier is for the transport of specimens from the centralized blood system to the field to reference laboratories. This can be overcome by drone transport mechanism for speeding delivery of vital samples.

Alternatives to transfusion
Refer pages 414-9.

Molecular techniques
Applications of molecular testing in the blood bank are given in Table 20.1.

Pretransfusion testing

The conventional pretransfusion testing techniques in immunohematology are quite cumbersome. The most commonly used conventional tube technique, though still considered as a gold standard has some limitations. These include elution of low affinity antibodies during washing, variability in the red cell concentrations, improper cell serum ratio, and lack of consistency in reporting the results due to inter observer

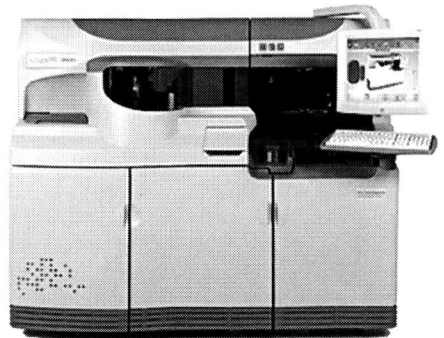

Fig. 20.4: Fully automated transfusion-transmitted infection (TTI) system.
Courtesy: Ortho-Clinical Diagnostics, Raritan, New Jersey 08869, United States of America.

Table 20.1: Applications of molecular testing in the blood bank.

Situations in blood bank	Uses
Transplantation • HPC and organ transplants • HPC transplants	• HLA antigen-level and allele-level typing • Engraftment studies
Transfusion • Red cell typing • To determine blood type • Rh typing • Screen for antigen-negative donor units	• In multiply transfused patients • When the DAT is positive • Complex Rh genotypes, weak D expression • When antisera are not available
Donor antigen screening	For prevention of alloimmunization
HDFN	Determine parental RhD zygosity Type fetal blood
Donor testing	Detect virus in donors that may be below detectable levels by antibody detection methods (NAT)
Relationship testing	Establish paternity and legal relationships

(DAT: direct antiglobulin test; HDFN: hemolytic disease of the fetus and newborn; HPC: hematopoietic progenitor cell; NAT: nucleic acid testing)

variability. Development in the molecular testing of blood groups on red cells and other cellular components can be also be applied to pretransfusion testing. Presently used serological tests to identify blood donor antigens and recipient blood groups and antibodies will probably be continued in hospital and donor center settings. However, these standard testing systems will be enhanced by automated methodology which reduces human testing errors and enhances turnaround time in transfusion services. In future, many blood banks and transfusion services will use molecular methods as adjunct to routine methods.

- **To resolve difficult patient problems:** Molecular method for detection of red cell antigen to screen blood donor and to resolve difficult patient problems where recent transfusions, autoantibodies or complicated transfusion histories make these testing systems a valuable adjunct to routine methods. The blood banks can perform routine **red cell genotype analysis** (one of the molecular techniques) which helps in more specific donor–patient matching and also help hospitals to find blood for difficult-to-match recipients.
- **Identify women who need Rh immune globulin:** Molecular methods can also be used to better identify women who need Rh immune globulin, avoiding the unnecessary treatment of many women with current testing methods. Similar systems may also be useful in platelet transfusion therapy.
- **Cellular antigen systems:** Increased antigen screening capability for cellular antigen systems (e.g. HLA) may prove to be important for cellular therapies which are likely to grow rapidly in the future. Prevention or reversal of alloimmunization to HLA will enhance solid organ transplantation or hematopoietic cell transplant.
- **To reduce adverse transfusion complications**: Better use of our evolving knowledge of immunohematology; it is possible to prevent or to detect persistent transfusion problems (e.g. delayed hemolytic transfusion reactions, TRALI) that are not caused by donor antibodies and allergic transfusion reactions.

VIRTUAL BLOOD BANK

Virtual blood bank is the computer-controlled, electronically linked information management system. It allows online ordering and remote delivery of blood for transfusion. It connects the site of testing to the point of care at a remote place through networked computers. Virtual blood bank can ensure that the right patient receives the right amount of the right blood component at the right time. It maintains the integrity of immunohematology test results. It takes the advantages of information and communication technologies to ensure the accuracy of patient, specimen and blood component identification and to enhance personnel traceability and system security. The built-in-logics can guide the selection of appropriate blood and minimize transfusion risk. Presently, computer crossmatch which is a combination of antibody screen, repeat ABO typing and electronic confirmation of ABO compatibility, can be done.

Blood Vending Machine

Components: Blood vending machine has two components:
i. Intelligent temperature-controlled blood storage and dispensing refrigerator with computerized controlled electromagnetic door lock.
ii. Attached kiosk that is a purpose-built computer terminal with identify card reader and barcode scanner for personnel login and patient identification, process control, and compatibility label printing.

Advantages:
- Only authorized personnel can gain access to the instrument.
- Checks the expiry date of donor unit.
- Confirms validity of reserved unit.
- Dispenses the oldest available donor unit.
- Monitors inventory and temperature continuously by the central blood bank.

Disadvantage: Very expensive.

RECENT ADVANCES IN THERAPY

Recombinant Coagulation Factors

Availability of recombinant coagulation factors and recently developed formulations with longer half-life has revolutionized the care of hemophilia.

Cellular Therapy

The cellular therapy in transfusion medicine includes the transplantation of hematopoietic stem cells, progenitor cells and whole organs. Mesenchymal stem cells (MSC) are multipotent, nonhematopoietic stromal cells present in the bone marrow and other tissues (e.g. adipose, peripheral blood, and placenta). MSC can differentiate into various other cells, including osteoblasts, myocytes, adipocytes, and chondrocytes. MSCs when injected intravenously, it was presumed that they can home in to sites of inflammation, post tissue injury; differentiate into various cell types, stimulate recovery of injured cells and inhibit inflammation. Current evidence suggests that some subsets of transplanted T-cells may persist in the patient for long periods of time. Cellular therapies, such as the use of T-regulatory (Tregs), natural killer (NK), and dendritic cells to treat tumors or graft-versus-host disease may provide future therapeutic promise.

CD34 cell expansion: There is increase in the use of cord blood for hematological transplantation, though the number of hematopoietic stem and progenitor cells obtained in one unit of cord blood is limited.

Manufacturing issues in cellular therapeutics: Cellular products from autologous and allogeneic donors are biological materials. To obtain licensure permission for their use, there is need of special facilities such as clean rooms, use of good manufacturing practices (GMPs), and maintenance of high levels of quality control.

SAFE BLOOD TRANSFUSION

Goal: It is essential to assure the quality and availability of safe blood and blood products for all who need transfusion, throughout the process beginning from the selection of blood donors through to their administration to the patient. Blood and blood products are necessary for numerous routine health care interventions and crucial in emergency situations.

WHO Strategy for Blood Safety

To achieve the above goal, it requires:
1. **A well-organized blood transfusion service** with quality systems and coordinated service throughout the country.
2. **Voluntary blood donors**: The blood should be collected only from voluntary, nonremunerated donors, and rigorous procedures for donor selection.
3. **Screening of donor's blood**: The screening of all donors blood for transfusion-transmissible infections such as HIV, hepatitis viruses B and C, syphilis, and malaria.
4. **Good laboratory practice** in all aspects of blood grouping, compatibility testing, component preparation, storage, transportation of blood and blood products.
5. **Rational use of blood**: A reduction in unnecessary transfusions through the appropriate clinical use of blood and blood products. Use of simple alternatives to transfusion, wherever possible.

Selection of Blood Donors

For details refer donor selection on pages 140-7.
- **Voluntary nonremunerated donors** are safer as the incidence of TTD is lower in these donors.
- **Counseling of donors:** Roles of counselors in blood bank are as follows:
  - To motivate voluntary blood donation and to assist to reach voluntary donors
  - To motivate donors at risk to undergo HIV testing and to promote AIDS awareness
  - To maintain a permanent, well indexed record of voluntary blood donors
  - To educate the community
- **Medical history**: It should be obtained as per standard questionnaire format
- **Clinical examination**: To detect any evidence of TTD.

Blood Grouping and Labeling

- Perform the ABO and RhD grouping of the blood drawn.
- Each unit should be labeled with correct ABO and RhD group.
- It is mandatory to perform all required tests before administrating blood or blood products.

Blood Products

- Safe blood or blood products, used correctly, can be life-saving. However, transfusion carries some risks. When standards are poor or inconsistent, transfusion may be very risky to the recipient.
- By preparing blood components, a single blood donated can be used to treat for two or three patients. The component also avoids the transfusion of elements of the whole blood that the patient may not require.
- Blood components can also be collected by apheresis.

Blood Group and Compatibility Testing (Crossmatch)

It is necessary to check for correct labeling of the blood sample for pretransfusion testing.

Crossmatch

- **Major crossmatch:** Donor's red cells are matched with patient's serum
- **Minor crossmatch:** Donor's serum matched with patient's red cells. If donor's serum has been screened for irregular antibodies and found negative, then there is no need for minor crossmatch.

Compatibility

- **If there is no incompatibility** (i.e. if compatible): Donor's blood or blood products can be transfused safely. In packed red cell transfusion, there must be ABO and RhD

compatibility between the donor's red cells and the recipient's plasma.
- **If incompatibility** (i.e. if incompatible): Do not transfuse which will be potentially dangerous. In such cases, identify antibodies.

Transport of Blood

Whole Blood and Red Cells

If the room temperature is more than 25°C or the blood will not be transfused immediately, it should be transported from the blood bank in a cold box or insulated carrier which will keep the temperature between 2°C and 6°C.
- Upper limit of 6°C minimize the growth of any bacterial contamination in the unit of blood.
- Lower limit of 2°C prevent hemolysis, which can cause fatal bleeding or renal failure.

Platelet

Platelets should be transported from the blood bank in a cold box or insulated carrier which will keep the temperature between 20°C and 24°C with constant agitation to prevent formation of platelet clumps.

Fresh Frozen Plasma and Cryoprecipitate

- Fresh frozen plasma should be stored in the blood bank at a temperature of –250°C or lower.
- It should be transported from the blood bank in a cold box or insulated carrier which will keep the temperature between 2°C and 6°C.
- It should be infused within 30 minutes of thawing.

Checking the Blood Bag

Check the blood bag for any discoloration or signs of any leakage. This may be the only warning sign that the blood has been contaminated by bacteria. Transfusion of this can cause a severe or fatal reaction. Check the blood bag for:
- **Any sign of hemolysis in the plasma**: This indicates that the blood has been contaminated, allowed to freeze or become too warm.
- **Any sign of contamination of RBCs**: Look for any change of color of the red cells, which often look darker or purple/black when contaminated.
- **Any clots or leakage of bag.**

Clinical Transfusion Procedures

- **Standard operating procedures**: Every hospital should have standard operating procedures (SOPs) for each stage of the clinical transfusion process. All the hospital staff should be trained to follow these SOPs.
- **Clear communication and cooperation**: There should be a clear communication and cooperation between staff of clinical departments and blood bank. This will be helpful in ensuring the safety of blood issued for transfusion.
- **Check the request form and label on blood sample**: The blood bank should not issue blood for transfusion unless a blood sample contains label and correctly completed blood request form.
- **Transportation and storage**: Blood products should be kept within the correct storage conditions during transportations and in the clinical area before transfusion. This is necessary to prevent loss of function or bacterial contamination.

Safe Administration of Blood

Final patient identity check: Before transfusing blood, the final check of the following details on the compatibility report given with the blood bag that they exactly match the details on the patient's documentation. Check the label attached to the blood bag for the following:
- **Accurate, unique identification of the patient**: All patients being transfused

must be positively identified. Name of the patient including middle name and surname; IP/hospital reference number and patient's ward or operating room.
- The name and IP no. should tally
- Patient's blood group
- Donor registration no.
- Date of collection and date of expiry.

At the bedside: A final identity check of the patient and the blood unit to ensure the administration of the right blood to the right patient. Confirm the patient's identity which should be checked from:
- The record of the patient
- In unconscious patients, identify the patient from wrist band
- Check that there are no discrepancies between the ABO and RhD group as well as unique blood bag number on:
  - Blood bag
  - Compatibility report
- Make sure that the expiry date on the blood bag has not been passed.

Monitoring the Transfused Patient

Monitoring: Do not infuse any other medication along with blood. For each unit of blood transfused, the patient should be monitored by a trained and competent staff who also administers the component. Monitoring of patient should be done as follows:
- **Before** starting the transfusion (pre-transfusion)
- **During transfusion:**
  - As soon as the transfusion is started
  - 15 minutes after starting the transfusion
  - At least every hour during transfusion
- **On completion** of the transfusion
- 4 hours **after** completing the transfusion.

Record the details: At each of the above stages, record the following information on the patient's chart:
- When transfusing blood, watch the patient's general appearance, temperature, pulse, blood pressure and respiratory rate till transfusion is completed.
- Fluid balance: Oral and IV fluid intake, urinary output
- Record about transfusion details:
  - Time of starting the transfusion
  - Time of completion of transfusion
  - Volume, number and type of blood/blood products transfused
  - Unique donation numbers of all products transfused
  - If there are any adverse effects
  - Transfusion, reaction, if any, should be immediately notified to the blood bank.
  - Testing of blood for TTD.

Rate of transfusion should be 1 mL/minute and transfusion should be completed within 4 hours.

Clinical Decision on Transfusion

- Used correctly, transfusion can be life-saving. Inappropriate use can be dangerous.
- Do not transfuse blood or blood components unless clear indication is present. The decision to transfuse blood or blood component should always be based on a careful assessment of clinical and laboratory indication that transfusion is necessary to save life or prevent significant morbidity.
- Blood transfusion is not without risks. Hence, overweigh the benefits for the patient. Transfusion is only one element in the patient's management.
- Prescribing decisions should be based on national guidelines on the clinical use of blood, taking individual patient needs into account. However, responsibility for the decision to transfuse ultimately rests with individual clinicians.

Transfusion in neonates and points to be remembered in transfusion are mentioned in Box 20.7 and Box 20.8 respectively.

■ PROTOCOLS IN BLOOD BANK

Standard operating protocols are prepared in blood bank and they include the following:

Box 20.7: Transfusion in neonates.

- In neonates, 10–20 mL/kg body weight blood is given and rate of transfusion should be less than 10 mL/kg/hour
- Blood less than 7 days is preferred for neonatal transfusion
- In neonates, only antigen grouping is done
- Blood transfused to neonates should be compatible with mother's serum
- If mother's and baby's group are the same use Rh negative blood of baby mother's ABO group. If not the same, use O Rh negative blood

Box 20.8: Points to be remembered in transfusion.

- One unit of whole blood will increase hemoglobin by 1 g/dL and PCV by 3%
- One unit of packed red cells has 250 mg of iron
- One unit of single donor platelets (SDP) will increase platelet count by 30,000–60,000 platelets/mm^3
- One unit of random donor platelets (RDP) will increase the platelet count by 4,000–6,000 platelets/mm^3
- Transfuse platelets if their count is less than 20,000. With antibodies to platelets, platelet transfusion may not be useful
- Platelet increase is observed after 1 hour and again at 12 and 24 hours of platelet transfusion
- Preserve the whole blood/PRBCS at 1–6°C
- Preserve the platelets at 22–24°C
- FFP once collected from the blood bank can be preserved at 1–6°C and has to be used within 12 hours

Donor selection:
- Criteria for donor selection
- Donor screening
- Hemoglobin estimation

Blood collection:
- **Selection of blood bags**
- **Traceability of blood bags**

Immunohematology:
- ABO grouping and Rh typing
- Preparation of RBC suspension
- Antibody screening
- Detection of incompatibility between recipient and donor
- Antiglobulin crossmatch
- Investigation of transfusion reactions

Screening for infectious diseases:
Tests for HIV, HBsAg, HCV, malaria and syphilis.

Separation of blood components

Labeling, preservation and storage of blood and its components:
- Labeling
- Preservation and storage

Issue of blood
Safe blood transfusion

Quality assurance
- Equipment maintenance-preventive maintenance, calibration
- Incident report

Clinical SOPs
- Patient identification
- Identification of blood and blood component
- Records of transfusion
- Records of monitoring the patient
- Record of adverse events/transfusion reactions.

SUMMARY

- Automation is the use of various control systems for operating equipment or processes requiring no, minimal, or reduced human intervention. Advances in test technologies and robotics are opening up new opportunities for automation in blood banks.
- The automation blood bank reduces the operating costs, increases productivity, and increases the quality.
- Automated testing systems are used for solid-phase, gel technology, and microtiterplates. Automated testing systems can perform ABO and Rh phenotyping, antibody detection, antibody identification and crossmatching.
- Future therapies will take benefit of recent advances in molecular testing of blood groups on red cells and other cellular components that are now applied to pretransfusion testing
- New technologies include pathogen reduction (PR) technology, photochemical treatment of plasma, and platelets.
- Virtual blood bank is the computer-controlled, electronically linked information management system.
- Safe blood transfusion: It is essential to assure the quality and availability of safe blood and blood products for all who need transfusion, throughout the process beginning from the selection of blood donors through to their administration to the patient.
- Protocols in blood bank: Standard operating protocols are prepared in blood bank and followed.

SELF-ASSESSMENT EXERCISE

Write short essays/notes on:
- Automation in blood bank
- Recent advances in blood banking
- Safe blood transfusion
- Protocols in blood bank
- Write an essay on "Modern trends in blood transfusion practice"
- Briefly discuss recent practices in blood transfusion
- Blood banking in 21st century
- Pathogen reduction technology

CHAPTER 21

Hemovigilance, National Blood Policy and Biomedical Waste

CHAPTER OUTLINE
- Hemovigilance
- National blood policy
- Medicolegal and ethical concerns in blood banking and transfusion services
- Biomedical waste

HEMOVIGILANCE

A system for reporting adverse events and learning from these events is a general requirement in all quality work today including in transfusion medicine. An adverse transfusion reaction is "an undesirable response or effect in a patient temporarily associated with the infusion of blood or blood component." The term hemovigilance is derived from the Greek word "hema" which means blood and the Latin word "vigilans" which means watchful.

Definition

Hemovigilance is defined as **set of surveillance procedures** covering the whole (entire) transfusion chain (from the collection of blood from donors and its components to the follow-up of recipients of transfusions), **intended to minimize** (or prevent) the occurrence or recurrence of **adverse events or reactions** (unexpected or undesirable effects) **in donors and recipients** (or vein to vein).

Hemovigilance includes the monitoring, reporting, investigation, and analysis of adverse events related to the donation, processing, and transfusion of blood. It also includes taking action to prevent their occurrence or recurrence. The reporting systems enhances patient safety by learning from failures and then putting in place system changes to prevent them in future.

Goal of the Hemovigilance

The ultimate goal of hemovigilance is **to promote or improve the** overall **safety** (of both patient and donor) **of blood transfusion** by detecting and analyzing all untoward effects of blood transfusion to correct their cause and to prevent recurrence. Hemovigilances for all blood components namely: Whole blood, erythrocytes concentrate, thrombocytes concentrate, and fresh frozen plasma. Hemovigilance is an essential component of quality management in a blood transfusion. It is useful for the continuous enhancement of quality and safety of blood products and transfusion process by monitoring and safeguarding the adverse events associated with the use of blood products.

Transfusion hazards: They can occur anywhere from donor selection to recipient transfusion to consequences beyond transfusion. Hence, it is necessary that a hemovigilance system should have a broad scope to capture, identify and define such risks, report, investigate, and analyze adverse events related to the donation, processing, and transfusion of blood. Only collecting data and obtaining information through hemovigilance without any action on it, does not produce any improvement in transfusion system. Hence, action should be taken to prevent their occurrence or recurrence. It is said that if you cannot measure it, you cannot improve it. However, measurement alone will not improve systems and corrective action to improve transfusion systems and reduce transfusion risks is necessary.

After obtaining data, it is necessary to establish problem frequency and document the process failures and determine priorities and allocate resources to provide opportunities for improvement in transfusion systems and patient outcomes. The information obtained through hemovigilance should be used to make necessary changes in transfusion policies, for amendments in transfusion practices in hospitals and blood services. This will help to enhance transfusion standards, transfusion guidelines, and improve quality and safety of entire transfusion process.

Biovigilance: It captures surveillance efforts in not only blood donor and transfusion recipient programs but also donors and transplant recipients of cellular therapies, tissues, and organs.

Historical Aspects

As early as 1980, it was realized that there is need for safe blood transfusion when many hemophilia patients (in UK, France, Canada, Japan, and USA) contracted *Hepatitis C* virus (HCV), *Hepatitis B* virus (HBV), and human immunodeficiency virus (HIV) from blood transfusions and factor concentrates. This emphasized the need for hemovigilance. The hemovigilance work was first started in France in 1991. Currently, on a global scale an International Hemovigilance Network (IHN) is functional. The aim of IHN is to develop and maintain a joint structure relating to the safety of blood and blood components and of hemovigilance in blood transfusion and transfusion medicine throughout the world. The IHN in coordination with International Society of Blood Transfusion (ISBT) working party on hemovigilance proposed standard definition for hemovigilance system (2011). Further, an international database— International Surveillance of Transfusion Associated Reactions and Events (ISTARE) has been formed to share hemovigilance data across the world. The World Health Organization (WHO) is actively involved in promoting development of hemovigilance by providing several resources including draft guidelines for adverse event reporting and learning systems.

International Hemovigilance Network (www.ihn-org.com)

Functions of IHN are listed in the Box 21.1.

International Society for Blood Transfusion (ISBT; www.isbtweb.org)

This is an international voluntary society and has individual professionals as its members. Its main objective is to promote and to maintain a high level of ethical, medical, and scientific practice in blood transfusion medicine, science, and related therapies throughout the world.

World Health Organization

World Health Organization is in formal relations with ISBT with regard to safe blood transfusion. It has a department of blood safety on implementing hemovigilance. Advantage of WHO is because of its direct links with governments and ministries of health. This can initiate activities to implement hemovigilance and improve the safety of blood transfusion.

Hemovigilance in India

As per the Ministry of Health and Family Welfare, Government of India, a need of a centralized hemovigilance system was established for

Box 21.1: Functions of International Hemovigilance Network (IHN).

IHN promote and engage in:
- Exchange of information among the members of the network
- Swiftly functioning alarm system or warning system among members of the network
- Joint activities among the members of the network
- Educational activities relating to hemovigilance

all authorized blood banks in India in 2012. The hemovigilance program is functional through a core group and an advisory committee. This committee coordinates the activities of hemovigilance between medical colleges (Department of Transfusion Medicine or the blood bank) and the National Coordinating Centre. It provides an expert opinion for analysis of the information generated and insights helpful in linking Hemovigilance Program of India with IHN. The Transfusion Reaction Reporting Form (TRRF) can be downloaded from these websites: www.nib.gov.in, www.ipc.gov.in, and www.cdsco.nic.in.

The hemovigilance system should cover processes throughout the entire transfusion chain, i.e. from blood donation, processing, and transfusion to patients for the monitoring, reporting, and investigation of adverse events and reactions and near misses related to blood transfusion. It should be coordinated well between the blood transfusion service, hospital clinical staff and transfusion laboratories, hospital transfusion committees, regulatory agency, and national health authorities. The modifications in transfusion policies, standards and guidelines, and improvements in blood services and transfusion practices in hospitals will provide improved patient safety.

Definitions and Terminology in Hemovigilance Systems

Hemovigilance systems are most effective when the data are reported consistently using standardized nomenclature and definitions. Analysis of transfusion reactions or incidents needs clear, precise definitions in order to decrease the misapplication of classification and misinterpretation of submitted data. The ISBT hemovigilance developed definition of transfusion reaction that may be useful for comparisons of data between countries. This incorporates transfusion adverse event definitions to define reaction, score its severity and determine the imputability or likelihood that the observed event is attributable to transfusion.

An example of an ISBT transfusion reaction definition is presented in Box 21.2.

■ RECIPIENT HEMOVIGILANCE

The "severity" of an adverse transfusion reactions when occur should be graded according to an internationally accepted scale. The ISBT has laid down criteria for "severity" of transfusion reactions. They should be investigated to establish the diagnosis and guide future treatment of the patient. The transfusion reactions in a recipient are subdivided as acute (within 24 hours) or delayed (after hours of transfusion) reaction (refer Chapter 14).

Hemovigilance Related to Blood Donors

The first part of the transfusion chain consists of collection of blood from the donor and is an essential element of hemovigilance. Donor hemovigilance aims at securing and improving the safety of both the donor and the recipient. The donor hemovigilance should include reporting of unexpected adverse events (reactions including errors, incidents, and failures) in whole blood and component donors along with action taken. These adverse reactions or complications may be the result of donation, selection, and management of donors. These may directly harm the donor or influence the quality of the product which may predispose the recipient to a risk or harm the recipient. Collection of blood from donors for the preparation of components for clinical use is most commonly by whole blood donation. Automated collection using apheresis technology may be used for the collection of plasma, platelets, and red blood cells. The less common donations of granulocytes, lymphocytes or peripheral blood stem cells are also collected by apheresis. Donor hemovigilance together with good clinical management of any complications will improve donor confidence and satisfaction. A joint working group from the ISBT and IHN (then, the EHN) has classified a set

Box 21.2: International Society for Blood Transfusion (ISBT) hemovigilance definition, severity score, and imputability grade examples.

Definition: Hypotensive transfusion reaction
- It is characterized by hypotension defined as a drop in systolic blood pressure of ≥30 mm Hg occurring during or within 1 hour of completing transfusion **and** a systolic blood pressure ≤80 mm Hg.
- Most reactions occur very rapidly after the start of the transfusion (within minutes). This reaction responds rapidly to cessation of transfusion and supportive treatment. This type of reaction appears to occur more frequently in patients on ACE inhibitors.
- Hypotension is usually the sole manifestation but facial flushing and gastrointestinal symptoms may occur.
- All other categories of adverse reactions presenting with hypotension, especially allergic reactions, must have been excluded. The underlying condition of the patient must also have been excluded as a possible explanation for the hypotension.

Severity
- **Grade 1 (nonsevere):** The recipient may have required medical intervention (e.g. symptomatic treatment) but lack of such would not result in permanent damage or impairment of a body function.
- **Grade 2 (severe):** The recipient may have required inpatient hospitalization or prolongation of hospitalization directly attributable to the event resulted in persistent or significant disability or incapacity; or the adverse event necessitated medical or surgical intervention to preclude permanent damage or impairment of a body function.
- **Grade 3 (life-threatening):** The recipient required major intervention following the transfusion (vasopressors, intubation, transfer to intensive care) to prevent death.
- **Grade 4 (death):** The recipient died following an adverse transfusion reaction.

Note: *Grade 4 should be used only if death is possibly, probably or definitely related to transfusion. If the patient died of another cause, the severity of the reaction should be graded as 1, 2 or 3.*

Imputability
Imputable means capable of being assigned or credited (i.e. attributable or ascribable). Imputability is the degree to which the reaction was caused by the transfusion. This is assessed, once the investigation of the adverse transfusion event (ATE) is completed, the assessment of the strength of relation to the transfusion of the ATE.
- **Definite (certain):** When there is conclusive evidence beyond reasonable doubt that the adverse event can be attributed to the transfusion.
- **Probable (likely):** When the evidence is clearly in favor of attributing the adverse event to the transfusion.
- **Possible:** When the evidence is indeterminate for attributing the adverse event to the transfusion or an alternative cause.
- **Unlikely (doubtful):** When the evidence is clearly in favor of attributing the adverse event to causes other than the transfusion.
- **Excluded:** When there is conclusive evidence beyond reasonable doubt that the adverse event can be attributed to causes other than the transfusion.

Note: *Only possible, probable and definite cases should be used for international comparisons.*

of definitions of complications related to blood donation. The reactions in a donor are discussed in Chapter 14.

Adverse Transfusion Incident/Event Detection and Reporting

Hemovigilance reporting systems: All hemovigilance systems should have a system to capture events directly from the site of transfusion or donation. The reporting system plays a fundamental role in hemovigilance. By learning from failures and then implementing system changes to prevent them in future will enhance patient safety. The hemovigilance system should involve all-involved in transfusion and it should be coordinated between the blood transfusion service, hospital clinical staff and transfusion laboratories, hospital transfusion committees, the national regulatory agency, and national health authorities. The staff/individual who first identifies the problems with a transfusion will report the occurrence is a critical first step in hemovigilance system.

Passive or active systems: In a passive system only the adverse events or near misses are reported to the system whereas in an active system, even an uncomplicated transfusion (or blood donation) is also reported.

Scope of reporting: The scope of hemovigilance systems varies. In some countries (e.g. UK), the system limits its focus to only *serious* hazards; others may include mild or moderate hazards. The more common approach is reporting all transfusion reactions, incidents ("deviation" or "error") not directly associated with a transfusion reaction or an untoward outcome. It is cumbersome system with numerous, less informative reports of nonsevere events that may obscure major, clinically significant events. But it is an important means of detecting problems in the transfusion system and preventing these from harming patients.

Most notable and dangerous incident/error has been due to the transfusion of an incorrect blood component. This occurs in pretransfusion testing often due to sample and patient identification errors. The "near miss" events/incidents in transfusion are the errors which are detected and remedied and/or where it does not cause harm to the recipient quickly. Inclusion of these "near miss" incidents in hemovigilance reporting provides insights into weak points of the transfusion process and opportunities to improve the system by reducing the potential for human error to cause harm.

Reporting requirements structure: Hemovigilance system reporting may be made voluntary or mandatory. In both, local preparations are a key success factor. Effective preparation includes detailed review of current processes and procedures for adverse reaction reporting and a gap analysis compared to what will be expected for the hemovigilance program. Such reviews optimally include representation from all involved in transfusion process including physicians, nurses, laboratory staff, and information system support staff.

Rapid alerts: Sometimes donors or patients report complications which are not one of the known complications. Rapid spread of information about these new risks may be difficult to handle/manage. Often, they are concluded as those not related to the donation or the transfusion. However, it is useful to collect the data because it can lead to the detection of complications that are **new or not previously recognized** (not aware of). Rapid spread of information about these rapid alerts is very useful. For example, when problems with disposables or reagents are discovered in one blood bank it may take some time before it is detected in other blood banks. It is necessary to verify the finding before an alert is circulated. The manufacturer must be informed and relevant advice or actions in response to the notification should be included in the alert.

Contact Persons

At the hospital level, it is necessary to have a point of contact for clinical staff to report reactions and adverse events. This may be a transfusion practitioner or safety officer, hematologist, transfusion medicine specialist, the blood transfusion laboratory, or a hospital blood bank manager.

Investigations and Assessment

Root cause analysis

It is necessary to perform root cause analysis. Many a times it may be due to several latent causes, such as lack of training, badly designed IT processes, or understaffing.

Risk Assessment

An in-depth root cause analysis requires considerable time and effort. Hence, it is usually done for selected reports of errors or incidents in the transfusion. When an event occurs, assessment of the potential harm (even though the worst did not happen) and the likelihood of recurrence can be combined.

This will support prioritization of a particular problem for detailed analysis and preventive measures. A prospective risk assessment can indicate possible improvement measures.

NATIONAL BLOOD POLICY

One of the vital components of any healthcare delivery system is having a well-organized blood transfusion service. It is necessary to provide safe and adequate blood transfusion services (blood and blood products) to the people. One of the requirements for blood safety is to prevent and eliminate transfusion transmitted infections (e.g. HIV, hepatitis virus and other blood-borne pathogens).

Challenges in Blood Banking in India

- **Highly decentralized blood banks:** In India, blood transfusion service is highly decentralized and there are not enough vital resources, such as manpower, adequate infrastructure, and financial base. The main in blood banking system in India is fragmented management (refer page 442).
- **No uniform standards:** The standards of blood bank vary in various blood banks running in the country. Many large hospitals and nursing homes do not have their own blood banks and this has resulted in proliferation of stand-alone private blood banks.
- **Limited availability of blood components:** The production/availability of blood component and utilization is extremely limited.
- **Shortage of trained healthcare professionals:** There are not enough trained healthcare professionals in the field of transfusion medicine. Well-equipped blood centers with adequate infrastructure and trained manpower is an essential need for quality, safety and efficacy of blood and blood products. For effective clinical use of blood, it is necessary to train clinical staff.
- **Total quality management:** It is a challenge to the organization and management of blood transfusion service to attain maximum safety, to follow a good manufacturing practices, and implementation of quality system moving toward total quality management.

To face the above challenges, there is a need for modification and changes in blood transfusion service. This has necessitated formulation of National Blood Policy (NBP). National Blood Policy was first published by the Government of India in 2002.

Aims under the National Blood Policy are:
- To ensure easily accessible and adequate supply of safe and quality blood and blood components.
- Blood is collected/procured from a voluntary nonremunerated regular blood donor in well-equipped premises.
- Blood or its product is free from transfusion-transmitted infections, and is stored and transported under optimum conditions.
- Reduce unnecessary transfusion.
- Transfusion under supervision of trained personnel for all who need it, irrespective of their economic or social status through comprehensive, efficient, and a total quality management approach will be ensured.

Objectives of the policy:
1. Government commitment to **provide safe and adequate quantity** of blood, blood components, and blood products.
2. To make available **adequate resources** to develop and reorganize the blood transfusion services (BTS) in the entire country.
3. To make **latest technology available** for operating the blood transfusion services and ensure its functioning in an updated manner.
4. To launch **extensive awareness programs** for donor information, education, motivation, recruitment, and retention in order to ensure adequate availability of safe blood.

5. To encourage **appropriate clinical use of blood** and blood products.
6. To **strengthen the manpower** through human resource development.
7. To **encourage Research and Development** in the field of transfusion medicine and related technology.
8. To take **adequate regulatory and legislative steps** for monitoring and evaluation of blood transfusion services and to take steps to eliminate profiteering in blood banks.

Some of the **main highlights of National Blood Policy** (2002) are as follows:
- Trading in blood, i.e. sale and purchase of blood shall be prohibited. The practice of replacement donors shall be gradually phased out in a time bound program to achieve 100% voluntary nonremunerated blood donation program.
- Efforts shall be directed to make the blood transfusion service viable through nonprofit recovery system.
- Standards, Drugs and Cosmetics Act/Rules and Indian Pharmacopoeia shall be updated as and when necessary.
- A Quality System Scheme shall be introduced in all blood centers. An External Quality Assessment Scheme (EQAS) through the referral laboratories approved by the National Blood Transfusion Council shall be introduced to assist participating centers in achieving higher standards and uniformity.
- Blood shall be used only when necessary. Blood and blood products shall be transfused only to treat conditions leading to significant morbidity and mortality that cannot be prevented or treated effectively by other means.
- Blood and its components shall be prescribed only by a medical practitioner registered as per the provisions of Medical Council Act, 1956.
- Transfusion medicine shall be treated as a speciality. A separate department of transfusion medicine shall be established in medical colleges. Medical colleges/universities in all states shall be encouraged to start PG degree (MD in transfusion medicine) and diploma courses in transfusion medicine.
- Computer-based information and management systems shall be developed which can be used by all the centers regularly to facilitate networking.
- Fresh licenses to stand-alone blood banks in private sector shall not be granted.

Role of National AIDS Control Organization:
- According to National AIDS Control Organization (NACO) of India, every person living with HIV should have access to quality care and is to be treated with dignity. NACO has taken measures such that patient with HIV have equal access to quality health services. NACO is involved in awareness of people of accurate knowledge about HIV and motivate them to protect themselves from the impact of HIV. It aims at building an India where every person is safe from HIV/AIDS.
- Presently, the National Blood Transfusion Council is housed within NACO. National Blood Transfusion Council together with NACO is involved in fulfilling the roles and responsibilities as the policy formulating apex body for all matters related to safe blood transfusion service for the country. NBTC has framed guidelines for the practice of transfusion medicine. NBTC has played a pivotal role in improving blood safety by infrastructure development, setting up component separation units, promoting voluntary blood donation, training staff and has also laid down standards for blood banks in India.

MEDICOLEGAL AND ETHICAL CONCERNS IN BLOOD BANKING AND TRANSFUSION SERVICES

If patients get injured during or as a result of transfusion, they may seek redress through legal channels. Blood transfusion services have high potential risk of adverse reactions to recipients and high-risk of legal liability to the blood bank. In blood banking and transfusion medicine there is the possibility of transmission of disease especially from previously unknown sources. This may even lead to death of the recipient. Hence, it is necessary to know some general principles and definitions so that ethically and legally sound practices continue within transfusion medicine.

Legal Issues

Legal issues play an important role in blood transfusion services. Legal issues for the transfusion medicine professional may arise due to several causes (e.g. ABO errors, acute lung injury, transfusion-transmitted diseases (e.g. dengue fever, babesiosis or other exotic diseases that are emerging globally, patient privacy), and issues regarding transfusion indications, informed consent, and other medically relevant topics. There were numerous litigations against blood centers, hospitals, and physicians because incidence of death and serious injury, such as those caused by transfusion-transmitted HBV and transfusion-transmitted acquired immunodeficiency syndrome (TTAIDS). The court after these litigations decided that transactions involving blood were not sales but were incidental to the provision of medical services. This precludes the application of commercial law, particularly that of warranties, to blood transfusions. The HBV cases stimulated legal courts to enact protection for blood banks through **blood shield statutes**. Because of these many lawsuits for TTAIDS and HBV, many TTAIDS have been either dismissed or unsuccessful for the person suing (the **plaintiff**). However, **blood shield statutes** do not apply whenever there are questions of appropriateness of transfusion, availability of blood components, and informed consent arise.

According to National Blood Policy (2002) trading in blood i.e. sale and purchase of blood shall be prohibited. The practice of replacement donors shall be gradually phased out in a time bound program to achieve 100% voluntary nonremunerated blood donation program.

Patients usually believe that medical treatment given to them (after obtaining their informed consent) will be beneficial. When transfusion causes harm (e.g. because of identification error, lung injury, and other causes), patients may seek redress in the courts. Such suits are generally civil (not criminal) and actions for them is by tort. Tort is defined as any wrongdoing for which action for damages may be brought.

Ethical Issues in Safe Blood Transfusion

- Ethical issues play a significant role in determining the quality of transfusion services.
- Hospital-based blood banks are compelled to practice replacement donations because they are not allowed to hold blood camps.
- All blood banks use blood judiciously as blood components. However, there is also demand for whole blood.
- The management and staff of blood banks need to implement ethical practices.
- Conflict of interest involving management and staff of blood banks need to be avoided, thereby ensuring ethical practices especially with reference to manufactures/suppliers of kits and reagents.

Licensing of Blood Banks by Drugs Controller

- Blood is considered as a "drug" under the Drugs and Cosmetic Act (D and C Act), 1940 and Drugs and Cosmetics Rules, 1945. Drugs controller is the regulatory authority in blood bank. India has a procedure for mandatory licensing under the drugs and cosmetics rules for blood banks.
- **Licensing of blood bank**: It is the first step towards quality. The procedure for licensing of blood banks is detailed in the D and C Act 1940 and Drugs and Cosmetics Rules, 1945. Blood bank can function only if it qualifies the criteria laid down by the organization. These range from quality and variety of the equipment used, to the qualification of the working staff, source of procurement of blood and blood components to labeling of blood units/

components license/renewal of license is necessary to run the blood bank.
- **Blood and/or its components request form:** As per the D and C Act "the blood and/or its components shall be supplied only on the prescription of a Registered Medical Practitioner".
- **Apheresis licensing:** Blood banks should obtain special permission for apheresis. It is necessary to show apheresis equipment, space, and staff available for apheresis. The various apheresis includes platelet apheresis, plasmapheresis, and leukapheresis on donors.
- **Therapeutic procedures**: Many blood banks can provide specialized procedures like therapeutic platelet apheresis, plasmapheresis, leukapheresis, peripheral blood stem cell (PBSC) collection, and red cell exchange. These procedures can be most competently performed by blood bank staff in conjunction with the clinicians.

PROBLEMS FACED BY THE BLOOD TRANSFUSION SERVICES IN INDIA

Fragmented Blood Transfusion Service
- In India, blood banks are opened for various reasons and some hospitals open blood banks as they are not permitted to open storage centers.
- Only regional blood transfusion centers (RBTC) are permitted to open storage centers and only very few blood banks are RBTCs.

Size of Blood Banks and Screening Methodologies
- Rapid tests are used in blood banks with small workloads (i.e. 5–10 donors/day). These rapid test compromise safeties and the antibody detection by these tests take time over 1 week.
- Quality control measures to guarantee safety in transfusion-transmitted infections testing (e.g. Levy-Jennings chart for ELISA)

is almost nonexistent, except in few blood banks.

No Standards for Safe Transfusion
National Aids Control Organization or NBTC standards address only safe donor and safe blood issues. It does not cover safe transfusion (the third element of blood safety).

Curbs on Conducting Blood Donation Camps
Drugs and Cosmetics Act permits to conduct blood donation camps only by licensed RBTCs, government blood banks, Indian Red Cross Society or licensed blood bank run by voluntary or charitable organization.

Failure to Incorporate New Technologies and Employ Centralized Testing
In the D and C Act, there is no mention about newer testing technologies, such as nucleic acid testing (NAT)/chemiluminescence immunoassay (CLIA)/enzyme-linked fluorescence assay (ELFA). Some of regulatory authorities are not aware of these new techniques.

Deficiencies in Documentation and Monitoring of Bedside Transfusions
Elements of Blood Safety
Refer 430-3.
National Blood Policy (NBP)
Refer page 441.

BIOMEDICAL WASTE
Definition: Biomedical waste means any waste that is generated during the diagnosis, treatment or immunization of human beings or animals or in research activities pertaining thereto or in the production or testing of biological material.

The rule of biomedical waste is prescribed by the Ministry of Environment and Forest, Government of India and applied on 28th

July 1998 and is called as Bio-Medical Waste (Management and Handling) Rules 1998. Bio-Medical Waste Management Rules was amended on 28th March 2016, 16th March, 2018 and 19th February 2019.

Categories

Biomedical waste consists of solid, liquid, sharps and laboratory waste. It includes human anatomical waste, animal waste, microbiology and biotechnology waste, waste sharps, discarded medicines and cytotoxic drugs, soiled waste, solid waste, liquid waste, incineration ash and chemical waste.

These may be **non-infectious** waste and **infectious** (potentially) or **dangerous waste** (may be hazardous to health). It differs from other types of hazardous waste such as industrial waste. The infectious waste carries a higher risk for infection.

Generation of Biomedical Waste

Biomedical waste is generated routinely and inevitably in hospitals, health clinics, nursing homes, medical research laboratories, offices of physicians, dentists and veterinarians in the course of healthcare activities.

Hazard/Risks of Poor/Inadequate Management

Poor/inadequate management of biomedical waste may have serious public health consequences and a significant impact on the environment. It may also create opportunities for the collection of disposable medical equipment (particularly syringes), its re-sale and potential re-use without sterilization. It also causes environmental, occupational and public health hazard.

Hazards to Humans

All individuals exposed to biomedical waste are potentially at risk of being injured or infected. These individuals include:
- **Medical staff:** Doctors, nurses, sanitary staff and hospital maintenance personnel.
- **Patients:** Both in-patients and outpatients receiving treatment in healthcare facilities.
- **Visitors** of hospitals/nursing home.
- **Workers involved in support services** linked to healthcare facilities such as laundries, waste handling and transportation services.
- **Workers involved in waste disposal** including scavengers.
- **General public** and more specifically the children playing with the biomedical waste if not properly disposed and are directly accessible to them.

Environmental Hazard

Inappropriate treatment and disposal of biomedical waste can cause environmental pollution. Uncontrolled incineration emission from formalin fumes and suspended particulate matter produces **pollution of air**, dumping in nallas, tanks and along the river bed chemical and liquid wastes disposed in the sewage or drainage system produces **pollution of water** and unscientific land filling (improper disinfecting and dumping of waste in landfills and incineration) produces **pollution of soil**.

Occupational Hazard

This involves individuals who generate, collect, segregate, handle, package, store, transport, treat and dispose biomedical waste.

Occupational exposure to blood may occur from percutaneous injury (needle prick or other sharps instrument injury), mucocutaneous injury (due to splash of blood or other body fluids into the eyes, nose or mouth) or blood contact with non-intact skin. The most common occupational hazard is infection due to needle prick injury. The needle prick injury occurs during poor recapping of disposable needle and the unsafe collection and disposal of sharps waste. Many blood borne diseases can be transmitted but most dangerous is spread of infectious/communicable diseases like Acquired immune deficiency syndrome (AIDS), hepatitis B and C, etc. Waste chemicals, radioactive substances and heavy metals, etc. are hazardous to health.

Public Health Hazard

Poor management of biomedical waste can lead to serious disease to healthcare personnel, to workers involved in disposal of waste, patients and to the general public. The greatest risk by infectious waste is accidental needle prick injuries (infectious syringes), which can cause hepatitis B and hepatitis C and HIV infection.

During the handling of biomedical wastes, injuries occur when syringe, needles or other sharps have not been collected in puncture proof containers. It can very likely happen when biomedical waste is dumped on an uncontrolled site which can be easily accessed by public.

Children and rag pickers are particularly at risk to come in contact with infectious waste.

Among unsafe practices, the reuse of syringes and/or needles without sterilization is of most particular concern.

Biomedical Waste Management

Necessity of biomedical waste management: It is an important challenge faced by all hospitals. Hence, it is necessary to know management of biomedical waste by all the hospital professionals and support staff and it is an integral part of health care. Biomedical waste management is important because biomedical waste:
i. May be highly infectious,
ii. Produces toxic substances, and
iii. Its unscientific disposal may cause highly infectious diseases.

Advantages of proper management of biomedical waste is:
- Prevents the exposure of healthcare workers, patients, waste handlers and the community to infections, toxic effects and injuries due to biomedical waste.
- Helps to control nosocomial diseases (hospital acquired infections), reduces transmission of hepatitis (B and C), HIV/AIDS from infected needles and other improperly cleaned/ disposed medical items, control zoonoses (diseases passed to humans through insects, birds, rats and other animals).
- Prevents illegal repackaging and resale of contaminated syringes/needles.
- Avoids long-term health effects like cancer, from the environmental release of toxic substances such as dioxin, mercury and others.

Objectives of biomedical waste management include:
- To reduce the health hazard due to waste
- Prevent misuse or abuse of waste
- For occupational safety.

Vital Steps for Safe and Scientific Management of Biomedical Waste (Flowchart 21.1)

Biomedical wastes are categorized into 4 (Table 21.1). Its handling, segregation, mutilation, disinfection, storage, transportation and final disposal are vital steps (Flowchart 21.1) for safe and scientific management of biomedical waste in any establishment.

Segregation and Identification

Rules to be followed as mentioned below:
- Biomedical waste **shall not be mixed with any other wastes**.
- All biomedical waste shall be **segregated/ sorted into color coded containers/bags** at the point of generation. These color coded containers (Table 21.1) include: 1) yellow, 2) red, 3) white translucent puncture proof or 4) puncture proof and leak proof blue depending on the disposal methodology planned.

Flowchart 21.1: Vital steps for safe and scientific management of biomedical waste.

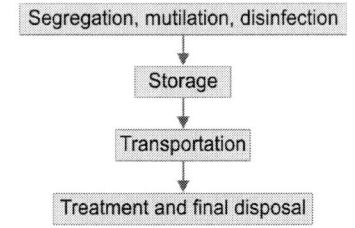

Table 21.1: Categories of bio-medical waste, color coding, treatment or disposal option for biomedical waste

Category	Types of bag or container to be used	Types of waste.	Treatment or disposal options
1.	Yellow colored non-chlorinated plastic bags	a. **Human anatomical waste:** Human tissues, organs, body parts b. **Animal anatomical waste:** Experimental animal carcasses, body parts, organs, tissues, including the waste generated from animals used in experiments or testing in veterinary hospitals or colleges or animal houses. c. **Soiled waste:** Items contaminated with blood, body fluids like dressings, plaster casts, cotton swabs and bags containing residual or discarded blood and blood components. d. **Expired or discarded medicines:** Pharmaceutical waste like antibiotics, cytotoxic drugs including all items contaminated with cytotoxic drugs along with glass or plastic ampoules, vials etc. e. **Chemical waste:** Chemicals used in production of biological and used or discarded disinfectants f. **Discarded linen**, mattresses, beddings contaminated with blood or body fluid routine mask and gown. g. **Microbiology, biotechnology and other clinical laboratory waste:** Blood bags, laboratory cultures, stocks or specimens of micro-organisms, live or attenuated vaccines, human and animal cell cultures used in research and industrial laboratories, waste from production of biological, toxins, dishes and devices used for cultures. **Note:** Autoclaving of Microbiology, Biotechnology and other clinical laboratory waste should be performed before disposal into yellow bags	Incineration, plasma pyrolysis/deep burial
2.	Red colored non-chlorinated plastic bags or containers	**Contaminated waste (recyclable):** Wastes generated from disposable items such as tubing, bottles, intravenous tubes and sets, catheters, urine bags, syringes (without needles and fixed needle syringes) and vacutainers with their needles cut) and gloves	Autoclaving/microwave/hydroclaving and then sent for recycling. Not to be sent for landfill
3.	White (translucent) puncture proof, leak proof, tamper proof containers-	**Waste sharps:** Needles, syringes with fixed needles, needles from needle tip cutter or burner, scalpels, blades, or any other contaminated sharp object that may cause puncture and cuts. This includes used, discarded and contaminated metal sharps	Autoclaving/dry heat sterilisation followed by shredding or mutilation or encapsulation
4.	Puncture proof and leak proof boxes or container with blue colored marking	a. **Glassware:** Broken or discarded and contaminated glass including medicine vials and ampoules except those contaminated with cytotoxic wastes. b. **Metallic body implants**	Disinfection or autoclaving/ microwaving/ hydroclaving, and then sent for recycling

 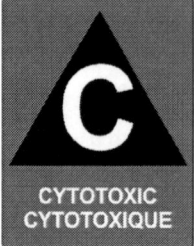

Fig. 21.1: Label for biomedical waste containers/bags

- The **containers shall be duly labelled**.
- Cytotoxic wastes should be collected in yellow container and should be clearly labelled as cytotoxic waste along with its specific logo (Fig. 21.1).
- Bags and containers for infectious waste should be marked with biohazard symbol (Fig. 21.1).
- Sharps should be collected in puncture proof containers. Needles and syringes should be destroyed with the help of needle destroyer and syringe cutters at the point of generation. Infusion sets, bottles and gloves should be cut with scissors and stored in blue bin/bag after disinfection. All disposable plastic should be subjected to shredding before disposing off to registered/authorized recycler of plastic waste. Shredding is essential to ensure that items are not used again.
- Disinfection is achieved by 1–2% sodium hypochlorite solution or any other equivalent chemical solution with minimum contact period of 1 hour. Fresh solution should be prepared in each shift.

Containers and Instructions

- **Place appropriate containers** or bag holders **in all locations** where particular categories of waste may be generated.
- **Instruction on waste separation and identification should be posted** at each waste collection point to remind all the staff about the procedures.
- **Remove the containers when they are three-quarter full**.
- **Collect the waste daily** (or as frequent as required).
- **Bags should be picked up from the neck** and placed in such a way that bags can be picked up by the neck again for further handling.
- **Minimize manual handling** of waste bags to reduce the risk of needle prick injury and infection.
- **Don't mix other forms of waste** with biomedical waste as different rules apply to the treatment of different types of waste.
- There **should be an easy access to waste collection vehicle**.

Temporary Central Storage

Ideally, all the hospitals and healthcare establishment should have a dedicated space to store the biomedical waste. This will act as a temporary central storage area before treatment and disposal of waste.

Final Treatment and Disposal

Various methods of disinfection and disposal options of biomedical waste are presented in Box 21.3 (refer Table 21.1).

Box 21.3: Methods of disinfection and disposal options for biomedical waste

- Incineration
- Deep burial
- Autoclaving
- Microwaving
- Plasma pyrolysis
- Hydroclaving/hydrolysis
- Encapsulation
- Mutilation
- Shredding
- Dry heat sterilisation
- Inertisation

SUMMARY

- Hemovigilance is a set of surveillance procedures covering the whole (entire) transfusion chain intended to minimize adverse events or reactions in donors and recipients to promote safe and effective use of blood components.
- Biovigilance captures surveillance efforts is not only blood donor and transfusion recipient programs but also donors and transplant recipients of cellular therapies, tissues, and organs.
- A centralized hemovigilance system was established for all authorized blood banks in India in 2012.
- One of the vital components of any healthcare delivery system is having a well-organized blood transfusion service. It is necessary to provide a safe and adequate blood transfusion services (blood and blood products) to the people.
- To face the challenges in transfusion services, it necessitated formulation of National Blood Policy. National Blood Policy was first published by the Government of India in 2002.
- Legal issues play an important role in blood transfusion services. Legal issues for the transfusion medicine professional may arise due to several causes.
- Biomedical waste consists of solid, liquid, sharps and laboratory waste. It should be properly disposed because it may have serious public health consequences and a significant impact on the environment.
- Biomedical wastes are categorized into 4. The vital steps involved in the management of biomedical waste consist of handling, segregation, mutilation, disinfection, storage, transportation and final disposal. All biomedical waste shall be segregated into four color coded containers/bags at the point of generation. These color coded containers include yellow/red/white translucent puncture proof/blue depending on the disposal methodology planned.
- Various methods of disinfection and disposal options of biomedical waste include incineration, deep burial, autoclaving, microwaving, plasma pyrolysis, hydroclaving/hydrolysis, encapsulation, mutilation, shredding, dry heat sterilisation and inertisation.

SELF-ASSESSMENT EXERCISE

Write short essays/notes on:
- Hemovigilance
- National blood policy (NBP)
- Medicolegal and ethical concerns in blood banking and transfusion services
- Biomedical waste and its management

CHAPTER 22

Quality Programs in Blood Banking and Transfusion Medicine

CHAPTER OUTLINE
- Quality program
- Quality assurance
- Quality control
- Quality assurance in the transfusion laboratory

INTRODUCTION

In the present era of medicolegal, regulatory, and public scrutiny, an effective quality program is very essential to blood banks/centers and transfusion services. The aim of sound quality program is to ensure the provision of safe and effective blood products and services.

Definition of Quality

Quality is defined as **"the degree to which a product or service meets requirements." Often quality is used for characteristic or conformance of a product or service.** The characteristics are usually further defined as satisfaction of needs or meeting requirements, standards or specifications. Thus, quality is a measure of how well a product or service does the job for which it is designed, i.e. conformity to specification.

The "product or service" in the **transfusion medicine** are blood, blood products, blood derivatives, and tissue. Thus, it is defined as **"the degree to which blood, blood products, blood derivatives, and tissue meets requirements.**

Requirements to achieve quality: Quality is essential in transfusion medicine. For achieving quality, the products and services must:

- Be consistent
- Meet previously established expectations
- Be free from defects.

Importance of quality: In transfusion medicine, even if one single product is unsuitable, it can harm the patient. Hence, quality must be built into each and every process employed to produce the blood component.

Compliance

Compliance means the action or fact of complying with a specification, policy, standard or law. It simply requires the correction of identified deviations and deficiencies of specification, policy, standard or law.

Compliance programs: Compliance program evaluates how effectively the facility meets the requirements. It is by detecting errors, deficiencies, and deviations.

Activities of a hospital blood bank/center (Box 22.1): Activities in blood banking and transfusion medicine begins with the collection of blood to the final step of transfusion to the patient. Blood bank/centere collects, processes, stores, and transports human blood intended for transfusion. Transfusion service performs testing and issues blood and blood components for transfusion.

Box 22.1: Activities of a hospital blood bank.

- Specimen collection, labeling, and quality
- Performing the correct tests in each situation for each specimen
- Correctly performing all tests according to the laboratory standard operating procedures (SOPs)
- Timely and accurately reporting all test results
- Maintaining complete, accurate, and legible records
- Preparing various blood components and accurately labeling them
- Providing an adequate supply of safe, high-quality blood components
- Storing the blood components to maintain optimum quality and effectiveness at the time of transfusion
- Timely and accurately providing blood components to patients

Box 22.2: Various interrelated building blocks of quality program.

- Quality management system (QMS)
- Quality system (QS)
- Quality assurance (QA)
- Quality control (QC)

QUALITY PROGRAM

The framework for quality program consists of several interrelated facets that constitute the building blocks of quality (Box 22.2).

Quality planning: It is the necessary activity which ensures the success of the quality management system (QMS). American Association of Blood Bank (AABB) defines quality planning as "a systematic process that translates quality policy into measurable objectives and requirements, and lays down a sequence of steps for realizing them within a specified time frame." There should be written quality plan which should be a living document which needs reviewing and edition whenever needed.

System: American Association of Blood Banks defines a system as, "An organized, purposeful structure that consists of interrelated and interdependent elements (components, processes, entities, factors, members, parts, etc.)". These elements continually influence one another, either directly or indirectly, to maintain their activity and the existence of the system, in order to achieve the goal of the system.

Quality system (QS): It is made up of a set of interrelated processes that work together to ensure quality (Fig. 22.1). QS includes everything that is utilized to ensure that products, processes, or services within a department or organization meet or exceed expectations. QS is also sometimes defined as the document that captures the quality program (e.g. the quality manual or quality plan of an organization). Quality functions of laboratory as per AABB are listed in Box 22.3.

Quality management (QM) refers to the overall process used to ensure that laboratory results/products meet the requirements for healthcare services to patients. QM is actively and continuously practiced by the blood bank's leaders, managers, and staff throughout all blood bank/center operations. QM validates its processes, monitors process performance, knows where the problems are, continuously takes action to determine root causes of problems and removes them, and documents its actions. Thus, with QM, the blood bank is always ready for an inspection. Laboratories/blood banks are required to develop procedures to monitor and ensure quality in all aspects of laboratory

Box 22.3: Quality functions of laboratory as per AABB.

- Review and approval of SOPs
- Review and approval of training plans
- Review and approval of validation protocols and results
- Review, validation, and approval of QMS software
- Audit of operational functions
- Development of evaluation criteria for systems
- Review and approval of suppliers and maintenance of an approved supplier list
- Review of products specifications
- Review of reports of adverse reactions, error reports, and complaints
- Determination of the suitability of products
- Monitoring and trending
- Inspection oversight and management
- Reporting to regulators, accrediting bodies, customers, or others as necessary

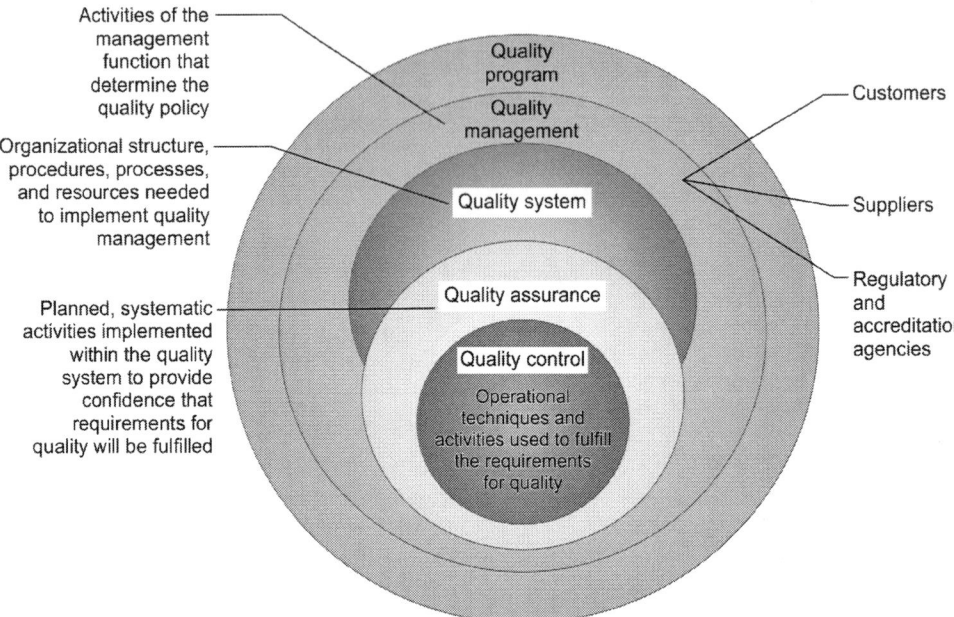

Fig. 22.1: Quality program activities with their interactions *(For color version, see Plate 4)*.

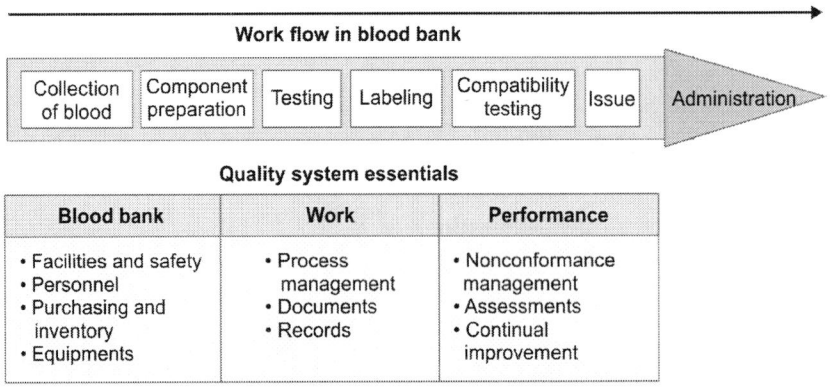

Fig. 22.2: Quality management system for the blood bank.

services. A QM program is a requirement for accreditation. Hence, it is necessary to have a good documentation of the review process and the improvements made. QMS for the blood bank is depicted in Figure 22.2.

Quality management system: A key goal of QMS is to ensure that quality laboratory services are provided. QMS is an integrated system that determine the quality policy and thereby quality assurance (QA). QMS is a collection of business processes that covers all matters which individually or collectively are focused on achieving quality (guarantee the quality) while meeting customer requirements. To accomplish quality, every laboratory should obtain modern equipment, to employ well-trained staff, to ensure a well-designed and safe physical environment, and to create a good management team. A strong and healthy QMS is important to provide the best possible service for the patient and clinicians.

Normally, the **QMS** includes three facets major components which includes **(i) the QS, (ii) QA (QA), and (iii) quality control (QC).**

It ensures that the overall quality program is effective and efficient with a continuous goal of process improvement and customer satisfaction. The quality program activities within each interact with the others as illustrated in Figure 22.2. For example, QC is a part of QA, which in turn is encompassed together with the QS document within QM. The International Organization for Standardization (ISO) established guidelines that reflect the highest level of quality.

The quality management system in practice
Several elements comprise a QMS. Basic AABB Standards elements of QMS are listed in Box 22.4.

Organization and Leadership

Organization

As per AABB, it is necessary that each blood bank or transfusion service should define and document its organization, policies, processes, and procedures related both to operational and quality functions. It is necessary to clearly document the responsibility for key operational and quality functions. All involved personnel must be trained in QS applications. Important organizational issues include the statement of the goals of the program and the organizational structure.

Premises

The design and construction of blood transfusion premises are important. Blood transfusion center premises must be located, designed, constructed, and adapted to suit the operation to be carried out. It should include the following (as per WHO):
- Adequate space for work and movement of the staff. Overcrowding must be avoided.
- Furnishing, fittings, and floor material must be carefully selected in such a manner that it can be cleaned, and is convenient for working.
- Adequate lighting throughout the premises. Proper lighting is necessary in bleeding room and the areas where tests are carried out.
- Should have proper ventilation.

Box 22.4: Basic AABB standards elements of quality management system (QMS).

- Organization and leadership
- Customer focus
- Human resources (personnel and hiring practices, training)
- Equipment management: Equipment and supplier qualification
- Supplier (vendor selection) qualification and materials management (purchasing and inventory) and customer issues
- Processes, process control, and management
  - Preanalytical
  - Analytical
    - Equipment validation/verification
    - Equipment calibration and maintenance
    - Quality control
  - Postanalytical
- Document and records (procedure manuals)
- Methods to detect errors, deviations, nonconformances, and adverse events
- Information management
- Management of nonconforming events and adverse events (occurrence management)
- Monitoring and evaluation:
  - Audits/Assessments
    - Internal (PT = Proficiency testing)
    - External (EQA = External quality assessment)
  - Quality indicators
- Process/Continual improvement
- Facilities, work environment, and safety

- Essential to have adequate power and water supplies, facilities for waste disposable, and strict adherence to standards of sanitation.
- Entire blood bank premises should be air-conditioned. If it is not possible, at least bleeding room, laboratories, and component preparation room should be air-conditioned.
- Essential to have provision of generator for continuous power supply.
- There should be separate areas for:
  - Donor registration, selection, and counseling
  - Blood collection and refreshment. Room for hemopheresis is optional.
  - Blood processing, storage, laboratory facilities, and auxiliary facilities.
  - Store and record room
  - Hand washing and toilet facility.

Leadership

An organization is only as good as its people, and people are guided by leaders and managers. For a quality program to be effective and successful, it is essential that the leaders of the organization should be committed to this and aim at continuous improvements. The senior management plays a fundamental role in the success of any QMS. It is the responsibility of the leadership to create an environment where individuals are fully engaged in the QMS and to monitor it to ensure that the system operates effectively. The director of the blood program activity should ensure the overall quality of the operation. Quality functions as per AABB are listed in Box 22.4.

Customer Focus

Customers: It can be defined as anyone who is affected by the processes of blood bank. Organizations which provide blood components or other cellular products and services have a variety of customers. Customers for transfusion services can be divided into internal and external customers.

External customers: These include organizations and individuals who use the product or service.

- **Recipients**: The real customers of these facilities are the person who receive the blood or blood component. The recipient must be satisfied with a product or service.
- **Donors**: The second type of customers are the donors, who want a safe and satisfying donation experience.

Internal customers: These include departments and employees within the organization.
- **Physicians and nurses**: Customers are the physicians who order the blood transfusions. They want the blood/blood products in a timely manner. The nurses are also customers who want the correctly issued blood components in a timely manner for administration to patients.
- **Employees**: For all types of facilities, the employees are the internal customers.

Feedback from customers: There should be a mechanism to receive feedback from the customer at regular intervals. Customer satisfaction data can be obtained by direct communication with the customer and by conducting anonymous or customer-specific surveys. These include both complaints and compliments. *Root-cause analysis* (described on page 483) of frequent or significant complaints is useful to prevent recurrences. Frequent review of customer feedback will help an organization to recognize the need for change before problems arise.

Human Resources (Personnel and Hiring Practices)

Selection Criteria

Good employees or the workforces are essential for the success of any organization. The human resources department is concerned with activities of its employees. These activities include recruiting (selecting the right individuals/personnel) and hiring of new employees, determining qualification requirements, adequate training for all blood bank jobs, position/job descriptions, monitoring competency, ongoing staff needs, employee benefits, and retention of qualified personnel and choosing the right people to move the gears of its operations. It is necessary to have adequate staff to perform the work and to support QMS. Hiring unqualified personnel not only incur significant expense to the organization but also create a demoralizing environment for coworkers who have to accommodate poor performance.

Selection: Successful personnel selection process must be done using minimal pre-established criteria identified for each type of position in the organization. These criteria include the careful analysis of each position to determine qualification requirements, responsibilities, and scheduling needs. These criteria should address the experience, background, skills, and credentials (e.g. degrees, licensure, and certification) that are necessary to perform the job. The selection criteria should not be stagnant and should be revised as changes in job duties or tasks occur.

Personnel: There must be professional and efficient adequate personnel/staff. Personnel involved in the department of blood transfusion services include laboratory staff, social workers, donor organizer and those involved in donor center. All categories of the staff should have all information about voluntary blood donation, need of blood and blood products, and scientific and technical advances in blood banking. Job description should exist for all personnel involved in blood transfusion service. The staff personnel should be courteous, interested, cheerful, and friendly.

Technical persons in blood bank:
- They must have basic educational qualification in medical laboratory technology and work experience in blood transfusion service.
- After their appointment, they should be given in-house training for laboratory procedures. They should have adequate training and experience to ensure competent performance of assigned duties.
- Periodically, evaluate and record the competence of personnel regarding the performance of their assigned job functions.
- Should be provided with continuous medical education (CME) program to upgrade the knowledge in recent techniques.
- Supervisory personnel must periodically review the results and evaluations of all persons. This will ensure that they adhere to testing standards. Corrective actions should be taken, if needed.

Hiring

Hiring includes activities such as contacting candidates, setting up interviews, and ensuring orientation of new employees. During hiring process, job qualifications are matched against applicant qualifications, and candidates are selected depending on their job qualifications including training, education, and experience.

Job Descriptions

Quality begins and ends with people. Well-written, criterion-based job description documents should be developed for each type of position and for all personnel in the organization. The criterion-based job descriptions include educational qualifications, experience, focus on roles, responsibilities, accountability, and internal and external organizational relationships, licensing requirements (where applicable), so that qualified persons can be hired. These documents should describe the tasks for which the employee is responsible and outline the areas of knowledge and skill that need to be acquired during training to perform the job. This provides a clear guide to expectations for both employee and employer. Current job descriptions defining qualifications for each position must be maintained.

Orientation and Training

All the quality policies, goals, and objectives in blood banking do not ensure safe and effective blood components and transfusions. Orientation and training are critical/important for a new employee to get the right start.

Orientation training usually includes an overview of the organization and its customers, knowing the work processes and procedures, benefits training, an introduction to regulations and safety training. Training and education benefit by reducing rework and inconsistency. Training is provided during new employee orientation and is needed whenever there are procedure changes or evidence of poor performance. By good training programs, the trainer explains all functions and demonstrates the task before employee performs it. Repetition of tasks in a "test" environment or with supervision is needed before the trainee is permitted to perform the procedure independently. Throughout the training process, the trainee must be given enough opportunities to ask questions, clarify doubts, and receive explanations. Finally, all training must be documented and initial and ongoing assessments of competence are needed by doing it right the first time, every time. The document is typically in the form of a checklist signed by the trainee, trainer, and supervisor.

Competency assessments

Competency assessment is the evaluation of the employee's knowledge and ability to perform a procedure or skill. Routine competency assessments should be conducted to ensure that the staffs maintain the ability to perform their jobs well and to determine the level of competency performing the work. It is necessary to have a written plan for the conduct of competency assessments and must include plan to be followed if an individual does not pass the assessment. Training is concluded only when there is documented evidence that the employee is able to demonstrate knowledge and application of the new procedure/skill. This demonstration is the aim of competency assessment. Various methods of competency assessment include direct observation of performance, written tests, review of results and records, or using blind samples. The procedures for assessments of competency of individuals who do not pass assessment are presented in Box 22.5.

- **Initial competency assessment:** It refers to the evaluation of the level of knowledge and skill of a trainee/employee gained during initial training. It will help to determine whether the trainee is ready to perform a procedure.
- **Periodic competency assessment:** It refers to the evaluation which determines whether the employee has maintained the level of knowledge and skill necessary to perform the job or task as described in the facility's standard operating procedure (SOP). It is required to conduct competency for testing personnel twice during the first year of employment and every year thereafter. It is necessary to have retraining for employees who fail to prove competency and they must not be allowed to perform the procedure (or procedures) until retraining is provided and subsequent competency assessment proves that competency is satisfactory or acceptable.
- **Actions to be taken when there is unacceptable performance:** Corrective actions should be taken. These include retraining and documenting performance and competency assessment.

Box 22.5: Procedures for assessments of competency of individuals who do not pass compliance assessment.

- Direct observation of routine patient job task performance/test performance (e.g. patient preparation, specimen handling, processing, and testing)
- Monitoring the recording and reporting of test results
- Reviewing the intermediate test results, QC records, etc.
- Direct observation of performance through testing previously analyzed specimens, or external proficiency testing samples
- Assessment of problem-solving skills
- Process/Continual improvement
- Facilities, work environment, and safety

Periodic evaluation and documentation of the continuing competence assessment of personnel to perform their assigned job functions and tasks is necessary. Documentation of the results of competency assessments should be available for inspection during accreditation.

Equipment Management

Selection of equipment: Equipment used in processes should be selected such that they must be optimally effective for its desired function. They should minimize the likelihood of microbial contamination, introduction of adventitious agents, or cross-contamination of cells among different individuals. The equipment must be maintained in a clean state. Other factors to be considered while purchasing the equipment include cost, service, and support. Workflow should be well defined before selection of equipment.

Unique equipment identification: Each equipment must have a unique identification and list of equipment should be maintained. The list should be kept updated, and if equipment is moved from one location to another or removed from service, the action taken should be recorded. Policies, processes, and procedures must be established such that the calibration, maintenance, and monitoring of equipment conform to requirements. New equipment should be qualified and validated before use. Equipment that is out of service should be removed from the operation areas and should be clearly labeled as out of service.

Installation: Equipment used in various processes in the blood bank must be installed as directed by the manufacturer and should be ensured that it works as stated or recommended by the manufacturer.

Validation: The Food and Drug administration (FDA) definition of validation "establishing documented evidence which provides a high degree of assurance that a specific process will consistently produce a product meeting its predetermined/pre-established quality and performance specifications." The validation is a good business practice and it includes procedures for validation, calibration, and preventive maintenance of equipment and records of this.
- **Type of validation:** Validation may be prospective, concurrent, or retrospective (Table 22.1)
- Validation is needed for both new equipment (including computer hardware and software), and new processes before being implemented. Validation consists of a series of checks, tests, and challenges which ensure the equipment and/or process function as desired.
- **Validation for new equipment:** Three types of validation are specific for new equipment (including computer systems).
  – **Installation qualification:** Equipment must be installed as directed by the manufacturer. Installation qualification should be according to written procedures and should be documented. Installation qualification ensures that manufacturer's specifications have been

Table 22.1: Validation definitions.

Type of validation and definition	Circumstances
Prospective: Performed before the equipment or process being implemented	It is the preferred type of validation and should be performed whenever possible
Concurrent: Performed during a live run of equipment or process	Perform when it is not possible to challenge the equipment or process in a test environment or if the previous equipment or process can no longer be used (e.g. cannot repair the equipment, reagents are not available)
Retrospective: Performed after implementation of equipment or process	If process, or less likely, equipment was not adequately validated in the past

met for installation within the proper environment.
- **Operational qualification:** The equipment must be operated as per the manufacturer's recommendation. Manufacturers may have requirements for temperature, humidity, surrounding space, or other specifications. Operational qualification ensures that the equipment is capable of operating as intended by the manufacturer. Installation and operational validation must be performed on-site and is usually performed by supplier personnel.
- **Performance validation:** It provides confidence in the equipment's capability when operated by the facility's own staff. The effectiveness and reproducibility of the process is confirmed by repeated testing.

Maintenance: Equipment should be maintained so that it is in proper working condition. A documented process (written program) for monitoring, cleaning, and maintenance of critical equipment must be placed at the equipment. Preventive maintenance should be established and documented. Procedures should describe the frequency, method, and acceptance criteria for monitoring and maintenance of equipment. Procedures should also mention the actions to be taken when unacceptable results are obtained. Records for this work should be available during assessment.

Revalidation: It should be done whenever there is failure of validation, when a change is made in a process or procedure, when equipment are moved or repaired, or if otherwise indicated.

Calibration: Routine calibration is needed as a routine for equipment used in measurements. Calibration is the process of standardization of an analytic instrument by comparing the instrument against a known accurate standard. If there is any error found during calibration, error can be corrected (adjusted) by determining deviation from the known standard and making adjustments to the instrument being calibrated.

Routine calibration is required for some equipment. There should be lists of equipment to be calibrated, frequency of calibration, and a written program for calibration. For example, a weighing scale is calibrated by weighing an object of known weight. If the scale measurement deviates from this weight beyond a predetermined specification, then adjustments or possibly repair are needed. All equipment should be calibrated before initial equipment use and after activities that may affect calibration. The calibration should be an ongoing program at prescribed intervals, to ensure that the equipment remains in a satisfactory performance range. The calibration can be outsourced to an approved outside vendor. The calibration record should be maintained and need to be available during assessment.

Storage Equipment

Storage temperature is very important for blood, its components, tissue, and its derivatives. Hence, it is necessary to have very specific standards for storage equipment. It is mandatory to continuously monitor and record temperature of refrigerators, freezers, and platelet incubators for at least every 4 hours. It is also necessary to record temperature every 4 hours in the ambient temperature of open areas where blood products are kept or stored. Most facilities use alarms to alert staff when significant variations in temperature occurs in refrigerator or freezer. These alarms must be set up in such a manner that they activate the alarm before the temperature reaches unacceptable level. In the event an alarm is being activated, there must be a process for immediate investigation and corrective action. It is also necessary to have procedures for periodic QC testing of alarms to make sure that alarms are functioning as expected.

Quality assurance essentials for equipment are outlined in Flowchart 22.1.

Computer Systems

Computer systems are being used in transfusion medicine and their important requirements in transfusion medicine are:

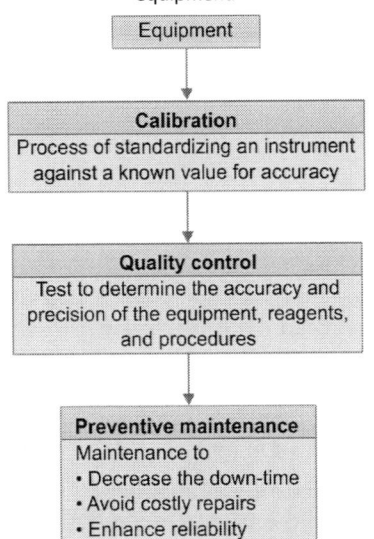

Flowchart. 22.1: Quality assurance essentials for equipment.

- Complete traceability of all products derived from blood or blood components. This includes from the collection of the donor through all preparation, distribution, and testing steps to transfusion to the recipient. The staff performing each significant step in a process must be identified.
- The software used should be thoroughly described, documented, and validated before using.
- The system must be described, documented, challenge-tested, and validated in the location where it will be used before implementation. Validation records should be maintained.
- Documented description of the system maintenance and operation.
- All users must be trained in the operation of the system before its use.
- System must be secure from unauthorized access and the confidentiality of donors and recipients should be maintained.
- Monitor the critical data integrity.
- Whenever the computer breaks down, there must be a plan to address the situation and alternate procedures during such periods must be available.
- Information stored in the system must be backed up. This is needed especially when there is loss of data due to an unexpected breakdown. There must be a documented plan for disaster recovery.

Supplier and Materials Management (Purchasing and Inventory)

The quality of any product depends on the quality of the raw materials that are used in its production. Hence, many blood banks and transfusion services use supplier qualification as a standard practice. Supplier qualification is an important concept. One of the critical aspects of QMS is that the supplier should meet pre-established specifications. By this process, it is determined whether the quality of critical products and services received from suppliers meets pre-established criteria. It is necessary to have a written agreement between blood banks and their suppliers. These agreements usually specify acceptable criteria, including expectations between the involved parties. In addition, there should be procedures for inspecting and testing incoming materials (when applicable). These procedures should also mention the course of action to be taken when the products do not meet the criteria.

Supplier Qualifications

The organization (or blood centers) should have a defined (specified) process for evaluation, selection, and approval of suppliers of critical materials, equipment, and services. Thus, organization determines whether the supplier can meet the requirements. Such requirements include the ability to meet the regulations, the availability of the supply, the timelines of delivery, responsiveness to issues and problems, cost, and support. Specifications or product requirements are provided to suppliers, and there should be a system to determine that suppliers meet these specifications continually. Supplier expectations should be defined in a written agreement. If a blood bank is referring specimens or products to another laboratory for testing, the referral laboratory must have all required accreditations, certifications, and registrations. In hospital-based blood banks and transfusion services, contract and purchasing issues are usually managed by the hospital's purchasing department. It is necessary to maintain a list of approved suppliers which should be reviewed routinely. Suppliers are added or removed from the list when necessary.

Contracts and Agreements

Usually, a written contract or agreement with a supplier that stipulates the organization's requirements and expectations is to be developed.

Receipt and inspection of incoming supplies and materials

Receipt of all products and materials (supplies and reagents) must be recorded (documented) and should be stored under proper conditions. Organization should develop written criteria for acceptance of all incoming supplies and same should be followed. Blood, tissue products, critical reagents, kits for testing, equipment, and materials must be inspected (both external packing and contents of that packing) on receipt and tested (where required such as blood bags and infectious disease testing kits). Collection sets, storage containers, and labels must be inspected to ensure they meet specifications. If the supplied materials do not meet the requirements, they should be returned to the supplier.

Process Control and Management (Fig. 22.3)

Process: It is defined as a set of interrelated resources and activities **that use resources to transform inputs to outputs.**

Example of process: Whole blood collection is a process.
- It has **many inputs** such as trained phlebotomist, an approved blood collection set, an approved arm-scrub solution, and phlebotomy SOPs.
- All inputs mentioned above, working together to produce the **output**, i.e. a unit of whole blood.

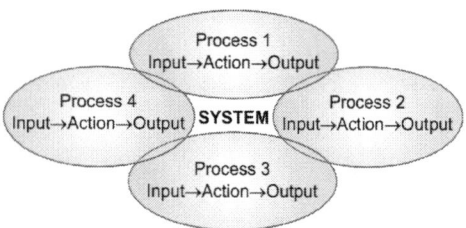

Fig. 22.3: Systems and processes.

- The **quality of output is determined by the quality and control** that is in place with the inputs and with the process itself.
- **Validation** of a process is key in ensuring that the process is consistent and produces the desired output.

Process control: It is a set (sum) of activities or tools that ensure a given work process and procedure is predictable, stable, and consistently operating at the target level of performance with only normal variations. Thus, process controls **standardize the processes,** or monitor process outcome. The goal of process controls is to produce a predictable outcome. It is continuously able to meet process goals without compromising the process itself. Many quality activities are process controls. Process controls in transfusion medicine are related to component preparation, such as end labeling and sterility checks. Process controls related to analytic testing, such as QC and proficiency testing, are similar in transfusion medicine and other medical laboratory disciplines.

Strategies for managing process should address all the components of the process. This includes inputs, outputs, resources, and its interrelated activities.
- **Strategies for inputs**: Suppliers qualification, formal agreements, supply verification, and inventory control are strategies for ensuring that the inputs to a process meet specifications.
- **Resources:** Personnel training and competency assessment, equipment maintenance and control, management of documents and records, and implementation of appropriate in-process

controls provide assurance that the process will operate as intended.
- **Strategies for outputs:** End-product testing and inspection, customer feedback, and outcome measurement provide data to evaluate product quality and improve the process. These output measurements and quality indicators are used to evaluate the effectiveness of the process and process controls.

For the effective management of a system of processes, it is necessary to understand how its processes interact and what cause-and-effect relationships exist between them.

Accepting a donor who is not eligible, will affect the almost every other process. For example:
- **Donor with a history of high-risk behavior:** If such as a donor is not identified during the donor selection process, the donated unit (s) may be positive for one of the viral makers.
- It **triggers follow-up testing, look-back investigations, and donor deferral and notification procedures. Components must be quarantined** and their discard documented.
- **Personnel involved** in collecting and processing the unit (s) are **at risk of exposure to infectious agents**.
- Part of quality planning is to identify these relationships so that quickly an appropriate corrective action can be taken when process control fails.

Total process control: It is the evaluation of the performance of a process, comparison of actual performance to a goal, and action taken on any significant difference. It is the concept which means to build quality, safety, and effectiveness into the product or service from the beginning. It is important to document the sequence of activities in a process and each step in the process must be controlled to meet quality standards. The procedures for each process should be written. Before actual use, the entire process should be validated to ensure that it works as expected. Total process control provides a predictable outcome or product from the process with a minimum of variability and as close as practical to the desired product every time it is produced.

Variation: Some degree of variation in processes and products is likely to occur due to variation of many factors such as reagents, operator technique, and resource materials. It is necessary that the expected outcome of processes must be pre-established in order for personnel to recognize when the process is not functioning as expected. The established, expected outcome may be determined by the manufacturer of a test kit, by regulating agencies, by validation testing, or by data collection.

Important components of process control are listed in Box 22.6.

A sequential flow of the elements of total process control is presented in Figure 22.3. **Figure 22.4** is an example of flowchart for the activities in the pre-transfusion testing process.

Standard Operating Procedures

Standard operating procedures are written procedures/ instructions which help to ensure the complete understanding of a process and to achieve consistency in performance from one individual to another. All procedures should be performed as per SOPs. It is the key to achieve consistency and control in operations. Every blood bank should have their own SOPs manual. It helps to maintain uniform standards of procedures, and QC. First of all, it is necessary to determine where SOPs are necessary and then decide who shall develop them. Thus, facilities need to say what they do (write SOPs) and do what they say (follow SOPs).

Box 22.6: Important components of process control.

- Standard operating procedures
- Process validation
- Computer system validation
- Test method validation
- Quality control
- Training
- Tracking and trending

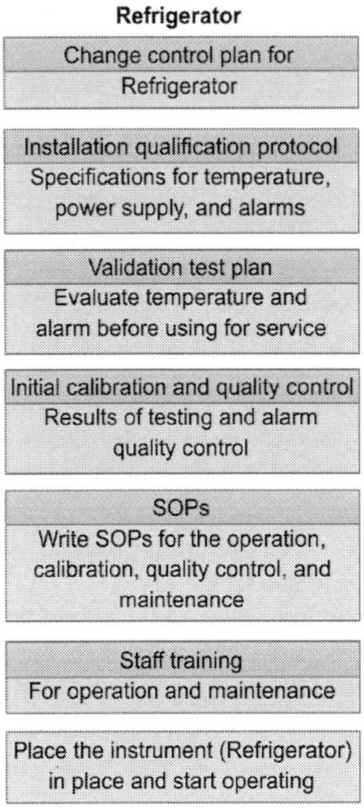

Fig. 22.4: Change control plan for a new refrigerator.

```
Refrigerator
    ↓
Change control plan for Refrigerator
    ↓
Installation qualification protocol
Specifications for temperature, power supply, and alarms
    ↓
Validation test plan
Evaluate temperature and alarm before using for service
    ↓
Initial calibration and quality control
Results of testing and alarm quality control
    ↓
SOPs
Write SOPs for the operation, calibration, quality control, and maintenance
    ↓
Staff training
For operation and maintenance
    ↓
Place the instrument (Refrigerator) in place and start operating
```

Salient features

Content: Well-written SOPs should contain steps/instructions in detail about process (a particular task or techniques), i.e. on how to perform each activity in the larger process, who does what and when it is done (in sequence or order).
- Principle or purpose of the test
- Specimen requirement
- Supplies, reagents, and equipment
- Procedure instructions: SOPs should be written in detail including all critical steps so that a trained staff can perform the task, but avoiding unnecessary or excessive description can cause confusion. For example, the process for providing a patient's ABO and Rh type involves: (i) ordering the test, (ii) collecting an appropriate specimen, (iii) delivering it to the laboratory, (iv) performing the test, and (v) reporting the results. In this process, a specific written procedure is necessary for ordering tests, collecting and labeling the blood specimen, delivering the specimen to the laboratory, performing and recording the ABO/Rh testing, and reporting the results.
- Quality control
- Interpretations and reporting
- References

Standard operating procedures should be written by subject experts and should be validated to ensure that they are effective. SOP validation usually involves an individual performing the task using the SOP as written. The individual will note whether the steps in the SOP make sense and whether steps can be performed as written. List of staff members with name, qualification, signature, experience, and training.

Language: SOPs should be written in language that can be easily understood and followed by workers.

Format: SOPs are important training tools for new employees and should be written in a systematic way using a standard format.

Placed at workplace: SOPs should be available at the place of work. SOPs must be readily available at all times to the concerned working staff.

Review and approval: Finalized SOPs should be reviewed and approved by concerned departmental personnel and medical director, before becoming effective and released. SOPs should be reviewed periodically and to update as and when required.

Performance: SOPs should be available at each working area. All steps should be carried out exactly and clearly accordingly to the written instruction specified in the SOPs.

Internal and external auditors carefully assess noncompliance with written SOPs, one of the most serious violations that can be identified during an inspection.

Usual contents of SOPs are listed in Box 22.7.

Standard operating procedures involved in blood banking are listed in Box 22.8.

Advantages of SOPs are outlined in Box 22.9.

Change control (Fig. 22.4): Blood banks and transfusion services are undergoing a constant state of change by development of new technologies and new regulatory and accrediting requirements. Hence, the blood banks and transfusion services need to develop or change existing processes or procedures. This process is known as change control and is a general element of process control. Change control is a system to plan and implement changes in procedures, equipment, policies, and methods. This will increase effectiveness and prevent problems. The change control needs the allocation of time, money, and manpower. For example, though addition of a new refrigerator for blood storage looks straightforward; a change control plan for it should address all critical steps in equipment installation to prevent potential problems.

- **Policy:** Blood bank should have a specific policy and procedure for changing procedures (change control), including definition of personnel authorized to make changes. The SOPs should be revised as often as necessary; and the date of revision should be clearly recorded. Obsolete operating procedures must be removed from circulation.
- A permanent record of all outdated SOPs should be maintained so that in the future there can be no doubt as to how each specimen was processed. The different contents of SOPs are listed in Box 22.7.

Box 22.7: Usual contents of standard operating procedures (SOPs).

- Title and an identification number
- Date of implementation
- Current version number or latest revision/review date
- Intent or purpose
- Scope or individual responsible for completing the steps
- List of required materials and equipment
- Detailed instructions including calculations
- Documentation requirements and result reporting steps (if required)
- References
- Name of the individual who prepared and his/her identity
- Identity and signature of approver
- Revision history

Box 22.8: Standard operating procedures manual required in blood banking (WHO).

- Donor selection questionnaire
- Donor registration and interview
- Donor selection and procedure of blood collection (phlebotomy)
- The title, and the brief explanation of the purpose of the procedure
- Procedures of testing and processing the blood donations
- Details of the methods and the example of work protocols
- Reporting procedure for results, and the action to be taken if errors/problem occurs
- Specification of reagents and equipment
- Procedures of preparations of blood components and their quality control
- Specific quality control procedures
- Quality monitoring of equipment
- Quality monitoring of laboratory techniques
- Training requirements of staff to perform the procedures
- Biosafety in the transfusion laboratory

Box 22.9: Advantages of standard operating procedures (SOPs).

- Established SOPs ensure the consistent quality of the final product or result. **It also** ensures that specified standards are met uniformly and at all times
- It helps:
  o to standardize and monitor the performance of all the staff members, especially technical personnel
  o in training the staff particularly newly appointed ones
  o the staff in performing assigned job
  o to standardize the training of staff
  o to reduce deterioration of performance when staff changes or absence occurs

Process Validation

Validation tests all activities in a new process/test to ensure that the new process will work as intended and consistently produce a desired result. Process validation is one of the most important aspects of process control and must be done before being put into use. Process validation is defined as the collection and evaluation of data, from the process design stage through commercial production, which establish scientific evidence that a process is capable of consistently delivering quality product. For example, when a new test for a transfusion-transmitted disease is added to those performed on donated blood units, the new test method with its associated instruments, test kits, computer functions, and procedures—the new test must be validated. Validation ensures that a new test/process will perform as expected (with consistent results) with that blood bank's instrumentation, written procedures, personnel, and computer systems. Validation should be done for all critical processes according to a written validation protocol. Important aspects of process control as per AABB are listed in Box 22.10.

Tracking and trending
Tracking is an integral part of record keeping and is discussed below. Trending is a concept embodied in many QS activities.

Computer system validation
A computer system consists of hardware, software, peripheral devices, networks, personnel, and documentation. Computer system validation ensures that the system can operate even when stressed.

Test method validation
The blood bank/laboratory must demonstrate that it can obtain performance specifications comparable to those manufacturers.

Different components of test system are listed in Box 22.11.

Box 22.10: Important aspects of process control as per AABB.

- System description
- Purpose of the validation
- Risk assessment
- Responsibilities
- Test cases
- Acceptance criteria
- Problem-reporting mechanism
- Approval signature
- Supporting documents

Box 22.11: Different components of test system.

- Accuracy
- Precision
- Reportable range of test results
- Reference intervals (normal values)
- Analytical sensitivity
- Analytical specificity (including interfering substances)

QUALITY ASSURANCE

The alternate term for QA is quality assessment. Laboratory services will improve the quality of health care only when it accomplishes QA. It consists of policies that maintain and control processes involving the patient and laboratory analysis of specimens. It also ensures for both staff and clinician that the data provided are reliable and relevant.

WHO definition: QA is the total process whereby the quality of laboratory reports can be guaranteed.

Quality assurance comprises the combined activities performed by an organization to ensure the quality of products and services, they offer.

Quality assurance is a **set of planned systematic activities** (actions) implemented within the QS **to provide confidence that requirements for quality will be fulfilled**. Thus, it is the monitoring performed that ensures that QSs and elements that influence the quality of the product or service are being adhered to and is working as expected, individually and collectively. Sometimes, terms QC and QA are used interchangeably. In this chapter, they are used as distinct processes.

Importance: QA is a sequence of activities that looks beyond the performance of a test method or equipment. It addresses how well an entire process is functioning. It helps to improve trust in laboratory results. This is especially important in those processes which are cross functional or at departmental lines. For example, blood bank can monitor the number of times and reasons why a set of collected whole blood units transported from the collection site to the component processing site did not arrive in time or is received not in an acceptable condition to make blood components. In the transfusion, it is essential to monitor the source, the number of times, and the reason why blood specimens collected for compatibility testing do not meet predetermined acceptance criteria.

Components of QA are given in Table 22.2. The basic components of a QA program are listed in Box 22.12.

Current Good Manufacturing Practices

Current good manufacturing practices (cGMPs) are performed in blood banks and transfusion services to manufacture blood components and plasma protein products as a part of QA and legal requirements. These regulations indicate "what" needs to be done without necessarily specifying "how." cGMPs are a form of process control that were initially used in the pharmaceutical industry and are now applied to blood banks. cGMPs will reduce error by staff members when affixing the end label to a blood product. Some commonly applied controls in this area include:

- The labeling area should be separate from other blood component preparation areas
- Physically segregating blood components that are at different steps along the testing and manufacturing process
- Automation of steps that are likely prone to human error (e.g. use of scanners to record numbers or check labels)
- Multiple independent reviews before the product is released.

Each blood bank must determine the best way to implement all these practices. The various elements of cGMPs are listed in Box 22.13.

Common QA indicators in most blood banks are listed in Box 22.14.

Box 22.12: Elements of quality assurance.

- Compliance with current Good Manufacturing Practices (cGMPs)
- Records and standard operating procedures (SOPs): Review and approval of all SOPs
- Personnel selection and training: Development, review, and approval of training programs
- Validation, specifications, calibration, preventive maintenance, proficiency testing
- Supplier qualification
- Error management: Review of error reports, review and approval of corrective action. Investigation of product recalls, errors, and complaints
- Process improvement
- Process control
- Label control
- Internal auditing: Coordination of internal quality auditing programs

Box 22.13: Various elements of good manufacturing practices

- write standard operating procedures (SOPs) and follow SOPs
- Record and document all work performed
- Training and education of qualify personnel
- Design and building of proper facilities and equipment
- Validate equipment, personnel, and processes
- Regularly perform preventive maintenance on facilities and equipment
- Control for quality
- Audit for compliance with all of the above

Table 22.2: Components of quality assurance (QA).

Components	Features
Planning	What will be done?
Retrospective review processes	What was done or not done? It includes monitoring, auditing, trend analysis, and *root-cause analysis* of errors
Analysis of performance data	Was it done the right way? It is done to measure how well processes and personnel are functioning through audits, competency assessments, and proficiency testing.

> **Box 22.14:** Common blood bank QA indicators.
>
> *Requisition forms:*
> - Number of donor forms with incomplete or incorrect information
> - Number and source of improper and incomplete requests for blood components
>
> *Specimen:*
> Number of, source of, and reasons for unacceptable specimens
>
> *Clerical:*
> - Number of and reasons for labeling check failures
> - Number and location of patients without proper identification at time of specimen collection or transfusion
>
> *Technical:*
> - Number of blood grouping/typing discrepancies in donors and patients
> - Number of and reasons for invalid tests
> - Number of times wrong component or ABO was selected for crossmatch or use
> - Number and types of unusable units and blood components
> - Number of and reasons for turnaround time failures
>
> *Transfusion complications:*
> Number and type of transfusion complications

QUALITY CONTROL

Quality control (QC) is one aspect of a quality assurance (QA) of quality program.

Definition: QC is **operational techniques** (routine testing often performed daily or during processing of each batch) **and activities used to fulfill the requirements for quality.**

Purpose: QC checks that the work process is functioning properly. Its purpose is to ensure that materials, reagents, and equipment are functioning as expected at any given stage of a process. It is determined through testing or observation to know if a process or particular task within a process is working as expected at a given time. It includes processes utilized in the laboratory to recognize and eliminate errors. Thereby, it ensures that the quality of work produced by the laboratory conforms to specified requirements before its release for delivery. Errors and/or deviations from expected results must be documented and the corrective action taken must be documented.

In the laboratory, QC is a component of accreditation requirements and should be performed as a daily practice.

Routine blood bank QC procedures: QC involves sampling and testing. Most blood bank technicians are familiar with routine blood bank QC procedures. These QC procedures include daily testing of the reactivity of blood typing reagents (reagent QC); clerical checks; visual inspections; calibrating serologic centrifuges; and regular measurements, such as monitoring temperatures of refrigerators, freezers, thawing devices, and volume or cell counts on finished blood components.

Type and frequency of QC: These are determined in regulations and accreditation standards, manufacturers' operator manuals, and package inserts.

Importance: Regular performance of QC indicates to operational staff members whether the method/process, piece of equipment, or procedure is not working as expected. Thereby, **indicate whether method/process, piece of equipment, or procedure should continue or stop.** If QC is not within specifications, it may indicate a problem. When QC results identify that a problem exists, the QC is said to be out of control. The problem may be either with the process itself or with how the process is being executed. This problem must be resolved before the process can continue.

Quality control is an important component of process control. It is the day-to-day activity and testing done to ensure that equipment, reagents, and materials are functioning as expected and that the method was performed correctly. For analytic procedures, QC solutions with an expected result range are tested by the same method as the patient or donor specimens. QC is routinely performed by testing a specified number of each type of manufactured components and products to ensure that they meet the regulatory and accreditation specifications.

QC versus validation: QC is an event that is different from validation and in contrast to validation; QC is not required to gain assurance of consistency. QC is repeated at a given frequency to ensure that the results are within acceptable ranges. QC also over-time determines if any trends are developing that might indicate something is eventually going to fail.

Frequency of QC testing: The frequency usually determined by the criticality of what is being tested. The method for performance of QC is determined by the manufacturer's requirements and/or accreditation requirements.

Documentation of QC: All QCs must be well documented immediately after QC is performed or concurrently. Components of QC documentation are listed in Box 22.15. Individual performing QC must be aware of acceptable results or ranges. This will help to know when a procedure is out of control and take appropriate steps for correction. The length of time for retaining the QC records is determined by regulatory and accreditation requirements.

Acceptable QC: Acceptable results or ranges for QC must be predetermined, usually by the kit or reagent manufacturer, by accrediting agencies and sometimes by internal data.

Unacceptable QC: When the results of QC are unacceptable, it is necessary to evaluate (perform immediate investigation), and the process should not be continued till the issue is resolved. Corrective actions may be needed before acceptable QC can be obtained. Results of the investigation and corrective action must be documented. Items which fail QC should be marked as "not for use" until the issue is resolved. Since QC is performed on a schedule, if a failure occurs, it is necessary to assess product produced since the last acceptable QC result.

Quality Control in Transfusion Medicine

Types: Laboratory QC may be of two types namely: (1) internal quality control and (2) external quality control.
- **Internal QC:** It is process in which the technical personnel in the laboratory check their performance by themselves and evaluate the reliability of their techniques.
- **External QC:** In this, the quality and standards of local laboratories is assessed and monitored by an external independent agency.

Various QCs in blood bank are listed in Box 22.16.

Quality Control in Collection of Blood

The quality, safety, and efficacy of the blood or its product transfused depend on several steps namely: (i) donor selection, (ii) blood collection, (iii) component preparation, and (iv) storage, issue, and transportation.

Donor Selection
- **Voluntary and nonremunerated donors:** It is recommended to collect blood from voluntary and nonremunerated donors. While selecting the donors, it is necessary to determine that the donor is in good health, in order to protect against damage to donor's own health, and to protect the recipient against transmission of disease or drugs which could be detrimental to the recipient.
- **Information collection and evaluation**: It is necessary to obtain a consent form filled by donor and donor is registered for permanent record. Donor must be checked for possible potential harm to both donor and recipient by providing a list of questionnaires.

Box 22.15: Components of quality control (QC) documentation.

- Date of performing QC
- Identification of individual performing QC
- Identification of reagent, material, or component (including manufacturer and lot number)
- Expiry date of above
- Identification of equipment
- Results and interpretation (acceptable or unacceptable)
- Corrective action taken when unacceptable results are obtained

> **Box 22.16:** Various quality controls in blood bank.
>
> - Quality control in collection of blood
> - Quality control of reagents: Daily reagent reactivity testing, use of autologous control in antibody identification tests
> - Quality control of kits used for testing blood transmissible infections
> - Quality control of equipment: Temperature checks, equipment calibration
> - Quality control of techniques: Positive and negative sample testing
> - Quality monitoring test: e.g. venepuncture
> - Quality control of storage and transport of blood
> - Quality control of blood components: Platelet counts in random or apheresis platelets, expiration date check
> - Quality control in transfusion practice
> - External quality assurance

Blood Collection

- **Preparation for collection:** Before collecting the blood, the equipment used must be cleaned, calibrated, and checked for performance (e.g. blood bags to be used should be inspected for any defect in anticoagulant solution, moisture or discoloration of the surface of the bag or leakage).
- **Blood collection:** For collection of blood, aseptic technique and seal closed method should be followed.
- **Labels and records:** Blood bags should be labeled with correct ABO and Rh grouping. Screening, expiratory date, and volume of the blood should be mentioned in the label.
- **Blood processing:** After collection, it should be immediately stored at 1-6°C. Components preparation has to be done within 6 hours after collection.

Quality Control of Reagents

Selection of good quality reagents ensures that the transfusion services are effective and correctly function. Most of the reagents in blood bank are obtained from commercial sources. Their standardization is mainly carried out by the manufacturers and meets the established requirements.

Reagents used

- Copper sulfate (if it us used for estimation of hemoglobin especially during blood camps)
- Reagent red blood cells
- Reagent antisera (antibody reagents)
- Test kits used for testing infectious disease

Quality Control of Reagents

- **Select the reagent with high specifications** for ABO, Rh and antihuman globulin (AHG). These reagents should have a minimum shelf life of 1 year.
- **All blood grouping reagents** (including antihuman globulin reagents—AHG) **should contain preservative.** This will minimize the growth of bacteria and fungus. These reagents should be refrigerated at a temperature of 2–8°C.
- **Label the reagents:** All reagents should be properly labeled with lot/batch number, date of manufacture, date of expiry, and storage temperature. Each reagent packing should be accompanied by instruction for its use.
- **Color codes:** Blue for anti-A, yellow for anti-B, and green for AHG.
- Use reagents as per manufacture's instruction.
- Routine QC of antibody reagents is based on running both positive and negative control with each batch of reagent. This will ensure that the reagents are specific and potent.
- Store reagents at the storage temperature specified in the manufacturer's instructions. The storage requirement for anti-A, anti-B, and anti-D reagents is between 2–8°C.

Quality control of main reagents used in blood bank is presented in Table 22.3.

Quality control of CuSO$_4$ used for hemoglobin estimation:
- Every batch of CuSO$_4$ solution should be checked with blood samples of known hemoglobin range around 12.5 g/dL.
- Blood with Hb of 12.5 g/dL or more will sink and those with Hb level below 12.5 g/dL will float.
- The containers must be covered when not in use.
- Discard CuSO$_4$ after 25 donors' blood has been tested.

Table 22.3: Quality control of main reagents used in blood bank.

Parameter	Quality requirements	Frequency of control
ABO reagents		
Appearance	No hemolysis, turbidity, precipitate or gel formation by visual inspection	Daily
Specificity	Clear cut reaction with corresponding red cell antigen without any reaction with negative control	Daily and with each new lot
Avidity	Macroscopic (gross) agglutination with 50% red cell suspension	Daily and with each new lot
Reactivity	No immune hemolysis, rouleaux formation, or prozone	Each new lot
Potency	Undiluted serum shows strong (+++) reaction with a 3% red cell suspension	Each new lot
Rh antisera		
Appearance	No hemolysis, turbidity, precipitate or gel formation by visual inspection	Each day
Specificity	Clear cut reactions with Rh+ve red cells without any reaction with Rh-ve control	Daily and with each new lot
Avidity	Visible agglutination with 40% red cell suspension in homologous serum	Daily and with each new lot
Reactivity	No immune hemolysis, rouleaux formation, or prozone	Each new lot
Potency	Undiluted serum shows strong (+++) reaction in designated test for each serum	Each new lot
Antihuman globulin reagent (AHG)		
Appearance	No turbidity, precipitate or gel formation by visual inspection	Each day
Reactivity and specificity	• No prozone phenomenon • No hemolysis or agglutination of unsensitized red cells	Each new lot
	Agglutination of red cells • Sensitized with anti-D serum containing not >0.2 mg/mL antibody activity • Sensitized with a complement binding antibody (e.g. anti-Le) • Coated with C3b and C3dm and no/weak agglutination with C4 coated red cells	
Normal saline		
Appearance	No turbidity, precipitate by visual inspection	Each day
NaCl content	154 mol/L (9 g/L)	Each new lot
pH	6–8	Each new lot
Hemolysis	Mix 0.1 mL saline and 0.1 mL of 5% red cell suspension and centrifuge for 10 minutes, must not show hemolysis	Each batch

Quality Control of Kits used for Testing Blood Transmissible Infections

Infectious disease test kits are used to detect blood transmissible infections thereby to reduce the blood-borne infectious disease in the recipient of transfusion. Following should be followed for QC of reagent kits used for screening testing for blood transmissible infections.

- Kits that are used for various serological tests such as hepatitis B, hepatitis C, HIV, and syphilis should be strictly used as per the manufacturers.
- Both positive and negative control should be provided with the kit and should be run along with the test.
- It is necessary to have some **internal and external QC samples** for monitoring the performance of various test kits and techniques both for sensitivity and specificity. Batch preacceptance testing (BPAT) of new batches of test kits should be performed as an additional QA measure. **External quality** checks, in confirmation of positive results should be carried out.
- **External proficiency exercise**, involving the testing of panel of sera circulated to blood bank by an approved reference institution.
- Implementation of any new technique should involve assessment on specificity and sensitivity.
- Collection of representative data may be useful to monitor performance test.

Quality Control of Equipment

Selection and Evaluation

- All equipment used in blood bank should meet mandatory technical, electrical, and safety standards.
- Equipment should be preferably purchased from manufacturer/supplier who have locally available expertise having the knowledge of maintenance and repair of the equipment.
- Installation should be done with the manufacturer's installation staff in conjunction with hospital engineering departments, to ensure compliance with electrical safety standards.
- After the installation and calibration of the equipment as per the supplier's specifications, it should be confirmed that its performance meets required standards. Only after this, it can be used for routine work.
- If any repair work is undertaken, the equipment should be checked and assessed for its proper working after repair and its record should be maintained.

General Quality Control of Equipment

- The performance of all equipment used in laboratory should be periodically monitored. The result must be recorded and if necessary, adjustment should be made.
- Preventive maintenance of equipment (which includes cleaning and recalibration) is mandatory.
- Laboratory staff must clean the equipment, and periodically verify the speed of the equipment (e.g. centrifuge) by using tachometer (an instrument used for measuring the speed of an engine) and temperature by thermometer.

Quality control and maintenance of equipment

Various equipment used in blood bank are given in Table 22.4.

Refrigerator for storage of blood

Blood refrigerator must be kept clean and well illuminated.

Temperature

- The proper temperature required is in the range of 2–6°C. Frequently (at least once a day) check the temperature chart and digital temperature.
- The temperature inside the cabinet should be counter checked periodically with the help of precision thermometer.

Alarm system

- It should be battery operated and independent of the main electric supply.

Table 22.4: Various equipment used in blood bank.

Collection equipment	Other equipment	
• Hemoglobin instrument • Hematocrit/Microhematocrit instrument • Apheresis equipment • Blood-weighing scales	• Refrigerators • Freezers • Heating instruments • Blood warmers • Water baths • Thawing devices for blood components • Centrifuges, refrigerated and serologic	• Cell washers • pH meters • Cell counters • Blood irradiators • Platelet incubators • Containers used for shipping

- It should be set in such a way so that it makes sound when the temperature is outside the required range of 2–6°C.
- It should be checked once a week by immersing the sensor in ice water (for low temperature) and in water at 15–20°C (for higher temperature). If alarm system is not properly functioning, corrective measures should be taken.

Freezers
- Similar to blood bank refrigerator, the temperature chart and digital temperature of freezers should be periodically checked (at least once a day). Periodically check the temperature of digital system by precision thermometer kept inside the cabinet.
- If there is no provision for automatic defrosting system, it should be defrosted whenever required.

Laboratory centrifuge (bench top)
- Check every 3–4 months for accuracy of the speed and time with the precision rpm meter using tachometer and stopwatch.
- Clean regularly.

Refrigerated centrifuge
- Should be checked every 3–4 months by the service engineer.
- Check the accuracy of speed and time for the precision rpm meter using tachometer and stopwatch.
- Record the temperature inside the centrifuge bowl by a temperature tester with the lid closed and the rotor stationery.

Water bath and incubator
- Keep them clean.
- Check the temperature daily. Periodically, check the accuracy of the thermometer.
- Change the water frequently.

Microscope
- Cover the microscope when not in use.
- Keep stage clean. Frequently clean the condenser and lenses with moistened lens paper. If accidentally the lenses become dirty, clean them immediately.
- Once in 6 months, lubricate coarse adjustment of rack and condenser.

Automated equipment for shaking and weighing blood bag
- Check them daily for its performance.
- Check its weighing system with a known weight in grams.

Quality Control of Techniques
- Objective of QC of techniques: To ensure a consistently high standard of performance of the common techniques. These techniques include ABO and Rh typing, antihuman globulin test, detection and identification of irregular antibodies of clinical significance and compatibility test.
- Techniques should be validated for accuracy, reliability, and sensitivity by the use of positive, negative and auto-controls.

Causes of Technique Errors
- Lack of proper reagents.
- Lack of attention to specific steps in procedure such as incubation time or temperature, or to centrifugation speed and time.
- Improper washing of cells.
- Preparation of too strong or too weak cells suspension and hemolysis may be read as a negative result
- Failure to confirm negative results without examining under microscope.

Quality Control of Blood and Blood Products

Quality control of blood and its products depends upon:
- Selection of proper donor: It is recommended to collect blood from voluntary and nonremunerated donors in good health. This will protect the donor against damage to his/her own health, as well as protect the recipient against transmission of disease or drugs which could be detrimental to the patient. Information collection and evaluation of donor includes getting consent in consent form, registration of donor with a permanent record, and checking the donor for any possible harm due to donation as well as potential harm to recipient (using list of questionnaires).
- Preparation for collection: Ensure the quality of the container (e.g. moisture or discoloration of the surface of the bag or leakage) used for blood collection and its anticoagulant preservative solution.
- Technique of phlebotomy: Technique of blood collection using aseptic technique and seal closed method.
- Blood processing: Immediately store blood at 1–6°C.
- Component preparation: Should be done within 6 hours after collection. There is the additional QC of the component preparation. These include residual white blood cell count in leukoreduced units, hemoglobin levels in apheresis red blood cell units, and bacterial detection of platelet units.
- Labels/records: Label correctly (ABO and Rh grouping), screening performed, expiratory date, and volume of the blood collected.
- Storage temperature of blood/blood components.
- Issue and transportation of blood/components.

Quality Control of Blood Components (Table 22.5)

- Red blood cell hematocrit
- Cryoprecipitated antihemophilic factor
- Residual leukocyte counts in leukocyte-reduced components
- Platelet counts in platelet units
- Bacterial contamination of platelet units

Quality Control in Transfusion Practice

This involves safety practices in: (i) transfusion transmitted diseases and (ii) donor compatibility.
- Compare the identity information received from recipient with data on the laboratory certificate of compatibility testing.
- Check the certificate of the recipient blood group against the blood group mentioned in the label on the donor blood unit.
- Check the expiry date of blood or blood components in the label attached to unit.
- Record the identity of the recipient.
- Sterility of the blood or blood components.
- Safe transfusion practice (refer pages 430-3).

Hospital Transfusion Committee

It consists of representatives of the blood transfusion center and the main clinical units with a significant transfusion activity. The committee includes clinicians, nurses, and administrative personnel. Its goals are to:
- Define blood transfusion policies
- Conduct regular evaluation of blood transfusion practices
- Analyze any transfusion reactions/undesirable events due to blood transfusion
- Take any corrective measures, if necessary

External Quality Assurance

- The internal QC should be complemented by regular external QA (e.g. participation in a proficiency testing program).
- In a proficiency testing program, coded "normal" and "problem" blood samples are distributed from national or regional reference laboratory to the participant blood banks usually 2–4 times in a year.
- The proficiency testing program is limited to compatibility testing. ABO-grouping, Rh-typing and phenotyping and alloantibody detection.

Table 22.5: Quality control of blood and blood products in blood bank.

Parameter	Quality requirements	Frequency of control
Whole blood		
Volume	350/450 ± 10%	1% of all units
Anticoagulants	49/63 mL	All units
PCV (Hct)	30–40%	4 units/month
HBs Ag	Negative by ELISA	All units
Anti-HCV	Negative by ELISA	All units
Anti-HCV I and II	Negative by ELISA	All units
Syphilis	Negative by screening test	All units
Sterility	By culture	Periodically
Red cell concentrate		
Volume	350 ± 20 mL	1% of all units
PCV (Hct)	55–65%	Periodically
Leukocytes poor red cells modified by centrifugation		
• White cells removed	<70% leukocytes of original quantity	4 units of month
• Residual red cells remaining	>70% of original quantity	
Washed red cells		
• Plasma removed	99%	
• RBCs loss	20%	
• Leukocytes removed	85%	
Leukocytes poor red cells modified leukocyte filter		
• White cells removed	99% removed	4 units a month
• Red cells remaining	90–95%	
Platelet concentrate		
Volume	50–70 mL	All units
Platelet count	>5.5 x 10^{10} in 75% of units tested	4 units per month
pH	>6.0	4 units per month
RBC contamination	0.5 mL	4 units per month
WBC contamination	5.5×10^7–5×10^8	4 units per month

Documents and Records

Documents: Document may be any type of recorded and approved information contained in a written or electronic format. Documentation is important in transfusion medicine and it provides evidence of what was done, as well as details about what was done. Good documentation can provide full traceability (details) and trackability (a logical sequence of steps) in the execution of processes. Examples of documents include written policies, process flowcharts, procedures and instructions, forms, manufacturers' package inserts, computer software and instrument operator manuals, and copies of regulations and standards.

Transfusion services involved in the production of blood and cellular products create many documents and records (Box 22.17).

Aims of Documentation

- To provide evidence that specified standard has been followed in donor selection, collection of blood, preparation of blood

> **Box 22.17:** Documents and record in blood bank as per AABB.
>
> - Quality manuals
> - Policies and process documents
> - Standard operating procedures (SOPs) and work instructions
> - Forms
> - Labels

components, and issue of blood and its products.
- It helps to trace each donation for any evidence of error and the staff involved in the exercise.
- It ensures consistency and reliability at each step in transfusion medicine.
- Provides an evidence for the investigation of any alleged products, adverse reactions or complaints, whether related to donor, transfusion recipient or staff.

Records

They capture the results or outcomes of performing procedures and testing on written forms or electronic media. These include manual worksheets, instrument printouts, tags, or labels. Records are the evidence of what was done. It proves that the procedures were followed and documentation of the work done was captured. Records should be created concurrent with the performance of the work, documenting each critical step. There should be written description of the records to be maintained and the length of retention. Good records provide the details (traceability—who, what, when, where, how) and logical sequences of steps taken (trackability). Since records are permanent, inedible ink should be used and if any corrections are needed, they should be made in such a manner that allows one to see what was the error. The common practice for correcting errors on paper documents is to draw a single line through the error, write the correction above it and then initial and date of correction. If any explanation is required for the correction, same can be written alongside the correction. If the space is not enough, an asterisk can be used and explanation written elsewhere on the document, even on the back.

Policies, process documents, procedures, and completed forms are examples of record in transfusion medicine and/or cellular therapy. They indicate how the work was being performed at any particular time. The records may be in paper or electronic form. It is necessary that record should have information or identity about the individual who created the record. Many of the records in transfusion medicine (especially those containing information of donor or patient) are confidential, they should never be left where they can be viewed by other individuals.

General requirements of records

- Each blood bank should maintain a record. The record should be clear, simple, easy to follow, and complete.
- Record should be legible and any correction should be initialized.
- Date of receiving the sample, performance of tests and interpretation should be recorded.
- A list of all staff members involved in record keeping should be maintained. It should contain the name, signature, and initials of each.
- Record should be retained for 5 years or as required by the National policy.

Protection of record: Records (both paper or electronic form) should be protected from unauthorized changes, from inadvertent destruction, and from damage which may be caused by rodents, fire or water. Storage of record should be designed to achieve these goals and also to easily retrieve them. Access to records should be restricted especially if the record contains information that are confidential.

Record retention

Organization should have a record retention policy (stored for possible future reference) as per the regulations and they should be retained as per the policy.

Retention of donor and blood unit records: Donors on permanent deferral and indefinite deferral lists for protection of the recipient should be maintained indefinitely. Other records need to be maintained for a minimum of 10 years.

Retention of patient records: Records concerned with difficulty in blood typing, clinically significant antibodies, significant adverse events to transfusions, and special transfusion requirements should be retained indefinitely.

Requests for blood and blood components, orders for blood, blood components, tests, and derivatives, recipient consent, and certification of patient identification before transfusion should be retained for a minimum of 5 years. Other records need to be maintained for a minimum of 10 years.

Records retention in blood bank helps to determine the source (donor) of the cells, donor-related information, all manipulations to which the blood or components were subjected, and key QC tests related to the safety, purity, and potency of the product. The records help in tracing all steps clearly. Record keeping should be done concurrently with the work and not after the work is completed. Some transfusion records must be stored indefinitely; others have a minimum retention period. Once the record reaches its "end of life," should be discarded in such a manner that it protects any confidential information. The destruction may be by shredding or burning.

Electronic records: Many records and documents are stored electronically. If records are stored electronically, they must be protected from unauthorized changes. The data should be stored in a manner that would not cause inadvertent loss of data from overwriting, physical damage, or system crashes. There must be a method for backing up all critical electronic data and back-up data files must be stored offsite. Computerized data integrity must be monitored. Backups should be routinely run, and there should be written procedures to restore any data that may be lost inadvertently.

Both documents and records must be controlled to provide evidence that regulations and standards are being met.

Various records/registers needed in blood bank

The various records:
- Must be legible hand written or typed
- Must be stored in such a way that they are protected from damage, unauthorized destruction or modification
- Should be retained for 5 years as per Drug and Cosmetics Act and Rules.

Minimum record keeping required in blood center/bank are listed in Box 22.18.

Record of donors (Donors selection and registration)
- This should contain record of all donors, those who have been deferred or rejected with reasons. This will be useful when the donor visits next time for donation. The following records are needed and include:
  - Blood donor registration: Donor registration form has following details to be entered namely blood donor consent for donation, donor's name, date of birth (age), gender and weight, father/husband name, donation—voluntary or replacement, address (office and residence) and telephone number. and history of illness
  - Donor deferral
  - Donor reaction
  - Voluntary donor panel
  - Rare donor panel
  - Donor recall system

Record of donor blood collection

This record should include:
- Date of collection of blood
- Donor identification or registration number

Box 22.18: Various minimum records needed in blood bank.

- Record of blood donors
- Record of donor blood collection
- Record of blood component preparation
- Record of recipients including requisition form
- Compatibility test record on the requisition form
- Record of infection markers tests
- Blood/blood component issue register
- Record of blood transfusion reactions and their investigations
- Other records

- Name, address, contact telephone/mobile number, email id
- Age and gender
- Details of physical examination such as weight, pulse, temperature, and blood pressure
- Laboratory test performed and their results. These include:
  - Hemoglobin/hematocrit value
  - ABO and Rh type
  - Irregular antibodies, if any
  - Results of HBsAg, anti-HCV, anti-HIV (1 and 2), syphilis (VDRL/RPR) test
- Disposal records or fate of collected blood units

Record of blood component preparation

This should contain:
- Name of component
- Donation number/serial number
- Donor registration or identification number
- ABO and Rh type
- Date and method of preparation
- Component prepared
- Result of testing
- Name of the staff involved in the preparation of the blood component
- Disposal or fate of the blood component

Record of recipients

This should have the following details
- Recipient's/patient's name, age and gender, father/husband's name
- Recipient's hospital registration or identification number
- Name of the hospital, ward, and bed number
- Name of the clinician or attending physician of the patient
- Previous history of transfusions, transfusion reactions, and pregnancy
- Indication for transfusion
- Number of units of blood or blood component needed
- Date and time when needed
- Whether routine or as an emergency basis

Compatibility test record
- Recipient's blood group (ABO and Rh)
- Antibody screening in patient's blood
- Identification of donor unit(s) and donation number
- Blood group (ABO and Rh) of donor unit(s)
- Technique used for crossmatching and the interpretation of test result: compatible or incompatible
- Initials of the staff performing the test

Record of infections markers tests

Anti-HIV 1 and 2 test, HBsAg test, anti-HCV test, VDRL/RPR, malaria

Blood/blood component issue register:
- Serial number, date and time of issue of blood/component
- Particulars of recipients (Name, age, gender, hospital registration number, room/ward number)
- Clinical diagnosis
- Date of collection and date of expiry
- Name/particulars of components supplied such as whole blood, packed red cells, fresh frozen plasma, platelet rich plasma, platelet concentrate, cryoprecipitate, etc.
- Number of units (quantity) issued
- Compatibility report, crossmatched by
- Issued by and time of issue
- Initials of issuing staff

Record of transfusion reactions and their investigations

Other records

These include:
- Stock register of consumable articles
- Register for nonconsumable articles
- Daily stock registers of blood and its components
- Quality control record

Document Creation

Documents should be created in a consistent manner. An SOP should be created to define the format of documents, for the review and approval process, both initially and at routine intervals. There should be a numbering system for documents and changes to documents should be made in a controlled manner.

Document Control

Document control is a structured **document control** system that standardizes facility documents. As per regulatory and accrediting agencies, the documentation should be thorough; well organized; appropriately stored; retrievable in a reasonable amount of time; and protected from unauthorized access, modification, and destruction. Document control is a key element of process control. The document control system includes instructions for creating documents in approved formats, assigning document identification and version designation, approving new and revised documents, preparing a master document list, and maintaining document history files. It links a facility's policies, processes, and procedures and ensures that only the latest (current) approved, copies of documents are available for use. It also protects documents from unauthorized access or modification. Document control systems may be in soft copy (electronic) form or a hard copy form. Elements of document control are listed in Box 22.19. A typical document control system is structured as a pyramid (Fig. 22.5). The following examples best illustrates how a blood bank should link its policies, processes, and procedures.

Document control system in blood bank (Fig. 22.5): The blood bank should have a system to control identification, approval, revision, and archiving of its policies, process descriptions, procedures, and related forms.

Policy document (What will be done): It is necessary for the blood bank to have a written policy document. This should indicate that the blood bank maintains a process and relevant procedures for correcting wrong entries or results on a paper record or in the computer.

Process document (How it happens): A second document (such as a process flowchart) is process document. It should describe the sequence of activities to identify the necessity for a correction, obtaining any necessary approvals for the changed information, making the correction in the computer or on paper (or both), and notifying all appropriate parties of the correction.

Procedure documents (How to do it): Features of procedure documents are presented in Box 22.20.

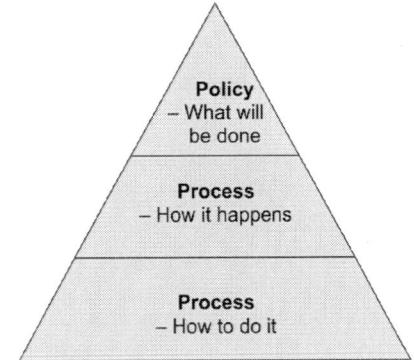

Fig. 22.5: Pyramid of documentation control system.

Box 22.19: Elements of document control.

- Master list of current documents (includes policies, processes, procedures, labels, and forms)
- Standardized format for policies, processes, and procedures
- Documented review and approval of new and revised documents before use
- Periodic review of documented policies, processes, procedures, and associated forms
- Distribution of new or revised documents to all areas that need the information
- Removal of obsolete documents from all areas
- Retention of obsolete documents for length of time as per accreditation policy

---

Box 22.20: Features of procedure documents.

Procedure documents instruct the staff how to:
- Record the need for a correction
- Obtain any necessary approvals for making the change
- Properly record a change to an entry on a paper record
- Properly record a change to an entry in a computer record
- Notify appropriate parties of the change and document the notification

The process and procedures should be written as per regulatory and accreditation requirements.

Quality Manual

Quality manual is the one of the most important documents in transfusion medicine (blood or cellular therapy). Quality manual describes the quality policy, quality objectives, and overall approach to quality by an organization. It defines how the organization is structured to ensure implementation of the QS and defines the role of staff and management.

Policies and process documents
- **Policies** describe the manner in which an organization operates. They are high-level documents which describe the position of an organization on a particular topic. For example, to avoid use of tobacco in the workplace.
- **Process documents** are also high-level documents which describe the inputs for a process, the conversion that takes place, and the output of a process.

Standard operating procedures (refer pages 462-3) and work instruments

Work instructions: They provide step-by-step instruction for performing the task. They are more specific and more detailed than procedures.

Forms

Forms are specially designed documents—either paper or electronic. Blank forms provide templates for obtaining information and on which the results or outcomes of performing procedure can be recorded. Forms should be designed by experienced individuals and often mistakes can be avoided by careful designing of form. If the form is not self-explanatory, it is necessary to provide the instruction for filling (completion) of the form and can be conveniently placed on the front or back side of the form. When a form (either paper or electronic) is filled out, it becomes a record.

Labels and Label Control

Though labels are not always considered as document, they need to be created and maintained within the document control system. Label control involves written procedures for handling labels, preventing mix-ups, revising labels, and discarding obsolete labels. Many blood product recalls are due to mislabeling of the product. When a unit of blood is incorrectly labeled, the product is called misbranded. Mislabeling errors are time-consuming and also embarrassing. Hence, blood banks should have a label control programs. Labeling is critical and should be done in areas designed only for that purpose.

Document Maintenance (Records Management)

Documents should be created and maintained in a controlled manner. Version control is important. When a document is revised, it should be approved and released. An archived copy of the original version should be retained for future reference. This helps in document control and also helps to ensure that the all old copies of the documents are removed and replaced by revised version.

There should be a master list of all the various types of documents in use. The list should define the most current version, how many are revised and where these copies are available.

Records (refer pages 474-6).

Information Management

As already discussed, documents provide information about what to do; records tell what happened, who did it, and when it was done.

Organizations have a large amount of information (most of them require confidentiality) which must be managed as part of QS (Quality System). Activities of information management system include using and manipulating the donor or patient information and test results in the facility's paper and electronic information systems. For example, maintaining the confidentiality of privileged donor and patient information and the facility needs to ensure its processes preserve that confidentiality. Access to information should be restricted to those who need the information for the work purposes. The facility must also ensure the integrity of any data or information sent inside or outside the facility, whether the medium used is paper or electronic. Unauthorized copying of information should not be allowed. Documents containing confidential information in a paper state should be in locked file cabinets. If it is electronic form, it should be protected by access rights.

Deviations, Nonconformances, and Adverse Events

One of the focuses of the quality program is proactive prevention of error. However, it is inevitable that errors will happen. Hence, the quality program should also include processes to detect, evaluate, investigate, and correct errors and accidents. Commonly used lists of terminologies of error used in blood banks and transfusion services are presented in Table 22.6. The term event (an unexpected or unintended incident or occurrence related to a process, procedure, or service) is often used which includes errors, accidents, nonconformances, deviations, and complaints.

Product Deviations

Whenever a nonconforming product is identified, it must be quarantined till the determination of the effect of the nonconformance on product quality is made. If a nonconforming blood product has been already distributed, the blood bank should attempt to recall (withdraw a distributed blood product that has been found to be unsuitable) the product. If a nonconforming blood unit has already been transfused, the blood bank should still notify the consignee (the person who accepted the blood product).

Nonconformance Management

It is necessary to provide safe and pure blood and blood components as per rules, standards, or laws (i.e. conformance). Any error is called noncompliance. The QMS should have processes and procedures for the blood banks to detect, document, investigate, correct, and report any error or accident in the manufacture of blood components that may affect the safety, purity, potency, identity, or effectiveness of the component or that compromises the safety of the blood donor or recipient. Each blood bank should have a process to detect, report, evaluate, and correct deviations and any nonconformance with its own procedures, products, or services. Various contents of nonconformance procedure are presented in Box 22.21.

Nonconformance management is one name for such a process. Other commonly used names include **occurrence, incident, or variation management**.

Definitions of terms used to classify occurrences of nonconformance in blood banks are presented in Table 22.6.

Donor or Recipient Adverse Events

Donor adverse events: It is mandatory that in the blood bank, the staff involved in the collection of blood staff must be educated to recognize and handle the adverse events related to donation. Any events occurring must

Box 22.21: Various contents of nonconformance procedure.

- Documentation of event (electronic or on paper)
- Determination of effect, if any, on the quality of products or services
- Evaluation of the effect
- Investigation and root cause analysis
- Selection of appropriate corrective action
- Implementation of corrective action
- Notification and recall
- Implementation of appropriate preventive action
- Reporting to external agencies when required
- Evaluation of the effectiveness of the corrective actions and preventive actions (CAPA) taken

Table 22.6: Nonconformance type and definition.

Definition of term	Blood bank*	Transfusion service**
Accident: Unexpected or unforeseeable adverse events. It is a nonconformance usually not due to a person's mistake	• Blood donor suffers a seizure during donation • Sudden malfunctioning of an age instrument	Transfusion recipient develops a transfusion-related acute lung injury (TRALI)
Adverse event/reaction: Unexpected complications that develop in the donor during or after the donation process or to the recipient of transfused blood components	Donor faints upon standing up after whole blood donation	Recipient develops symptoms of a suspected immediate hemolytic transfusion reaction
Complaint: A statement or expression of dissatisfaction from internal customers (physicians, employees) or external customers (donors, patients)	Transfusion service states that an emergency blood delivery ordered after hours did not arrive within the time indicated in the customer agreement	Operating room states that plasma units were issued instead of the request for platelet units
Error: Nonconformance due to a human or system problem. Deviation from applicable regulation, applicable standards, or established specifications	Problem from failure to follow established procedure or a part of a process that did not work as expected. Stock of obsolete labels is found in the back of a shelf in the room set aside for final labeling of products	Rh (D)-positive red blood cell unit is issued and transfused to a Rh (D)-negative female of child-bearing age with no prior approval from medical director when this contradicts the facility's written policy
Deviation: Departure from policies, processes, procedures, applicable regulations, standards, or specifications	During investigation into a batch of products which failed QC, it is observed that the processing staff adjusted settings of centrifuge to below optimal relative centrifugal force specified in the standard operating procedure (SOP)	During investigation into a proficiency test failure, it is found that the testing staff did not incubate antibody screen for the minimum time specified in the SOP
Biological product deviation: It is the event that affected the safety, purity, or potency of a distributed product	Bacterial detection system shows the bacterial growth after a platelet unit was issued to the transfusion service	Transfusion service irradiates a unit, applies a new label with an incorrect expiration date, and issues the unit after the correct expiration date
Nonconformance: Failure to meet requirements; often specific to an accreditation assessment	During a routine inspection, assessor of accreditation agency finds that monthly QC testing on manufactured platelets was outside limits and was not investigated on two different occasions	Accreditor finds that multiple procedures do not have medical director approval documented
Discrepancy: Difference or inconsistency in the outcomes of a process, procedure, or test result		
Postdonation: The receipt of information (call or information letter) from a donor with additional details regarding his or her donation, such as subsequent illness or neglecting to mention an illness or medication		

*Blood Bank = blood collection and processing center.
**Transfusion service = laboratory area responsible for pre-transfusion testing and blood product distribution (typically located in a hospital).

be documented, evaluated, and monitored. It is also necessary to follow-up on the donor. After this, method to reduce such occurrence must be implemented.

Recipient adverse events: Similar to donor adverse reactions, nursing and other clinical staff members who are involved in administering blood products must be educated to recognize potential reactions in transfusion recipients. If the adverse reaction resulted in discontinuance of the transfusion, it must be informed to the transfusion service. Immediate investigation is carried out to rule out the possibility of immediate hemolytic transfusion reactions. Further investigation may be performed to identify the type of reaction. If there is suspicion that reaction is due to a donor or manufacturing process [e.g. suspected bacterial contamination, transfusion-related acute lung injury (TRALI), or transfusion-associated infection], the transfusion service must report the event to the collection facility. This will help collection facility to investigate possible sources. It is necessary to document (electronic or written) all adverse reactions. The contents of an adverse event form should include particulars listed in Box 22.22.

Traceback and Lookback

Transfusion-transmitted infections can produce immediate transfusion reactions or infections which may not be detected for months or even years.

Bacterial infections: Usually, transfusion of bacterially contaminated products produces an immediate reaction. In such cases, investigation should be carried out which includes ruling the other causes of the symptoms, culturing the remaining blood product, and culturing a post-transfusion blood specimen from the recipient. If bacterial contamination is suspected, transfusion services must report it to the collection facility as soon as possible so that other products from the same collection can be immediately quarantined. When the transfusion service identifies that the recipient's symptoms are due to exposure to bacteria or bacterial toxins, it should be notified immediately without waiting for culture results. However, the culture results are used to confirm or rule out a case of bacterially contaminated product and also to decide the final disposal of any quarantined products.

Viral infections: In contrast to bacterial infections, many viral infections do not cause symptoms in the recipient for months or years after the causative transfusion. If a transfusion recipient notifies the transfusion service or blood bank that he/she has developed a viral infection and suspects it to be due to transfusion, it is necessary to investigate to identify and test all the donors implicated in his/her treatment. This investigation is usually known as a **traceback**. If one or more donors are presently found to be carriers of the same virus, this can trigger a lookback. A **lookback** is the process to track the disposition of blood products from previous donations when supplemental/confirmatory tests on a donor are found to be positive for anti-HIV, anti-HCV, or anti-*Trypanosoma cruzi* (parasite causing Chagas disease). The lookback need not follow from a complaint from a recipient, but can be a result of testing when a donor returns to donate again. Main purpose of the lookback process is to notify all blood recipients that he or she may be at risk for exposure to infectious disease. The other aim is to retrieve and prevent further distribution of the donor's other blood products.

Nonconformance Reporting

In the blood bank, information about events that deviate from accepted policy, process, or procedure should be captured and acted upon. Hospitals usually have a risk management program which captures information about events involving patients and visitors that could result in financial loss to the facility. In blood

> **Box 22.22:** Basic contents of an adverse event form.
>
> - Identity of individuals involved in the event and its investigation
> - Location, date, and time and description of the event
> - Component identification number(s) and volume involved
> - Donor/patient identification and their signs and symptoms
> - Treatment or actions taken
> - Donor/patient outcome
> - Investigation results
> - Follow-up and corrective actions
> - Notification to other facilities

bank, an internal blood bank nonconformance management does this work. This system captures and analyzes information about events that occurred across the entire path of workflow for blood collection and transfusion service activities whether or not a patient was involved. In blood bank, nonconformances include errors and accidents, and adverse reactions in donors and recipients. The program should be written and appropriate portions should have SOPs and be part of the laboratory's SOP system.

All employees should participate in nonconformance reporting. Staff should be trained to find and report nonconformances. It is necessary to convince the staff that nonconformance reporting is not a tool for finger-pointing or disciplinary action. Instead, all staff must be realized that nonconformances represent blood bank processes that do not work as they should. This knowledge of these problems is used to identify shortcomings in the operation and provides opportunities for improvement. Nonconformances may be identified either by staff in the course of routine activities or by supervisors during review of records. Complaints received in the blood bank are also considered nonconformances. The facility requires to capture information about all nonconformances and including those identified before blood components are distributed or issued. In the reporting process, staff must describe who, where, and when and then briefly describe what happened and what they did at the time to remediate the problem. A standard report form may be used to capture information on all occurrences of nonconformance. It is advisable for supervisors and quality function personnel to record the nonconformances in a spreadsheet or database so that the resolution process can be tracked.

Impact of nonconformance on product/service: Once a nonconformance is discovered, it is very important to determine its impact on products and/or services as soon as possible. If the nonconformance has a **negative impact on the product quality**, it is necessary to **quarantine the product(s) or to perform a recall** if the product has been already distributed or issued for patient use. This activates a product recall or withdrawal and it is necessary to gain control of the product as early as possible. These are complex but rather rigid processes.

The reporting process of nonconformance must be clearly defined so that information is tracked and acted upon and feedback is provided. The individual responsible for the quality function in the blood bank (usually called quality manager) reviews all nonconformance reports, assigns an accession number, and forwards the report form to the sections or departments that will be involved in the investigation.

Investigation and Corrective Action

Nonconforming events that occur during donor selection, blood collection, testing or cell processing should be documented.

Classification of nonconformances: As part of a QA plan, there should be mechanisms for the detection and management of errors and their consequences. The nonconformances are errors that can be classified as, accidents, incidents, deviations, complaints, variances or any another nonconformances. Whenever any nonconformance occurs, they should be thoroughly documented, reviewed, and investigated.

Remedial action: Once a problem is identified, an immediate response follows to correct the problem. This immediate action (i.e. the initial quick-fix solution) is called as remedial action. These remedial actions do not address the real cause of the problem. The real cause can be determined only through investigation.

Error Management

For the process to be successful, it is necessary to actively involve employees in the problem-solving stages. Investigation of complaints or errors: Not all nonconformances need full investigation. However, some level of investigations is needed for most nonconformances to determine whether this indicates any shortcoming in the processing method. Investigations help to identify underlying factors that contributed to the problem. A thorough investigation consists of interviewing the staff, reviewing training records, and reviewing SOPs.

Identification of errors: Errors can be identified either internally by employees or externally by customers. Errors must be logged, and their frequencies must be tracked and monitored.

Root cause analysis and problem solving:
- Root cause analysis is defined as systematic process of investigation and subsequent identification/determination of the factors that contributed to an imperfection/error at the cores of a problem. It is a powerful tool to prevent recurrence of error. It is a collective term which describes a wide range of approaches, tools, and techniques used to know the causes of problems. It is often necessary when there are nonconformances. It is important to initiate a root cause analysis to identify what factors contributed to the occurrence of the problem. Root causes are specific underlying causes for problems/errors, which are apparent, reasonably identifiable and can be easily fixed. For example, QC results are beyond acceptable limits and when investigated, it is found that the test was run using expired reagents. Other times what can be seen on the surface is not really the cause. It is important to understand that the root cause analysis is necessary to find the true cause(s) of a nonconformance. If the true cause is not identified, the problems will recur. In order to truly correct a problem and bring a process back in line, the *root cause* (flaw at the core of the problem) must be found and corrected. If the root cause is fixed, the problem should not recur. Not every event needs to be subjected to a full root cause analysis.

Corrective actions: Once the root cause is identified, an appropriate corrective action should be taken. This action should fix the issue, but this corrective action should be reasonable. For example, if the true fix for a problem is a new computer system to accurately capture specific data, it cannot be immediately implemented, so a more reasonable alternative may need to be chosen till the implementation of new computer system. Most corrective action involves making changes in the process. There should be a documentation of these corrective actions. All staffs involved in performing that process must be informed of the changes and retrained when necessary. Sometimes, the corrective action involves retraining only specific staff who may not have been adequately trained initially or who have been taking unapproved deviations from the established processes or procedures. The completed report is returned to the quality officer, who reviews it for completeness and appropriateness of remedial and corrective action.

In addition to any action in response to a particular event, it is necessary to periodically review these events to determine whether systemic or process changes are indicated. Thus, there should be a system of corrective action that will define the actions to be taken as a result of nonconforming vents or adverse reactions.

Hemovigilance reporting will help to detect, investigate, and respond to adverse transfusion reactions and events that result in nonconformances.

Preventive actions: Once the cause is identified, prepare a proposed plan for its prevention. After changes are made and the process is fine-tuned or adjusted, it is necessary to have a subsequent review to evaluate the effectiveness of the preventive corrective action. If the error recurs, another root cause analysis should be performed. This strategy ensures a continuous quality improvement of all processes. Errors should be considered as an opportunity for improvement, and employees should be encouraged to report errors without concern for act of retaliation.

Recalls

Recalls are removal of products from the market usually by manufacturers' that may compromise the safety of the recipient. Recalls can be classified depending on the degree of danger or hazard they impose. Sometimes, recalls are issued months or years after the product has been transfused or has expired. In such situation, the purpose of the recall notification is to alert the client of possible hazards or adverse consequences the recipient might have incurred by receiving the product.

Monitoring and Evaluation

Organizations should have a system to monitor and evaluate the effectiveness of the organization's processes. This should be a part of QMS.

Monitoring: It can be done at various levels such as in process activities, the result or the process, or even the system in which the process resides. Record review and analysis is an ongoing form of monitoring. The internal and external assessments of the process are a very useful way of monitoring. Assessments include comparison of actual or expected results, quality assessments, peer-reviews, self-assessment, and proficiency testing.

In organizations, there should be process that describes the method of conducting the internal assessments. Each assessment should be well planned and conducted accordingly. Assessors look at data such as quality indicators and other quality records or observe processes as they are performed. If any issues are found during assessment, the process should include a mechanism to respond to these issues.

Quality Indicators

These are statistical measures that give an indication of output quality. They are useful in the evaluation of customer requirements, personnel, inventory management and process control, and stability. They are measurable facets of a process or data collected as a result of a process or service. Quality indicators may be based on outcomes (e.g. quantity not sufficient-QNS rates) or they may be based on the process' ability to deliver an expected result consistently. Organization should identify quality indicators that can be used to evaluate the effectiveness of the system. Organization should establish alert limits for quality indicators. Thresholds (acceptable or unacceptable limit) for each quality indicator should be established. Thresholds are determined from regulatory or accreditation requirements or data derived internally. Quality indicator data is collected over a defined period of time and periodically reported. Examples of common quality indicators are listed in Box 22.23.

Internal and External Assessments

Assessments are carried out to find objective evidence that policies, processes, and procedures are being followed and are achieving the intended results (includes consistently high quality). When the finding show evidence of nonconformance or ineffectiveness, assessments highlight areas where quality initiatives would be most effective.

Internal Audits

Internal audits are conducted by the QA unit or others within the same organization. These are the most valuable tools in assessing the organization's QS. Internal audits are planned and performed periodically (at least annually) to assess the effectiveness of the total/entire QS (to assess the QS of each operation). They should be considered as an opportunity for improvement. Each facility should have written audit policies and procedures. If

Box 22.23: Examples of common quality indicators.

- Turnaround time between specimen check-in and completion of test
- Number of specimens incorrectly labeled and rejected by the laboratory
- Number of incomplete donor records
- Number of donor adverse reactions

nonconformances or areas of concern were found during previous audit, these areas should carefully review to assess the effectiveness of corrective and preventive actions.

Blood-utilization monitoring: It is a type of audit specific to transfusion services. As well known, transfusion practice may be associated with known risk. Appropriate blood utilization is a key factor in limiting risk by ensuring that patients do not receive unnecessary transfusions and conversely that patients receive blood products when needed.

External Assessments

External assessments are those assessments that are conducted by agencies or organizations which are not affiliated (outside the organization) with the facility being assessed. These assessments may be voluntary or mandatory and are conducted by regulating and accrediting agencies. Though any assessment or inspection creates some level of anxiety, it is to be borne in mind that these assessments are usually beneficial to the facility and are opportunities for learning and improving operations. All staff should be trained on how to conduct themselves during inspection or assessment including about what an assessor/ inspector can and cannot do. All staff should be aware that inspectors may ask front-line staff questions and/or directly observe their work performance. Internal audits can help employees become familiar with the types of questions asked by assessors. During assessment, records should be readily available for the inspector. If issues are discovered during assessment/inspection, these are usually documented and provided to the facility in an exit meeting. The facility should perform the root cause analysis and take corrective actions.

Corrective and preventive action: In response to a reported event, corrective action should be taken to prevent recurrence. **Near-miss events** are unexpected occurrences where an error was identified and corrected before a patient or product was adversely affected (refer corrective action on page 483).

Proficiency Testing

Definition: Proficiency testing is the testing of samples, previously unknown to the laboratory, that are sent by an organization approved by proficiency testing program.

Purpose: Proficiency testing is a program designed to ensure that test methods and equipment are working as expected and that laboratory staff have mastered the skills and tasks related to processing, performing, and interpreting accurate laboratory tests. Proficiency testing is a required component of the QA program for testing laboratories. PT samples should be managed as any other sample that the laboratory tests. The testing should be rotated among staff so that different staff is tested. When failures occur, an investigation is carried out to find out the root cause and implements the corrective action.

Process Improvement

Continuous improvement is essential for quality program. Hence, organization that manufacture blood component or cellular therapy products should have processes that allow for continuous improvement in operations and safety of patient. Information gained from nonconformance management system should be used to improve operations and is the primary benefit of effective nonconformance management process. Other sources for improvement opportunities include complaints, QC records, proficiency testing, internal audits, quality indicators, external assessments, etc.

Facilities, Work Environment, and Safety

It is necessary to address the adequacy of the facility (Fig. 22.6) and equipment used in the blood bank and transfusion service.

Adequate facilities must be provided to the staff for performing the work and there should be a safe environment for staff, patients, donors, and visitors. There should be sufficient/adequate space to allow proper storage of materials and to prevent mix-ups during

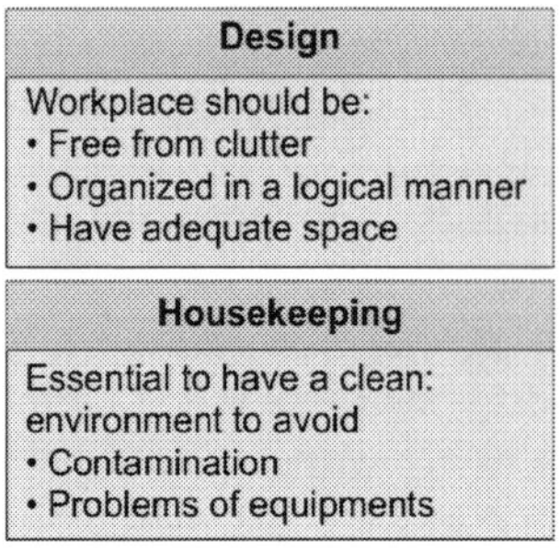

Design
Workplace should be: • Free from clutter • Organized in a logical manner • Have adequate space
Housekeeping
Essential to have a clean: environment to avoid • Contamination • Problems of equipments

Fig. 22.6: Essentials of quality assurance for facilities.

performance of processes. Adequate building utilities, ventilation, sanitation, trash, and disposal of hazardous substance must be provided by the organization. There should be procedures for responding to spills or accidents. Safety includes providing nonslip surfaces, fire safety, radiation safety, chemical safety and disaster preparedness, response, and recovery.

Biosafety Precautions and Guidelines in the Transfusion Laboratory

The personnel working in blood banks and transfusion services (like any other laboratory professionals) should be aware of common terminology used in biosafety standards. Staff in blood transfusion laboratories is constantly at risk of infection from the blood that they handle every day. They should follow biosafety guidelines and safe working measures for the protection against diseases transmissible through blood (e.g. HIV, HbsAg, and HCV). The risk of laboratory-acquired infection with blood-borne diseases is mainly due to contamination of hand, mucosa of eyes, mouth and nose by infectious blood and other body fluids. Though the risk is low, it is necessary to know that the consequences of infection of blood-borne diseases are extremely serious.

Universal/general safety precautions (Box 22.24) for the personnel in blood bank should be strictly followed:

Separate room for microbiological tests: Microbiological test such as for HBsAg, antibodies to HIV and HCV must be carried out in a separate room.

Disinfection: The disinfectant of choice for disinfection of viral and bacterial contamination in blood bank is **1% hypochlorite solution**. The hypochlorite solution needs at least 30 minutes to disinfect the infected material.

- All used glass tube and slides before washing, must be disinfected in hypochlorite solution.
- Used plastic tubes must be soaked in hypochlorite before disposal.
- For blood spillage and heavily soiled equipment, the hypochlorite solution of 10 times (10%) normal strength (1%) should be used.
- Before disposal or incineration of infected material, they should be decontaminated by autoclaving.

Box 22.24: Universal precautions in blood bank.

- Entry to the laboratory will be restricted
- At all times while working in the laboratory, wear gowns or full aprons or closed laboratory coats with long sleeves, often closed at wrists and at neck. They should cover front and must be fluid resistant. These should be removed before leaving the laboratory. Contaminated clothing should be removed promptly, placed in a suitable container and laundered or discarded as potentially infectious
- Wear gloves (latex, nitrile or polyvinyl chloride) when performing phlebotomy and at all times in the laboratory or when handling specimens
- Use safety goggles, face shields, fume hood sashes, and biological safety cabinets. This is needed to prevent a splash risk (e.g. opening specimens, pouring specimens)
- Any cut, puncture wounds or skin eruption must be kept covered with waterproof dressing
- Prohibit eating, drinking, gum-chewing, smoking, application of cosmetics or manipulation of contact lenses and mouth-pipetting all the time in the in the work area of the laboratory
- After removing gloves, after handling specimens, before using a laminar flow, between medical examination, before leaving the laboratory or restricted work area; and after using toilet, handwashing is mandatory

Guidelines for safe use of gloves
- Securely apply bandage or cover open skin lesions on hands and arms of laboratory personnel before using gloves.
- Use gloves only when required and avoid touching clean surfaces such as telephones, door knobs or computer terminals with glove hands.
- Routine use of gloves is not necessary by phlebotomists while working with healthy prescreened donors. If gloves are worn, unsoiled gloves need not be changed between donors.
- Immediately change gloves if they are torn, punctured or contaminated, or after handling high-risk samples.
- Remove gloves by keeping their outside surfaces in contact only with the outside and by turning the glove inside out while taking it off.
- Wash hands with soap or other suitable disinfectant after removing gloves
- Do not wash/disinfect surgical gloves if they are reused.

Work area
- **Disinfection:** The work surface should be disinfected after the procedures and also at the end of each working day with 0.1% sodium hypochlorite solution.
- **Spillage**: In case of any spill, the work area should be covered with 0.1% sodium hypochlorite solution using gloved hands. The area will be left for 10–15 minutes and only cleaned after this. The surface should be wiped again with the disinfectant. If sharp objects are involved in the spill, the gloves should be puncture resistant, and a broom should be used during cleanup to avoid injury.
- **Equipment**: It must be repaired or submitted for preventive maintenance. If it is potentially contaminated with blood, it must be decontaminated before its release to a repair technician.
- **Accidental exposure** to suspected or actual hazardous material is reported to the laboratory director or responsible person immediately.

Hospital Transfusion Committees
Each blood transfusion center should have a hospital transfusion committee which deals with transfusion activity. The committee includes physicians, nurses, and administrative personnel. Main goals hospital transfusion committee are listed in Box 22.25.

QUALITY ASSURANCE IN THE TRANSFUSION LABORATORY
The QMS for a hospital transfusion laboratory are important because errors can lead to patient morbidity and mortality. This should include the following:
- **Quality control:** There should be appropriate internal QCs and should participate in external quality assessment exercises.
- **Validation:** Validation of automated equipment and computer systems should be done. This will ensure that they function as specified. There should be back up procedures to cover the failure of automated equipment and computers.
- **Policies and procedures:** The SOPs should be available. They should cover all aspects of the laboratory work, and these must be reviewed and updated regularly.
- **Reagents, calibrators, and control materials:** They should be used according to the manufacturer's instructions.
- **Preventative maintenance:** The regular checking and maintenance of all laboratory equipment must be documented.
- **Training and competency testing:** Laboratory procedures should only be performed by properly trained staff. A documented program for training laboratory staff should be conducted.

Box 22.25: Main goals of hospital transfusion committee.
- To define blood transfusion policies
- To conduct regular evaluation of blood transfusion practices
- To analyze any undesirable events due to blood transfusion
- To take any corrective measures, if necessary

This should cover all SOPs in use which fulfill the documented requirements of the laboratory. There must be a documented program for assessing staff proficiency. This should include details of the action limits for retraining.
- **Quality incidents and exceptions:** There should be a system in place for documenting and reviewing all incidents of noncompliance with procedures. Independent audits should be conducted to assess compliance with documented "in-house" procedures.

Indicators for Monitoring of Blood Transfusion Services (BTS)

Each blood bank should have the following information for continuous monitoring of basic operational quality:
- Units of blood transfused during a definite period.
- No. of patients transfused compared with total no. of in-patients.
- No. of units of each component transfused per transfused patients.
- **Whole blood:** Red cell concentrate.
- **No. of units transfused:** No. of units requested.
- Number of date expired units of components.
- Components used without clear cut indications.
- No. and type of transfusion reactions.
- No. of units issued without crossmatch (urgent transfusion).
- **Urgent requests:** Routine requests.
- No. of unused units returned.
- No. of surgical operations cancelled because of lack of blood.
- No. of late preoperative requests.
- No. of units issued to other hospitals.
- Replacements versus voluntary donors.

Quality Assurance Audits

Audit: It is a systematic investigation to determine if an organization's actual activities and practices are being performed according to its approved and written policies and procedures.

Performing audits is an important function of the QA and serves as an internal self-assessment tool. It provides confidence that systems and processes are in control.
Audit may be general or focused.
- **General audit:** It is more comprehensive and is used to assess overall operations of a department.
- **Focused or process audit:** It is used to assess a specific problem.

Audits in blood bank: It should be used to monitor transfusion, testing, component preparation and distribution practices, and other processes (e.g. record reviews).

Audits should be conducted by individuals not directly involved in the activity being audited.

There must be a written procedure on how to conduct an audit. Audit should be well planned with follow-up action to correct any problem discovered during the audit.

Accreditation

Laboratory accreditation is a procedure by which an authoritative body gives formal recognition that a laboratory is competent to carry out specific tasks based on Third Party Assessment.
- Drugs and Cosmetic Rules under Government of India provide accreditation services for blood bank.
- National Blood Policy (NBP) of the government takes step towards improving transfusion services in the country.
- National Aids Control Organization (NACO) plans for an accreditation program for blood banks, blood storage centers, and other centers involved in providing transfusion services.

Worldwide Regulatory and Accrediting Agencies for Quality and Safety for Blood Banks

There are many regulatory and accrediting agencies for controlling the blood industry. They focus on ensuring product quality and blood donor and patient safety. They address similar issues regarding QA and quality improvement.

Food and Drug Administration
The Food and Drug Administration (FDA) enforces regulations to ensure the safety and efficacy of biologics, drugs, and devices, blood and blood components, and diagnostic reagents used or manufactured by blood establishments.

American Association of Blood Banks
AABB, formerly known as the American Association of Blood Banks, is a voluntary accrediting agency. It publishes guidelines for members seeking accreditation. These guidelines include the Standards for Blood Banks and Transfusion Services (outlines minimal standards of practice in areas relating to transfusion medicine), the Technical Manual (provides a reference to current acceptable practices in blood banking), and others.

International Society of Blood Transfusion
The International Society of Blood Transfusion (ISBT) is not a regulatory or accrediting agency. However, the goal of the society is to improve the safety of blood transfusion worldwide.

The ISBT provided a standard for worldwide terminology, identification, and labeling of medical products of human origin (i.e. blood, cell, tissue, and organ products). This standard provides international consistency to support the transfer, traceability, and transfusion/transplantation of blood, cells, tissues, and organs.

College of American Pathologists
The College of American Pathologists (CAP) was established in 1946 and issued the first CAP accreditation certificates in 1964. CAP conducts on-site inspection every second year and complete a self-inspection during the intervening year.

External Quality Assessment

External quality assessment (EQA) is an important component of QSs for blood transfusion services. It is the external assessment of a laboratory's overall performance in testing exercise.

In blood banks, there are several processes involved. These processes include the selection of blood donors, the collection, processing and testing of donated blood, the testing of specimens from potential transfusion recipients, and the issue of compatible blood and its administration to the recipient. There is a risk of error in each process. Hence, for the transfusion of safe, compatible blood and blood products it needs prevention of errors in all the processes. For example, failures in screening donated blood for transfusion-transmitted infection (TTI) can produce serious effects in the recipients of blood and blood products.

Causes of errors:
- Inadequate procedures for identification of donor specimens
- Use of inappropriate reagents
- Poor testing practices
- Inadequate maintenance of equipment
- Inaccuracies in recording or transcription
- Incorrect storage of blood and its products
- Inadequate staff training

Steps:
- In EQA, EQA program provider sends testing sets of exercise materials of known, but undisclosed content for testing by the laboratory participating in EQA. Each participating laboratory receives same/identical set of exercise materials, which should be processed in the same way as routine blood donor specimens to ensure that the laboratory's performance in EQA accurately reflects its usual performance.
- After the EQA exercise materials are tested, participating laboratories will send the test results obtained back to the EQA program provider.
- EQA program provider analyzes the results of each laboratory. It sends to all laboratories participating in EQA, a feedback on its own results, together with the anonymized results and the reference results. It will help the participating laboratory to compare its performance with that of other participants.

Benefits to Participating Laboratories (Box 22.26)

The assessment of performance of blood bank through EQA helps the participating laboratory to determine whether their systems are operating effectively or whether there are any deficiencies that require correction. Information obtained by EQA, provides an opportunity for continual quality improvement. This will help to identify the laboratory errors and the implement measures to prevent their recurrence. Thus, EQA plays an important role in making safer blood transfusion. For example, in blood banks that screen donated blood for TTI, participation in EQA helps to monitor and raise standards of performance. Thus, information obtained by EQA helps to improve the overall quality of the laboratory and the safety of its blood and blood products. Even if there is no availability of complete quality system, EQA can still be used as part of a process of continual quality improvement.

Box 22.26: Benefits of external quality assessment (EQA) to participating laboratories.

- Opportunities for improvement relating to laboratory processes
- Compare laboratory's own performance with that of other participating laboratories
- Compare performance between different testing systems
- Encouragement of best practice

SUMMARY

- Quality management refers to the overall process used to ensure that laboratory results/products meet the requirements for healthcare services to patients.
- The QMS includes three facets major components which have an internal focus namely: i) QS, ii) QA, and iii) QC.
- Quality organization should understand and meet the customer needs and expectations.
- Quality management should provide adequate staff and address staff selection, orientation, training, and competency assessment.
- The blood industry is regulated by multiple regulatory and accrediting agencies. All these agencies require compliance with QA and quality improvement concepts.
- Current Good Manufacturing Practices (cGMP) requires the safety, potency, purity, and quality of blood products. They include SOPs, record keeping, training, facilities, maintenance, equipment, validation, QC, change control, and audits.
- Quality assurance consists of planned activities that ensure the quality of the products or services offered. These include record keeping and SOPs, personnel selection and training, validation, supplier qualification, calibration, preventive maintenance, proficiency testing, error management, process improvement, process control, label control, and internal auditing.
- Quality control procedures in blood bank include daily testing of the reactivity of blood typing reagents, positive and negative controls in infectious disease testing, calibration of serologic centrifuges, and temperature monitoring of refrigerators, freezers, and thawing devices.
- Process control consists of a set of activities that ensures that a given process will keep operating in a state that is continuously able to meet process goals without compromising the process itself.
- Process validation challenges all activities in a new process before implementation. It provides a high degree of assurance that the process will work as intended.
- Routine QC procedures, review of records, and capture of nonconformances when the process does not perform as expected. These are routine process control measures and monitor whether a process is functioning as needed.
- Documents include policies, process description, procedures, work instructions, forms, and labels. Records provide evidence that the process is being performed as intended.
- Nonconformance management is a process that detects, report, evaluate, and correct events in blood bank operations that do not meet the facility's or other requirements. Deviation from facility defined requirements, standards, and regulations must be addressed.
- An internal audit reviews a specific facility process. It is determined by examining documents and records, interviews, and observations and intends to know whether the facility is meeting the requirements and its own policies, processes, and procedures.

Contd...

Contd...

- Assessment of facility processes includes internal and external assessments.
- Safety in blood bank is needed to decrease infection risk and physical and chemical hazards in the workplace. Safety programs should address fire, electrical, biological, chemical, and radioactive hazards in the workplace.
- Laboratory safety policies and procedures should be followed by individual employees for their own health and safety, and the safety of coworkers.

SELF-ASSESSMENT EXERCISE

Long essay on:
- Discuss quality assurance in blood banks or blood transfusion services
- Discuss quality control in blood banking /blood transfusion
- Discuss quality assurance and quality control of various blood components

Write short essays/notes on
- Quality control in blood bank
- Records in blood bank
- Write short note on standard operating procedures in blood banking

CHAPTER 23

Major Histocompatibility Complex Molecules

CHAPTER OUTLINE

- Classification of HLA
- Techniques of histocompatibility testing and matching
- Techniques for detection of HLA (HLA typing)
- Donor-recipient crossmatch
- Techniques for detection of HLA antibodies
- HLA and transplantation

INTRODUCTION

Survival of an individual depends on defense mechanism consisting of immune system. The immune system recognizes and responds to various microorganisms and foreign substances (antigens). However, the same defense system has a negative impact when tissue is transplanted from one individual to another, or its malfunctioning may trigger autoaggressive reactions.

Cells with HLA Antigens

All human nucleated (e.g. leukocytes and tissue) cells have a series of inherited molecules on their surfaces (cell surface) that are recognized by other individuals as foreign antigens. The surface antigens or receptors responsible for the recognition and elimination of foreign tissues are **coded by genes in the human leukocyte antigen (HLA) region/complex.** **HLA system is composed** of a complex array or series of closely linked genes located within the major histocompatibility complex (MHC). Hence, the HLA system (region/complex) is also referred to as the MHC. It was named HLA because in humans, MHC-encoded proteins were initially detected on leukocytes by the binding of antibodies.

Major histocompatibility complex molecules were discovered as **products of genes that evoke rejection of transplanted organs** and are responsible for tissue compatibility between individuals.

Antibodies to HLA: HLA antigens, similar to red cell antigens can elicit antibodies from transfusion of blood products, pregnancy, and transplantation. Significance of HLA antibodies in transfusion are as follows:

- **Poor response to platelet transfusion**: HLA antibodies may be responsible for poor platelet response or refractoriness, in patients requiring platelet transfusions. Thus, to improve platelet response, it may be necessary to do HLA matching of donor platelets with the recipient. Refractoriness is a condition in which there is unresponsiveness to platelet transfusions. This is due to HLA-specific or platelet-specific antibodies or platelet destruction from fever or sepsis. The platelet responsiveness is measured by platelet counting following transfusion (post-transfusion).
- **Transfusion reaction**: HLA antibodies can cause reactions and produce chills and fever in some patients receiving red cell transfusions. In such cases, use of

"leukocyte reduced" blood products will be useful to prevent further reactions.

Human leukocyte antigen testing is not routinely performed in the transfusion service or blood bank. However, an understanding of its inheritance, nomenclature, and application is useful for optimal patient support.

MHC genes are codominantly expressed in each individual, i.e. for a given MHC gene, each individual expresses the alleles which are inherited from both parents.

- The **human** MHC, commonly called the **HLA complex** is the name of the **loci of genes** that are densely packed (clustered) on a **small segment** in the short arm of **chromosome 6** (6p21.3). They were named HLA because in humans, MHC-encoded proteins were initially detected on leukocytes by the binding of antibodies. They contain genes that determine membrane molecules (class I and class II) that bear HLA antigens.
- **Physiologic function of MHC molecules:** To **display peptide fragments of proteins for recognition by antigen-specific T-cells**.
- The MHC molecules are products of MHC gene. The best known of these genes are the HLA class I and class II genes. Their products are important for immunologic specificity and transplantation histocompatibility, and they play a major role in susceptibility to a number of autoimmune diseases.
- **Polymorphism of MHC gene:**
  - **MHC gene is highly polymorphic:** Polymorphism means that there are many alleles of each MHC gene resulting in extreme (high degree) variation in the MHC in human population (genetic diversity). Each person inherits one set of these alleles that is different from the alleles in most other persons. The possibility of two different individuals having the same combination of MHC molecules is very remote. Therefore, grafts exchanged between individuals are recognized as foreign and attacked by the immune system. **Polymorphism is an important barrier in organ transplantation.**
  - **HLA haplotype:** It is the combination of HLA alleles in each individual. Each individual inherits one set of HLA genes from each parent and thus, typically expresses two different molecules for every locus.
- **Importance of MHC:** (1) In **organ/tissue transplantation,** (2) HLA is **linked to many autoimmune diseases**.

Function and importance of MHC/HLA molecules (Box 23.1).

- **In immune response**: MHC system was first recognized and named from experiments in tissue transplantation. However, MHC play an essential role in the recognition of self and nonself, the coordination of cellular and humoral immunity, antigen presentation, and initiation of the immune response to antigens. The normal function of MHC/HLA molecules is to **display peptide fragments of proteins for recognition by antigen-specific T-cells (CD4+ and CD8+ T lymphocytes)**. In each individual, T cells recognize only peptides displayed by that individual's MHC/HLA molecules. This phenomenon is called *MHC restriction*.
- **In organ/tissue transplantation**: HLA system is considered as second important only to ABO antigens which influence the survival of solid organ transplant.

Box 23.1: Applications of HLA Testing.

Transplantation
- Hematopoietic progenitor cell transplants
- Solid-organ transplants

In transfusion: Platelet selection for refractory patients

Disease association
- Ankylosing spondylitis HLA-B27
- Celiac disease HLA-DQ2

Pharmacogenomic applications to optimize certain drug therapy regimens
- Abacavir sensitivity (for HIV treatment) and B*57:01 allele

Forensic investigations

- **In hematopoietic progenitor cell (HPC) transplantation:** HLA system is important with regard to graft rejection and graft-versus-host disease (GVHD). Best outcome of organ and HPC transplants depends on HLA matching.
- **In transfusion:** HLA antigens and antibodies are important in complications of transfusion therapy such as **platelet refractoriness, febrile nonhemolytic transfusion reactions** (FNHTRs) **transfusion-related acute lung injury** (TRALI) and **transfusion associated GVHD** (TA-GVHD).
- **To assess risk factors for disease susceptibility:** HLA testing is useful to assess risk factors for disease susceptibility. Though, they are not diagnostic for the associated diseases but are useful to assess relative risk. HLA is linked to many autoimmune diseases.
- **Pharmacogenomic applications:** Certain HLA antigens are associated with optimal drug therapy regimens for certain diseases.
- **In forensic investigations (paternity):** In relationship testing, genetic markers from the mother, child, and alleged father are analyzed to determine whether the tested man could be the biological father of a child.

CLASSIFICATION OF HLA

Protein products of HLA system consists of HLA antigens (MHC molecules). The HLA complex contains about 35–40 genes. The genes encoding the expression of the HLA antigens are part of the MHC gene system located on the short arm of chromosome **6 (6p21.3)**. **HLA/MHC** gene product is classified based on their structure, cellular distribution, and function into **three groups** (regions) **namely: class I, class II, and class III regions** (refer Fig. 23.2). MHC class I and class II gene products are critical for immunologic specificity and transplantation histocompatibility, and they play a major role in susceptibility to a number of autoimmune diseases.

Class I MHC Molecules (HLA antigens)

Expression class I antigens: Class I MHC molecules are the products of MHC class I genes and are **expressed on all nucleated cells and platelets** (neurons, corneal epithelial cells, and trophoblasts). On mature red cells, only vestigial amounts remain, with certain allotypes better expressed than others. The class I region encodes genes from the classic transplantation molecules: HLA-A, HLA-B, and HLA-C.

Structure of class I molecules (Fig. 23.1): Class I HLA molecule is a heterodimer (a protein formed by two different proteins) and consists of **two protein chains: i)** a polymorphic **glycoprotein, α heavy chain** (44-kD) encoded on the short arm of chromosome 6 **and ii)** a smaller (12-kD) non-polymorphic protein/polypeptide called $β_2$-**macroglobulin** (light chain).

- **α chains:** These chains are **encoded by three closely linked genes, designated *HLA-A, HLA-B,* and *HLA-C*** in the MHC locus. The extracellular (external) portion of α chain is divided into three domains namely: $α_1$, $α_2$, and $α_3$. Of these, outermost domains $α_1$ and $α_2$ contain majority of polymorphic regions which confer serologic HLA antigen specificity. Between $α_1$ and $α_2$ domains, there is a cleft (peptide binding cleft) or groove where the foreign peptides (antigens) bind to the MHC molecules for presentation to T cells. The polymorphic amino acid residues that line the sides and the base of the peptide-binding groove are responsible for binding of different peptides (antigens) at class I alleles. It ensures that only CD8+ T cells can respond to peptides displayed by class I molecules
- $β_2$-**microglobulin** polypeptide is not encoded within the MHC but is encoded by a separate gene on chromosome 15. The non-variable $α_3$ is bound to $β_2$-macroglobulin. The α heavy chain

penetrates the cell membrane, whereas β_2-macroglobulin does not.

Antigen presentation and functions of class I MHC:

- **Cells with class I antigens:** Class I antigens are found on the surface of platelets, leukocytes, and most nucleated cells in the body. There are no HLA antigens in mature red cells. However, reticulocytes express HLA class I antigens.
- **Endogenous antigens:** All cells with class I MHC proteins on their surface can bind, display, and transport peptides/antigens to the cell surface. These cell-associated antigens on their surface are synthesized within the cells. Hence, these antigens are referred to as *endogenous* antigens. These endogenous antigens are derived from proteins produced within the cells such as normal cellular proteins, tumor proteins, or viral and bacterial proteins produced within infected cells. These antigens are degraded intracellularly within the cytosol by *proteasomes*, large complexes containing enzymes that cleave peptide bonds, thereby converting proteins to peptides. Then these peptides/antigens become associated with class I MHC proteins. This process, in which most T cells recognize antigens only after they have been degraded and become associated with MHC molecules, is often referred to as **MHC restriction**.
- These peptides/**antigens can be presented** to cytotoxic (CD8+) T lymphocytes. This process, in which **CD8+ T lymphocytes** recognize antigens associated with self-class I molecules are referred to as **class I MHC-restricted**.
- **Immune response:** Products of MHC class I gene are integral participants in the **immune response to intracellular infections, tumors and allografts**. When cells bearing class I molecules and peptides can be recognized and potentially killed by cytotoxic (CD8+) T lymphocytes, they are often known as *target cells*. Thus, class I molecules are **involved in cyto-toxic reactions**. Almost all nucleated cells expressing class I MHC proteins can function as a *target cell* presenting **endogenous antigens** to cytotoxic (CD8+) T lymphocytes.
- **Target cells:** These include: i) cells infected with a virus or some other intracellular microorganism, ii) altered self-cells such as cancer cells and aging body cells, and iii) *allogeneic* cells introduced via skin grafts or organ transplantation (between genetically nonidentical individuals).

Other features:

- The class I region encodes genes for the classic transplantation molecules.
- **Highly polymorphic** in the population and most highly polymorphic segment known within the human genome.
- **Functions:** Products of MHC class I gene are integral participants in the **immune response to intracellular infections, tumors, and allografts**.
- Class I molecules present antigen to cytotoxic (CD8+) T lymphocytes and are **involved in cytotoxic reactions**. **CD8+ T lymphocytes** recognize antigens only in the context of self-class I molecules, they are referred to as **class I MHC-restricted**.

Diagrammatic representation of the HLA complex and the structure of class I and class II HLA molecules is presented in Figure 23.1.

Class II MHC Molecules

Expression of class II antigens: Their expression is more restricted than that of class I antigens. Class II antigens (HLA-D and -DR, D-related) **are expressed only on professional antigen-presenting cells (B lymphocytes, monocytes/macrophages, Langerhans cells, and dendritic cells)**, intestinal epithelium, and early hematopoietic cells. Many other cells may express class II molecules after immune stimulation. Class II antigens are not found on platelets. Hence, there is no need to match class II antigens when HLA-compatible platelets are requested. In the circulation, the number of cells expressing class I antigens is greater than the number of cells with class II antigens.

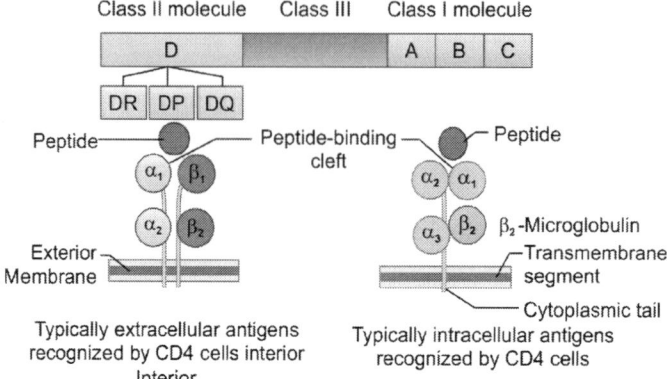

Fig. 23.1: Diagrammatic representation of the human leukocyte antigen (HLA) complex and the structure of class I and class II HLA molecules (not to scale). The class I MHC-encoded chain has three globular domains α_1, α_2, and α_3. A non-MHC-encoded peptide, β_2-microglobulin, is closely associated with the α_3 domain. Alloantigens occur on the α_1 and α_2 domains. The HLA-DR antigen consists of an α and a β peptide, noncovalently bound together. Each peptide has two globular domains, which are structurally related to immunoglobulin (Ig) domains.

Structure of class II molecules: Class II antigens are encoded in a region called **HLA-D**. There are three subregions in HLA-D namely: **HLA-DP, HLA-DQ and HLA-DR**. These molecules are the classic transplantation antigens. Each class II antigen/molecules are a heterodimer which consists of two noncovalently associated structurally similar glycoprotein chains (α and β), both of which traverse the cell membrane. The extracellular (extramembranous) portion of each chain has two amino acid domains designated as α_1 and α_2, and β_1 and β_2. Similar to class I molecules, they have a peptide binding cleft facing outward. This cleft is formed by α_1 and β_2 domains. This peptide binding cleft is this outermost portion which contains the variable regions of the class II alleles and it is in this portion that most class II alleles differ.

Antigen presentation and functions of class II MHC: Antigens that are captured by endocytosis or phagocytosis are called as *exogenous* antigens. The exogenous antigens are **internalized into vesicles, and are usually derived from extracellular microbes and soluble proteins.** The internalized exogenous proteins/antigens are proteolytically digested in endosomes or lysosomes, where they go through several increasingly acidic compartments and encounter hydrolytic enzymes including proteases. Peptides resulting from proteolytic cleavage then associate with class II heterodimers in the vesicles and form stable peptide-MHC complexes.

Function: The class II MHC locus contains genes that **encode many proteins involved in antigen processing and presentation**. **Class II MHC proteins** that bind peptides are then transported to the cell surface and presented to helper T (CD4) lymphocytes. The **class II peptide complex is recognized by CD4+ T-cells** (function as helper cells) and in this interaction, these CD4 molecule acts as the coreceptor. In this process because **CD4+ T lymphocytes can** recognize antigens associated with self-class II molecules, these are referred to as **class II MHC-restricted**.

Soluble HLA Class I and Class II antigens shed from cells are present in blood and body fluids. They may play a role in modulating immune reactivity.
- **Increased levels:** The levels of these soluble HLA antigens increase with infection (including HIV), inflammatory disease and transplant rejection.
- **Decreased levels:** With progression of some malignancies.

Class III MHC Molecules

Their gene **encode some** components of the **complement system** (C2, C4, and Bf), 21-hydroxylase (CYP21), **cytokines,** heat-shock protein (HSP) 70, and **tumor necrosis factor (TNF), lymphotoxin** and some proteins without apparent role in the immune system.

HLA haplotype: The combination of HLA alleles in each individual is termed as the HLA haplotype.

Patterns of inheritance: Each individual inherits one set of HLA genes from each parent and thus, typically expresses two different molecules for every locus. Because of the polymorphism of the HLA genes, innumerable combinations of HLA molecules exist in the population. Each individual expresses an MHC profile on their cell surface that is different from the haplotypes of most other individuals.

Nomenclature for HLA antigens: HLA antigens are designated by a number following the letter that denotes the HLA series, e.g. HLA-A1 or HLA-B8.

Polymorphism of MHC gene: MHC gene is highly polymorphic. Polymorphism means that there are many alleles of each MHC gene resulting in extreme (high degree) variation in the MHC in human population (genetic diversity). Each individual inherits one set of these alleles that is different from the alleles in most other individuals. The possibility of two different individuals having the same combination of MHC molecules is very remote. Therefore, grafts exchanged between individuals are recognized as foreign and attacked by the immune system. **Polymorphism is an important barrier in organ transplantation.**

HLA haplotype: It is the combination of HLA alleles in each individual. Each individual inherits one set of HLA genes from each parent and thus, typically expresses two different molecules for every locus. The expression of gene products constitutes the phenotype of an individual. The phenotype can be determined by typing for HLA antigens or alleles.

Major histocompatibility complex (HLA complex) showing location of genes is presented in Figure 23.2.

Note: It is important to point out that the proper format used when referring to genes in written documents is *italics*.

HLA Inheritance

Codominant expression of HLA: The MHC genes that encode HLA antigens are inherited as haplotypes. A haplotype (haploid genotype) is a group of alleles in an individual that are inherited together from a single parent. Each individual has two alleles for each locus. Both alleles of a locus are expressed codominantly. Codominant expression is characterized by equal expression of both alleles and the presence of one allele does not suppress the expression of the other allele. If there are two different alleles on one locus, the individual is heterozygous and if both alleles on that locus are the same, the individual is homozygous. Each child could potentially share at least one haplotype with the other and has a 25% chance of having the same HLA typing (Fig. 23.3). This

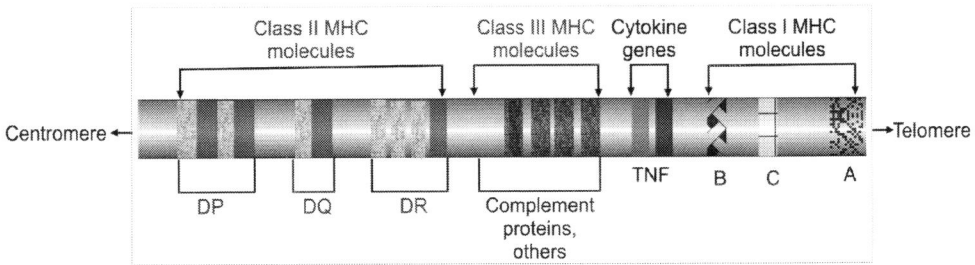

Fig. 23.2: Major histocompatibility complex (human leukocyte antigen complex) showing location of genes.

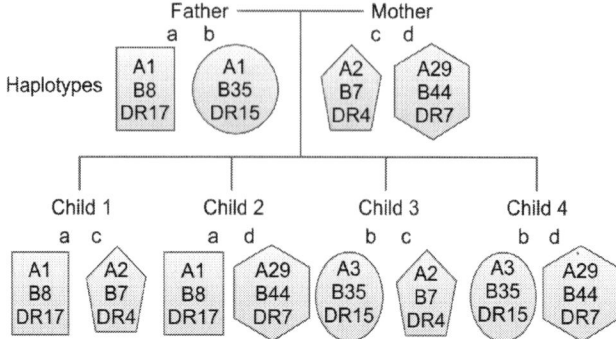

Haplotype is a group of alleles on the same chromosome that are transmitted together

Fig. 23.3: Example of the inheritance pattern of class I and class II HLA antigens (only A, B and DR is shown in figure). Each child inherits a complete set of HLA alleles (a, b, c, d in figure) as a unit from chromosome of each parent. There is 25% chance that two children in a family will inherit the same sets and have identical HLA typing.

is the reason for likely matching of organ or bone marrow transplants in siblings (having one or both parents in common).

Each individual inherits one haplotype from each parent, and both haplotypes are expressed. There are hundreds of possible alleles at each locus (Table 23.1).

The expression of each HLA antigen is identified with a unique number that is determined by either serologic (antigen-antibody reactions) or molecular methods. The MHC region is the most polymorphic system of genes in humans and several alleles exist at each locus. This is responsible for the many possible alleles at each location. Thus, obtaining any two individuals with the same HLA antigens is extremely difficult.

Table 23.1: MHC class I and class II, their nomenclature, and number of antigens.

Genetic locus	Antigen	Number of antigens
Class I molecules		
A	A1 to A80	26
B	B5 to Bw6	62
C	Cw1 to Cw10	10
Class II molecules		
DR	DR1 to DR18	24
DQ	DQ1 to DQ9	9
DP	DP1 to DP6	6

Nomenclature of HLA

The HLA antigens are named by a letter designating the locus for both class I (i.e. A, B, C) and class II regions (DR, DQ, and DP). This is followed by a number which indicates the antigen, for example A2, B27, Cw7, DR1, and DQ5. For the C locus, the "w" is included in the nomenclature to distinguish HLA C locus antigens from complement components. HLA nomenclature was standardized by World Health Organization (WHO).

Techniques of Histocompatibility Testing and Matching

Before any organ transplantation and in patients who are refractory to platelet therapy (of random donor platelets), it is necessary to evaluate the HLA antigen composition in prospective donor-recipient pairs. It is also important to evaluate and identify HLA antibodies in the serum of recipients before transplantation and transfusion.

Laboratory test methodologies: Laboratories involved in histocompatibility performs various techniques (Box 23.2).

TECHNIQUES FOR DETECTION OF HLA (HLA TYPING)

HLA typing: The principles used in **histocompatibility testing or HLA typing or tissue**

> **Box 23.2:** Various laboratories techniques in histocompatibility testing and matching.
>
> - Type for HLA
> - Screen for HLA antibodies
> - Crossmatch donor and recipient samples
> - Monitor recipient status post-transplant

typing are similar to those used for red blood cell (RBC) testing.

Testing to Identify HLA

The protein products of HLA system are called HLA antigens. The evaluation of the HLA antigen composition in prospective donor-recipient pairs is necessary before organ transplantation and in patients for platelet therapy refractory to random donor platelets. Testing HLA antigen is also used in disease correlation, relationship testing, and anthropologic studies.

Methods: Red cell antigens and antibodies are mainly identified by agglutination reactions or hemagglutination test methods. However, agglutination techniques are not effective for HLA antigens and antibodies. Methods used for identification of HLA antigens and alleles can be categorized into two groups:
1. **Serological (antibody based) assays**
2. **DNA-based molecular typing (molecular technology):** In this method, recipient serum is screened for the presence of HLA antibodies using immunoassays.

Serological Typing (HLA Antigen Detection)

Principle: In this method, HLA antigens are identified by using antigen-specific sera with known anti-HLA antibodies to determine an individual's HLA type. The sera react to a specific HLA antigen expressed on white blood cells. An individual's HLA tissue type is determined by noting which type of sera react with the individual's white blood cells and which sera do not react. The white blood cells are incubated with the specific sera and complement is added. If the HLA antigen is present in the white blood cell, it will bind to specific antibody in the sera. The complement in turn will cause cell lysis. The reaction is then viewed under the microscope and graded accordingly depending on the amount of cell lysis. The HLA type is assigned after reviewing the reaction patterns for the various sera. Serological based HLA typing is less specific than molecular-based tissue typing.

Complement-dependent Microlymphocytotoxicity Typing

Serologic identification of HLA antigens requires the lymphocytotoxicity test method. Complement-dependent microlymphocytotoxicity is abbreviated as complement-dependent cytotoxicity (CDC). It was also called as *microlymphocytotoxicity/* **lymphocytotoxicity or lymphocyte microcytotoxicity test/assay** and is used for detection of HLA antigens. It detects the complement fixing antibodies reacting with the HLA antigen present on the cell surface, leading to the activation of complement via the classical pathway and in cell death. This test is sensitive and reproducible. The most important use of this test is to detect specific donor-reactive HLA antibodies present in a potential recipient prior to transplantation. This test is used also in cadaver transplantation. However, this test does not discriminate between HLA and non-HLA cytotoxic lymphocyte-reactive antibodies such as IgM autoantibodies, although these antibodies are not clinically significant in solid organ transplant recipients or in patients immunologically refractory to random donor platelet transfusions.

Sample required: Cytotoxicity techniques need only 1–2 µL of serum. The acid-citrated dextrose or phenol-free heparinized blood is used for the test. The cell used for determination of HLA phenotype is unseparated lymphocyte preparation peripheral blood lymphocytes (PBL) or T lymphocytes (for HLA-A, HLA-B, and HLA-C antigens) or the enriched B lymphocytes (for HLA-DR and HLA-DQ typing). These cells are tested against a panel of well-characterized HLA alloantisera.

Lymphocyte preparation: Lymphocytes are used for the test because of their excellent expression of HLA and are comparatively easy to isolate than many other tissues. Lymphocytes are separated from other blood cells by differential centrifugation or by magnetic beads.

- **Differential centrifugation (Fig. 23.4):** A purified lymphocyte suspension used routinely in HLA serologic typing is prepared by layering peripheral whole blood on a Ficoll-Hypaque gradient to separate the blood cells by density centrifugation. Residual RBCs and granulocytes are forced to occupy the bottom of the gradient, and platelets remain in the supernatant. The separated peripheral blood lymphocytes (PBLs) collect at the gradient's interface. These lymphocytes can be harvested, washed, and adjusted to appropriate test concentrations. They can be used for HLA-A, HLA-B, and HLA-C typing. To test for HLA-DR, -DQ serologic specificities, it is necessary to enrich B lymphocytes, or to use a special two-color fluorescent technique to simultaneously differentiate between unseparated B cells and T cells.

- **Magnetic beads** can also enrich a lymphocyte preparation for T or B cells. Purified enriched B-lymphocyte suspensions can be prepared by nylon wool separation. The B cells adhere preferentially to nylon wool and from the nylon wool they can be eluted.

Method for HLA typing (Fig. 23.5)

It can be performed on recipients or donors and consists of following stages:

- **Sensitization stage:** The CDC method consists of incubating T or B lymphocytes with a panel of well-characterized HLA antisera. First, a suspension of T or B **lymphocytes is added to the wells of a** commercial **microtiter tray containing** one microliter of **antiserum** (known

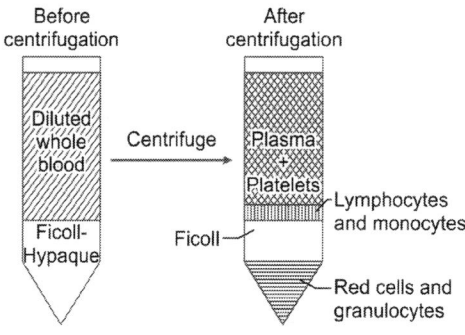

Fig. 23.4: Lymphocyte separation.

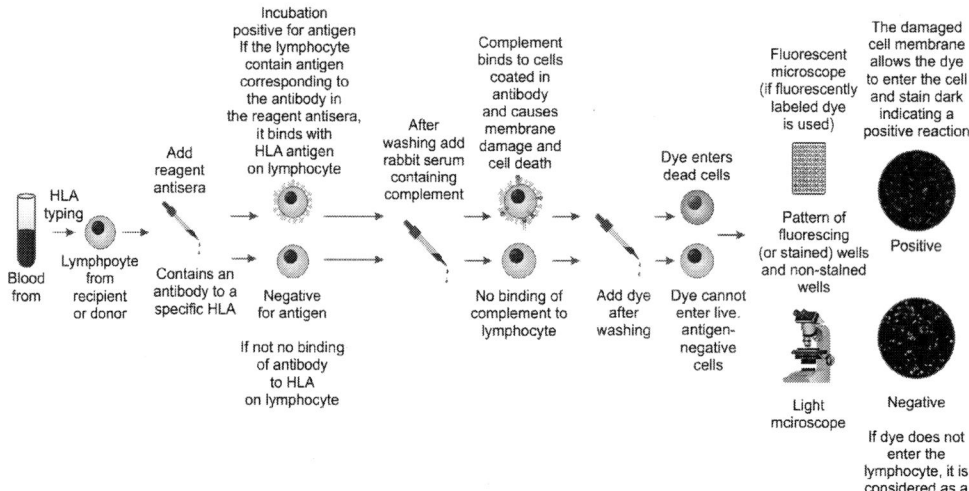

Fig. 23.5: Main steps in complement-dependent microlymphocytotoxicity.

antibody specificities). The antisera contain antibodies which may or may not be directed to specific HLA antigens on the lymphocytes. After incubation at room temperature, unbound antibodies are removed by washing. **If the antiserum contains an antibody specific to an HLA** (class I or class II) antigen on the lymphocytes, the antibody in the antiserum **will bind to this HLA on the lymphocytes.**
- **Adding complement:** The prescreened and standardized rabbit serum containing complement is added in excess to the cells and the mixture is incubated at room temperature for an additional period.
- **Lysis of lymphocytes:** If the antibody (in the antiserum) on the plate matches the HLA antigen (complimentary) on the lymphocyte. Rabbit complement will react with antibodies bound to the lymphocyte surface HLA antigen resulting in activation of complement. This activated complement causes cell membrane damage/injury and lysis (complement mediated lysis by C5b-9) of lymphocytes. The lymphocytes with damaged membrane are called **positive cells**.
- **Vital staining:** Cell damage is detected by the addition of a dye. The damaged lymphocytes are not completely undergoing lysis but the membrane damage is sufficient to allow **uptake of vital stains** (for dye visualization methods) **such as eosin** and formalin or trypan blue and ethylene diamine tetra acetic acid. Microscopic (phase-contrast microscopy) **identification of the stained lymphocytes indicates** the presence of **specific HLA antibody.** Thus, it is a visual means to distinguish the positive cells from nonreactive cells.
OR
- **Fluorescently labeled dyes/stains such as ethidium bromide** or fluorescein diacetate **can be used instead of vital stains** for fluorescent detection procedures. Fluorescent microscope similar to the vital stains can differentiate live and dead cells.

Inference
- **Positive cells:** If the lymphocyte **sample is positive for the HLA** corresponding to the antiserum in the **microtiter** well, the **cells in that well will take up the dye**. The, dead cells will not refract the light. Hence, they appear as large and nonrefractile, or dull and dark. Reaction is read for percentage lysis and is numerically graded (Table 23.2).
- **Negative cells:** If the lymphocyte **sample is negative for the HLA** corresponding to the antiserum in the **microtiter** well, the antigen-negative lymphocytes will be live and unstained. They will look small and refractile, or shiny when compared to dead lymphocytes.

HLA typing sera trays: HLA typing reagents are obtained from the sera of alloimmunized individuals such as multiparous women, transplant recipients, multitransfused patients, and planned immunization of humans. Multiwell plates of human alloantisera (i.e. HLA typing trays) are available commercially. These commercial HLA typing trays have 60 or 72 wells, each containing a different antiserum. The reaction pattern is analyzed to determine the HLA alleles.

Immunomagnetic Beads

Immunomagnetic beads can be used to positively select (target cells rosetted on beads) lymphocyte subpopulations (T or B cells) for HLA typing. This can be used for both class I and II antigens. Either T or B cells can be isolated by coating the surface of the bead by

Table 23.2: Scoring pattern in complement-dependent cytotoxicity (CDC).

Description	Score
All live cells	1
Maximum live cells and small number of dead cells	2
50% of cells are live and 50% are dead cells	3
Maximum cells are dead and small number of cells are live	4
All cells are dead	5

surface capture monoclonal antibody. These techniques can rapidly isolate cells with a high degree of purity and use immunofluorescence lymphocytotoxicity.

Isolation of B cells: B cells can also be identified by fluorescent labeling. In fluorescent labeling, lymphocytes are incubated with fluorescein isothiocyanate (FITC)-labeled anti-immunoglobulin. B lymphocytes develop distinct fluorescent caps. This is produced due to the binding of the labeled anti-immunoglobulin to the cell surface immunoglobulin found on B cells and not on T cells. A major advantage of the fluorescent labeling technique is that it does not need the physical separation of T and B cells.

DNA-based Molecular Typing (HLA Molecular Techniques)

Histocompatibility testing or HLA typing or tissue typing is performed only in few laboratories because it uses specialized procedures and reagents.

HLA class I (HLA-A, HLA-B, HLA-C) and class II (HLA-DR, HLA-DQ, HLA-DP) typing can be performed by DNA analysis techniques. DNA-based molecular typing has replaced serologic typing in many laboratories. Polymerase chain reaction (PCR) methods are used to type.

Advantages of DNA-based techniques/ assays: When compared to serological assays, it has certain advantages which are listed in Box 23.3.

Use: Molecular typing for class I and II alleles is needed in hematopoietic stem cell transplantation. This is because serologic typing cannot adequately determine HLA compatibility.

Molecular-based tissue typing assays target nucleic acid of a gene rather than to detect a synthesized gene product such as antigen or protein. Molecular-based typing determines an individual's HLA tissue type by using standard synthetic probes and primers.
- A **nucleic acid probe** is a short strand of DNA or RNA of a known sequence. It is well characterized and complementary for the base sequence on the test target. Probes may be fragments of genomic nucleic acids, cloned DNA (or RNA), or synthetic DNA.
- **PCR primer:** The primers are short segment of oligonucleotides (usually about 15–20 nucleotides in length) of single-stranded DNA (or RNA) required for use in PCR. Primers are synthesized based on prior knowledge of the genome by a gene machine.

These probes and primers do not react to the gene product such as proteins/antigens but react with genes (DNA) expressed on an individual's white blood cells. This gene specifies which antigens to be synthesized. Production of an amplicon (amplicon is an amplified product obtained by PCR) indicates in the DNA sequence encoding that a specific allele is present in the patient's sample.

Polymerase Chain Reaction Testing

With the molecular genetics, the genes encoding many of red cell and HLA antigens are sequenced and cloned. This provides "maps" for the specific nucleotide differences that occur at each allele. Most HLA and red cell antigen differences are due to the substitutions of single nucleotide in the coding sequence of each unique allele. DNA-based assays detect single-nucleotide polymorphisms (SNPs) in the gene by amplifying the part of the DNA where the SNPs are located. This amplification is achieved by an in vitro technique called polymerase chain reaction (PCR). PCR is

---

Box 23.3: Advantages of DNA-based techniques/ assays.

- High sensitivity and specificity
- Sample:
  - Required volume of sample is small
  - Any source of cells can serve as sample for tissue typing.
  - No need for cell-surface antigen expression
  - No living/viable cells are required to perform HLA class I and II typing
- Flexible: Can identify all known alleles as well as antigens. Thus, provides higher level of HLA typing detail.
- Easier than serological typing and can often resolve blanks and ambiguities that would occur with cytotoxic methods.

used to rapidly multiply/amplify and precise specific DNA sequences of interest.

Principle and steps of PCR are discussed on pages 375-6 of Chapter 17.

Polymerase chain reaction (for details refer pages 372-7) uses repeated cycles of denaturation, primer annealing, and extension by DNA polymerase to produce an exponential increase in the HLA allele flanked by the primers.

PCR methods are the most common methods used for HLA typing. These methods have largely replaced complement-dependent microlymphocytotoxicity in a many laboratories.

Preparation and Amplification of DNA

Provided that some sequence of the DNA molecule is known, PCR can be used to amplify a defined/particular target segment (defined region) of genomic DNA several million times. The amplification of DNA-encoding HLA genes by the PCR technique greatly increases the sensitivity of detection of HLA types. The term amplification means that many copies of the DNA region of particular interest have been made. In other words, the region between the two primers has been cloned.

Source of DNA: Good source of DNA includes:
- **Any cell with a nucleus can be used as a source of DNA.** Usually nucleated blood cells such as **lymphocytes are used.** RBCs do not contain nuclei. Hence, cannot be used.
- Cell lines such as Epstein-Barr virus transformed B lymphocytes.

Sample needed: DNA is usually prepared from a small quantity (0.2-1 mL) of whole blood.

Isolation of DNA: Many different protocols can be used to isolate DNA from cells, and commercial kits are available for the preparation of DNA.

Types of assay: To generate millions (large of amounts) of copies of HLA genes (i.e. DNA in a defined region) needed for HLA typing by PCR, a pair (two) of synthetic oligonucleotides (primers). These two primers are complementary to sequences of a specific HLA gene. Some HLA typing procedures use primer sequences that are shared by all alleles at an HLA locus; other typing reactions utilize primer sets that are shared by only a subset of alleles at a locus. During the PCR reaction, annealing of the primers to sample DNA uses reaction conditions which guarantee that the primers will bind to perfectly matched sequences (target sequences). The reaction condition prevents binding of primers to sequences of other loci or other alleles that are not matched or not complimentary to the primer. By adjusting the temperature of the annealing component of the PCR reaction, the specificity of the amplification can be controlled.

Polymerase Chain Reaction-based Human Leukocyte Antigen Typing Procedures

Human leukocyte antigen typing procedures depend on the amplification by PCR of one or more alleles. The test methods vary in the techniques used to detect and identify the amplified products.

The three most common molecular PCR-based variations in HLA DNA typing/assays are used in the laboratory depending on the primer used. These are: i) **sequence-specific oligonucleotides** (SSO) probe hybridization, ii) **sequence-specific primer** (SSP) typing, and iii) **sequence-based typing** (SBT).

PCR Sequence-Specific Oligonucleotides Hybridization/ Probing (Fig. 23.6)

In sequence-specific oligonucleotides probes (SSO or SSOP) typing, the target DNA [chosen HLA nucleotide sequence (gene of interest)] is amplified by PCR using a group-specific primer (**designed to anneal with DNA sequences common to all alleles**) in separate wells (e.g. A, B, C, DR, DQ, DP specific for HLA loci). The amplified HLA gene to be typed is then immobilized on an inert support membrane. Then HLA gene is hybridized with selected mixture of complementary set of labeled sequence-specific oligonucleotide

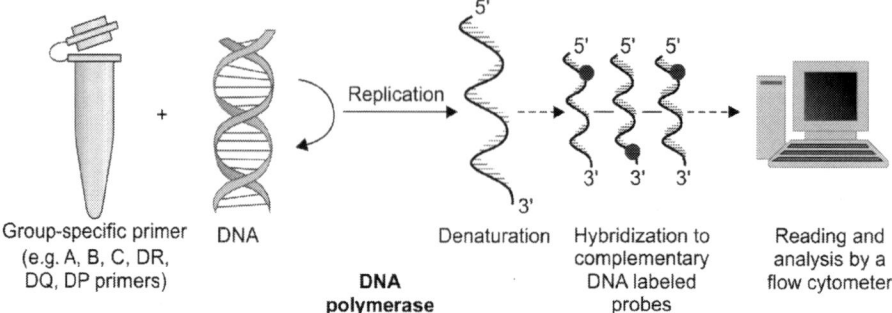

Fig. 23.6: Diagrammatic representation of steps of the SSOP process.

probes (SSOPs). These SSOPs are designed to bind to complementary specific HLA sequences of interest using the properties of complementary base pair sequencing. These oligonucleotide probes detect HLA alleles (nucleotide sequence). It needs use of one or a combination of several different allele-specific oligonucleotide probes to define a specific HLA allele or the use of sequence-specific priming coupled with hybridization with panels of probes. Hybridization conditions are adjusted in such a way that the probes will anneal to denature DNA containing the HLA alleles from which the oligonucleotide sequence was derived.

Detection: The probes are short sequence of DNA complementary to the area being identified and are attached to a marker (usually fluorescent). Detection of hybridization and analysis of reaction patterns is largely automated. The oligonucleotides are labeled with a tag (e.g. oligonucleotide coupled with an enzyme such as alkaline phosphatase) for detection of hybridization. Following addition of a substrate, alkaline phosphatase cleaves the substrate to yield a colored compound or to produce light (chemiluminescence). There can be 30–70 probes per locus to characterize various alleles. The hybridized solution is read and evaluated by an instrument such as a flow cytometer. The intensity of fluorescent is measured and the software analyzes the reaction pattern. The pattern obtained is compared with patterns associated with published HLA gene sequences and read to determine the HLA alleles present. Thus, assignment of the HLA typing is determined.

The SSOP typing test provides both serologic and allele-level evaluations. The SSOP method is highly accurate, specific, and reliable. All known HLA alleles can be identified. It can perform typing of large numbers of samples. This method has been widely accepted and is utilized in laboratories with low throughput.

Reverse SSOP: In a related procedure, which is reverse of the above technique is called **reverse format** or reverse SSO (rSSO). In this technique, the sequence-specific probe DNA, also called oligonucleotide probes (called oligonucleotide probes because the probes are less than 20 nucleotides long) are immobilized by binding to membranes (solid-phase matrix in which each probe may be attached to a different microbead). DNA from the samples to be tested for a target DNA/locus (in this case the DNA at the HLA gene sites) is then amplified by PCR using labeled (e.g. biotinylated on their 5′ end) primers. Biotin is a small molecule that can be attached to protein or nucleic acids. Biotin binds to streptavidin and avidin; hence, it is usually used in biochemical procedures to separate out a protein or nucleic acid of interest. The amplified DNA is then hybridized/added to the immobilized (in the past nylon membranes were used; more recently beads are commonly used for immobilization) oligonucleotide probes, which contain sequences found in the alleles present in the DNA. Beads allow for multiplex testing (e.g. Luminex described on page 511), where multiple amplifications and detections occur simultaneously. The amplified sample DNA will bind only to complimentary (exactly matched) sequences of the oligonucleotide probe. Binding is detected after addition of streptavidin to the biotin primer probe complex and subsequent visualization with substrate (e.g. phycoerythrin). Using an avidin-linked detection system, the pattern of hybridization can be read to determine the HLA alleles present. Commercially available microbead array assays use rSSO method for HLA class I and class II low to high resolution tissue typing. This procedure is useful for typing both small and large numbers of samples. The beads can also have different fluorescent markers incorporated to identify them. Flow cytometry is used to determine which beads are reactive and software analyzes the results and reports the HLA type.

PCR Sequence-Specific Primers Typing (Fig. 23.7)

Sequence-specific PCR is another major method of identifying HLA alleles. The SSP technique/typing, uses sequence-specific (allele-specific) primer pairs that are specific for unique sequences (SSP) within an exon. The SSPs are specific (HLA antigen specific) for a particular sequence in the DNA to be evaluated. The SSPs in the PCR reaction designed to only anneal with DNA in the area of interest initiating DNA synthesis. **SSP target and amplify a particular DNA sequence** (i.e. specific alleles or groups of alleles and **not all alleles** as in SSOP technique described above). The specificity of the genetic material being amplified is determined by the primer. Each primer pair can amplify one or several alleles.

Amplification only takes place if the primer can bind. HLA system is very polymorphic. Hence, SSP method requires large number of specific primers to obtain a low resolution HLA type. It is necessary to perform multiple PCR assays in which each reaction is selected for a particular allele or groups of alleles. HLA typing by this method is based on the principle that a completely matched primer will be more efficiently used in the PCR reaction than a primer with one or more mismatches. These primers anneal to denature DNA containing HLA alleles from which the primer sequences were derived. In the subsequent PCR reaction, only these selected alleles are amplified.

Visualization: After PCR, the specificity of the amplified DNA by the primers (i.e. the product of amplification) or amplicons, is directly visualized and assessed using agarose gel electrophoresis or if the DNA is labeled with a dye during amplification, by fluorescence. Amplicon is a short sequence of amplified DNA flanked on either end by the primer. Determination of HLA allele(s) depends on the presence or absence of PCR amplified product. Because SSPs have specific targets, the amplified material indicates the presence of the allele or alleles that have that sequence. Primer pair sets are commercially available that can determine HLA-A, -B,-C, -DR,-DQA1, -DQB1, and DPB1 phenotypes and may be combined to determine common alleles. This procedure allows for rapid identification of the HLA types and is useful in HLA typing of small number of samples within a short time period. PCR SSP requires prior knowledge

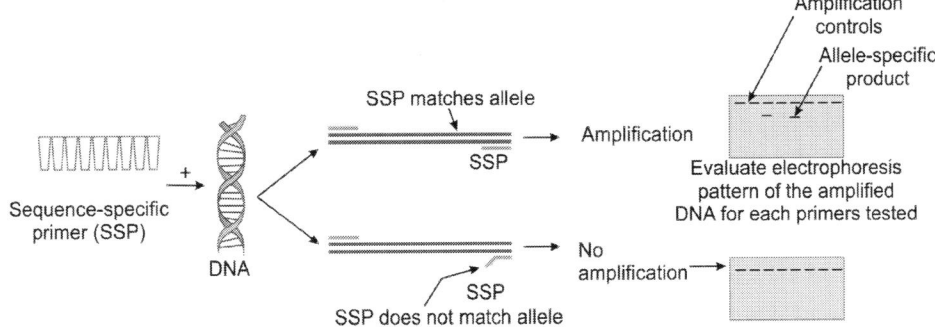

Fig. 23.7: Diagrammatic representation of steps of sequence specific PCR.

of the sequence to be detected and may not detect novel/new HLA types.

DNA Sequence-based Typing/Nucleic Acid Sequencing

As already discussed, HLA alleles may be identified following PCR amplification to separate the alleles based on SSPs, or as a mixture of two alleles. Both SSO and SSP methods evaluate known polymorphisms in variable regions, but assume that constant regions are conserved.

For HPC transplants, donor and recipient typing need high-resolution typing at the allele level. High resolution is most accurately performed by SBT.

Third method of identification of HLA alleles is by **direct determination of the DNA sequences of the HLA alleles** by SBT. SBT is a high-resolution method which determines the nucleotide sequence of the entire exon, including the regions that are usually constant. SBT is labor-intensive and highly complex process. SBT uses two rounds of PCR. In the first round PCR, consensus primers amplify a specific exon. In the second cycle of PCR, it uses cycle sequencing, resulting in DNA fragments of different sizes, each tagged with a fluorescent-labeled nucleotide.

Procedure: This method of direct nucleotide sequencing of HLA genes involves the denaturation of the DNA to be analyzed to provide a single-strand template.
- Sequencing primers, exon or locus specific, are then added. The DNA extension is performed by the addition of Taq polymerase in the presence of excess nucleotides.
- The sequencing mixture is divided into four tubes, each of which contains specific dideoxyribonucleoside triphosphate (ddATP). When these are incorporated into the DNA synthesis, elongation is interrupted with chain terminating inhibitors.
- In each reaction, there is random incorporation of the chain terminators and therefore products of all sizes are generated.

Detection: The sequencing products of SBT are detected by labeling the nucleotide chain inhibitors with fluorescent dyes during PCR reaction. The fluorescently tagged DNA fragments (products) of the four reactions are sorted by capillary electrophoresis and interpreted by computer software (using an automated DNA sequencer) to provide a DNA sequence. Generated DNA sequences are then compared to the known DNA sequences of HLA alleles to find a match, identifying the HLA allele.

Results: In HLA SBT, some ambiguous results can be obtained with heterozygous samples. These may be retested using PCR SSP or reverse PCR SSOP.

Uses: SBT permits high resolution HLA typing. In this technique, HLA detection is not dependent on the use of sequence-specific oligonucleotide probe, and prior knowledge of the nucleotide sequences is not needed. Therefore, SBT can be used to identify known alleles and can detect and characterize/define a previously undefined new allele. Since high-resolution typing is known to be important in the selection of HLA matched HSC unrelated donors, SBT is the preferred method used to determine the HLA match at an allele level between hematopoietic progenitor/stem cell transplant patients and their prospective donors.

Short Tandem Repeats

Most of our DNA is similar to the DNA of others. However, inherited regions of DNA can vary from individual to individual. These variations in DNA sequence between individuals are termed polymorphisms. Sequences with the highest degree of polymorphism are used for relationship testing, forensics, and determining engraftment after HPC transplants.

Short tandem repeats (STRs) are short sequences of DNA that are repeated 4 to more than 50 times. Normally STRs are two to five base pairs in length. The number of times the STRs present varies between individuals and is genetically determined. Thus, STR identification can be used to establish genetic relationships between individuals.

DONOR-RECIPIENT CROSSMATCH

To detect sensitization of recipient to donor antigens, tests are performed to detect the presence of donor-specific antibodies in recipient serum. These antibodies to donor antigens may be detected by crossmatching the recipient serum with donor lymphocytes. There are three methods for conducting such testing.

Complement-Dependent Microlymphocytotoxicity (Fig. 23.8)

The complement-dependent microlymphocytotoxicity (CDC) crossmatch is similar to the CDC method used for HLA typing, except that in a crossmatch the recipient's serum is used rather than reagent antisera.
- Donor lymphocytes are incubated with the recipient's serum. The washing, addition of complement, and staining steps are the same as in the CDC antigen typing method (refer pages 499-501).
- If antibody is present in the recipient's serum, there will be lysis of donor lymphocytes.
- The addition of an antihuman globulin (AHG) reagent prior to complement increases the test's sensitivity. This can detect some low-level class I antibodies.

AHG increases the binding efficiency of complement, allowing antibodies that normally cannot fix complement to lyse cells.

Flow Cytometry

It is known that the adding AHG to the CDC crossmatch increases the sensitivity, but sometimes it fails to predict antibody-mediated rejection. Crossmatch by flow cytometry is more sensitive than CDC.

Method:
- In the flow cytometry crossmatch, unseparated donor lymphocytes are incubated with patient serum.
- After the incubation, unbound antibody is washed away.
- Goat antihuman IgG labeled with fluorescein isothiocyanate (FITC) is added. FITC fluoresces green and binds to the antibodies on the donor lymphocytes.
- An antibody to CD3, labeled with peridinin-chlorophyll-protein (PerCP) will fluoresce orange. PerCP is used to identify T lymphocytes.
- B lymphocytes are labeled with an antibody to CD19 that has been complexed with phycoerythrin. Phycoerythrin will fluoresce red.

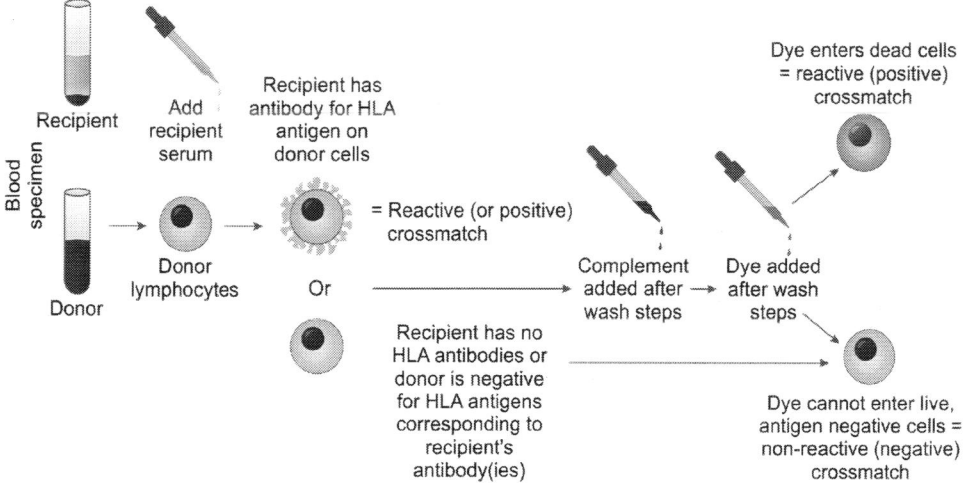

Fig. 23.8: Complement-dependent microlymphocytotoxicity for HLA crossmatching.

- The lymphocytes are suspended in isotonic media and passed single file in front of a laser. Detectors determine the proportion of cells exhibiting the various combinations of fluorescence, green and orange or green and red.
- The resulting semiquantitative measure of the recipient's serum reactivity is compared to reactivity of antibody-negative serum. This will determine the immune status of the recipient specific to the donor.

Differentiation of HLA and Non-HLA Antibodies

A positive crossmatch indicates the presence of an antibody in the recipient which is reactive with any antigen on the donor cells. Though, these reactive antibodies are usually directed against HLA class I or class II molecules, it might be reactive with non-HLA antibodies. These include other lymphocyte membrane antigens or a foreign antigen processed by the lymphocyte which is presented by the HLA molecules on the surface of lymphocyte. The antibody may be an alloantibody or an autoantibody. Crossmatching alone cannot differentiate whether the antibody is IgG or IgM type.

Methods to distinguish HLA antibodies from non-HLA antibodies: To distinguish HLA antibodies from non-HLA antibodies, solubilized HLA molecules adhered to a solid matrix may be used.
- **ELISA or flow cytometry**: The antigen may be bound to microtiter plate wells, such as in enzyme linked immunoassay (ELISA), or microbeads, such as in flow cytometry.
- **Removal of class I antigens**: Platelets can be used to remove antibodies against class I antigens, leaving only antibodies to class II antigens in the adsorbed serum.
- **Autoantibody**: A crossmatch using autologous lymphocytes will reveal if autoantibody is present. Autoantibody in recipient serum can be removed by adsorption using autologous tissue.
- **Alloantibody**: The adsorbed serum can be tested for alloantibodies.

- **IgG and IGM**: Similar to RBC antibody identification, the recipient serum is treated with dithiothreitol (DTT) which will destroy IgM antibodies. This allows in differentiation of IgG and IgM. Antibodies to HLA are generally IgG.

Specimen required: HLA class I molecules are widely distributed and are present on platelets and almost all nucleated cells. HLA class II molecules are expressed on only a few cell types, including B lymphocytes. Because of ease in obtaining blood specimens are used for most routine HLA tests.

Compatibility is directly determined by crossmatching of potential donor's cells and recipient sera in the solid organ transplant setting. The **Luminex technique** is the main technique used for HLA antibody detection and definition. HLA crossmatching is done by two main techniques namely: i) complement dependent cytotoxicity (CDC) test (refer page 506) and ii) flow cytometric techniques.

Enzyme-linked immunosorbent crossmatch assays are also been used.

Detection and identification techniques of HLA antibodies are similar to those for RBC antibodies. The unknown serum is tested against a panel of cells or soluble antigen of known HLA phenotype. If antibodies to all HLA specificities are to be detected, it is necessary to select targets from a large panel of donors. It is necessary to have a panel of at least 30 carefully selected targets for initial screening in the determination of panel reactive antibody (PRA), and a panel of at least 60 cells is needed for accurate antibody identification.

The level of HLA match is important for the outcome in transplantation.

Criteria and strategies for histocompatibility matching differ depending on the various factors (Box 23.4).

HLA evaluation: Matching is usually done to evaluate at least three loci: HLA-A, HLA-B, and HLA-DR.

Terminology used:
- If individuals are matched for all three loci mentioned above, it is called **6/6 matches**

Box 23.4: Factors deciding the criteria and strategies for histocompatibility matching.

- Type of graft, e.g. solid vascularized organ vs hematopoietic progenitor cell
- Disease, e.g. chronic myelogenous leukemia vs aplastic anemia
- Clinical protocol, e.g. marrow vs umbilical cord blood, T cell depletion of marrow vs non-T cell depletion
- Age of the patient

or *0 mismatches*. Zero mismatches are a term used in solid organ transplantation. It also means that donor/recipient pairs in which the donor has no detectable HLA differences from the recipient.
- If individuals matched for 4 of 6 alleles or antigens, they are called as *4/6 matches*.

Matching for classical HLA molecules at the allele level is necessary for the optimal outcome for all grafts (both vascular organs and hematopoietic progenitor cells). Multiple mismatches are detrimental to outcome.

Clinical Relevance of HLA Antigens and Antibodies

HLA molecules play the main role to present antigenic peptides to T cells. However, HLA molecules can themselves be recognized as foreign by the host T cells by a mechanism known as allorecognition. Two pathways of allorecognition have been identified: direct and indirect.

TECHNIQUES FOR DETECTION OF HLA ANTIBODIES

Formation of HLA Antibodies: Before transplantation and transfusion, it is more important to evaluate and identify HLA antibodies in the serum of recipients. Pre-sensitization to HLA antigens may cause rapid rejection of transplanted tissue or poor platelet survival following transfusion. The majority of HLA alloantibodies are of IgG type.

HLA system antigens and antibodies play a major role in number of transfusion-related reactions such as platelet refractoriness, FNHTRs, TRALI, and TA-GVHD. HLA antigens are highly immunogenic. In an immunologically competent individual, HLA-specific antibodies to HLA antigens are likely to be induced by pregnancy, transplantation, blood transfusions, and planned immunizations. The affinity, avidity, and class of HLA-specific antibodies produced depend on various factors. These factors include the route of immunization, the persistence and type of immunological challenge, and the immune status of the host.

- **HLA-specific antibodies in pregnancy:** Cytotoxic HLA antibodies induced in human pregnancies are normally multispecific, high titer, high affinity and of the IgG class. These HLA IgG antibodies can cross the placenta. But they are not harmful to the fetus.
- **HLA-specific antibodies in transplantation:** Antibodies produced following transplantation are mostly IgG and rarely HLA IgM type.
- **HLA-specific antibodies in transfusion:** Majority of HLA antibodies found in multitransfused patients are multispecific IgM and IgG, and are mostly directed at public epitopes. The use of leukocyte reduced blood components may reduce alloimmunization in naive recipients, but this may not be very effective in preventing alloimmunization in already sensitized recipients (i.e. women who have become immunized as a result of pregnancy).
- **HLA-specific antibodies after immunization:** The deliberate immunization of healthy individuals to produce HLA-specific reagents is not ethically justified.

Preformed antibodies to the tissue of the donor and recipient may produce significant complications in transplantation or transfusion. The clinical management of transplant patients includes screening for and determining the specificity of anti-HLA class I and class II antibodies both in pre- and post-transplant. There are two groups of antibodies to HLA molecules:

1. **Private antibodies:** These antibodies **detect a single HLA gene product** and bind to an epitope unique to one HLA gene product.

2. Antibodies that **detect more than one HLA gene product.**

Types of antibodies:
- **Lymphocytotoxic HLA antibodies** to donor antigens in recipient will **accelerate graft rejection** and cause **poor response to platelet transfusion.**
- **Leukocyte antibody**: Antibody to recipient leukocytes in donor plasma can produce severe pulmonary infiltrates and respiratory distress following transfusion. This is called as TRALI. Crossmatching involves serologic and cellular procedures.

Methods of detecting HLA antibodies (antibody screen) and their identification: ABO compatibility is required for the success of all solid-organ transplants. After ABO compatibility, next it is essential to carefully match HLA antigens in patients with existing antibodies for long-term graft survival for all solid organ transplants (e.g. kidney, heart, and lung transplants). HLA antibody screening identifies all HLA antibodies in the recipient serum. The crossmatch detects only donor specific antibody. There are many techniques to detect HLA antibodies. These include the complement-dependent lymphocytotoxicity (LCT) test, ELISA and flow cytometry and Luminex-based technique (recent technique).

HLA antibody screening is performed to identify all HLA antibodies in the recipient serum. In contrast, crossmatch detects only donor specific antibody.

Identification of HLA antibodies: It is done by the use of solubilized HLA molecules adhered to a solid matrix or microparticle. The antibody screening may predict crossmatch results. The antibodies expressed by a sensitized potential recipient can change with time or if the patient experiences another sensitizing event. Hence, at the time of transplant, previous antibody screens may not reflect the recipient's antibody status.

Complement-Dependent Microlymphocytotoxicity (Fig. 23.9)

The CDC antibody screen is similar to HLA typing or crossmatching using the CDC technique. In the antibody screen, recipient serum acts as the unknown and is tested against a panel of previously HLA typed lymphocytes. Antibody screen results in HLA are usually expressed as a percentage of the cells that reacted, called a PRA level. A higher PRA means that the recipient has many reactions and was less likely to be compatible with available organs.

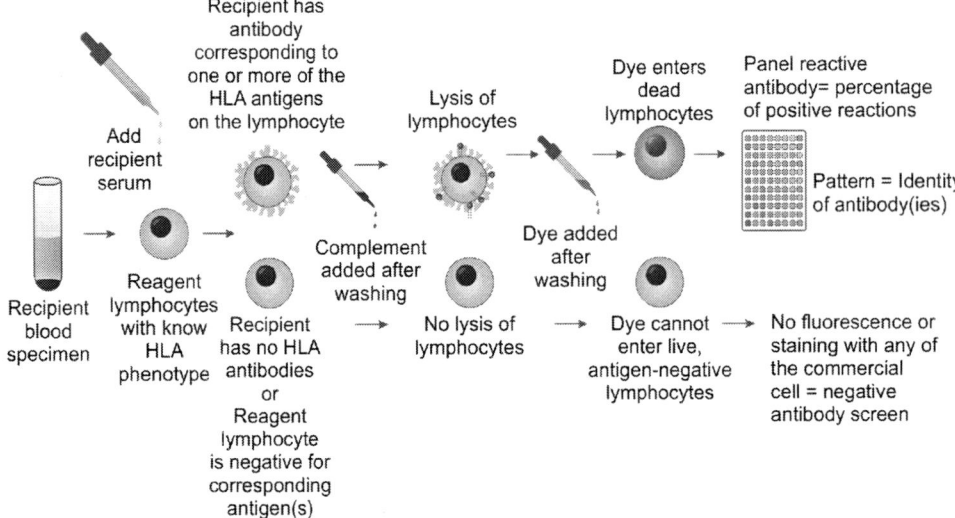

Fig. 23.9: Complement-dependent microlymphocytotoxicity for antibody screening.

Solid-Phase Assays

Cells may express numerous antigens in addition to HLA. CDC screens detect any antibodies (both HLA and non-HLA) bound to intact cell. In contrast, solid-phase assays detect antibodies specific to the HLA system and use HLA class I or class II molecules purified from human cell cultures. The culture usually used includes Epstein-Barr virus-transformed human B lymphocytes or transfected HLA-deficient human lymphoid cells. The purified antigens are used in ELISA and flow cytometry assays to detect antibodies specific to the HLA system.

Calculated panel-reactive antibody (CPRA): The newer solid-phase methods have increase in sensitivity and specificity. Hence, PRA determined by serologic methods has been replaced with a CPRA. CPRA estimates the percentage of donors that would be incompatible with a transplant candidate, based on the candidate's antibodies to HLA antigens. Unacceptable antigens are antigens that the potential graft recipient is reacting against. The antibodies to these antigens can reduce the survival of a graft.

Enzyme-Linked Immunosorbent Crossmatch Assays

In the ELISA test, purified HLA antigens are used instead of lymphocytes or cells as targets for antibodies that may be present in the patient's sera. Purified HLA antigens may be pooled for detection of HLA antibodies or derived from specific donors to allow the definition of HLA-specific antibodies. This assay has increased specificity. This is because the purified HLA antigens used recognizes false-positive non-HLA reactions and it distinguishes class I and class II specificities.

Uses: ELISA can be used as a screening assay for the detection of anti-HLA antibodies and also to determine antibody specificity.
- **Screening assay:** It uses a pool of purified HLA antigens. Results are interpreted as either positive or negative.
- **Specificity determination assay:** It uses a **panel of purified HLA antigens**, rather than a pool. It permits the evaluation of PRA and HLA antibody specificity.

Detection of HLA antibodies: Purified HLA class I and class II antigens are obtained from either transformed cell lines or from platelets with known HLA phenotypes.
- The purified HLA antigens, i.e. HLA class I or class II molecules, (pooled or specific) are bound/coated directly to wells of microtiter plates/plastic trays (i.e. immobilized on a microwell plate).
- The test serum or plasma sample under investigation is added to the wells of microtiter plates. After incubation, the unbound antibodies are washed away. The specific binding of antibody with any of the antigens is detected by subsequent incubation with enzyme-linked anti-human immunoglobulin (i.e. alkaline phosphatase-conjugated antihuman IgG/antibody) that recognizes human IgG. This is followed by second incubation.
- The microtiter plate is washed again and p-nitrophenyl phosphate substrate (enzymes substrate) is added. A quantitative measure of the reaction can be obtained by spectrophotometry.

Interpretation

If the recipient serum contains HLA antibody, it will result in a sandwich of HLA antibody-goat antihuman IgG conjugate–p-nitrophenyl phosphate substrate, all bound to the antigen, which in turn is fixed to the plate well. The alkaline phosphatase will react with the p-nitrophenyl phosphate and produces a color change which can be read by a spectrophotometer.

Advantage of ELISA technique: It detects both complement fixing and non-complement fixing HLA antibodies and is specific for HLA.

Flow Cytometry

In flow cytometry, the bound antibody is detected by using an antibody against human immunoglobulin labeled with a fluorescent marker (e.g. fluorescein isothiocyanate or R-phycoerythrin).

- **HLA antibody screen** by the flow cytometry **directly detects antibody binding.** Hence, there is no need for complement activation as required in the lymphocytotoxicity assay.
- Similar to ELISA assays, flow cytometry HLA antibody screening:
  - **Can distinguish between IgG and IgM antibodies** with the use of either anti-IgG or anti-IgM secondary antibodies.
  - May be used to **screen for the presence of HLA antibodies** and **determine antibody specificity.**
  - Uses either pooled or specific HLA antigen-coated microparticles as targets.
- Flow screening **can also detect non-complement-fixing antibodies.** This is because flow screening identifies binding of the antibodies rather than complement fixation.
- Flow cytometric antibody screens **uses T and B lymphocytes as targets or,** in a newer technique, **uses purified HLA antigens coated onto microparticles** 2–4 μm in diameter.
- One of the disadvantages of flow cytometry is that they also detect non-HLA lymphocyte-reactive antibodies that are of unclear clinical relevance.

Method
- In HLA antibody screening by flow cytometry, the **recipient serum is incubated with microbeads coated with class I or class II molecules.** Each microbead can be coated with a single HLA antigen or with a combination of HLA antigens (depending on the assay and the level of differentiation desired). The microbeads with class II molecules attached are also coated with a phycoerythrin label.
- After incubation, unbound antibody is washed away. FITC-labeled antihuman IgG is then added. The microbeads are transferred from the microtiter tray wells (where the reactions have taken place) into plastic tubes, which are loaded onto the flow cytometer.
- In the flow cytometer, microbeads will pass in a single file in front of a laser and the fluorescence is measured.

Inference
- If the recipient has an antibody against class I molecule or molecules coated on the microbeads, it will demonstrate FITC fluorescence. If the recipient has antibody against class II molecules, the microbeads coated with a class II molecule or molecules will display both phycoerythrin and FITC fluorescence.
- The fluorescence of the recipient serum is compared with that of a serum known to be negative for HLA antibody to determine if the antibody is present.
- The pattern of positivity is analyzed to assign HLA specificity and PRA level.

Disadvantages of use of lymphocytes as targets:
- Difficulty to distinguish between HLA-specific and non-HLA antigens on lymphocytes.
- B lymphocytes express both class I and class II markers. Hence, it is not possible to distinguish class I or II antibody specificity.

The above problems due to use of lymphocytes can be resolved by the use of microparticles/beads coated with purified class I or II antigens. HLA antibodies present in patient sera react specifically with the beads. After incubation of serum with beads, staining is done with a fluorescently labeled antihuman IgG antibody. The serum with the anti-HLA IgG-positivity shows a fluorescent channel shift as compared with the negative serum. Percent PRA is represented by the percentage of pooled beads that react positively with the serum.

Multiplex Immunoassay (Luminex)

HLA has a highly polymorphic nature. Hence, detection of HLA antibody requires a large number of cell types to accurately screen for alloantibodies by either serologic, lymphocytotoxicity crossmatching or by ELISA with cell lysate techniques. The determination of anti-HLA specificity was simplified by the development of the **multiplex flow assay**. This increases assay throughput and sensitivity. Luminex assay/technique uses fluorochrome-dyed polystyrene beads coated with specific recombinant soluble HLA antigens called as **Luminex single antigen**. The precise ratio of the fluorochromes creates 100 distinctly colored microbeads, each of which is coated with a single antigen. The beads are then incubated with the patient's serum. The reaction due to anti-HLA antibody binding to specific HLA antigen is detected using a phycoerythrin-conjugated antihuman IgG (Fc-specific) antibody and measured on a specialized flow cytometer (Lumex analyzer). The Luminex analyzer has two lasers: i) to detect the internal fluorescence of the bead and ii) to detect PE-labeled antihuman IgG indicating the presence of antibodies directed against the specific HLA antigen on that specific bead. Positive reactions are described as the mean fluorescence intensity (MFI) of positive beads.

The increased sensitivity of the Luminex assay is clinically relevant. Thus, detection of **donor-specific antibody** (DSA) by multiplex immunoassay is a strong predictor of antibody-mediated rejection.

POST-TRANSPLANT IMMUNOLOGICAL MONITORING

Graft rejection in either solid organ or HPC transplants can occur at any time following transplant (post-transplant). HPC transplant recipients also have a risk of developing GVHD, where the immunocompetent donor transplanted cells attack the recipient's cells. Immunosuppressive drugs are given permanently to prevent both graft rejection and GVHD, even in HLA-matched recipients. These antirejection drugs can predispose recipient to infection, cancer, and drug toxicity. The regulation of drug dosage to minimize toxic side effects and recognition of graft rejection or GVHD is the goal of post-transplant monitoring. Detection of injury to the graft or the host by the immune system is the standard post-transplant monitoring technique. Ideally, immunosuppressive therapy should be adjusting before injury occurs. Hence, assays should identify immune activation even before injury has occurred. These assays include the detection of signal transduction, DNA synthesis, gene activation, cytokine production or antibody production.

Signal Transduction

One method used for signal transduction is to detect adenosine triphosphate (ATP) levels in CD4-positive T lymphocytes. ATP is a nucleotide that provides energy for signal transduction. Signal transduction is the process in response to a stimulus and activates series of biochemical pathways. For example, activation of T-lymphocyte after interaction with an antigen-presenting cell that is presenting a foreign antigen.

Method: The recipient's whole blood is incubated with phytohemagglutinin (PHA). PHA will stimulate immunocompetent CD4-positive T lymphocytes. Using monoclonal anti-CD4-coated magnetic beads, CD4-positive cells are selected. The CD4 cells are lysed and ATP is released. A luminescent reagent namely luciferin is added and the ATP emits light which is proportional to the amount of ATP released. The light emission is measured with a luminometer. A parallel testing of the recipient's blood without the addition of PHA is done to determine the baseline ATP level in unstimulated T lymphocytes. Ranges of ATP concentration predicts whether there is underimmunosuppression or overimmuno-suppression. Underimmunosuppression can lead to rejection and overimmunosuppression can lead to infection.

DNA Synthesis

DNA synthesis can be measured with mixed lymphocyte culture (MLC), also called as mixed lymphocyte reaction (MLR). In this assay, lymphocytes from two different individuals are mixed and cultured together. If there are differences in the class II molecules, the lymphocytes will activate and proliferate. This is characterized by increase in the level of DNA synthesis. Radioactive thymidine is added to the culture and its uptake is proportional to the amount of lymphocyte proliferation.

Gene Activation

Many genes screen at once as well as it can be determined the genes that are currently active and which are not by using microarray technology. There is correlation of gene expression with acute rejection, chronic rejection, organ dysfunction, and well-functioning transplants. Both peripheral blood lymphocytes and biopsies samples can be tested by microarray technology. Active genes produce messenger RNA. In the microarray analysis, first step is reverse transcription, which produces complementary DNA from the messenger RNA, if present. The detectable number of copies of complimentary DNA is produced by PCR. The amount of messenger RNA produced as measured by the number of copies of complimentary DNA formed is proportional to the amount of protein expressed by the gene. When the gene is active, it produces more protein than when it is inactive. In microarray technology, fluorescently labeled DNA probes attached to a solid glass matrix are used and each DNA probe represents a specific gene or a functional group of genes. The amplified patient DNA is added and "reacts" with the probes, causing them to fluoresce. One color indicates an upregulation of a gene and a second color indicates downregulation. The groups of genes expressed are determined by computer analysis.

Cytokine Production

Cytokines are molecules produced and secreted by activated cells. Immune response such as graft rejection also produces specific cytokines. An increase of cytokines in serum or biopsy may predict acute or chronic rejection. The cytokine-producing cells are detected by enzyme-linked immunosorbent spot (ELISPOT) assay. It measures specific cytokine levels, including interleukins, tumor necrosis factors, transforming growth factors, interferons, and colony-stimulating factors.

Antibody Detection

In the HLA laboratory, antibody detection is the most common/most important post-**transfusion monitoring technique performed. The post-transplant development of HLA antibodies can be detected by CDC and solid-phase assays.** To determine donor specific antibody, the detected antibodies are compared to the donor's HLA type. HLA crossmatch techniques can also be performed to detect donor-specific antibody, if donor cells are available.

■ HLA AND TRANSPLANTATION

HLA and Tissue/Organ Transplantation

- An important factor that determines the outcome of solid organ transplantation (particularly renal transplants) is the matching for HLA-A, -B and -DR antigens between donor and recipient. PCR-based techniques can identify the molecular differences between otherwise serologically identical HLA types of donor and recipient pairs (especially in the HLA-DRβ1 chain).
- The graft survival rate is higher in kidney graft survival when recipients and donors are HLA-DR identical by serological and molecular techniques, compared to HLA-DR identical by serological but not molecular methods.
- In renal and cardiac recipients, the presence of circulating HLA-specific antibodies directed against donor antigens will produce hyperacute rejection of the graft. Hence, these antibodies should be detected and identified to ensure that incompatible donors are not considered for transplantation.
- The development of donor-specific antibodies after transplantation is associated with graft rejection. This indicates the importance of post-transplant antibody monitoring for some groups of patients.

The donor HLA class I and class II molecules are recognized by the recipient's immune system as foreign antigens. Hence, it is beneficial to ensure that donor and recipient are histo- (i.e. tissue) compatible (i.e. HLA matched). To increase success rates of transplant, **histocompatibility testing or HLA typing or tissue typing** is done to identify alleles at important MHC loci (in lymphocytes) so that potential donors can be sought with a closely matching MHC profile, and drugs are administered that can suppress immune responses. However, MHC polymorphism (i.e. having two or more common distinct genotypes maintained in a population) remains a challenge for successful transplantation.

Transplantation mainly consist of solid organ (e.g. renal, heart, lung, liver, and pancreas) and HPC transplants. Long-term survival of transplants/grafts is one of the most challenging goals in medical science. Renal transplantation is the therapy of choice for most patients with end-stage renal disease.

Rejection of transplant: A **major barrier for transplantation** in both solid organ and HPC transplantation is immunologically-mediated rejection of the foreign tissue. This is because the recipient's immune system recognizes the graft as being foreign and mounts the immunological reactions against it. Hence, the success of allografting depends on the ability to deter the immune reaction.

Mechanism of Immune Recognition and Rejection of Allograft

- Transplantation **rejection is a complex phenomenon** and it is **mainly due to antigenic differences between a donor and recipient's MHC molecules**.
- Graft survives when MHC antigens of recipient closely matches with the donor.
- Both cell-mediated immunity and circulating antibodies play a role in transplant rejection.

T-cell Mediated Graft Rejection

- T-cells are the most important cells involved in allograft rejection.
- Host immune recognizes and responds to graft tissue by two pathways—direct and indirect.

Direct recognition (direct pathway)

Direct recognition is the **major pathway** in acute cellular rejection. In this pathway, **MHC antigens on** donor/**graft APCs** (e.g. tissue dendritic cells and endothelial cells) are directly **recognized by host CD8+ cytotoxic cells (class I MHC) and CD4+ helper T-cell (class II MHC)**, followed by their activation.

Consequences

- **Killing of graft cells by CTLs:** Host CD8+ T-cells which **recognize class I MHC antigen on the APCs in the graft** → differentiate into **cytotoxic T-cells** (CTLs) → **kills parenchymal and endothelial cells** in the graft tissue. The endothelial damage results in thrombosis and ischemia of graft tissue.
- **Inflammatory reaction:** Host **CD4+ helper T-cells** which **recognize class II MHC antigens** → **proliferate** → **produce cytokines (e.g. IFN-g)** → stimulate **delayed type hypersensitivity inflammatory reaction** (local accumulation of lymphocytes and macrophages) → damage to the graft. CD4+ T-cells may also be activated by indirect pathway.

Indirect recognition (indirect pathway)

- **MHC molecules and antigen of the graft cell** may be taken up and **processed by the host's APCs** (similar to other foreign antigens such as microbial antigens).
- **Recognition of APCs with graft antigen by the host's CD4+ T-cells** → activates CD4+ T-cells. This has two effects:
  i. **Stimulation of B lymphocytes** which transform into **plasma cells** and **produce antibodies against graft alloantigens**→ mediate rejection through to a lesser extent. These alloantibodies bind to graft endothelium → causing endothelial damage → thrombosis and vascular injury.
  ii. **Stimulation of delayed hypersensitivity reaction** in the tissue and blood vessel

by **producing cytokines (e.g. IFN-g)** as mentioned under direct pathway.

Antibody-mediated Graft Rejection

- T-cells play main role in the rejection of organ transplants. However, **antibodies produced against alloantigens** in the graft also mediate rejection and this is called **humoral rejection.**
- **Forms:** It can develop in two forms:
  i. **Hyperacute rejection**
  ii. **Acute humoral rejection** sometimes referred to as rejection vasculitis.

Methods of preventing transplant rejection: This may be accomplished by the methods listed in Box 23.5.

HLA and Hematopoietic Stem Cell Transplantation

Acute graft-versus-host disease (aGVHD):
- One of the main factors associated with the **development of acute** aGVHD is **HLA incompatibility.** This is particularly important when using matched unrelated donors.
- **HLA-identical siblings:** HSC transplantation between HLA-identical siblings ensures matching for all HLA-A, -B, -C, -DRB1 and -DQB1 genes. However, **aGVHD still develops in about 20–30% of these patients**. This may be due to the effect of untested HLA antigens, such as DP, or minor histocompatibility antigens which activate donor T-cells. However, there is higher risk of developing GVHD in patients receiving grafts from HLA-matched unrelated donors than those transplanted using an HLA-identical sibling.

HLA matching by DNA-based techniques for patients and unrelated donors has reduced the development of GVHD.

Box 23.5: Methods of preventing transplant rejection.

- Histocompatibility matching between the donor and recipient
- Immunosuppressive therapy of the recipient
- Achieving specific unresponsiveness to donor alloantigen(s) (i.e. tolerance)

HLA and graft-versus-leukemia:
- Increased GVHD due to HLA mismatch is also associated with lower relapse rates, probably due to a graft-versus-leukemia (GVL) response associated with the graft-versus-host response.
- **Use of T-cell depleted marrow and leukemia:** It decreases the incidence of GVHD. But it is associated with increased incidence of leukemia relapse. It suggests that the cells in the bone marrow which are responsible for GVHD, may also be involved in the elimination of residual leukemic cells.

Other features:
- **Cord blood:** Hematopoietic stem cell transplantation using cord blood from both HLA-matched and HLA-mismatched donors is associated with a **reduced risk and severity of GVHD** and with **no increase in relapse rates**. It may be due to the immaturity of the immunological effectors presents in cord blood.
- Graft failure is mediated by residual recipient T- and/or NK cells reacting with major or minor histocompatibility antigens present in the donor marrow cells. They are also associated with antibodies reacting with donor's HLA antigens. Thus, rejection is particularly high in HLA-alloimmunized patients.
- During the post-transplant period in a highly immunized patient, HLA antibodies can produce immunological refractoriness to random platelet transfusions. Such patients need transfusions of HLA-matched platelets.

HLA and Blood Transfusion

- White cells and platelets present in transfused products express high concentration of HLA antigens. Hence, transfusion of platelets or leukocytes is associated with the risk of immunizing the patient. If patients with intact immune system need multiple transfusions of whole blood, platelets or leukocytes concentrates, they develop antibodies to HLA antigens. This risk can be minimized by washing or filtering the red cell preparations and by reducing leukocyte contamination as far is possible.

Transfusion reaction in recipients:
- **Due to activation of T cells in recipient:** When HLA antigens of blood donor are not identical to those antigens expressed by the recipient, the donor HLA antigens can **activate T-cells in the recipient.** This in turn may lead to the development of **antibodies and/or effector cells in the recipient against donor HLA antigens.** These can result in some of the serious complications of blood transfusion.
- **Due to antibodies and T cells in donor blood product:** The antibodies (and T cells) present in the transfused (donor) blood product may react directly with the relevant HLA antigens in the recipient. This also can lead to the development of a transfusion reaction.

Types of transfusion reaction: The types of transfusion reactions due to the presence of HLA antibodies in the recipient are as follows:
- **Febrile nonhemolytic transfusion reaction:** FNHTR is most commonly due to the presence of **HLA antibodies** and to a lesser extent due to human platelet antigen (HPA) or human neutrophil antigen (HNA) antibodies in the recipient. These antibodies react with white blood cells or platelets present in the transfused blood product. However, FNHTRs may also be produced due to the direct action of cytokines (e.g. IL-1β, TNF-α, IL-6) and/or by chemokines (e.g. IL-8) which are found in transfused products.
- **Platelet refractoriness: Immunological refractoriness to random platelet transfusions** is mainly due to the presence of HLA and, to a lesser extent, HLA and high titer ABO alloantibodies in the patient (recipient) reacting with the transfused incompatible donor platelets. The refractory state is identified when a transfusion of suitably preserved platelets fails to increase the recipient's platelet count. The incidence and proportion of HLA alloimmunization and platelet refractoriness has been substantially reduced by implementation of nearly universal leukocyte-reduced cellular donor blood components in multitransfused patients with HLA antibodies, previously sensitized transplanted or transfused recipients and multiparous women. It has to be noted that platelet refractoriness may be caused by clinical factors such as sepsis, high fever, disseminated intravascular coagulation (DIC), bleeding medications, hypersplenism, and complement-mediated platelet destruction.
- **Transfusion-related acute lung injury:**
  – **HLA and HNA antibodies in blood component:** The development of TRALI is associated with the **transfusion of blood components containing HLA and HNA antibodies.** These antibodies are able to recognize the relevant antigen(s) on recipient white cells triggering an immunological reaction. This leads to the accumulation of neutrophils in the lungs and edema.
  – **HLA and HNA antibodies in recipient:** Sometimes TRALI may be associated with the presence of **HLA or HNA antibodies in recipients.** These antibodies in the recipient **react with transfused leukocytes** and/or to **interdonor antigen-antibody reactions in pooled platelets.**
- **Transfusion associated (TA) GVHD:** It is a rare but often severe and fatal transfusion reaction. It is produced due to **immunocompetent HLA-matched T lymphocytes** present in **donor blood or blood components reacting with HLA and/or minor histocompatibility antigens** present on the **recipient cells.** TA GVHD mainly occurs in immunosuppressed individuals, but can also occur in immunocompetent recipients. The diagnosis of TA GVHD depends on finding evidence of donor-derived cells, chromosomes or DNA in the blood and/or affected tissues of the recipient.

SUMMARY

- The HLA genetic region consists of a series of closely linked genes located on the short arm of chromosome 6. The genes producing HLA are part of the MHC and are responsible for recognizing and eliminating foreign tissues.
- MHC genes are inherited as haplotypes. The HLA system is polymorphic, i.e. there are multiple alleles for each HLA gene in humans.
- The HLA class I region encodes genes for the classic transplantation molecules HLA-A, HLA-B, and HLA-C. The class II region encodes genes for the molecules HLA-DR, HLA-DP and HLA-DQ.
- The class III region encodes genes for C2, C4, Bf (complement factors), 21-hydroxylase, and tumor necrosis factor.
- Human leukocyte antigen class I and class II molecules play a critical role in the adaptive immune system.
- The main use of HLA typing is to match potential transplant donors and recipients.
- Techniques of histocompatibility testing include HLA typing, HLA antibody detection and identification (recipient serum is tested against a panel of cells or a panel of single antigens), and crossmatching (specific donor cells and recipient sera are tested for compatibility).
- Human leukocyte antigen or allele typing is performed using serologic techniques (complement-based microlymphocytotoxicity [CDC] or DNA-based techniques (reverse SSO probe hybridization, sequence-specific primer [SSP] typing, and SBT).
- Human leukocyte antigen crossmatches are performed using CDC methodology or flow cytometry.
- Human leukocyte antigen antibody screens are performed using CDC methodology or solid-phase techniques such as ELISA, flow cytometry, and Luminex®-based assays.
- Human leukocyte antigen typing also done in patients with platelet refractoriness which is manifested by the failure to achieve a rise in circulating platelet count by 1 hour after infusion of adequate numbers of platelets.

SELF-ASSESSMENT EXERCISE

Write short essays/notes on:
- Role of HLA in transfusion and transplantation
- Methods of HLA typing, HLA antibody screening and HLA crossmatching

CHAPTER 24

Hematopoietic Progenitor Cell Transplantation

CHAPTER OUTLINE

- Hematopoietic progenitor cell (HPC) collection
- Processing HPC products
- Cryopreservation of hematopoietic grafts
- Transplanting the recipient
- Complications of hematopoietic stem cell transplantation
- Transfusion therapy for HPC transplantation
- Ex vivo manipulation of hematologic cells
- Autologous transplantation

INTRODUCTION

As treatment and possible cure for certain malignant disorders, high doses of chemotherapy and/or radiotherapy are administered in order to destroy the malignant cells. The dose may exceed the tolerance limit of bone marrow and eliminates or nearly eliminates (ablates) the patient's marrow.

Hematopoietic cells contain stem cells capable of self-renewal. Progenitor cells have the ability to differentiate into committed blood cell lineages. Both cell lines are collectively termed as hematopoietic progenitor cells (HPCs).

Cellular therapy consists of using a wide variety of cells for transplantation. The bone marrow contains primitive pluripotent cells called as **hematopoietic stem cells** (HSCs). Hematopoietic stem cells are capable of self-renewal and differentiation into any of hematopoietic lineage from which all the cells of the blood are formed (lymphocytes, monocytes, granulocytes, RBCs, and platelets) as well as committed and lineage-restricted progenitor cells. Once differentiated into a blood cell lineage, the hematopoietic stem cells lose their capability for self-renewal and are called as hematopoietic progenitor cells.

In common usage, both cell types are often referred to as HPCs. The hematopoietic stem cells in the bone marrow constitute only a small portion of about 0.01%. These cells are not a uniform population but are in varying stages of development. As HSCs mature, the daughter cells commit (differentiate) to specific cell lines and are known as **hematopoietic progenitor cells (HPCs)**. HPCs are committed to specific cell lines namely:

- *Myeloid line:* It differentiates into RBCs, platelets, neutrophils, basophils, eosinophils, monocytes, and macrophages.
- *Lymphoid line:* It forms dendritic cells (DCs) and lymphocytes, including T cells, B cells, and natural killer (NK) cells.

Hematopoietic progenitor cells are capable of fully reconstituting the marrow function when transplanted into conditioned recipients. Hence, HPC transplantation is performed to treat diverse hematological as well nonhematological diseases. Features of stem cell are mentioned in Box 24.1.

Box 24.1: Stem cell.

Stem cells are characterized by their ability of self-renewal and capacity to generate differentiated cell lineages (asymmetric replication)

Hematopoietic progenitor cells (HPCs) transplantation **formerly called as hematopoietic stem cells transplantation** is the process of collection and infusion of hematopoietic progenitor cells obtained from bone marrow or peripheral blood or umbilical cord blood (UCB). The source may be either from other individual or own hematopoietic progenitor cells. Progenitor cell transplants can be allogeneic (genetically unrelated), syngeneic (identical twin), or autologous (self). The pluripotential hematopoietic progenitor cells (HPCs) are capable of both replication and differentiation into all lineages of blood cells. Hematopoietic stem cells (HSCs) are characterized by their ability to self-renewal and differentiate into committed hematopoietic progenitors.

Terminology of hematopoietic progenitor cells products are provided in Box 24.2.

The **purpose and goals of collecting and transplanting HPC are listed in Box 24.3.**

Marker for HPCs: CD34 is a cell surface antigen. Though it is not specific to HPCs, it is used to identify and quantify HPCs by flow cytometry in cellular products used in transplantation.

HEMATOPOIETIC PROGENITOR CELL (HPC) COLLECTION

Sources of Hematopoietic Stem Cells are listed in Box 24.4.

The HPCs for transplantation are collected in one of three ways:
1. Bone marrow collection, known as HPC-marrow (HPC-M)
2. Peripheral blood progenitor cell (leukapheresis) collection, called HPC-apheresis (HPC-A)
3. Umbilical cord blood collection, referred to as HPC-cord (HPC-C).

Bone Marrow-derived Hematopoietic Progenitor Cells (HPC, Marrow/HPC[M])

They are concentrated where mesenchymal elements (e.g. osteogenic progenitor cells, osteoblasts, adipocytes, mesenchymal stem/stromal cells, and endothelial cells) interact with hematopoietic precursors to generate a niche that supports and regulates hematopoiesis.

Prior to the procedure, a full medical examination is done to confirm fitness for anesthesia. Routine hematological and biochemical tests are performed along with chest X-ray and ECG.

Box 24.3: Purpose and goals of hematopoietic progenitor cell (HPC) transplantation.

- To replace bone marrow following total body irradiation or chemotherapy given to treat primary marrow and non-marrow disorders
- To provide a graft-versus-leukemia (or tumor) reaction
- To replenish diseased or destroyed bone marrow

Box 24.4: Sources of hematopoietic stem cell transplantation.

1. Bone marrow transplantation (BMT): Bone marrow is the richest source of hematopoietic stem cells
2. Peripheral blood stem cell transplantation: Few hematopoietic stem cells are present in the circulation, but these can be mobilized from bone marrow by administering G-CSF or GM-CSF
3. Umbilical cord blood stem cell transplantation: It is easily available following delivery and is a rich source of hematopoietic stem cells

(G-CSF: granulocyte colony-stimulating factor; GM-CSF: granulocyte-macrophage colony-stimulating factor)

Box 24.2: Terminology of various hematopoietic progenitor cells products.

- Hematopoietic progenitor cells (HPC)
- Hematopoietic progenitor cells, apheresis (HPC, apheresis HPC A), i.e. cells mononuclear cell fraction separated by apheresis equipment] formerly called as peripheral blood progenitor cells, or peripheral blood stem cells (PBSC). This is the most common type of HPC at the present time
- Bone marrow-derived hematopoietic progenitor cells (HPC, marrow/HPC[M])
- Umbilical cord blood-derived hematopoietic progenitor cells (HPC, umbilical cord blood/HPC[C])

Collection site
Bone marrow of the donor is harvested/gathered from the both posterior iliac crests in the operating theater/room. Other sites are occasionally used, namely—sternum and anterior iliac crest. It is performed under sterile conditions and either under general or spinal/regional anesthesia by trained medical personnel.

Amount of marrow to be collected
It depends on the recipient size. Aspiration of 10–15 mL/kg recipient weight (maximum 20 mL/kg donor weight) is usually sufficient. Usually, sufficient marrow is collected to provide $3\text{–}5 \times 10^8$ nucleated cells per kilogram of recipient body weight. For example, an adult of 70-kg weight generally needs collection of about 700 mL of marrow. Because of the volume collected is significant, some donors may require RBC transfusion. Many donors donate their own blood days to weeks before the HPC-M collection and transfuse the same during or after the collection.

Technique
Bone marrow is harvested similar to a diagnostic bone marrow aspiration, except the needle used is stronger and longer than used for marrow aspiration.
- **Collection:** Bone marrow is usually gathered by using especially designed stainless steel needles. About 3–5 mL per aspiration at each position in iliac crest is collected into a heparinized syringe. It is possible to take marrow at several different depths from one site. Multiple aspirations are performed, moving the needle within the skin puncture to various points within the marrow, and making additional bone marrow punctures. Aspirating too large a volume from one site will dilute the marrow with peripheral blood. Generally, two individuals will harvest marrow at the same time from each side of the donor iliac crest.
- **Adding anticoagulant:** Aspirated marrow is collected; the anticoagulant [acid-citrate-dextrose (ACD), citrate-phosphate-dextrose (CPD), or heparin] is added to the collected fresh product.

Processing HPCs discussed on pages 527-9.

Risks of HPC-M collection
These include anesthesia, pain (acute and chronic), bruising, allogeneic blood transfusion, and rarely nerve damage.

Presently, HPCs for transplantation are collected from the peripheral blood of both patients and normal donors, as well as from placental or umbilical cord blood.

Peripheral Blood Progenitor Cells (Leukapheresis [HPC-A])
Hematopoietic progenitor cell collection by apheresis (HPC-A) was developed in 1980. Since then, the collection of HPCs from peripheral blood increasingly used both in the autologous and allogeneic transplantation. It has replaced the bone marrow harvest (HPC-M) in many donors and patients. Approximately, 50% of allogeneic hematopoietic transplants use HPCs from peripheral blood, about 30% use umbilical cord blood-derived HPCs, and the remaining 20% use from marrow.

Normally, HPCs circulate in the peripheral blood in very low numbers (less than 0.1% of the total white blood cell count). To obtain adequate graft, it is necessary to mobilize HPCs from the marrow into the peripheral circulation. On healthy donors, granulocyte colony-stimulating factor (G-CSF) is used for mobilization, whereas G-CSF and/or chemotherapy such as cyclophosphamide or disease-specific combination are used for mobilization of HPCs from patients undergoing autologous HSCT.

Benefits of hematopoietic progenitor cell collection by apheresis
Hematopoietic progenitor cell collection by apheresis (HPC-A) has replaced the collection of hematopoietic progenitor cells by bone marrow harvest (HPC-M) for many donors and patients. It has certain advantages and disadvantages (Box 24.5) over marrow harvest.

Hematopoietic Progenitor Cell Dose
An important factor, which determines the success of HPC transplantation, is the dose

Box 24.5: Advantages and disadvantages of collection of hematopoietic progenitor cells (HPCs) from peripheral blood by apheresis (HPC-A) over bone marrow collection/harvest (HPC-M).

Advantages of Collection of HPCs from Peripheral Blood
- **Advantages to donors:**
  - **Better tolerated:** Donors tolerate hemapheresis better than bone marrow harvest, since it is an outpatient procedure and does not require general anesthesia
  - **Quick recovery:** Donor recovers more quickly from the procedure without the pain and temporary disability that often accompany bone marrow harvest
  - **Advantages for the autologous HPC donor:** Shorter period of cytopenias, decreased transfusion requirements, lesser infectious complications, and decreased length of hospitalization
- **Collection:**
  - Relatively easy to collect by hemapheresis and more convenient
  - Less expensive and safer
- **Quality of HPCs:**
  - Increased number of HPCs collected through hemapheresis compared to traditional bone marrow harvest
  - No contamination with tumor cells (if patient's marrow is involved by malignant tumor) in autologous transplantation
- **Advantages to recipients:**
  - Restore hematopoietic and immune function more rapidly than bone marrow HPCs
  - Increased rate and reduced time required for engraftment (neutrophil and platelet engraftment), progenitor cells obtained from the peripheral blood. The engraftment of white cells and platelets occurs about a 1 week earlier.
  - Less number of days of immune suppression required and less exposures to allogeneic blood products in the recipient
  - In autologous transplantation, collection of peripheral HPCs by hemapheresis can be performed even when marrow is involved by malignancy or with prior pelvic irradiation. This cannot be done in bone marrow harvest.

Disadvantages of Collection of HPCs from Peripheral Blood
- Adverse effects of mobilization regimens:
- More time required for collection
- Requires larger volume of component to be transfused at the time of transplantation
- Needs central venous access in many cases, which has accompanying risks and complications (e.g. pneumothorax, hemothorax, thrombosis, bleeding, vascular injury, and infection)
- Requires to process large volume (20–30 liters) of blood

of HPCs infused. Unfortunately, there is no definite method available for estimating dose of HPCs. Following methods can be used to measure the dose of HPCs:

1. **Mononuclear cell count (MNC):** HPCs are found within the mononuclear cell component of blood. Hence, the mononuclear cell count (MNC) can be used as an indicator of when to discontinue HPC collection.
2. **Assessment of colony-forming unit (CFU) granulocyte-macrophage (CFU-GM) colonies** grown on soft agar.
3. **Measurement of CD34+ cell count:** The CD34 is the surface antigen restricted to primitive cells of all lineages. It is expressed on hematopoietic progenitor cells and vascular endothelium throughout the body. Quantitation of the number of cells bearing the CD34 antigen by flow cytometry using antibody to the CD34 antigen is the most widely used method for determining the quantity of HPCs harvested by bone marrow, apheresis, or cord blood collection. This is better indicator of HPC dose than MNC and also correlates with CFU-GM.

Hematopoietic progenitor cell mobilization

Peripheral circulating blood contains only few (0.05%) HPCs. HPCs collection during steady state (i.e. without mobilization) needs more number of procedures (about 12) and many days to collect sufficient quantities (acceptable "dose") for a successful transplant. Each collection procedure needs 4 to 6 hours, since very large blood volumes are processed in order to obtain the required yield. Use of "mobilization therapies" increases the numbers of circulating HPCs and thus improves the efficiency of hemapheresis collection. The mobilization of HPCs from the marrow to the peripheral blood reduces the number of leukapheresis procedures to one or two. HPCs can be mobilized from bone marrow by pharmacological methods using chemotherapy (e.g. cyclophosphamide and etoposide), cytokines, or a combination of chemotherapy and cytokines (e.g. G-CSF and granulocyte-macrophage colony-stimulating factor [GM-CSF]). The effects of combination of chemotherapy and cytokines are better than either regimen is used alone. The mobilization with chemotherapy can be applied only to autologous transplants.

Cytokines such as G-CSF and granulocyte-macrophage colony stimulating factor (GM-CSF) increase HPCs within the peripheral blood and beneficial because of its minimum short-term toxicity. In contrast to use G-CSF in the routine granulocyte donor, four to five daily injections of GCSF are usually needed. Hence, it is not uncommon for individuals to develop headache and musculoskeletal pain.

HPCs express the cell surface glycoprotein CD34. The measurement of CD34+ cells in the peripheral blood prior to collection is usually done to ensure that the adequate mobilization has occurred.

Autologous versus allogeneic hematopoietic progenitor cell harvest

- Initially, chemotherapy was used as a mobilizing agent for HPCs. Hence, HPC-A collections were initially limited to autologous transplantation and restricted to patients with Hodgkin lymphoma (HL), non-Hodgkin lymphoma (NHL), multiple myeloma (MM), and leukemias.
- Present methods for mobilization do not depend upon chemotherapy and HPC-A collection has included allogeneic donations as well.

Hematopoietic progenitor cell collection procedure

Method: HPCs are more commonly harvested from peripheral blood by **leukapheresis**.

Time to initiate the collection of HPC:
- **In allogeneic donors:** Initiate collection on the **5th day** after the start of G-CSF administration.
- **For autologous donors:** Many criteria can be used, which are as follows:
  - Myelocytosis and rising monocyte levels
  - A two-fold rise in total white blood cell count in 24 hours
  - Time of first platelet count increase
  - Day 14 after initiation of chemotherapy
  - White blood cell count of 10,000/µL
- Serial CD34+ cell counts by flow cytometry—to detect a rise in CD34+ cells and to trigger HPC harvest.

Hematopoietic progenitor cell donor concerns

Side effects of HPCs mobilization in donor:

- **Central venous access:** It is needed when large volume (20–30 liters) of blood is processed to obtain HPC donation especially for pediatric donors (a need which is inversely related to age). The central venous access is associated with complications such as pneumothorax, hemothorax, catheter thrombosis, bleeding, vascular injury, and infection.
- Mobilization tumor cells into the peripheral blood following chemotherapy in patient with malignancy (e.g. multiple myeloma).
- **Citrate toxicity:** If large amount of blood is processed in HPC collection, there is the greater exposure to citrate anticoagulant. This increases the risk of hypocalcemia, hypomagnesemia, hypokalemia, and metabolic alkalosis (refer citrate toxicity page 326).
- Side effects of cytokines on the donor are as follows:
  - Bone pain due to the marrow expansion, headache, myalgia (muscle pain), nausea and vomiting, fatigue, and insomnia. These signs and symptoms resolve after cytokines are discontinued.
  - G-CSF can produce several changes in hematologic parameters such as increase in the leukocyte count, an

increase in the lymphocyte count, and a decrease in the platelet count.
- Decrease in platelet count and few donors may need platelet transfusions. Rarely, chronic thrombocytopenia and splenic bleeding may occur.

Umbilical Cord Blood-derived HPC

Umbilical cord blood (UCB) was once considered biological waste. It was known that it contains high numbers of CFU cells or progenitor cells (HPCs) and is an important donor source of HSCs for transplantation. Though HPCs presence in umbilical cord blood was known for many years, it was, in 1989, the first attempt made to use cells recovered from placenta umbilical cords for hematopoietic transplantation. The cord blood transplantation is most appropriate for children requiring transplantation. In children UCB is used for a wide range of malignant and nonmalignant conditions. Advantages of umbilical cord HPCs are listed in Box 24.6.

Harvesting
Cord blood collection: It is similar to those of whole blood collection.

After the baby's delivery, the umbilical cord is clamped, cut, and separated from the infant in a manner that does not interfere with routine delivery practice. It can be collected either after caesarean section or vaginal delivery.

Box 24.6: Advantages of umbilical cord hematopoietic progenitor cells (HPCs).

- The progenitor cells of cord blood have greater degree of tolerance and high degree of engraftment
- Cord blood is banked and more immediately available for use. Thus, it reduces the time to transplantation.
- Cord blood is immunologically naïve
- Less risk of graft-versus-host disease than with adult HPCs
- HLA mismatches are better tolerated by the recipient
- Cord blood is collected at or after delivery without any risk to the mother or infant

(HLA: human leukocyte antigen)

Umbilical cord blood can be collected/harvested by cannulation of the placental vessels (using a cannula or needle) either before (while the placenta is still in utero) or more commonly after (*ex utero*) the delivery of the placenta. There are advantages and disadvantages to each method, but neither seems to be better overall.

Features of umbilical cord blood (HPC-C) Collection are presented in Box 24.7.

Ex utero collection: In this method, the placenta is removed during the delivery and transported to a nearby sterile room for the collection. Usually, the placenta is suspended in a device to allow collection of blood by gravity. The advantage of *ex utero* collection is that the placenta and cord are more accessible. Hence, more manipulation, such as "milking" of the cord, can be used to increase the volume collected. Speed is important in this process because the blood begins to clot and the volume and number of HPCs obtained will be inadequate, if the collection is not done quickly.

In utero collection: After the newborn is delivered and assessed, the umbilical cord is clamped and cut. UCB is collected by the obstetrician or nurse/midwife. Care should be taken to maintain a relatively clean field.

The collections are done either in the sterile delivery room or a separate sterile room. As in whole blood collection, the venipuncture needle is integral to the bag. After identifying the umbilical vein, prior to venipuncture, the site is cleaned with aseptic precaution. The HPC-C is collected by gravity into a collection bag containing CPD anticoagulant. Usually, only 100–150 mL are collected. The collection is of no risk to the mother or infant. While the UCB is being collected (a 3–5-minute process),

Box 24.7: Features of umbilical cord blood (HPC-C) collection.

- After the mother delivers infant, clamp the umbilical cord of placenta
- Collect cord blood from placenta through cord blood vessel
- Collect only about 100–150 mL of cord blood
- No risk for mother or infant

the collected blood should be gently mixed with the anticoagulant to prevent clotting. When the collection is complete, the umbilical cord will appear collapsed. During collection, place the bag on a laboratory scale. This allows monitoring the volume and also helps in determining when collection is completed.

Number and volume of HPCs collected: The number of HPCs collected is directly proportional to the volume of cord blood collected. This in turn varies with the size of the infant/placenta and the experience of the individual performing the collection. Usually, a volume of 40–150 mL is collected. This will harvest about $4–11 \times 10^8$ nucleated cells. If the collected volume is inadequate (<40 mL), they are usually discarded. Usually, UCB collections are not processed further to reduce their volume but they are frozen directly with dimethyl sulfoxide (DMSO) and liquid nitrogen storage.

Careful screening and testing of the mother are necessary to ensure the safety of the cord blood product, as well as the absence of genetic disease. Tests should be done for serologically transmissible disease and confirmation by nucleic acid testing (NAT) on a maternal sample, bacteriologic testing on a sample of the umbilical cord blood.

Testing to be done on umbilical cord blood is listed in Box 24.8.

Umbilical cord blood processing
Umbilical cord blood needs special processing:
- Both the mother's blood sample and the cord blood are tested for ABO, Rh, and, for the mother's sample, antibodies (Box 24.8).
- Test for the total nucleated cell (TNC) count and the CD34 content.
- Test for **hemoglobinopathies**.
- Serologic and DNA testing for human leukocyte antigen (HLA) A, B, and DRB1 is performed on both mother and cord to assure no mix-ups occurred.
- Mother's sample is tested for human immunodeficiency virus (HIV)-1, -2; hepatitis B virus (HBV); hepatitis C virus (HCV); and human T-lymphotropic virus (HTLV)-I, -II. Also, for surface antigen of hepatitis B (HBsAg), anti-hepatitis B core (HBc) antigen, and syphilis.
- Cord blood is cultured for *Cytomegalovirus* (*CMV*).
- West Nile virus (WNV) by nucleic acid tests (NAT) is performed in some cases.

Processing the cord blood product: The cord blood is diluted with dextran and albumin or hetastarch (to improve the viability of the HPCs). The cells are allowed to sediment, and the buff coat and plasma are transferred to another bag. It is centrifuged to separate and then remove plasma. The final volume is about 20 mL. Then 5 mL of 50% DMSO is slowly added for a final content of 10%. At the end of processing, a sample from the product is tested for viability and cell count. Bacterial and fungal cultures are performed.

Types/Categories of Hematopoietic Progenitor Cell Transplant (Box 24.9)

Comparison of hematopoietic progenitor cell sources and products with collection and complications are mentioned in Table 24.1.

Indications for Hematopoietic Progenitor Cell Transplantation

Indications for HPCs transplantation range from non-neoplastic immune disorders to malignant conditions (Box 24.10).

Donor/Patient Selection

It is important to have a close allele-level HLA matching between the donor and the recipient of HPC transplants to avoid transplant rejection and graft-versus-host

---

Box 24.8: Testing to be done on umbilical cord blood.

- ABO and Rh typing
- CD34+ cells and TNC
- Hemoglobinopathies
- HLA A, B, DRB1
- Infectious diseases
- Antibody screen—mother

(HLA: human leukocyte antigen; Rh: Rhesus; TNC: total nucleated cell)

Box 24.9: Categories of HPCs for transplantation.

Autologous:
- From self: The patient's own HSCs are removed, cryopreserved and reinfused

Allogeneic ("from different genes"): HSCs are obtained from another individual—
- From one human to another
- Related or unrelated

Syngeneic ("from same genes"):
- HSCs are obtained from an identical twin or triplet. **Syngeneic HPC transplantation** is used infrequently due to the relative rarity of identical twins or triplets

Xenogeneic (from different species): HSCs are obtained from a nonhuman species. Not clinically feasible

(HPC: hematopoietic progenitor cell; HSC: hematopoietic stem cell)

Box 24.10: Indications for hematopoietic progenitor cell transplantation.

Red blood cell disorders:
- Aplastic anemia
- Thalassemia major
- Sickle cell anemia
- Fanconi anemia
- Paroxysmal nocturnal hemoglobinuria

WBC disorders:
- Leukemia:
  - Acute myeloid leukemia—relapse following initial remission
  - Acute lymphoblastic leukemia—relapse after initial chemotherapy-induced remission
  - Chronic myeloid leukemia
- Myelodysplastic syndromes
- Myeloproliferative neoplasms
- Lymphomas: Hodgkin lymphoma, non-Hodgkin lymphoma
- Multiple myeloma

Immunological disorders:
- Severe autoimmune disorders: Scleroderma, lupus erythematosus
- Congenital immune deficiencies: Severe combined immunodeficiency (SCID)

Solid tumors:
- Neuroblastoma
- Ewing's sarcoma
- Rhabdomyosarcoma

Inborn error of metabolism

disease (GVHD). When compared with solid-organ transplants, preformed HLA antibodies and ABO compatibility are less important in HPC transplants.

Donor's workup: It includes a complete history and physical, laboratory tests, ECG, chest X-ray, donor health history, and extensive informed consent.
- **Testing for markers of infectious diseases:** These include tests for HBsAg, anti-HBc, hepatitis C virus nucleic acid testing (HCV NAT), anti-HCV; HIV-1, -2 NAT, anti-HIV-1, -2; HTLV-I, -II NAT; and syphilis.
- **Other tests:** These are performed when indicated and include WNV NAT, HBV NAT, anti-CMV, and others.

The type of HPCs transplantation depends on the type of disease being treated and the availability of the donor.

Autologous Donors/Patients

Autologous bone marrow or peripheral blood HPCs are used for most patients,

Table 24.1: Comparison of hematopoietic progenitor cell sources and products with collection and complications.

Features	Cord blood (HPC, UCB)	Autologous (HPC, Apheresis + Marrow)	Allogeneic (HPC, Apheresis + Marrow)
Source	Umbilical cord blood	Patient	Related or unrelated matched donor
Product	Cord blood progenitor/stem cells	Bone marrow or peripheral blood progenitor cells	Bone marrow or peripheral blood progenitor cells
Method of collection	Placenta (umbilical cord at birth)	Intraoperative marrow or hemapheresis	Intraoperative marrow or hemapheresis
Major drawback or complication	Insufficient progenitor cells	Recurrence of original disease	Graft-versus-host disease

(HPC: hematopoietic progenitor cell; UCB: umbilical cord blood)

especially patients with hematologic/marrow malignancies or metastatic solid tumors. The patient should be in clinical remission to decrease the risk of collecting malignant cells with the HPCs. Pulmonary function tests and cardiac stress tests are performed along with the tests mentioned. Testing for infectious disease is important because of their possible reactivation after the transplantation. If patient is found positive for infectious disease, the HPC product should be stored in such a way as to prevent cross-contamination of other products.

Allogeneic HPC Transplantation

It is used for patients who cannot donate their own cells. This may be due to multiple cycles of chemotherapy, irradiation of bone marrow, disease of marrow (e.g. aplastic anemia), or genetic disease.

- **Unrelated donors:** They should undergo initial screening and more testing, including high-resolution (DNA) HLA typing. HPCs express HLA, but not ABO blood group antigens.
- **Related donors:** Siblings or other related donors are screened and tested as mentioned above.

PROCESSING HPC PRODUCTS

After the laboratory receives the HPC products, it is necessary to assure the quality and quantity of the product before storage, transportation, and dispensing. Careful labeling should be done to prevent mix-ups during processing and storage.

Initial Testing

Upon receipt of HPC at the laboratory, it is examined for proper labeling, clumps of platelets, hemolysis, and integrity of the collection container.

- Test the sample for complete blood count (CBC), platelets, WBC differential; CD34+ cells (HPCs) and viability. Sampling is done in a laminar flow hood, using a sterile connecting device or integral sampling tubes attached to the collection set. Usually, cell counts are performed on automated instruments. The differential count is performed manually to confirm mononuclear cells, which contain the HPCs. CD34+ cells are determined by flow cytometry, and viability is also determined by flow, using markers for **apoptosis**. Viability is determined by dye exclusion, because dead cells cannot exclude the dye from their cytoplasm.
- Bacterial and fungal culture: If a culture is positive, antibiotic sensitivity is determined so that appropriate antibiotic(s) can be given to the recipient when the product is infused.

Initial Processing

The HPC processing methods can be divided into—(i) routine methods and (ii) specialized methods.

Routine Methods

These are usually centrifuge based and include volume (plasma) reduction, red cell reduction, buffy-coat preparation, thawing/washing, and filtration.

- **Volume reduction:** It is performed in the setting of minor-ABO-mismatched allograft (marrow or peripheral blood) transplantation. The purpose is to reduce the amount of incompatible plasma and to prevent fluid balance/overload in small patients and/or patients with renal disease and cardiac failure. The larger products need to be volume reduced before freezing (cryopreservation) to limit the aliquots for freezing (e.g. for UCB banking where storage space is limited).
  - **Centrifugation:** The hematopoietic progenitor cells are contained within the nucleated cell fraction. Hence, the collected marrow is further processed to reduce the volume by centrifuging to separate the plasma from cellular elements. An automated cell separator device can be used to separate the buffy coat (nucleated WBC) from the large proportion of RBCs and plasma.
  - **Using sedimentation agents:** Another method to concentrate the buffy coat is

by using a sedimenting agent such as Ficoll, dextran, or hydroxyethyl starch (HES). These agents form a density gradient using centrifugation, with the plasma or supernatant on top, the RBCs on the bottom, and the **buffy coat** (containing WBC, HPCs, and platelets) in-between. The buffy coat is resuspended in autologous plasma or a balanced salt solution and dextrose. This process will remove all RBCs and plasma for major and minor ABO incompatibility and reduce volume for frozen storage. Thus, this method is used to prevent hemolytic transfusion reactions when major ABO incompatible marrow HPC allografts and allografts with other clinically relevant red cell antigens (e.g. Kell and Kidd) are transplanted.
- **Red cell reduction:** RBCs are removed from bone marrow products, because freezing and thawing causes the cells to lyse and release **nephrotoxic** free hemoglobin and RBC stroma. Thus, red cell reduction before freezing reduces the amount of lysed red cell fragments, especially in patients with renal failure. Red cell reduction is also useful when there is limited storage space.
- **Buffy-coat concentration:** It involves centrifugation and harvesting of the white cell fraction and can be performed with apheresis of cell-washing device. When the volume of product is too low for apheresis or cell washing, manual centrifugation may be used. Usually, buffy-coat preparation is used to reduce the unit volume for cryopreservation or as a method to reduce red cell before further manipulation (e.g. immunomagnetic selection).
- **Thawing:** Procedure for thawing is same for all HPCs irrespective of the source. It should be done with utmost care because frozen plastic containers are prone to break for several reasons. The product should be handled with care while verifying to determine the product's identity and make sure about the integrity of the bag. The product is then placed into a clean or sterile plastic bag and submerged in a water bath at 37°C.
- **Washing of HPCs:** It removes lysed RBCs, hemoglobin, and cry precipitant [i.e. dimethyl sulfoxide (DMSO)]. However, there may be some loss of HPCs. Routine washing is done with UCB and involves slow, sequential addition of a wash solution (e.g. 10% dextran followed by 5% albumin), transfer into a bag for centrifugation and resuspension of the cell pellet(s) before infusion. Automatic methods are also available.
- **Filtering:** Immediately, after mixing with anticoagulant, the bone marrow product is filtered by passing through large-pore (500 and 200 μm) filters to remove bone spicules, clots, fat, fibrin, and other debris prior to infusion or further processing.

Contaminating granulocytes are higher in HPC-A products and can cause febrile reactions with chills in the recipient because of lysing during thawing.

Specialized HPC Processing Methods

These can produce pure and potent HPCs product than obtained by routine methods. However, they need unique reagents and instruments.

Elutriation

Elutriation is a process for separating particles based on their size, shape, and density, using a stream of gas or liquid flowing in a direction usually opposite to the direction of sedimentation. Counterflow centrifugal elutriation separates cell populations depending on two physical properties, namely—(i) size and (ii) density (sedimentation coefficient). It can also be used to enrich monocytes for preparing dendritic-cell vaccines.

Cell Selection Systems

Cell depletion/enrichment may be performed using immunomagnetic cell selection systems. In these methods, cell type of interest are isolated either by positive selection (i.e. by

retaining target cells) or negative selection (i.e. by depletion of target cells).
- **Cell enrichment:** CD34+ cells can be separated from the other cells in the product by using magnetic beads attached with anti-CD34 antibodies. The cell suspension is passed through a column in which magnetic field is generated. Unlabeled cells pass through the column and are collected in a negative fraction bag. The magnetic beads separate the CD34+ cells from the column by magnetic force and allow the passage of cells into a separate collection bag. Thus, it gives an enriched CD 34+ product. The enrichment may also be achieved by fluorescent cell sorting.
- **Cell purging and reduction:** In patient with leukemia, the leukemic cells also are mobilized from the marrow by **cytokine** therapy and are collected by HPC-A. Bone marrow can also contain leukemic precursors. The process of removing (purging) the malignant cells from the HPCs is called *cell purging*. This can be done by using antibodies specific for the malignant cell antigen, which bind and then remove (purge) the malignant cells. T, B, and NK cells can also be reduced by using antibodies to specific antigens and this will reduce the risk of graft-versus-host disease, but the rate of relapse may be increased.

Cell Expansion

The dose of HPCs is positively correlated with patient outcome. The expansion of HPCs increases hematopoietic engraftment and reduces transfusion-dependent risk of infection and duration of hospital stay. Cell expansion is used in UCD HPCs because the cell quantity in a UCB collection is limited as well as because it has both higher proliferative and self-renewal capacity. Most expansion cultures use cytokine cocktail consisting of stem cell factor, FLT-3 ligand, and thrombopoietin along with novel and/or proprietary ingredients.

Transplantation (Shipping) Fresh Products

Allogeneic and syngeneic HPCs collected from bone marrow or peripheral blood are usually transplanted fresh. If not, they are stored 24–72 hours at 20–24°C or at 4°C.

CRYOPRESERVATION OF HEMATOPOIETIC GRAFTS

Usually, bone marrow from allogeneic marrow donations is collected immediately before transplantation. HPC grafts collected from all autologous and many allogeneic are cryopreserved and stored for weeks to years before transplantation. The cryopreservation process directly affects the efficacy and quality of HPC transplants.

Preparation for Freezing HPCs

Cryopreservation

Freezing: Routinely, after processing, the products (PBSC) are cryopreserved in a saline solution mixture and supplemented with a protein (usually albumin or autologous plasma), and cryoprotectants (cryoprotective chemicals) such as dimethyl sulfoxide (DMSO) or DMSO and hydroxyethyl starch (HES) without or with 1% dextran-40. The cryoprotective chemicals are slowly added to produce a final concentration of 5–10% DMSO. The cryoprotective chemicals cross the cell membrane and protect the cells from ice damage and cell dehydration during the freezing and thawing process. DMSO provides significant improvement in post-thaw viability. However, the amount of DMSO added should be limited because of toxicities, which are associated with the post-thaw infusion of progenitor cell products containing DMSO. Washing of products following thaw to reduce the amount of DMSO present causes significant loss of progenitor cells. Freezing is performed after transferring the products to freezing bags in small aliquots of about 45–70 mL.

Thawing and Preparing Products for Transplant

Thawing of the HPCs for transplant should be followed by testing the product for TNC count, CD34 count, and viability and culturing for contamination. Each bag must be thawed quickly at 37°C and infused through the recipient's IV within 1–2 hours. There will be significant loss of HPCs, if the product is kept at room temperature even if for a short time. The thawed products may be washed, especially if DMSO toxicity is a problem for the recipient.

■ TRANSPLANTING THE RECIPIENT

Conditioning Regimens for Hematopoietic Graft Recipients

- **Conditioning (myeloablative transplants):** Before the HSC transplant, classically the recipient is given a high-dose chemotherapy and/or gamma radiation therapy, sometimes total-body irradiation (TBI). This procedure is called conditioning. The purpose is to eradicate/ablate/eliminate the recipient's hematopoietic marrow and immune system and to eliminate cancer/tumor cells, if any, in patients with malignant disease. In nonmalignant conditions, its purpose is to restore normal function in patients with defects of hematopoiesis (aplastic anemia and sickle cell anemia). Conditioning also makes physical space available for HPCs to engraft (accept). Most conditioning regimens completely ablate the bone marrow and immune system. Once this conditioning has occurred, the recipient must receive a transplant or patient will die. Thus, the transplant is a "rescue". However, bone marrow ablative conditioning regimens prior to transplants is not always successful in eliminating cancer cells before HPC transplant. In contrast, these high-dose regimens increase morbidity and mortality. These factors, and demonstration of greater benefit from allogeneic versus autologous HPC grafts, have led to the utilization of nonmyeloablative transplant protocols discussed below.
- **Nonmyeloablative conditioning** (reduced intensity-conditioning regimens): Recently, nonmyeloablative conditioning was used in some recipients. These are more commonly referred to as reduced intensity conditioning regimens. This allows survival of part of their bone marrow and immune system. The aim of this is to establish a stable **chimerism** (two cell populations), so that donor cells recognize malignant cells as foreign cells and destroy them. It is used in patients who are not suitable for **myeloablative** conditioning such as those who have serious comorbidity or are elderly. In the reduced intensity conditioning of HPC grafts, recipient's tumor is controlled by donor T-cells, which recognize host residual tumor cells. The morbidity and mortality associated with the conditioning regimen in nonmyeloablative HPC grafts are lower. However, the risk of GVHD is the same as that follows high-dose conditioning regimens.

T-Cell Depletion

The reduction in the incidence and severity of GVHD can be achieved by techniques that reduce the numbers of T lymphocytes in allogeneic hematopoietic grafts. These techniques either target the HPCs (positive selection) or the T-cells (negative selection).

Techniques Targeting T-Cells (Negative Selection)

The various techniques used are soybean lectin agglutination, E-rosette formation, combinations of the two, counterflow elutriation, monoclonal antibodies, and the application of monoclonal antibodies in vivo in the recipient post-transplant to reduce donor T-cells.

Disadvantage of T-cell Depletion

It is associated with increase in the incidence of disease relapse. Patients who develop mild GVHD have a lower incidence of relapse of neoplastic disease than do those patients who have no GVHD. The presence of the donor T-cell population is important for "graft-versus-leukemia effect". The donor T cells recognize host antigens and generate an immune response, which eliminates residual host tumor cells.

Reinfusion of HPCs

- **Process similar to blood transfusion:** HPCs, regardless of the source, are infused to the recipient in a manner similar to that transfusion of any blood product. These pluripotent progenitor cells have unique membrane receptors. They will home to the marrow space, engraft, and replicate.
- **Cryopreserved HPCs:** HPC products that are cryopreserved with DMSO are usually thawed and immediately reinfused, without washing. Few wash HPCs prior to infusion for patients who are at higher risk of toxicity (e.g. neonatal). HPCs collected by hemapheresis, if they are not further processed, may contain large numbers of RBCs. Cryopreservation in DMSO does not maintain integrity of mature RBC membrane. When these products are thawed, they will contain a large amount of free hemoglobin. The severity of reaction in the recipient to both the free hemoglobin and DMSO varies from mild to severe. The mild reactions include nausea, chills, or headache; and more severe reactions include hypotension, vomiting, systemic inflammatory response syndrome (SIRS), renal failure, cardiac arrest, and neurologic ischemia/toxicity. Usually, the recipients of cryopreserved progenitor cell products are given antihistamines and/or antiemetics before HPC transplantation. The renal toxicities associated with free hemoglobin and larger volume infusions can be reduced by maintaining adequate hydration and the use of diuretics.

Infusion

- Fresh HPCs products (allogeneic) are infused slowly to avoid/minimize volume overload and adverse reactions.
- Leukapheresis products can be infused over an hour or two than those of bone marrow products.
- If volume is larger, it can be infused over 2–4 hours.

ABO Incompatibility (Table 24.2)

If there is ABO incompatibility between recipient and the HPCs products, it needs special care.

- **Major incompatibility** occurs when the recipient has ABO antibody against the donor. For example, the recipient is group O and the donor is A. The group A recipient's plasma contains anti-A. This can hemolyze the donor RBCs in the product.
    - Usually, HPC-A and HPC-C products contain only a few milliliters of RBCs. Hence, it is likely to develop a **serious hemolytic reaction**.
    - Bone marrow HPCs contain a much higher portion of RBCs and it is necessary to remove most of the RBCs to prevent a serious acute hemolytic reaction.
    - **Delayed RBC engraftment:** The recipient may also have delayed RBC engraftment, if group O RBCs containing anti-A are selected for transfusion.
- **Minor ABO incompatibility:**
    - **Hemolysis:** It is less likely to produce adverse reaction. For example, if the recipient is A group and the donor is O group, the donor may have high-titered anti-A or anti-A, -B. This may cause hemolysis of the recipient's group A cells.
    - **Passenger lymphocyte syndrome:** Donor's T lymphocytes are primed to

Incompatibility	Recipient	Donor	Possible outcome
Major	O	A	Hemolysis of donor RBCs Delayed RBC engraftment
Minor	A	O	Hemolysis of recipient RBCs Passenger lymphocyte syndrome

Table 24.2: ABO incompatibility.

make anti-A. This can produce ongoing hemolysis of the recipient's RBCs and may also attack other cells bearing the A antigen. This is called **passenger lymphocyte syndrome**.

Adverse Recipient Reactions

Similar to blood transfusion, to reduce or avoid reactions, the recipient may receive premedication.
- **Odor of DMSO:** It has an odor like the sulfur in garlic or rotten eggs. Hence, if it is used in HPCs, the recipient may have this odor.
- **Flushing and nausea** are the most common adverse reaction.
- **Other reactions:** Vomiting, changes in heart rate, and blood pressure.
- **Fever and chills:** It may be due to contamination of HPCs with granulocytes. These granulocytes release their cytoplasmic granules and their content by freezing and thawing.
- **Renal damage:** RBCs are not preserved by DMSO. Hence, free hemoglobin and red blood cell stroma may cause renal damage.
- **Other transplant-related complications:** These include liver or lung toxicity caused by myeloablative chemotherapy. In the autologous recipient, it may mimic graft-versus-host disease.

Engraftment

Engraftment should occur after the infusion of HPC products. The standard measurement of success is engraftment of all three cell lines, namely, RBCs, WBCs and platelets, in 100 days.
- **Early engraftment:** It is defined as the interval from transplant to the rise of absolute neutrophil count greater than 500/μL. It occurs usually in 9–30 days.
- **Platelet engraftment:** It is defined as the rise of platelet count greater than 20,000/μL without transfusion. It requires 15 or more days.
- **RBC engraftment and immune reconstitution:** It occurs 90 days or longer.

Factors Affecting the Rate of Engraftment

It varies depending on the source of the HPCs, the number and viability of CD34+ cells, cellular processing, the conditioning regimen of the recipient, and other variables. Examples are as follows:
- **Engraftment of neutrophils and platelets:** They occur earlier when the CD34 counts in the HPC product are higher.
- **Cord blood and leukapheresis products:** It usually engraft earlier than bone marrow products. CD34+ cell dose in cord blood is lower. Hence, engraftment may be delayed or, in about 20% of cases, it never occurs.
- **Children weighing less than 45 kg:** In these children, cord blood transplantation is most successful.
- Children weighing more than 45 kg and in adults—transplanting two or three HPC-C products may be successfully used.

The longer the engraftment takes, the higher the risk of severe viral or fungal infection. Major ABO mismatch can also delay RBC engraftment.

Autologous Transplantation

In autologous HPC transplantation, HPCs are obtained from the patient before the high-dose antineoplastic therapy. They are used for rescuing hematopoietic tissue from high-dose chemotherapy. The HPCs collected are frozen (cryopreserved) and then reinfused after the high-dose therapy to reconstitute marrow function. Indications for autologous HPC transplant are mentioned in Box 24.11.

Different steps of autologous stem cell transplantation are mentioned in Figure 24.1 and Box 24.12.

Box 24.11: Indications for autologous hematopoietic progenitor cell (HPC) transplant.

- Multiple myeloma
- Non-Hodgkin lymphoma
- Hodgkin lymphoma
- Other cancers
- Acute myelogenous leukemia (AML)

Allogeneic Stem Cell Transplantation

The HPCs are obtained from an HLA-matched or HLA-mismatched family member (usually a sibling) or an unrelated donor.

Box 24.12: Different steps of autologous stem cell transplantation.

- Harvesting
- Processing of HPCs
- Conditioning
- HPC transplant
- Post-transplant engraftment

(HPC: hematopoietic progenitor cell)

Different steps of allogeneic stem cell transplantation are mentioned in Box 24.12 and Figure 24.2.

COMPLICATIONS OF HEMATOPOIETIC STEM CELL TRANSPLANTATION

Autologous HSC transplants have fewer immunologic complications but have higher rates of relapse of the disease after transplant. Allogeneic HSC transplants have lower rates of relapse but have more immunologic

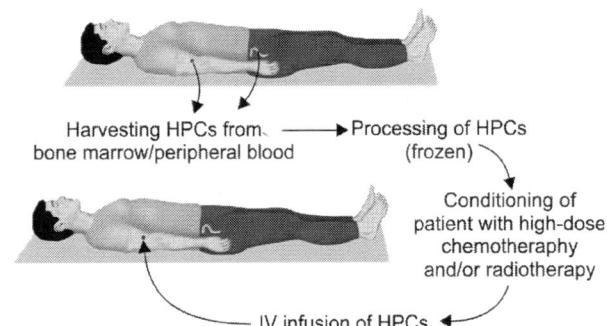

Fig. 24.1: Autologous stem cell transplantation.
(HPC: hematopoietic progenitor cell; IV: intravenous)

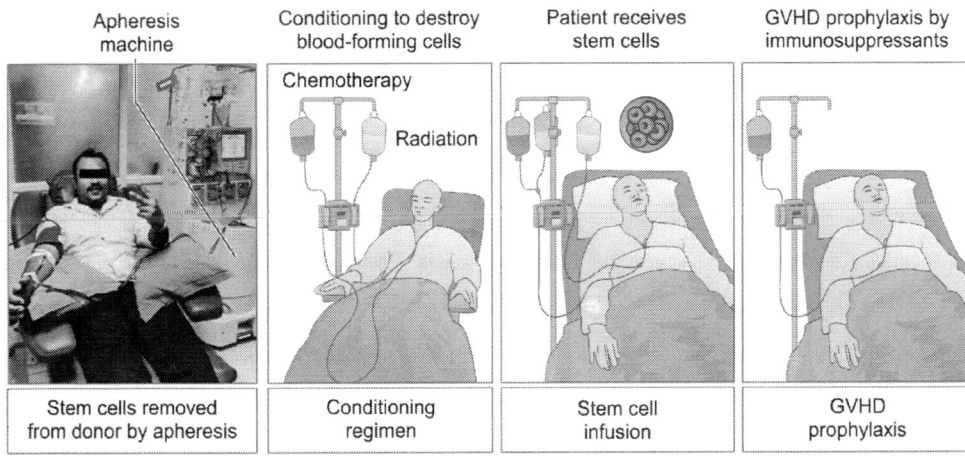

Fig. 24.2: Different steps in allogeneic hematopoietic stem cell (HSC) transplantation. (A) Collection of allogeneic HSCs: They are collected by apheresis or from the bone marrow of the donor. (B) Conditioning (preparatory) regimen: The patient receives a conditioning regimen of chemotherapy or radiation therapy (or both). Its purpose is to both eliminate the underlying malignancy and suppress the immune system of recipient to prevent rejection of the allogeneic HSCs. (C) The collected HSC is infused intravenously into the donor. (D) Immunosuppressant drugs: After the infusion of the HSCs, the patient is given immunosuppressant drugs to prevent the development of graft-versus-host disease (GVHD).

complications, including GVHD, which can be fatal.

Infections

Patients are susceptible to a variety of infections (bacterial, viral, and fungal) due to lack of granulocytes, as well as lack of a functioning immune system.

Graft Rejection

- **Nonmyeloablative transplant:** Graft rejection may occur in the nonmyeloablative transplant. In these cases, recipient/host cells may mount an immunological response to the graft. Graft rejection is mediated by T cells or NK cells.
- A graft **mismatched for HLA and sex** has a higher risk of graft rejection.

Graft-versus-Host Disease

Graft-versus-host disease (GVHD) is the major complication of allogeneic HSC transplants. It is mediated by the donor T lymphocytes that are transplanted with allogeneic HPC products. Three conditions are necessary for the development of GVHD:
1. An immunocompetent graft (i.e. one containing T cells).
2. HLA mismatch (minor or major) between donor and recipient.
3. An immunosuppressed recipient who cannot mount an immune response to the graft.

Cord blood transplants (even with HLA mismatch) are less likely to produce severe GVHD than other sources of HPCs.
- **Acute GVHD** is defined as **GVHD** occurring within the first 100 days after transplant.
- **Chronic GVHD** is defined as **GVHD** occurring after 100 days after transplant. It develops in about 25–50% of allogeneic recipients. It mostly affects skin, gastrointestinal tract, liver, lung, and eyes. Since, **immunosuppressive** drugs are needed to treat GVHD; they increase the risk of infection.

Relapse of Disease and Donor Lymphocyte Infusion

- **Relapse or recurrence of leukemia and lymphoma** can occur following HPCs transplantation. It is **due to inadequate conditioning or contamination of the autologous graft.** The incidence of relapse is lower in recipients with chronic GVHD.
- **Donor leukocyte infusion (DLI):** A "graft-versus-leukemia effect" was observed in patients transplanted with HPCs for acute leukemia and this correlated with the development of chronic graft-versus-host disease in the recipient. This effect was dependent on donor T lymphocytes and was found to have the high-relapse rate of leukemia in patients receiving T-cell-depleted HPC grafts. If there is relapse of leukemia or lymphoma following allogeneic transplants, the donor can be asked to donate another leukapheresis. The aim behind this is to collect donor T lymphocytes to attack the relapse of malignancy in patients. The technique or process of infusion donor T cells after HPC grafting in a patient with relapse is called **donor leukocyte infusion (DLI).** The T cells in DLI induce graft-versus-leukemia, which can control the leukemia or lymphoma relapse. For DLI collection, the donor should not be stimulated with cytokines (e.g. G-CSF). DLI is used for relapse of chronic myeloid leukemia (CML) and it not so useful for other hematologic malignancies.

Outcomes

- **Autologous HPC transplantation:** Following myeloablative therapy, autologous HPC transplantation provides an improved quality of life and increased disease-free survival for patients with multiple myeloma, acute myelogenous leukemia (AML), non-Hodgkin's lymphoma, and Hodgkin's disease. For patients with multiple myeloma, it was found beneficial of giving two sequential autologous transplants.

- **Allogeneic transplants:** The outcome is less successful, mainly because of development of acute GVHD and infections caused by immunosuppressive therapy.

TRANSFUSION THERAPY FOR HPC TRANSPLANTATION

Once a patient is chosen for an HPC transplant, it is necessary for the blood bank to provide blood products, which prevent alloimmunization to HLA antigens, *CMV* infection, or graft-versus-host disease. This can be achieved by providing cellular products that have been leukocyte reduced, gamma-irradiated, and, in special circumstances, *CMV* seronegative.

HLA Alloimmunization

Leukocyte-reduced cellular products will reduce the incidence of **alloimmunization** to HLA antigens.

Consequences of HLA alloimmunization:
- It can **interfere with platelet transfusion** needed during the critical pre- and post-transplantation periods.
- **Delayed platelet engraftment:** Platelet engraftment may be delayed by weeks. This can lead to increased risk of hemorrhage, if the patient is refractory to platelet transfusion.

CMV Transmission

Cytomegalovirus seronegative or leukocyte-reduced is beneficial in HPC transplantation recipients because it reduces the risk of transfusion transmitted *CMV* infections. Allogeneic recipients are immunosuppressed and are at risk for acquiring a life-threatening *CMV* infection from a *CMV*-infective blood component.

Transfusion-associated Graft-versus-Host Disease

Transfusion-associated graft-versus-host disease (TA-GVHD) is uncommon, but the mortality rate is above 90%. TA-GVHD is produced by donor T lymphocytes engrafting in a susceptible immunosuppressed host. Donor T lymphocytes can cause **microchimerism** and can survive for months to years in the recipient's circulation. The clinical features may start 1–4 weeks after transfusion and include fever, **maculopapular** rash, bloody diarrhea, or **pancytopenia.** If a patient is considered for HPC transplant, it is recommended that gamma irradiation of all transfused cellular blood components should be done in the pre-HPC transplantation period. Irradiation is needed, beginning at conditioning. Usually, the patient is given irradiated blood products for life.

EX VIVO MANIPULATION OF HEMATOLOGIC CELLS

Majority of adult B-cell malignancies, including acute lymphoblastic leukemia (ALL), chronic lymphocytic leukemia (CLL), and non-Hodgkin lymphoma, are incurable by the currently available therapies, even with HPC transplant.

Immunotherapy

Immunotherapy is a treatment that uses your body's own immune system to help fight cancer.

Immunotherapy is another approach to treat patients having hematological malignancies. This is by engineering of the patient's own immune cells to recognize and attack their tumors. Two primary strategies may be used:
1. **Sensitization in vivo or ex vivo of a patient's T-cells** through their dendritic cells (similar to a vaccination for infectious disease)
2. **Genetically engineering the patient's T-cells ex vivo** to target the tumor cells.

Use of Dendritic Cells in Cancer Immunotherapy

Dendritic cells (DCs) are special immune cells in the body that help the immune system to recognize cancer cells. The purpose of the

DC immunotherapy approach is to induce antigen-specific expansion of effector and memory CD8+ T-cells against cancer cells by utilizing the patient's own immune system. The effector and memory CD8+ T-cells will directly reduce the tumor mass and can also induce an immunological memory to control relapse of the tumor. For an optimal functioning vaccine, the vaccine-elicited CD8+ T-cells should meet several criteria as listed in Box 24.13.

Dendritic cells are at the center of the immune system owing to their ability to control both tolerance and immune responses. Because of these key properties of DCs, they are used for antigen delivery and vaccination, including therapeutic vaccination against cancer.

Mechanism of Action

- Dendritic cells break down cancer cells into smaller pieces (including antigens) and present/deliver the captured antigen to naïve cells.
- Naïve cells in turn induce antigen-specific expansion of effector and memory CD8+ T-cells against cancer cells.

Box 24.13: Criteria required for dendritic cell vaccine to elicit CD8+ T-cells.

- Should be of high avidity
- Able to recognize peptide-MHC class I complexes on tumor cells
- Able to express high levels of granzyme and perforin, which are essential proteins required for cytotoxic activity against cancer cells
- Able to enter a tumor microenvironment
- Able to overcome the immunomodulatory mechanisms operational in a tumor cell.

(MHC: major histocompatibility complex)

- The T cells then start an immune reaction against any cells in the body that contain these antigens.

Methods: There are two approaches used with DCs:
1. **Vaccination approach:** In this approach, DC is utilized in which the antigen is provided together with an adjuvant to elicit a therapeutic T-cell response in vivo. The DCs can be used as therapeutic vaccines for a variety of neoplastic conditions. The dendritic cell-based vaccines are safe and can induce the expansion of circulating CD4+ T-cells and CD8+ T-cells that are specific for tumor antigens.
2. **Autologous antigen-specific dendritic cells:** Dendritic cells are isolated and expanded ex vivo by culturing hematopoietic progenitor cells or monocytes with cytokine combinations. These are then reinfused into the patient.

Adoptive Cell Transfer/Chimeric Antigen Receptors

Another method of treatment of cancer cells is by genetic engineering of T-cells to target tumor-associated antigens. It is achieved through the introduction of genes encoding artificial T-cell receptors, called chimeric antigen receptors (CARs), specific to cancer-associated antigens. CARs are proteins that allow the T-cells to recognize a specific protein (antigen) on tumor cells. After antigen binding, it activates T-cells. Thus, by using CARs, it may be possible to treat wide range of hematologic and nonhematologic malignancies (e.g. advanced melanoma, colon cancer, and B-cell lymphomas).

SUMMARY

- Hematopoietic progenitor cells (HPCs) can be obtained from three sources, namely—bone marrow aspiration, peripheral blood mobilization followed by collection by apheresis, and umbilical cord blood collection.
- Granulocyte colony-stimulating factor with/without chemotherapy is currently the gold standard for HPC mobilization.
- The types of HPCs transplantation include autologous ("from self"), allogeneic ("from different genes"), or syngeneic (from identical twin).
- Clinical indications for stem cell transplants (both autologous and allogeneic) are increasing.
- After obtaining HPCs, they are cryopreserved. Accurate nucleated cell counting, CD34+

(Contd...)

(Contd...)

- enumeration, and sterility analysis should be done before and after cryopreservation.
- Hematopoietic progenitor cells can be used for the treatment of many malignant and nonmalignant conditions.
- Hematopoietic stem cells transplants can be a curative treatment for patients with hematological malignancies.
- Autologous HPCs are usually used to rescue marrow function for patients undergoing high-dose chemotherapy and/or radiotherapy.
- A major complication of mainly allogeneic transplant is GVHD.

SELF-ASSESSMENT EXERCISE

Write short essays/notes on:
- Application of hematopoietic stem cell transplantation.
- What are the indications for hematopoietic stem cell transplantation? What are its short- and long-term complications?
- Stem cell collection.
- Stem cell transplantation.
- Hematopoietic stem cells.
- Compare bone marrow stem cell transplantation with cord blood stem cell transplantation.
- Cord stem cell banking.
- Indication of allogeneic bone marrow transplantation.
- Hematopoietic stem cell banking.
- Biological bias and indications of stem cell transplantation.

CHAPTER 25

Transfusion Regulation and Legislation

CHAPTER OUTLINE
- Blood bank regulations and legal framework in India
- Licensing procedure
- Evolution of blood safety program in India

INTRODUCTION

Blood transfusion service (BTS) is a vital part of National Health Service. There is no substitute for human blood or its components. The aim of blood transfusion services should be to provide safe, adequate, and effective blood and blood products to meet the patient's needs. Increased awareness about transfusion-transmitted diseases has necessitated the enforcement of stricter control over the quality of blood and its components. It is impossible to achieve zero risk with blood products. However, blood transfusions have become increasingly safe with advances in testing, production, and storage. Successful blood services depend on legally empowered regulatory services and/or other voluntary standards defined by professional organizations. The voluntary non-governmental organizations (NGOs) working on a nonprofit basis (e.g. Red Cross Society). Blood banks and transfusion services have to comply with state or other regionally defined requirements. The Government has the full responsibility for the blood program.

BLOOD BANK REGULATIONS AND LEGAL FRAMEWORK IN INDIA

Drugs and Cosmetics Act and Rules

Regulatory affairs in the Indian blood banking system are controlled by central and provincial Drug Control Authority under Drug Controller General of India. In order to improve the standards of blood and its components, the Central Government has regulated blood transfusion services in India by the **Drugs and Cosmetics Act, 1940** and its subsequent amendments. Drugs Controller General of India has formulated a comprehensive legislation to ensure better quality control system on collection, storage, testing, and distribution of blood and its components. Ministry of Health and Family Welfare (Department of Health and Family Welfare) New Delhi, on 29th November, 2018 notified in the Drugs and Cosmetics Rules, 1945, in Part X B, that the heading "Blood Banks", should be substituted by "Blood Centers".

Human blood is covered under the definition of "Drug" under Section 3 (b) of Drugs and Cosmetics Act, 1940. Hence, it is imperative that Blood Centers (Banks) need to be **regulated under the Drugs and Cosmetics Act** and rules there under. The Central Government amends the rules from time to time.

National AIDS Control Organization (NACO) acts as a facilitator to Indian blood transfusion services on behalf of the Ministry of Health and Family Welfare, Government of India, especially to the government sector. The National Blood Policy (Refer Chapter 21) was published by the Government of India in 2002 and it provides objectives to provide safe and adequate quantity of blood, blood components, and products.

Under the direction of the Supreme Court, a National Blood Transfusion Council (NBTC) was formed under the Ministry of Health and Family Welfare at Delhi. The NBTC was started with the objective to strengthen the blood bank system in country and to cover the entire blood bank services including voluntary blood donor motivation program, proper storage and utilization of blood, quality control program, education training, and research.

In the year 1967, Central Government (Ministry of Health) enacted a separate provision in Schedule F Part XIIB of Drugs and Cosmetics Rules. This included **various requirements such as accommodation, technical staff, equipment, etc. for operation of blood center** (bank). State Drugs Controllers were authorized to issue the licenses for blood centers (banks). The standards for "Whole Human Blood" were prescribed in Indian Pharmacopoeia.

Due to prevalence of AIDS virus, the Ministry of Health and Family Welfare (Government of India) issued a notification in the year 1989 under the Drugs and Cosmetics Rules and made the **test HIV 1 and 2 antibodies** of Whole Human Blood as mandatory requirement before transfusion. Three laboratories, viz. National Institute of Communicable Disease (NICD), Delhi; National Institute of Virology (NIV), Pune; and Christian Medical College (CMC), Vellore, were notified to function as laboratory under 3A of Drugs and Cosmetics Rules to test HIV antibodies in respect of human blood and human blood products.

The requirement of a blood bank is inserted in Part X-B of the Drugs and Cosmetics Rules, 1945. The rules from 122F to 122P explain the various procedure of making applications by a blood bank, fees to be paid for grant/renewal of license by the applicant and conditions of license to be followed by the applicant after grant/renewal and conditions of license to be followed by the applicant after grant/renewal of license.

As per the Supreme Court order, blood center (bank) legislation was extensively revised on April 5, 1999 to include good manufacturing practices, standard operating procedure and validation of equipment, etc. (refer Chapter 22).

The salient features of the amended Drugs and Cosmetic Rules, 1945 along with the brief requirements for grant/renewal of blood center/bank licences are discussed in this chapter. Tare also discussed.

Part XB: Requirements for the Collection, Storage, Processing, and Distribution of Whole Human Blood, Human Blood Components by Blood Banks, and Manufacture of Blood Products

122-EA. Definitions: (1) In this Part and in the Forms Contained in Schedule A and in Part XIIB and Part XIIC of Schedule F, Unless there is Anything Repugnant in the Subject or Context

a. "Apheresis" means for the process by which blood drawn from a donor, after separating plasma or platelets or leukocytes, is retransfused—simultaneously into the said donor.
b. "Autologous blood" means the blood drawn from the patient for retransfusion unto himself later on.
c. "Blood" means and includes whole human blood, drawn from a donor and mixed with an anticoagulant.
d. "Blood center (bank)" means a place or organization or unit or institution or other arrangements made by such organization, unit or institution for carrying out all or any of the operations for collection, apheresis, storage, processing, and distribution of blood drawn from donors and/or for preparation, storage, and distribution of blood components.
e. "Blood component" means a drug prepared, obtained, derived, or separated from a unit of blood drawn from a donor
f. "Blood product" means a drug manufactured or obtained from pooled plasma

or blood by fractionation, drawn from donors.
g. "Donor" means a person who voluntarily donates blood after he has been declared fit after a medical examination, for donating blood, on fulfilling the criteria given hereinafter, without accepting in return any consideration in cash or kind from any source, but does not include a professional or a paid donor.
h. 'Leucapheresis' means the process by which the blood drawn from a donor, after leukocyte concentrates have been separated, is re-transfused simultaneously into the said donor.
i. 'Plasmapheresis' means the process by which the blood drawn from a donor, after plasma has been separated, is re-transfused during the same sitting into the said donor.
j. 'Plateletpheresis' means the process by which the blood drawn from a donor, after platelet concentrates have been separated, is re-transfused simultaneously into the said donor.
k. 'Professional donor' means a person who donates blood for a valuable consideration, in cash or kind, from any source, on behalf of the recipient – patient and includes a paid donor or a commercial donor.
l. 'Replacement donor' means a donor who is a family friend or a relative of the patient –recipient.

122-F. Form of Application for License for Operation of Blood Bank/Processing of Whole Human Blood for Components/Manufacture or Blood Products for Sale or Distribution

1. Application for the grant and/or renewal of license for the operation of blood bank/processing of human blood for components/manufacture of blood products shall be made to the Licensing Authority appointed under Part VII in Form 27-C or Form 27-E as the case may be and shall be accompanied by license fees of rupees 6,000 and an inspection fees of rupees 1,500 for every inspection thereof or for the purpose of renewal of license.
Provided that if the applicant applies for renewal of license after the expiry but within 6 months of such expiry, the fee payable for the renewal of the license shall be rupees 6,000 and inspection fees of rupees 1,500 plus an additional fees at the rate of rupees 1,000 per month or a part thereof in additional to the inspection fee.
Provided further that a licensee holding a license in Form 28-C or Form 28-E as the case may be for operation of blood bank/processing of whole human blood for components/manufacture of blood products shall apply for grant of license under sub-rule (1) before the expiry of the said license on Form 27-C or Form 27-E as the case may be and he shall continue to operate the same till the orders on his application are communicated to him.
2. A fee of rupees 1,000 shall be paid for a duplicate copy of license issued under this rule, if the original is defaced, damaged, or lost.
3. Application by licensee to manufacture additional drugs listed in the application shall be accompanied by a fee of rupees 300 for each drug listed in the application.
4. On receipt of the application for the grant or renewal of such license, the Licensing Authority shall:
   i. Verify the statements made in the application form.
   ii. Cause the manufacturing and testing establishment to be inspected in accordance with the provisions of rules 122-I; and
   iii. In case, the application is for renewal of license, call for information of past performance of the licensee.
5. If the Licensing Authority is satisfied that the applicant is in position to fulfill the requirements laid down in the rules, he shall prepare a report to that effect and forward it along with the application and the license (in triplicate) to be granted or

renewed, duly completed to the Central License Approving Authority:

Provided that if the Licensing Authority is of the opinion that the applicant is not in a position to fulfill the requirements laid down in these rules, he may, by order, for reason to be recorded in writing, refuse to grant or renew the license, as the case may be.

6. If, on receipt of application and the report of the Licensing Authority referred to in sub-rule 5 and after taking such measures including inspection of the premises, by the inspector, appointed by the Central Government under Section 21 of the Act, and/or along with expert in the field concerned if deemed necessary, the Central License Approving Authority is satisfied that the applicant is in a position to fulfill the requirement laid down in this rule. He may grant or renew the license, as the case may be:

Provided that if the Central License Approving Authority is of the opinion that the applicant is not in a position to fulfill the requirements laid down in these rules he may, notwithstanding the report of the Licensing Authority, by order, for reason to be recorded in the writing, reject the application for grant or renewal of license as the case may be and shall supply the applicant with a copy of the inspection report.

122-G. Form of License for the Operation of a Blood Bank/Processing of Whole Human Blood for Components and Manufacture of Blood Products and the Conditions for the Grant or Renewal of Such License

A license for the operation of a blood bank or for processing whole human blood for components and manufacture of blood products shall be issued in Form 28-C or Form 28-E or Form 26-G or Form 26-I as the case may be. Before a license in Form 28-C or Form-28-E or Form 26-G or Form 26-I, as the case may be, is granted or renewed, the following conditions shall be compiled with by the applicant:

i. The operation of the blood bank and/or processing of whole human blood for components/manufacture of blood product shall be carried out under the active direction and personal supervision of component technical staff consisting of at least one person who is whole-time employee and who is a Medical Officer, and possessing:
   a. Postgraduate degree in Medicine—MD/DNB (Pathology/Transfusion Medicines); or
   b. Degree in Medicine (MBBS) with Diploma in Pathology or Transfusion Medicines having adequate knowledge in blood group serology, blood group methodology, and medical principles involved in the procurement of blood and/or preparation of its components; or
   c. Degree in Medicine (MBBS) having experience in blood bank for 1 year during regular service and also has adequate knowledge and experience in blood group serology, blood group methodology, and medical principles involved in the procurement of blood and/or preparation of its components, the degree or diploma being from a university recognized by the Central Government.

ii. The applicant shall provide adequate space, plant, and equipment for any or all the operations of blood collection or blood processing. The space, plant, and equipment required for various operations are given in Schedule "F", Part XIIB and/or XIIC.

iii. The applicant shall provide and maintain adequate technical staff as specified in Schedule "F", Part XIIB and/or XIIC.

iv. The applicant shall provide adequate arrangements for storage of whole human blood, human blood components, and blood products.

v. The applicant shall furnish to the licensing authority, if required to do so, data on the stability of whole human blood, its components or blood products, which are likely to deteriorate, for fixing the date of expiry, which shall be printed on the labels of such products on the basis of the data so furnished.

122-H. Duration of License

An original license in Form 28-C or Form 28-E or a renewed license in Form 26-G or Form 26-I unless sooner suspended or cancelled shall valid for a period of 5 years and from the date on which the year in which it is granted or renewed.

122-I. Inspection Before Grant or Renewal of License for Operation of Blood Bank, Processing of Whole Human Blood for Components and Manufacture of Blood Products

Before a license in Form 28-C or Form 28-E is granted or a renewal of license in Form 26-G or Form 26-I is made, as the case may be, the Licensing Authority or Central License Approving Authority, as the case may be, shall cause the establishment in which blood bank is proposed to be operated/whole human blood for component is processed/blood products are manufactured to be inspected by one or more inspectors, appointed under the Act and/or along with the expert in the field concerned. The inspector or inspectors shall examine all portions of the premises and appliances/equipment and inspect the process of manufacture intended to be employed or being employed along with the means to be employed or being employed for operation of blood bank/processing of whole human blood for components/manufacture of blood products together with their (testing) facilities and also enquire into the professional qualification of the expert staff and other technical staff to be employed.

122-J. Report by Inspector

The inspector or inspectors shall forward a detailed descriptive report giving his finding on each aspect of inspection along with his recommendation in accordance with the provisions of Rule 122-I to the Licensing Authority or to the Central License Approving Authority.

122-K. Further Application After Rejection

If within a period of 6 months from the rejection of application for a license, the applicant informs the Licensing Authority that the conditions laid down have been satisfied and deposits an inspection fee of rupees 250, the Licensing Authority, if after causing further inspection to be made is satisfied that the conditions for the grant of a license have been complied with, shall grant or renew a license in Form 28-C or Form 28-E:

Provided that in case of drug notified by the Central Government under rule 68-A, the application, together with the inspection report and the form of license (in triplicate to be granted or renewed), duly completed shall be sent to the Central License Approving Authority who may approve the same and return it to the Licensing Authority for issue of the license.

122-L. Delegation of Powers by the Central Licensing Approving Authority

The Central Licensing Approving Authority may, with the approval of the Central Government, by notification, delegate his power of signing licenses and any other power under rules to persons under his control having same qualifications as prescribed for Controlling Authority under Rule 50-A, for such areas and for such periods as may be specified.

122-M. Provision for Appeal to the State Government by a Party Whose License has not been Granted or Renewed

Any person who is aggrieved by the order passed by the Licensing Authority or Central License Approving Authority, as the case may be, may within 30 days from the date of receipt of such order appeal to the State Government or Central Government, as the case may be, after such enquiry, into the matter as it considers necessary and after giving the said person an opportunity for representing his view in the matter may pass such order in relation thereto as it thinks fit.

122-N. Additional Information to be Furnished by an (Applicant) for License or by a Licensee to the Licensing Authority

The applicant for the grant of license or any person granted a license under the part shall, on demand, furnish to the Licensing Authority, before the grant of the license or during the period, the license is in force as, as the case may be, documentary evidence in respect of the ownership or occupation, rental or other basis of the premises, specified in the application for license or in the license granted, constitution of the firm or any other relevant matter, which may be required for the purpose of verifying the correctness of the statement made by the applicant or the licensee, while applying for or after obtaining the license, as the case may be.

122-O. Cancellation and Suspension of Licenses

1. The Licensing Authority or Central License Approving Authority may, for such licenses granted or renewed by him after giving the licensee an opportunity to show cause by such an order should not be passed by an order in writing stating the reason thereof, cancel a license issued under this part or suspend it for such period as he thinks fit, either wholly or in respect of some of the substances to which it relates, [or direct the licensee to stop collection, storage, processing, manufacture, and distribution of the said substances and (thereupon order the destruction of substances and) stocks thereof in the presence of an inspector] if in his opinion, the licensee has failed to comply with any of the conditions of the license or with any provision of the Act or Rules thereunder.
2. A licensee whose license has been suspended or cancelled within 3 months of the date of the order under sub-rule (1) prefers an appeal against that order to the State Government or Central Government, which shall decide the same.

122-P. Conditions of License

A license in Form 28-C, Form 28-E, Form 26-G, or Form 26-I shall be subjected to the special conditions set out in Schedule F, Part XIIB, and Part XIIC, as the case may be, which relate to the substance in respect of which the license is granted or renewed and to the following general conditions, namely:
  i. a. The licensee shall provide and maintain adequate staff, plant, and premises for the proper operation of a blood bank for processing whole human blood, its components, and/or manufacture of blood products.
  b. The licensee shall maintain staff, premises, and equipment as specified in Rule 122-G. The licensee shall maintain necessary records and registers as specified in Schedule F, Parts XIIB, and XIIC.
  c. The licensee shall test in his own laboratory whole human blood, its components, and blood products and (maintain records and) registers in respect of such tests as specified in Schedule F, Part XIIB, and Part XIIC. The records and registers shall be maintained for a period of 5 years from the date of manufacture.
  d. The licensee shall maintain/preserve reference (sample and) supply to the Inspector the reference sample of the whole human blood collected by him in adequate quantity to conduct all the prescribed tests. The licensee shall supply to the Inspector the reference sample for the purpose of testing.
  ii. The licensee shall allow an inspector appointed under the Act to enter, with or (without) prior notice, any premises where the activities of the blood bank are being carried out, for the processing of whole human blood and/or blood products, to inspect the premises and

plant and the process of manufacture and the means employed for standardizing and testing the substance.

iii. The licensee shall allow an Inspector appointed under the Act to inspect all registers and records maintained under these rules and to take samples of the manufactured product and shall supply to Inspector such information as he may require for the purpose of ascertaining whether the provisions of the Act and Rules thereunder have been observed.

iv. The licensee shall from time to time report to the Licensing Authority any changes in the expert staff responsible for the operation of a blood bank/processing of whole human blood for components and/or manufacture of blood products and any material alterations in the premises or plant used for that purpose, which have been made since the date of last inspection made on behalf of the Licensing Authority before the grant of the license.

v. The licensee shall on request furnish to the Licensing Authority, or Central License Approving Authority or to such Authority as the Licensing Authority, or the Central License Approving Authority may direct, from any batch unit of drugs as the Licensing Authority or the Central License Approving may from time to time specify, sample of such quantity as may be considered adequate by such Authority for any examination and, if so required, also furnish full protocols of the test, which have been applied.

vi. If the Licensing Authority or the Central License Approving Authority so directs, the licensee shall not sell or offer for sale any batch/unit in respect of which a sample is, or protocols are furnished under the last preceding subparagraph until a certificate authorizing the sales of batch/unit has been issued to him by or on behalf of the Licensing Authority or the Central License Approving Authority.

vii. The licensee shall, on being informed by the Licensing Authority or the Controlling Authority that any part of any batch/unit of the substance has been found by the Licensing Authority or the Central License Approving Authority not to conform with the standards of strength, quality, or purity specified in these Rules and on being directed so to do so, withdraw from sales and so far as may in the particular circumstances of the case be practicable recall all issues already made from that batch/unit.

viii. No drug manufactured under the license shall be sold unless the precautions necessary for preserving its properties have been observed throughout the period after manufacture. Further, no batch/unit manufactured under this license shall be supplied/distributed to any person without prescription of Registered Medical Practitioner.

ix. The licensee shall comply with the provisions of the Act and of these Rules and with such further requirements, if any, as may be specified in any Rules subsequently made under Chapter IV of the Act, provided that where such further requirements are specified in the Rules, these would come in force 4 months after publication in the Official Gazette.

x. The licensee shall maintain an Inspection Book in Form 35 to enable an Inspector to record his impressions and defects noticed.

xi. The licensee shall destroy the stocks of batch/unit, which does not comply with standard tests in such a way that it would not spread any disease/infection by way of proper disinfection method.

xii. All biomedical waste shall be treated, disposed off, or destroyed as per the provisions of The Bio-Medical Wastes (Management and Handling) Rules, 1996.

xiii. The licensee shall neither collect blood from any professional donor or paid donor nor shall he prepare blood components and/or manufacture blood products from the blood drawn from such a donor.

Various forms used for licensing in blood bank and their purpose are mentioned in Table 25.1.

Table 25.1: Various forms used for licensing in blood bank and their purpose.

Form	Purpose
Form 27-C (See Rule 122-F) (Application for grant or renewal of license)	Application for grant/renewal of license for the operation of a blood bank for processing of whole blood and/or preparation of blood components
Form 28-C (See rule 122-G) (Original license)	License to operate a blood bank for collection, storage, and processing of whole human blood and/or its components for sale or distribution
Form 26-G (See Rule 122-F) (Renewal license)	Certificate of renewal of license to operate a blood bank for processing of whole human blood and/or for preparation for sale or distribution of its components
Form 26-I (See Rule 122-I)	Certificate of renewal of license for manufacture of blood products
Form 27-E (See Rule 122-F)	Application for grant/renewal of license to manufacture blood products for sale or distribution
Form 28-E (See Rule 122-G)	License to manufacture and store blood products for sale or distribution

Part XIIB: Requirements for the Functioning and Operation of a Blood Bank and/or for Preparation of Blood Components

I. Blood Banks/Blood Components

A. General

1. **Location and surroundings:** The blood bank shall be located at a place, which shall be away from open sewage, drain, public lavatory, or similar unhygienic surroundings.
2. **Building:** The building(s), used for operation of a blood bank and/or preparation of blood components, shall be constructed in such a manner so as to permit the operation of the blood bank and preparation of blood components under hygienic conditions and shall avoid the entry of insects, rodents, and flies. It shall be well lighted, ventilated, and screened (mesh), wherever necessary. The walls and floors of the rooms, where collection of blood or preparation of blood components or blood products is carried out, shall be smooth, washable, and capable of being kept clean. Drains shall be of adequate size and, where connected directly to a sewer, shall be equipped with traps to prevent back siphonage.
3. **Health, clothing, and sanitation of staff:** The employees shall be free from contagious or infectious diseases. They shall be provided with clean overalls, headgears, footwears, and gloves, wherever required. There shall be adequate, clean, and convenient handwashing and toilet facilities.

B. Accommodation for a blood bank

A blood bank shall have an area of 100 square meters for its operations and an additional area of 50 square meters for preparation of blood components. It shall be consisting of a room each for:

1. Registration and medical examination with adequate furniture and facilities for registration and selection of donors
2. Blood collection room (air-conditioned)
3. Blood component preparation (this shall be air-conditioned to maintain temperature between 20°–25°C)
4. Laboratory for blood group serology (air-conditioned)
5. Laboratory for blood transmissible diseases like hepatitis, syphilis, malaria, HIV-antibodies (air-conditioned)
6. Sterilization-cum-washing
7. Refreshment-cum-rest room (air-conditioned). Refreshments to the donor after phlebotomy shall be served, so that he is kept under observation in the blood bank.
8. Store-cum-records.

C. Personnel

Every blood bank shall have following categories of whole time competent technical staff:

a. Medical officer, possessing the qualifications specified in condition of rule 122-G.
b. Blood bank technician(s), possessing:
   i. Degree in Medical Laboratory Technology (MLT) with 6 months of experience in the testing of blood and/or its components; or
   ii. Diploma in Medical Laboratory Technology (MLT) with 1 year of experience in the testing of blood and/or its components, the degree or diploma being from a University/Institution recognized by the Central Government or State Government.
c. Registered nurse(s).
d. Technical Supervisor (where blood components are manufactured), possessing:
   i. Degree in Medical Laboratory Technology (MLT) with 6 months of experience in the preparation of blood components; or
   ii. Diploma in Medical Laboratory Technology (MLT) with one year of experience in the preparation of blood components, the degree or diploma being from a University/Institution recognized by the Central Government or State Government.

Staffing pattern: It depends on the workload (Table 25.2).

D. Maintenance

The premises shall be maintained in a clean and proper manner to ensure adequate cleaning and maintenance of proper operations. The facilities shall include:

1. Privacy and thorough examination of individuals to determine their suitability as donors.
2. Collection of blood from donors with minimal risk of contamination or exposure to activities and equipment unrelated to blood collection.
3. Storage of blood or blood components pending completion of tests.
4. Provision for quarantine, storage of blood, and blood components in a designated location, pending repetition of those tests that initially give questionable serological results.
5. Provision for quarantine, storage, handling, and disposal of products and reagents not suitable for use.
6. Storage of finished products prior to distribution or issue.
7. Proper collection, processing, compatibility testing, storage and distribution of blood and blood components to prevent contamination.
8. Adequate and proper performance of all procedures relating to plasmapheresis, plateletpheresis, and leukapheresis.
9. Proper conduct of all packaging, labeling, and other finishing operations.
10. Provision for safe and sanitary disposal of:
    i. Blood and/or blood components not suitable for use, distribution, or sale.
    ii. Trash and items used during the collection, processing, and compatibility

Table 25.2: Staff requirement in blood center/bank for whole blood.

Staff required	Annual blood collection (units)				
	Up to 5,000	Up to 10,000	Up to 20,000	>20,000	>50,000
Medical director/in charge	1	1	1	1	1
Medical personnel	1	2	4	6	10
Counselor	1	2	2	2	3
Nurse	1	1	1	1	2
Senior technical assistant	1	1	1	1	2
Laboratory technologist	3	6	10	12	20
Laboratory attender	1	3	4	4	8

testing of blood and/or blood components.

E. Equipment
Equipment used in the collection, processing, testing, storage, and sale/distribution of blood and its components shall be maintained in a clean and proper manner and so placed as to facilitate cleaning and maintenance. The equipment shall be observed, standardized, and calibrated on a regularly scheduled basis as described in the Standard Operating Procedures Manual and shall operate in the manner for which it was designed so as to ensure compliance with the official requirements (the equipment) as stated below for blood and its components. Equipment that shall be observed, standardized, and calibrated with at least with frequencies mentioned in Table 25.3.

F. Supplies and reagents
All supplies and reagents used in the collection, processing, compatibility, testing, storage, and distribution of blood and blood components

Table 25.3: Equipment and frequency of their calibration.

Sl. No.	Equipment	Performance	Frequency	Frequency of calibration
1.	Temperature recorder	Compare against thermometer	Daily	As often as necessary
2.	Refrigerated centrifuge	Observe speed and temperature	Each day of use	As often as necessary
3.	Hematocrit centrifuge	—	—	Standardize before initial use, after repair or adjustments, and annually
4.	General laboratory centrifuge	—	—	Tachometer (an instrument for measuring the rotation speed), every 6 months
5.	Automated blood typing	Observe controls for correct results	Each day of use	—
6.	Hemoglobinometer	Standardize against cyanmethemoglobin standard	Each day of use	—
7.	Refractometer or urinometer	Standardize against distilled water	Same as above	—
8.	Blood container-weighing device	Standardize against container of known weight	Same as above	As often as necessary
9.	Water bath	Observe temperature	Same as above	Same as above
10.	Rh view box (wherever necessary)	Same as above	Same as above	Same as above
11.	Autoclave	Same as above	Each time of use	Same as above
12.	Serologic rotators	Observe controls for correct results	Each day of use	Speed as often as necessary
13.	Laboratory thermometers	—	—	Before initial use
14.	Electronic thermometers	—	Monthly	—
15.	Blood agitator	Observe weight of the first container of blood filled for correct results	Each day of use	Standardize with container of known mass or volume before initial use, and after repairs or adjustments

shall be stored at proper temperature in a safe and hygienic place, in a proper manner and in particular:

a. All supplies coming and contact with blood and blood components intended for transfusion shall be sterile, pyrogen-free, and shall not interact with the product in such a manner as to have an adverse effect upon the safety, purity, potency, or effectiveness of the product.

b. Supplies and reagents that do not bear an expiry date shall be stored in a manner that the oldest is used first.

c. Supplies and reagents shall be used in a manner consistent with instructions provided by the manufacturer.

d. All final containers and closures for blood and blood components not intended for transfusion shall be clean and free of surface solids and other contaminants.

e. Each blood-collecting container and its satellite container(s), if any, shall be examined visually for damage or evidence of contamination prior to its use and immediately after filling. Such examination shall include inspection for breakage of seals, when indicated, and abnormal discoloration. Where any defect is observed, the container shall not be used or, if detected after filling, shall be properly discarded.

f. Representative samples of each lot of the following reagents and/or solution shall be tested regularly on a scheduled basis (Table 25.4) by methods described in the Standard Operating Procedures Manual to determine their capacity to perform as required.

G. Good manufacturing practices (GMPs)/ standard operating procedures (SOPs)

Written standard operating procedures shall be maintained and shall include all steps to be followed in the collection, processing, compatibility testing, storage, and sale or distribution of blood and/or preparation of blood components for homologous transfusion, autologous transfusion, and further manufacturing purposes. Such procedures shall be available to the personnel for use in the concerned areas. The standard operating procedures shall inter alia include:

1. a. Criteria used to determine donor suitability.
   b. Methods of performing donor-qualifying tests and measurements including minimum and maximum values for a test or procedure, when a factor in determining acceptability
   c. Solutions and methods used to prepare the site of phlebotomy so as to give maximum assurance of a sterile container of blood

Table 25.4: Various reagents and solutions and their frequency of testing with controls.

Reagents and solutions	Frequency of testing along with controls
Antihuman serum	Each day of use
Blood grouping serums	Each day of use
Lectin	Each day of use
Antibody screening and reverse grouping cells	Each day of use
Hepatitis test reagents	Each run
Syphilis serology reagents	Each run
Enzymes	Each day of use
HIV-I and -II reagents	Each run
Normal saline (LISS and PBS)	Each day of use
Bovine albumin	Each day of use

(HIV: human immunodeficiency virus; LISS: low ionic strength saline; PBS: phosphate buffered saline)

d. Method of accurately relating the product(s) to the donor
e. Blood collection procedure, including in-process precautions taken to measure accurately the quantity of blood drawn from the donor
f. Methods of component preparation including, any time restrictions for specific steps in processing
g. All tests and repeat tests performed on blood and blood components during processing
h. Pre-transfusion testing, wherever applicable, including precautions to be taken to identify accurately the recipient blood components during processing
i. Procedures of managing adverse reactions in donor and recipient reactions
j. Storage temperatures and methods of controlling storage temperatures for blood and its components and reagents
k. Length of expiry dates, if any, assigned for all final products
l. Criteria for determining whether returned blood is suitable for reissue
m. Procedures used for relating a unit of blood or blood component from the donor to its final disposal
n. Quality control procedures for supplies and reagents employed in blood collection, processing, and retransfusion testing
o. Schedules and procedures for equipment maintenance and calibration
p. Labeling procedures to safeguard its mix-ups, receipt, issue, rejected and in-hand
q. Procedures of plasmapheresis, plateletpheresis, and leukapheresis, if performed, including precautions to be taken to ensure reinfusion of donor's own cells
r. Procedures for preparing recovered (salvaged) plasma, if performed, including details of separation, pooling, labeling, storage, and distribution.
s. All records pertinent to the lot or unit maintained pursuant to these regulations shall be reviewed before the release or distribution of a lot or unit of final product. The review or portions of the review may be performed at appropriate periods during or after blood collection, processing, testing, and storage. A thorough investigation, including the conclusions and follow-up, of any unexplained discrepancy or the failure of a lot or unit to meet any of its specification shall be made and recorded.
2. A licensee may utilize current standard operating procedures, such as the manuals of the following organizations, so long as such specific procedures are consistent with, and at least as stringent as, the requirements contained in this part, namely:
   a. Directorate General of Health Services manual
   b. Other organizations or individual blood bank's manuals, subject to the approval of State Licensing Authority and Central License Approving Authority.

H. Criteria for blood donation
Conditions for donation of blood

1. **General:** No person shall donate blood and no blood bank shall draw blood from a person, more than once in 3 months. The donor shall be in good health, mentally alert, and physically fit and shall not be inmates of jail, persons having multiple sex partners and drug addicts. The donors shall fulfill the following requirements, namely:
   a. The donor shall be in the age group of 18–60 years.
   b. The donor shall not be less than 45 kilograms.
   c. Temperature and pulse of the donor shall be normal.
   d. The systolic and diastolic blood pressures are within normal limits without medication.
   e. Hemoglobin, which shall not be less than 12.5 grams.
   f. The donor shall be free from acute respiratory diseases.

g. The donor shall be free from any skin diseases at the site of phlebotomy.
h. The donor shall be free from any disease transmissible by blood transfusion, insofar as can be determined by history and examination indicated above.
i. The arms and forearms of the donor shall be free from skin punctures or scars indicative of professional blood donors or addiction of self-injected narcotics.
2. **Additional qualifications of a donor**: No person shall donate blood, and no blood bank shall draw blood from a donor, in the conditions mentioned in Table 25.5 before the expiry of the period of deferment.
3. No person shall donate blood and no blood bank shall draw blood from a person, suffering from any of the diseases mentioned in Box 25.1.

I. General equipment and instruments
1. **For blood collection room (Box 25.2)**
2. **For hemoglobin determination (Box 25.3)**
3. **For temperature and pulse determination (Box 25.4)**
4. **For blood containers:**
   a. Only disposable polyvinyl chloride (PVC) blood bags shall be used (closed system) as per the specifications of IP/USP/BP.

Box 25.1: Diseases that contraindicate donation of blood.

- Cancer
- Heart disease
- Abnormal bleeding tendencies
- Unexplained weight loss
- Diabetes—controlled on insulin
- Hepatitis infection
- Chronic nephritis
- Signs and symptoms, suggestive of AIDS
- Liver disease
- Tuberculosis
- Polycythemia vera
- Asthma
- Epilepsy
- Leprosy
- Schizophrenia
- Endocrine disorders

Box 25.2: Equipment required for blood collection room.

- Donor beds, chairs, and tables: These shall be suitably and comfortably cushioned and shall be of appropriate size
- Bedside table
- Sphygmomanometer and stethoscope
- Recovery beds for donors
- Refrigerators, for storing separately tested and untested blood, maintaining temperature between 2°C and 6°C with digital dial thermometer, recording thermograph and alarm device, with provision for continuous power supply.
- Weighing devices for donor and blood containers

Table 25.5: Deferment of blood donation.

Conditions	Period of deferment
Abortions	6 months
History of blood transfusion	6 months
Surgery	12 months
Typhoid	12 months after recovery
History of malaria and duly treated	3 months (endemic) 3 years (nonendemic area)
Tattoo	6 months
Breastfeeding	12 months after delivery
Immunization (cholera, typhoid, diphtheria, tetanus, plague, gamma globulin)	15 days
Rabies vaccination	1 year after vaccination
History of hepatitis in family or close contact	12 months
Immunoglobulin	12 months

> **Box 25.3:** Equipment required for hemoglobin determination.
>
> - Copper sulfate solution (specific gravity 1.053)
> - Sterile lancet and impregnated alcohol swabs
> - Capillary tube (1.3–1.4 × 65/96 mm or Pasteur pipettes)
> - Rubber bulbs for capillary tubing
> - Sahli's hemoglobinometer/colorimetric method

> **Box 25.4:** Equipment required for temperature and pulse determination.
>
> - Clinical thermometers
> - Equipment and materials for aseptic cleaning of the thermometer
> - Watch (fitted with a seconds-hand needle) and a stopwatch

b. Anticoagulants: The anticoagulant solution shall be sterile, pyrogen-free, and of the following composition that will ensure satisfactory safety and efficacy of the whole blood and/or for all the separated blood components.
   - Citrate phosphate dextrose adenine (CPDA) solution or citrate phosphate dextrose adenine-1 (CPDA-1)—14 mL solution shall be required for 100 mL of blood.

Note 1:
- In case of single/double/triple/quadruple blood collection bags used for blood component preparations, CPDA blood collection bags may be used.
- Acid citrate dextrose solution (ACD with Formula-A). IP—15 mL. Solution shall be required for 100 mL of blood.
- Additive solutions such as SAGM (saline, adenine, glucose, and mannitol), ADSOL (adenine, dextrose, sorbitol, sodium chloride and mannitol), and NUTRICEL may be used for storing and retaining red blood corpuscles up to 42 days.

Note 2:
The licensee shall ensure that the anticoagulant solutions are of a licensed manufacturer and the blood bags in which the said solutions are contained have a certificate of analysis of the said manufacturer.

5. **Emergency equipment/items (Box 25.5)**
6. **Accessories (Box 25.6)**
7. **Laboratory equipment (Box 25.7)**

J. Special reagents
1. Standard blood grouping sera Anti-A, Anti-B, and Anti-D with known controls. Rh typing sera shall be in double quantity and each of different brands or if from the same, supplier each supply shall be of different lot numbers.
2. Reagents for serological tests for syphilis and positive sera for controls.
3. Antihuman globulin serum (Coombs' serum)
4. Bovine albumin 22% enzyme reagents for incomplete antibodies.
5. Enzyme-linked immunosorbent assay (ELISA) or reversed passive hemagglutination (RPHA) test kits for hepatitis and HIV-I and -II.
6. Detergent and other agents for cleaning laboratory glassware.

> **Box 25.5:** Emergency equipment/items required.
>
> - Oxygen cylinder with mask, gauge, and pressure regulator
> - About 5% glucose or normal saline
> - Disposable sterile syringes and needles of various sizes
> - Disposable sterile IV infusion sets
> - Ampoules of adrenaline, noradrenaline, mephentine, betamethasone or dexamethasone, and metoclopramide injections
> - Aspirin and spirit ammonia aromatic

> **Box 25.6:** Accessories required.
>
> - Such as blankets, emesis basins, hemostats, set clamps, sponge forceps, mouth gauze, dressing jars, solution jars, and waste cans
> - Medium cotton balls, 1.25 cm adhesive tapes
> - Denatured spirit, tincture iodine, green soap or liquid soap and injection of procaine or xylocaine
> - Paper napkins or towels
> - Autoclave with temperature and pressure indicator
> - Incinerator
> - Standby generator

> **Box 25.7:** Laboratory equipment required in blood bank/center.
>
> - Refrigerators, for storing diagnostic kits and reagents, maintaining a temperature between 4°C and 6°C (plus/minus 2°C) with digital dial recording thermometer having provision for continuous power supply. The refrigerator shall have temperature recording and alarm device
> - Compound microscope with low- and high-power objectives
> - Centrifuge table model
> - Water bath—having range between 37°C and 56°C
> - Rh-viewing box in case of slide technique
> - Incubator with thermostatic control
> - Mechanical shakers for serological tests for syphilis
> - Hand-lens for observing tests conducted in tubes
> - Serological graduated pipettes of various sizes
> - Pipettes (Pasteur)
> - Glass slides
> - Test tubes of various sizes/micrometer plates (U or V type)
> - Precipitating tubes 6 mm × 50 mm of different sizes and glass beakers of different sizes
> - Test tube racks of different specifications
> - Interval timer electric or spring wound
> - Equipment and materials for cleaning glasswares adequately
> - Insulated containers for transporting blood, between 2°C and 10°C temperatures, to wards and hospitals
> - Wash bottles; filter papers
> - Dielectric tube sealer
> - Plain and EDTA vials
> - Chemical balance (wherever necessary)
> - ELISA reader, washer and micropipettes for HIV-antibodies testing (in case HIV-antibodies testing is done by ELISA kits).
> - RPHA/ELISA test kits with reader for hepatitis
> - Shipping containers
> - Ice box for transport of blood units
> - Hot air oven

(EDTA: ethylenediaminetetraacetic acid; ELISA: enzyme-linked immunosorbent assay; RPHA: reversed passive hemagglutination)

K. Testing of whole blood

1. It shall be responsibility of the licensee to ensure that the whole blood collected, processed, and supplied conforms to the standards laid down in the Indian Pharmacopoeia and other tests published, if any, by the government.
2. Freedom from HIV antibodies (AIDS) tests: Every licensee shall get samples of every blood unit tested, before use, for freedom from HIV-I and HIV-II antibodies either from laboratories specified for the purpose by the Central Government or in his own laboratory. The results of such testing shall be recorded on the label of the container.
3. Each blood unit shall also be tested for freedom from hepatitis B surface antigen, and hepatitis C virus antibody VDRL (Venereal Disease Research Laboratory) and malarial parasite, and results of such testing shall be recorded on the label of the container.

Note:
- Blood samples of donors in pilot tube and the blood samples of the recipient shall be preserved for 7 days after issue.
- The blood intended for transfusion shall not be frozen at any stage.
- Blood containers shall not come directly in contact with ice at any stage.

L. Records

The records which the licensee is required to maintain shall include inter alia the following particulars, namely:

1. **Blood donor record:** It shall indicate serial number, date of bleeding, name, address, and signature of donor with other particulars of age, weight, hemoglobin, blood grouping, blood pressure, medical

examination, bag number, and patient's detail for whom donated in case of replacement donation, category of donation (voluntary/replacement) and deferral records, and signature of Medical Officer in-charge.
2. **Master records for blood and its components:** It shall indicate bag serial number, date of collection, date of expiry, and quantity in mL. ABO/Rh group, results for testing of HIV-I and HIV-II antibodies, malaria, VDRL, hepatitis B surface antigen and hepatitis C virus antibody, and irregular antibodies (if any), name and address of the donor with particulars, utilization issue number, components prepared or discarded, and signature of the Medical Officer in-charge.
3. **Issue register:** It shall indicate serial number, date and time of issue, bag serial number, ABO/Rh group, total quantity in mL, name and address of the recipient, group of recipients, unit/institution, details of cross-matching report, and indication for transfusion.
4. **Records of components supplied:** Quantity supplied; compatibility report, details of recipient and signature of issuing person.
5. **Records of ACD/CPD/CPDA/SAGM bags** giving details of manufacturer, batch number, date of supply, and results of testing.
6. **Register for diagnostic kits and reagents used:** Name of the kits/reagents, details of batch number, date of expiry, and date of use.
7. **Blood bank must issue the cross-matching report** of the blood to the patient together with the blood unit.
8. **Transfusion adverse reaction records.**
9. **Records of purchase, use, and stock** in hand of disposable needles, syringes, blood bags shall be maintained.

Note: The above said records shall be kept by the licensee for a period of 5 years.

M. Labels

The labels on every bag containing blood and/or component shall contain the following particulars, namely:

1. The proper name of the product in a prominent place and in bold letters on the bag
2. Name and address of the blood bank
3. License number
4. Serial number
5. The date on which the blood is drawn and the date of expiry as prescribed under Schedule P to these rules.
6. A colored label shall be put on every bag containing blood. The color scheme for the labels used for different groups of blood is presented in Table 25.6.
7. The results of the tests for hepatitis B surface antigen, and hepatitis C virus antibody, syphilis, freedom from HIV-I and HIV-II antibodies and malarial parasite.
8. The Rh group
9. Total volume of blood, the preparation of blood, and nature and percentage of anticoagulant
10. Keep continuously temperature at 2–6°C for whole human blood and/or components as contained under III of Part XIIB.
11. Disposable transfusion sets with filter shall be used in administration of equipment
12. Appropriate compatible cross-matched blood without a typical antibody in recipient shall be used.
13. The contents of the bag shall not be used, if there is any visible evidence of deterioration like hemolysis, clotting, or discoloration.
14. The label shall indicate the appropriate donor classification like "Voluntary Donor" or "Replacement Donor" in no less prominence than the proper name.

Table 25.6: Blood group and corresponding color of label.

Blood group	Color of the label
O	Blue
A	Yellow
B	Pink
AB	White

Notes:
- In the case of blood components, particulars of the blood from which such components have been prepared shall be given against item numbers (5), (7), (8), (9), and (14).
- The blood and/or its components shall be distributed on the prescription of a Registered Medical Practitioner.

II. Blood Donation Camps

A blood donation camp may be organized by:
a. A licensed designated Regional Blood Transfusion center; or
b. A licensed Government Blood Bank; or
c. The Indian Red Cross Society; or
d. A licensed blood bank run by registered voluntary or charitable organizations recognized by State or Union Territory Blood Transfusion Council.

Note:
- "Designated Regional Blood Transfusion center" shall be a center approved and designated by a Blood Transfusion Council constituted by a State Government to collect, process, and distribute blood and its components to cater to the needs of the region and that center has also been licensed and approved by the Licensing Authority and Central License Approving Authority for the purpose.
- The designated Regional Blood Transfusion center, Government Blood Bank, and Indian Red Cross Society shall intimate within a period of 7 days, the venue where blood camp was held and details of group-wise blood units collected in the said camp to the Licensing Authority and Central License Approving Authority.

Requirements for holding a blood donation camp

For holding a blood donation camp, the following requirements shall be fulfilled/complied with, namely:

A. *Premises, personnel, etc.*
   a. Premises under the blood donation camp shall have sufficient area and the location shall be hygienic so as to allow proper operation, maintenance, and cleaning.
   b. All information regarding the personnel working, equipment used, and facilities available at such a camp shall be well documented and made available for inspection, if required, and ensuring:
      i. Continuous and uninterrupted electrical supply for equipment used in the camp
      ii. Adequate lighting for all the required activities
      iii. Handwashing facilities for staff
      iv. Reliable communication system to the central office of the controller/organizer of the camp
      v. Furniture and equipment arranged within the available place
      vi. Refreshment facilities for donors and staff
      vii Facilities for medical examination of the donors
      viii. Proper disposal of waste.

B. *Personnel for outdoor blood donation camp*
To collect blood from 50–70 donors in about 3 hours or from 100–120 donors in 5 hours, the following requirements shall be fulfilled/complied with:
i. One medical officer and two nurses or phlebotomists for managing 6–8 donor tables
ii. Two medicosocial workers
iii. Three blood bank technicians
iv. Two attendants
v. Vehicle having a capacity to seat 8–10 persons, with provision for carriage of donation goods including facilities to conduct a blood donation camp.

C. *Equipment (Box 25.8)*

III. Processing of Blood Components from Whole Blood by a Blood Bank

The blood components shall be prepared by blood banks as a part of the blood bank services. The conditions for grant or renewal of license to prepare blood components shall be as follows:

Transfusion Regulation and Legislation

Box 25.8: List of equipment needed for conducting blood donation camps.

1. BP apparatus
2. Stethoscope
3. Blood bags (single, double, triple, and quadruple)
4. Donor questionnaire
5. Weighing device for donors
6. Weighing device for blood bags
7. Artery forceps and scissors
8. Stripper for blood tubing
9. Bedsheets, blankets/mattress
10. Lancets, swab stick/toothpicks
11. Glass slides
12. Portable Hb meter/copper sulfate
13. Test tube (big) and 12 mm × 100 mm (small)
14. Test tube stand
15. Anti-A, anti-B and anti-AB, antisera, and anti-D
16. Test tube sealer film
17. Medicated adhesive tape
18. Plastic waste basket
19. Donor cards and refreshment for donors
20. Emergency medical kit
21. Insulated blood bag containers with provisions for storing between 2°C and 10°C
22. Dielectric sealer or portable sealer
23. Needle destroyer (wherever necessary)

A. Accommodation

1. Rooms with adequate area and other specifications, for preparing blood components depending on quantum of workload shall be as specified in item B under the heading "*1. Blood Banks/Blood Components (page 545)*" of this part.
2. Preparation of blood components shall be carried out only under closed system using single, double, triple, or quadruple plastic bags except for preparation of red blood cells concentrates, where single bags may be used with transfer bags.

B. Equipment

1. Air conditioner
2. Laminar air flow bench
3. Suitable refrigerated centrifuge
4. Plasma expresser
5. Clipper and clips and/or dielectric sealer
6. Weighing device
7. Dry rubber balancing material
8. Artery forceps, scissors
9. Refrigerator maintaining a temperature between 2°C and 6°C, a digital dial thermometer with recording thermograph and alarm device, with provision for continuous power supply
10. Platelet agitator with incubator (wherever necessary)
11. Deep freezers maintaining a temperature between −30 to −40°C and −75 to −80°C
12. Refrigerated water bath for plasma thawing
13. Insulated blood bag containers with provisions for storing at appropriate temperature for transport purposes.

C. Personnel

The whole time competent technical staff meant for processing of blood components (that is Medical Officer, Technical Supervisor, Blood Bank Technician, and Registered Nurse) shall be as specified in item C, under the heading "I. BLOOD BANKS/BLOOD COMPONENTS" of this part.

D. Testing facilities

General: Facilities for A, B, AB, and O groups and Rh (D) grouping.

Hepatitis B surface antigen and hepatitis C virus antibody, VDRL, HIV-I and HIV-II antibodies, and malarial parasites shall be mandatory for every blood unit before it is used for the preparation of blood components. The results of such testing shall be indicated on the label.

E. Categories of Blood Components

1. Concentrated human red blood corpuscles:

The product shall be known as "packed red blood cells" that is packed red blood cells remaining after separating plasma from human blood.

General requirements:
a. Storage: Immediately after processing, the packed red blood cells shall be kept at a temperature maintained between 2°C and 6°C.
b. Inspection: The component shall be inspected immediately after separation of the plasma, during storage, and again at

the time of issue. The product shall not be issued, if there is any abnormality in color or physical appearance or any indication of microbial contamination.

c. Suitability of donor: The source blood for packed red blood cells shall be obtained from a donor who meets the criteria for blood donation as specified in item H under the heading "*1. Blood Banks/ Blood Components (page 545)*" of this part.

d. Testing of whole blood: Blood from which packed red blood cells are prepared shall be tested as specified in item K relating to testing of whole blood under the heading "*1. Blood Banks/Blood Components (page 545)*" of this part.

e. Pilot samples: Pilot samples collected in integral tubing or in separate pilot tubes shall meet the following specifications:
   i. One or more pilot samples of either the original blood or of the packed red blood cells being processed shall be preserved with each unit of packed red blood cells, which is issued.
   ii. Before they are filled, all pilot sample tubes shall be marked or identified so as to relate them to the donor of that unit or packed red blood cells.
   iii. Before the final container is filled or at the time the final product is prepared, the pilot sample tubes accompanying a unit of packed red blood cells shall be attached in a tamper-proof manner that shall conspicuously identify removal and reattachment.
   iv. All pilot sample tubes, accompanying a unit of packed red blood cells, shall be filled immediately after the blood is collected or at the time the final product is prepared, in each case, by the person who performs the collection of preparation.

f. Processing:
   i. Separation: Packed red blood cells shall be separated from the whole blood—
      a. If the whole blood is stored in ACD solution within 21 days, and
      b. If the whole blood is stored in CPDA-1 solution, within 35 days, from the date of collection. Packed red blood cells may be prepared either by centrifugation done in a manner that shall not tend to increase the temperature of the blood or by normal undisturbed sedimentation method. A portion of the plasma, sufficient to ensure optimal cell preservation, shall be left with the packed red blood cells.
   ii. Packed red blood cells frozen: Cryophylactic substance may be added to the packed red blood cells for extended manufacturer's storage not warmer than −65°C provided the manufacturer submits data to the satisfaction of the Licensing Authority and Central License Approving Authority, as adequately demonstrating through invivo cells survival and other appropriate tests that the addition of the substance, the material used, and the processing methods results in a final product meets the required standards of safety, purity and potency for packed red blood cells, and that the frozen product shall maintain those properties for the specified expiry period.
   – Testing: Packed red blood cells shall conform to the standards as laid down in the Indian Pharmacopoeia.

2. Platelets concentrate

The product shall be known as "platelets concentrates" that is platelets collected from one unit of blood and resuspended in an appropriate volume of original plasma.

General requirements:
i. Source:
   The source material for platelets shall be platelet-rich plasma or buffy coat, which may be obtained from the whole blood or by plateletpheresis.

ii. Processing:
   a. Separation of buffy coat or platelet-rich plasma and platelets and resuspension of the platelets shall be in a closed system by centrifugal method with appropriate speed, force, and time.
   b. Immediately after collection, the whole blood or plasma shall be held in storage between 20°C and 24°C. When it is to be transported from the venue of blood collection to the processing laboratory, during such transport action, the temperature as close as possible to a range between 20°C and 24°C shall be ensured. The platelet concentrates shall be separated within 6 hours after the time of collection of the unit of whole blood or plasma.
   c. The time and speed of centrifugation shall be demonstrated to produce an unclamped product, without visible hemolysis, that yields a count of not less than 3.5×10^{10} (3.5×10 raised to the power of 10) and 4.5×10^{10} (4.5×10 raised to the power ten), i.e. platelets per unit from a unit of 350 mL and 450 mL blood, respectively. 1% of total platelets prepared shall be tested of which 75% of the units shall conform to the above said platelet count.
   d. The volume of original plasma used for resuspension of the platelets shall be determined by the maintenance of the pH of not less than 6 during the storage period. The pH shall be measured on a sample of platelets, which has been stored for the permissible maximum expiry period at 20–24°C.
   e. Final containers used for platelets shall be colorless and transparent to permit visual inspection of the contents. The caps selected shall maintain a hermetic seal to prevent contamination of the contents. The container material shall not interact with the contents, under the normal conditions of the storage and use, in such a manner as to have an adverse effect upon the safety, purity, potency, or efficacy of the product. At the time of filling, the final container shall be marked or identified by number so as to relate it to the donor.
iii. Storage: Immediately after resuspension, platelets shall be placed in storage not exceeding for a period of 5 days, between 20°C and 24°C, with continuous gentle agitation of the platelet concentrates maintained throughout such storage.
iv. Testing: The units prepared from different donors shall be tested at the end of the storage period for:
   a. Platelet count
   b. pH of not less than 6 measured at the storage temperature of the unit
   c. Measurement of actual plasma volume
   d. One percent of the total platelets prepared shall be tested for sterility
   e. The tests for functional viability of the platelets shall be done by swirling movement before issue
   f. If the results of the testing indicate that the product does not meet the specified requirements, immediate corrective action shall be taken and records maintained.
v. Compatibility test: Compatible transfusion for the purpose of variable number of red blood cells, A, B, AB, and O grouping shall be done, if the platelets concentrate is contaminated with red blood cells.

3. Granulocyte concentrates
a. Storage: It shall be kept between 20°C and 24°C for a maximum period of 24 hours.
b. Unit of granulocytes shall not be less than 1×10^{10} (i.e. 1×10 raised to the power of 10) when prepared on cell separator.
c. Group specific tests/HLA test wherever required shall be carried out.

4. Fresh frozen plasma
Plasma frozen within 6 hours after blood collection and stored at a temperature not warmer than –30°C shall be preserved for a period of not more than 1 year.

5. Cryoprecipitate
Concentrate of antihemophiliac factor shall be prepared by thawing of the fresh plasma frozen stored at –30°C.

a. Storage: Cryoprecipitate shall be preserved at a temperature not higher than −30°C and may be preserved for a period of not more than 1 year from the date of collection.
b. Activity: Antihemophiliac factor activity in the final product shall be not less than 80 units per bag. 1% of the total cryoprecipitate prepared shall be tested of which 75% of the unit shall conform to the said specification.

f. Plasmapheresis, plateletpheresis, leukapheresis using a cell separator

An area of 10 square meters shall be provided for apheresis in the blood bank. The blood banks specifically permitted to undertake the said apheresis on the donor shall observe the criteria as specified in item H relating to criteria for blood donation under the heading "*1. Blood Banks/Blood Components (page 545)*" of this part. The written consent of the donor shall be taken and the donor must be explained, the hazards of apheresis. The Medical Officer shall certify that donor is fit for apheresis and it shall be carried out by a trained person under supervision of the Medical Officer.

1. Plasmapheresis, platelet apheresis, and leukapheresis

The donors subjected to plasmapheresis, platelet apheresis, and leukapheresis shall, in addition to the criteria specified in item H relating to the criteria for blood donation under the heading "I. BLOOD BANKS/BLOOD COMPONENTS" of this part being observed, be also subjected to protein estimation on postapheresis/first sitting whose results shall be taken as a reference for subsequent apheresis/sitting. It shall also be necessary that the total plasma obtained from such donor and periodicity of plasmapheresis shall be according to the standards described under validated standard operating procedures.

Note:
- At least 48 hours must elapse between successive apheresis and not more than twice in a week.
- Extracorporeal blood volume shall not exceed 15% of donor's estimated blood volume.
- Platelet apheresis shall not be carried out on donors who have taken medication containing aspirin within 3 days prior to donation.
- If during plateletpheresis or leukapheresis, RBCs cannot be retransfused then at least 12 weeks shall elapse before a second cytapheretic procedure is conducted.

2. Monitoring for apheresis

Before starting apheresis procedure, hemoglobin or hematocrit shall be done. Platelet count, WBC counts, and differential count may be carried out. In repeated plasmapheresis, the serum protein shall be 6 g/100 mL.

3. Collection of plasma

The quantity of plasma separated from the blood of a donor shall not exceed 500 mL per sitting and once in a fortnight or shall not exceed 1,000 mL per month.

Part XIIC: I. Requirements for Manufacture of Blood Products

The blood products shall be manufactured in a separate premise other than that meant for blood bank. The requirements that are essential for grant or renewal of license to manufacture blood products, such as albumin, plasma protein fraction, immunoglobins, and coagulation factor concentrates, shall be as follows, namely:

A. General Requirements

1. Location and surroundings, buildings, and water supply

The requirements as regards location and surrounding, buildings and water supply as contained in paragraphs 1.1.1, 1.1.2, and 1.1.3 of Part I of Schedule M, shall apply mutatis mutandis to the manufacture of blood products.

2. Disposal of waste and infectious materials

i. The requirement as regards disposal of waste and infectious materials as contained in paragraph 1.1.4 of Part I of Schedule M shall apply mutatis mutandis to the manufacture of blood products.

ii. Proper facility shall also be provided for potentially infectious materials, particularly HIV-I and HIV-II, hepatitis B (surface antigen and hepatitis C virus antibody) through autoclaving, incineration, or any other suitable validated methods.

3. Health, clothing, and sanitation of personnel

i. The requirement as contained in paragraph 3 of Part I of Schedule M shall be complied with.

ii. The personnel working in the manufacturing areas shall be vaccinated against hepatitis B virus and other infectious transmitting diseases.

4. Requirements for manufacturing area for blood products

i. For the manufacture of blood products, separate enclosed areas specifically designed for the purpose shall be provided. These areas be provided with air locks for entry and shall be essentially dust free and ventilated with an air supply. Air supply for manufacturing area shall be filtered through bacteria retaining filters (HEPA filters) and shall be at a pressure higher than in the adjacent areas.

The filters shall be checked for performance on installation and periodically thereafter, and records thereof shall be maintained.

ii. Interior surfaces (walls, floors, and ceilings) shall be smooth and free from cracks; they shall not shed matter and shall permit easy cleaning and disinfection. Drains shall be excluded from aseptic areas.

Routine microbial counts of the manufacturing area shall be carried out during manufacturing operations. The results of such counts shall be checked against well-documented in-house standards and records maintained.

Access to the manufacturing areas shall be restricted to a minimum number of authorized personnel. Special procedures for entering and leaving of the manufacturing areas shall be prominently displayed.

iii. Sinks shall be excluded from aseptic areas. Any sink installed in other clean areas shall be of suitable material such as stainless steel, without an overflow, and be supplied with water of potable quality. Adequate precautions shall be taken to avoid contamination of the drainage system with dangerous effluents and airborne dissemination of pathogenic microorganisms.

iv. Lighting, air-conditioning, and ventilation shall be designed to maintain a satisfactory temperature and relative humidity to minimize contamination and to take account of the comfort of personnel working with protective clothing.

v. Premises used for the manufacture of blood products shall be suitably designed and constructed to facilitate good sanitation.

vi. Premises shall be carefully maintained and it shall be ensured that repair and maintenance operations do not present any hazard to the quality of products. Premises shall be cleaned and, where applicable, disinfected according to detailed written validated procedures.

vii. Adequate facilities and equipment shall be used for the manufacture of blood products derived from blood plasma.

viii. All containers of blood products, regardless of the stage of manufacture, shall be identified by securely attached labels. Cross-contamination shall be prevented by adoption of the following measures, namely:

a. Processing and filling shall be in segregated L areas
b. Manufacture of different products at the same time shall be avoided
c. Simultaneous filling of the different products shall be avoided

d. Ensure transfer, containers/materials by means of airlocks, air extraction, clothing change and careful washing, and decontamination of equipment
e. Protecting containers/materials against the risk of contamination caused by recirculation of untreated air or by accidental re-entry of extracted air
f. Using containers that are sterilized or are of documented low "bioburden".
ix. Positive pressure area shall be dedicated to the processing area concerned
x. Air-handling units shall be dedicated to the processing area concerned
xi. Pipe work, valves, and vent filters shall be properly designed to facilitate cleaning and sterilization. Valves on fractionation/reacting vessels shall be completely steam-sterilizable. Air vent filters shall be hydrophobic and shall be validated for their designated use.

5. Ancillary areas
i. Rest and refreshment rooms shall be separated from other areas.
ii. Facilities for changing and storing clothes and for washing and toilet purposes shall be easily accessible and appropriate for the number of users. Toilets shall not be connected directly with production or storage areas.
iii. Maintenance workshops shall be separated from production areas. Wherever parts and tools are stored in the production area, they shall be kept in rooms or lockers reserved for that use.
iv. Animal houses shall be well isolated from other areas, with separate entrance.

5. Collection and Storage of Plasma for Fractionation

A. Collection
1. Plasma shall be collected from the licensed blood banks through a cold chain process and stored in frozen condition not warmer than −20°C
2. Individual plasma shall remain in quarantine till it is tested for hepatitis B surface antigen and hepatitis C virus antibody HIV-I and HIV-II.
3. A sample from pooled -lot plasma of about 10–12 units of different donors shall be tested for hepatitis B surface antigen and hepatitis C virus antibody, HIV-I and HIV-II, and, if the sample found negative, only then it shall be taken up for fractionation.

B. Storage area
1. Storage areas shall be of sufficient space and capacity to allow orderly storage of the various categories of materials, intermediates, bulk and finished products, products in quarantine, released, rejected, returned, or recalled products.
2. Storage areas shall be designed or adopted to ensure good storage conditions. In particular, they shall be clean, dry, and maintained within temperature required for such storage and where special storage conditions are required (e.g. temperature and humidity); these shall be provided, checked, and monitored.
3. Receiving and dispatch bays shall protect materials and products from the weather and shall be designed and equipped to allow containers of incoming materials to be cleaned, if necessary, before storage.
4. Where quarantine status is ensured by storage in separate areas, these areas shall be clearly marked and their access restricted only to authorized personnel.
5. There shall be separate sampling area for raw materials. If sampling is performed in the storage area, it shall be conducted in such a way so as to prevent contamination or cross-contamination.
6. Segregation shall be provided for the storage of rejected, recalled, or returned materials or products.
7. Adequate facility shall be provided for supply of ancillary material, such as ethanol, water, salts, and polyethylene glycol. Separate facilities shall be provided for the recovery of organic solvents used in fractionation.

C. Personnel

1. Manufacture

The manufacture of blood products shall be conducted under the active direction and personal supervision of competent technical staff, consisting of at least one person who shall be a whole-time employee, with 1-year practical experience in the manufacture of blood products/plasma fractionation and possesses:

a. Postgraduate degree in Medicine—MD (Microbiology/Pathology/Bacteriology/Immunology/Biochemistry); or
b. Postgraduate degree in Science (Microbiology); or
c. Postgraduate degree in Pharmacy (Microbiology), from a recognized University or Institution.

2. Testing

The head of the testing unit shall be independent of the manufacturing unit and testing shall be conducted under the active direction and personal supervision of competent technical staff consisting at least one person who shall be a whole-time employee. The head of the testing unit shall have 18 months practical experience in the testing of drugs especially the blood products and possesses:

a. Postgraduate degree in Pharmacy or Science—(Chemistry/Microbiology/Biochemistry); or
b. Postgraduate degree in Medicine—MD (Microbiology/Pathology/Biochemistry), from a recognized University or Institution.

D. Production control

1. The production area and the viral inactivation room shall be centrally air-conditioned and fitted with HEPA filters having Grade C (Class 10,000) environment as given in the Table 25.7.
2. The filling and sealing shall be carried out under aseptic conditions in centrally air-conditioned areas fitted with HEPA filters having Grade A or, as the case may be, grade B (Class 100) environment as given in Table 25.6.
3. The physical and chemical operations used for the manufacture of plasma fractionation shall maintain high yield of safe and effective protein.
4. The fractionation procedure used shall give a good yield of products meeting the in-house quality requirements as approved by the Licensing Authority and Central License Approving Authority reducing the risk of microbiological contamination and protein denaturation to the minimum.
5. The procedure adopted shall not affect the antibody activity and biological half-life or biological characteristics of the products.

E. Viral inactivation process

The procedure used by the licensee to inactivate the pathogenic organisms such as enveloped and nonenveloped virus, especially infectivity from HIV-I and HIV-II, hepatitis B surface antigens, and hepatitis C virus antibody—the viral inactivation and validation methods adopted by the licensee, shall be submitted

Table 25.7: Air classification system for manufacture of sterile products. Maximum number of particles permitted per m^3.

Grade	Maximum number of particles permitted per m^3		Maximum number of viable microorganisms permitted per m^3
	0.5–5 micron	Less than 5 microns	
A (Class 100) (Laminar-airflow workstation)	3,500	None	Less than 1
B (Class 100)	3,500	None	Less than 5
C (Class 10000)	350,000	2,000	Less than 100

for approval to the Licensing Authority and Central License Approving Authority.

Notes:
1. No preservative (except stabilizer, to prevent protein denaturation such as glycine, sodium chloride, or sodium caprylate) shall be added to albumin, plasma protein fraction, intravenous immunoglobulins, or coagulation factor concentrates without the prior approval of Licensing Authority and Central License Approving Authority.
2. The licensee shall ensure that the said stabilizers do not have deleterial effect on the final product in the quantity present so as not to cause any untoward or adverse reaction in human beings.

F. Quality control
Separate facilities shall be provided for quality control such as hematological, biochemical, physicochemical, microbiological, pyrogens, instrumental, and safety testing. The Quality Control Department shall have inter alia the following principal duties, namely:
1. To prepare detailed instructions, in writing for carrying out test and analysis.
2. To approve or reject raw material, components. Containers, closures, in-process materials, packaging material, labeling, and finished products.
3. To release or reject batch of finished products, which are ready for distribution.
4. To evaluate the adequacy of the conditions under which raw materials, semifinished products, and finished products are stored.
5. To evaluate the quality and stability of finished products and when necessary of raw materials and semifinished products.
6. To review production records to ensure that no errors have occurred or if errors have occurred that they have been fully investigated.
7. To approve or reject all procedures or specifications impacting on the identity, strength, quality, and purity of the product.
8. To establish shelf life and storage requirements on the basis of stability tests related to storage conditions.
9. To establish and when necessary revise control procedures and specifications.
10. To review complaints, recalls, returned or salvaged products and investigations conducted there under for each product.
11. To review master formula records/cards periodically.

G. Testing of blood products
The products manufactured shall conform to the standards specified in the Indian Pharmacopoeia and where standard of any product is not specified in the Pharmacopoeia, the standard for such product shall conform to the standard specified in the United States Pharmacopoeia or the British Pharmacopoeia. The final products shall be tested for freedom from HIV-I and HIV-II antibodies, hepatitis B surface antigen, and hepatitis C virus antibody.

H. Storage of finished product
i. The final products shall be stored between 2°C and 8°C, unless otherwise specified by the Central License Approving Authority.
ii. The shelf life assigned to the products by the licensee shall be submitted for approval to the Licensing Authority and Central License Approving Authority.

I. Labeling
The products manufactured shall be labeled as specified in the Indian Pharmacopoeia, the British Pharmacopoeia, or the United States Pharmacopoeia, which shall be in addition to any other requirement stated under Part IX or Part X of these rules. The labels shall indicate the results of tests for hepatitis B surface antigen and hepatitis C virus antibody, freedom from HIV-I and HIV-II antibodies.

J. Records
The licensee shall maintain records as per Schedule U and also comply with batch manufacturing records as specified in Paragraph 9 of Part I of Schedule M and any other requirement as may be directed

by Licensing Authority and Central License Approving Authority.

K. Master formula records

The licensee shall maintain Master Formula records relating to all manufacturing and quality control procedures for each product, which shall be prepared and endorsed by the competent technical staff, i.e. head of the manufacturing unit. The Master Formula Records shall contain:

i. The patent or proprietary name of the product along with the generic name, if any, strength and the dosage form;
ii. A description or identification of the final containers, packaging materials, labels, and closures to be used;
iii. The identity, quantity, and quality of each raw material to be used irrespective of whether or not it appears in the finished product. The permissible overage that may be included in a formulated batch shall be indicated;
iv. A description of all vessels and equipment and the sizes used in the process;
v. Manufacturing and control instructions along with parameters for critical steps such as mixing, drying, blending, sieving, and sterilizing the product;
vi. The theoretical yield to be expected from the formulation at different stages of manufacture and permissible yield limits;
vii. Detailed instructions on precautions to be taken in the manufacture and storage of drugs and of semifinished products; and
viii. The requirements in-process quality control tests and analysis to be carried out during each stage of manufacture including the designation of persons or departments responsible for the execution of such tests and analysis.

Part XIIC: II. Requirements for Manufacture of Blood Products from Bulk Finished Products

Where the blood products, such as albumin, plasma protein fraction, immunoglobulins, and coagulation factor concentrates, are manufactured through the manufacturing activities of filling and sealing the blood products from bulk powder or solution or both, the requirements as they apply to the manufacture of blood products from whole blood shall apply mutatis mutandis to such manufacture of blood products, unless other requirements have been approved by the Central License Approving Authority.

Guidelines for Approval of Blood and/or its Components to Storage Centers and First Referral Unit, Community Health Center, Primary Health Center or Any Hospital

Ministry of Health and Family Welfare (Department of Health) vide Notification No. GSR 909(E) dated 20th December, 2001 exempted blood storage centers run by First Referral Unit (FRU), Community Health Center, Primary Health Center (PHC), or any hospital from the purview of obtaining license for operation. This notification has been inserted under Schedule K of Drugs and Cosmetics Rules, 1945 under serial no. 5B. The main aim of this notification is to make abundant availability of whole human blood or its components to the said hospitals without taking license. However, this exemption is applicable to those centers, which are transfusing blood and/or its components less than 2,000 units per annum.

In order to ensure the safety and quality of blood and/or its components to be stored in such blood storage centers, the following conditions are applicable before getting exemption from the purview of taking of a license from the respective State Drugs Controllers.

The provisions of Chapter IV of the Act and the rules made there under which require obtaining of a license for operation of a blood bank or processing whole human blood and/or its components, subject to the following conditions, namely:

1. The First Referral Unit, Community Health Center, Primary Health Center, and/or any hospital shall be approved by the State/Union Territory Licensing Authority after satisfying the conditions and facilities through inspection.
2. The captive consumption or whole human blood IP or its components in the First Referral Unit, Community Health Center, Primary Health Center, and/or any hospital shall not be more than 2,000 units annually.
3. The whole human blood and/or its components shall be procured only from Government Blood Bank and/or Indian Red Cross Society Blood Bank and/or Regional Blood Transfusion Center duly licensed.
4. The approval shall be valid for a period of 2 years from the date of issue unless sooner suspended or cancelled and First Referral Unit, Community Health Center, Primary Health Center, or the hospital shall apply for renewal to the State Licensing Authority 3 months prior to the date of expiry of the approval.
5. The First Referral Unit, Community Health Center, Primary Health Center, and/or any hospital shall have the following technical staff for storage of blood or its components:
   a. A trained Medical Officer for proper procurement, storage, and cross-matching of blood and/or its components. He/she shall also be responsible for identifying hemolyzed blood and ensure nonsupply of date expired blood or its components.
   b. A blood bank technician with the qualification and experience as specified in Part XII B of Schedule F or an experienced laboratory technician trained in blood grouping and cross-matching.
6. The First Referral Unit, Community Health Center, Primary Health Center, and hospital shall have an area of 10 square meters. It shall be well lighted, clean, and preferably air-conditioned. Blood bank refrigerator of appropriate capacity fitted with alarm device and temperature indicator with regular temperature monitoring shall be provided to store blood units between 2°C and 8°C and if the components are proposed to be stored, specified equipment as specified in Part XII B of Schedule F shall also be provided.
7. The First Referral Unit, Community Health Center, Primary Health Center, and hospital shall maintain records and registers including details of procurements of whole human blood IP and/or blood components, as required under Part XII B of Schedule F.
8. The First Referral Unit, Community Health Center, Primary Health Center, and Hospital shall store samples of donor's blood as well as patients' sera for a period of 7 days after transfusion.

Guidelines before Grant of Approval for Operation of Whole Human Blood and/or its Components Storage Centers Run by First Referral Unit, Community Health Center, Primary Health Center, or Any Hospital

The following guidelines may be followed before exempting the said institutions for obtaining of a license for operation of a blood bank or processing whole human blood or its components:

1. The applicant shall be First Referral Unit, Community Health Center, Primary Health Center, or any hospital.
2. The applicant shall furnish an undertaking to the licensing authority that the captive consumption of whole human blood or components shall not be more than 2,000 units annually.
3. The applicant shall enclose list of equipment needed for storage, viz. blood bank refrigerator with alarm system and temperature indicator. A separate list of equipment for blood components would be enclosed, if proposed to be stored.

4. The applicant shall furnish the following:
   a. Name of the medical officer responsible for conducting operation of blood storage center.
   b. Attested certified copies of MBBS or MD qualification
   c. Name, certified copies of qualification, and experience of the blood bank technician.
   d. Name, attested certified copies of qualification, and experience of the blood bank technician having non-DMLT qualification.
5. The applicant shall furnish the source of procurement of whole human blood or blood components, namely the name and address of the blood banks.
   a. The source of procurement of blood/components shall be from licensed blood banks run by Government Hospitals/Indian Red Cross Society/Regional Blood Transfusion Centers only.
   b. A letter of consent from the above blood banks who intend to supply whole human blood/blood components to the blood storage centers shall be furnished along with the application.
6. The applicant shall submit the plan of the premises. A minimum area of 10 square meters is essential for the blood storage center.
7. In order to satisfy the conditions and facilities, an inspection of the proposed blood storage center may be carried out by the respective State Drug Control Department.
8. The inspection team shall also inspect the blood banks who have given consent letters for supply of whole human blood/components. The inspection team may verify whether the blood banks have sufficient quantity of blood units to be supplied to the blood storage centers and also verify the mode of shipper or containers used for supply of blood units/components to ensure that the proper storage condition is maintained as per the pharmacopeia. The blood bank shall label the blood units/components as per the Drugs and Cosmetics Rules, 1945.
9. The blood banks who intend to supply the blood units/components shall test the following mandatory tests before supplying to blood storage centers:
   a. Blood grouping
   b. Antibody testing
   c. Hemoglobin content
   d. HIV-I and -II antibodies
   e. Hepatitis B surface antigen
   f. Hepatitis C antibody
   g. Malarial parasite
   h. Syphilis or VDRL

   The label of the tested blood unit shall contain the above particulars with date of testing before supplying to blood storage centers.

   The blood bank shall maintain a separate register for supply of blood units/components to blood storage centers with all necessary details.
10. The validity of approval shall be for a period of 2 years from the date of issue of the approval.
11. The State Licensing Authority shall forward the approved Blood Storage centers to the concerned Zonal Officer immediately.

Amendments and Notification 2018

Ministry of Health and Family Welfare (Department of Health and Family Welfare)
New Delhi, the 29th November, 2018

G.S.R. 1152(E): The following draft of certain rules further to amend the Drugs and Cosmetics Rules, 1945, which the Central Government proposes to make, in exercise of the powers conferred by Section 12 and Section 33 of the Drugs and Cosmetics Act, 1940 (23 of 1940).

Draft Rules

1. i. These rules may be called the Drugs and Cosmetics Amendment) Rules, 2018.

ii. They shall come into force on the date of their final publication in the Official Gazette.
2. In the Drugs and Cosmetics Rules, 1945 (hereinafter referred to as the said rules), in Part XB, in the heading, for the words "Blood Banks", the words "Blood Centers" shall be substituted.
3. In the said rules, in rule 122EA, in sub-rule (1):
   i. For clause (d), following shall be substituted, namely:
   "(d) 'Blood Center' is an authorized premise in an organization or institution, as the case may be, for carrying out all or any of the operations including collection, processing, storage, and distribution of blood drawn from donors or received from another licensed blood center and for preparation, storage, and distribution of blood components."
   ii. After clause (m), the following clauses shall be inserted, namely:
   "(n) 'Voluntary Blood Donor' means a person who voluntarily donates blood upon being declared fit for donation without accepting in return any remuneration in cash or kind or in any manner whatsoever.
   (o) 'Erythrocyt apheresis' means selective collection of one or two units of red cells from a donor or patient using a cell separator and retransfusing the remaining blood into the donor or patient."
4. In the said rules, in rule 122EA, rule 122F, rule 122G, rule 122I, and rule 122P, for the words "Blood Bank", the words "Blood Center" wherever they occur shall be substituted.
5. In the said rules, in rule 122G, in sub-rule (1), for condition (i) the following shall be substituted, namely:
   "(i) The operation of Blood Center or processing or both of whole human blood for components shall be conducted under the active direction and personal supervision of competent technical staff consisting of at least one person who is whole time employee and who is Medical Officer, and possessing:
   a. Degree in Medicine MBBS having experience of working in Blood center, not less than 1 year during regular service and also has adequate knowledge and experience in blood group serology, blood group methodology, and medical principles involved in the procurement of blood or preparation of its components or both; or
   b. Degree in Medicine MBBS with Diploma in Clinical Pathology or Diploma in Pathology and Bacteriology with 6 months of experience in a licensed Blood Center; or
   c. Degree in Medicine MBBS with Diploma in Transfusion Medicine or Diploma in Immunohematology or Blood Transfusion with 3 months of experience in a licensed Blood Center; or
   d. Doctor of Medicine Pathology or Diplomat of National Board Pathology with 3 months of experience in a licensed Blood Center; or
   e. Postgraduate degree in Transfusion Medicine—Doctor of Medicine in Transfusion Medicine or Diplomat of National Board Transfusion Medicine, Doctor of Medicine Immunohematology and Blood Transfusion, the degree or diploma being from a University recognized by the Central Government.
   Explanation: For the purposes of this condition, the experience in blood center shall not apply in the case of persons who are approved by the Licensing Authority or Central License Approving Authority or both prior to the commencement of the Drugs and Cosmetics (Second Amendment) Rules, 1999."
6. In the said rules, in rule 122G, for sub-rule (2), the following shall be substituted, namely:
   "(2) Applications for grant or renewal of license for operation of blood center or processing of human blood components shall be made by the blood center run by the Government, Indian Red Cross Society,

hospital, charitable trust, or voluntary organization and blood center run by charitable trust or voluntary organization need to be approved by a State or Union Territory Blood Transfusion Council as per procedure laid down in this regard by the National Blood Transfusion Council."

7. In the said rules, in Schedule A, in Form 26G, Form 27C and Form 28C, for the words "Blood Bank", the words "Blood Center" wherever they occur shall be substituted.
8. In the said rules, in Schedule F, in Part XIIB:
   1. a. For the words "Blood Bank", the words "Blood Center" wherever they occur shall respectively be substituted.
      b. For the words "Blood Banks", the words "Blood Centers" wherever they occur shall respectively be substituted.
      c. For the words "Blood Banking", the words "Blood Centers" wherever they occur shall respectively be substituted.
      d. For the words "Blood Bank's", the words "Blood center's" shall be substituted.
   2. Under the heading "*1. Blood Banks/Blood Components (page 545)*", under sub-heading "B. ACCOMMODATION FOR A BLOOD CENTERS" so amended:
      i. After serial number (8), the following shall be inserted, namely:
         "(9) Counseling area with adequate privacy;
         (10) Identified Quality Control area with component preparation area may be provided."
      ii. Under subheading "C. PERSONNEL":
         a. For clause (b), the following shall be substituted, namely, "(b) Blood Center Technician(s) possessing—
            i. Diploma in Medical Laboratory Technology (DMLT) or Transfusion Medicine or Blood Bank Technology after 10+2 with 1-year experience in the testing of blood and/or its components in licensed blood center; or
            ii. Degree in Medical Laboratory Technology (MLT) or Blood Bank Technology with 6 month's experience in the testing of blood and/or its components in licensed blood center; or
            iii. BSc in Hematology and Transfusion Medicine with 6 months of experience in the testing of blood and/or its components in licensed blood center; or
            iv. MSc in Transfusion Medicine with 6 months of experience in the testing of blood and/or its components in licensed blood center; or
            v. Postgraduate Diploma in Medical Laboratory Technology (PGDMLT)/Postgraduate Diploma in Medical Laboratory Science (PGDMLS) with 6 months of experience in the testing of blood and/or its components in licensed blood center."
         b. For clause (d), the following clause shall be substituted, namely:
            "(d) Technical supervisor (where blood components are manufactured), possessing—
            i. Diploma in Medical Laboratory Technology or Transfusion Medicine or Blood Bank Technology after 10+2 with 1-year experience in the testing of blood or its components or both in licensed blood center; or
            ii. Degree in Medical Laboratory Technology or Blood Bank Technology with 6 months of experience in the testing of blood or its components or both in licensed blood center; or
            iii. BSc in Hematology and Transfusion Medicine with 6 months of experience in the testing

of blood or its components or both in licensed blood center; or

iv. MSc in Transfusion Medicine with 6 months of experience in the testing of blood or its components or both in licensed blood center; or

v. Postgraduate Diploma in Medical Laboratory Technology or Postgraduate Diploma in Medical Laboratory Science with 6 months of experience in the testing of blood or its components or both in licensed blood center."

c. After clause (d) so amended, the following paragraph shall be inserted, namely:

"Blood center organizing blood donation camps shall have following whole time or part time counseling staff:

a. Counselor or Medical Social Worker, possessing—
   (i) Master's degree in social work, sociology, psychology with 6 months of experience; or
   (ii) Degree in Science or Health Science with 1 year of experience; or
   (iii) Person with 10+2 having 3 years of experience in the field of counseling in the blood centers collecting blood less than 3,000 units per annum can share counselor medical social worker within the institution."

iii. Under subheading "E. EQUIPMENT", after serial number 15 in Table 25.3, the following entries shall be inserted namely:

16.	Standard Certified Weight(s)	—	—	Once in a year
17.	Equipment for transfusion-transmitted infection (TTI), laboratory like ELISA plate reader, if ELISA is used (or) chemiluminescence immunoassay (CLIA) or enzyme-linked fluorescence assay (ELFA)	—	Each run / Each day of use	Once in a year
18.	Micropipettes, if ELISA is used	—	—	Once in a year

iv. For subheading H, the following shall be substituted, namely:

"H. CRITERIA FOR BLOOD DONATION"

Blood donor Selection Criteria

Sl. No.	Condition	Criteria
1.	Well-being	The donor shall be in good health, mentally alert, and physically fit and shall not be inmates of jail or any other confinement. Differently abled or donor with communication and sight difficulties can donate blood provided that clear and confidential communication can be established and he/she fully understands the donation process and gives a valid consent
2.	Age	• Minimum age 18 years • Maximum age 65 years • First time donor shall not be over 60 years of age, for repeat donor upper limit is 65 years • For apheresis donors age 18–60 years
3.	Whole blood volume collected and weight of donor	• 350 mL—45 kg • 450 mL—more than 55 kg • Apheresis—50 kg

Contd...

Contd...

Sl. No.	Condition	Criteria
4.	Donation interval	• For whole blood donation, once in 3 months (90 days) for males and 4 months (120 days) for females. • For apheresis, at least 48 hours interval after platelet/plasma-apheresis shall be kept (not more than 2 times a week, limited to 24 in 1 year). • After whole blood donation a plateletpheresis donor shall not be accepted before 28 days. • Apheresis platelet donor shall not be accepted for whole blood donation before 28 days from the last platelet donation provided reinfusion of red cell was complete in the last plateletpheresis donation. If the reinfusion of red cells was not complete then the donor shall not be accepted within 90 days. • A donor shall not donate any type of donation within 12 months after a bone marrow harvest, within 6 months after a peripheral stem cell harvest.
5.	Blood pressure	• 100–140 mm Hg systolic; 60–90 mm Hg diastolic with or without medications • There shall be no findings suggestive of end organ damage or secondary complication (cardiac, renal, eye, or vascular) or history of feeling giddiness, fainting made out during history and examination. Neither the drug nor its dosage should have been altered in the last 28 days
6.	Pulse	60–100 Regular
7.	Temperature	Afebrile; 37°C/98.4°F
8.	Respiration	The donor shall be free from acute respiratory disease.
9.	Hemoglobin	>or = 12.5 g/dL Thalassemia trait may be accepted, provided hemoglobin is acceptable
10.	Meal	The donor shall not be fasting before the blood donation or observing fast during the period of blood donation and last meal should have been taken at least 4 hours prior to donation. Donor shall not have consumed alcohol and show signs of intoxication before the blood donation. The donor shall not be a person having regular heavy alcohol intake
11.	Occupation	The donor who works as air crew member, long distance vehicle driver, either above sea level or below sea level or in emergency services or where strenuous work is required, shall not donate blood at least 24 hours prior to their next duty shift. The donor shall not be a night shift worker without adequate sleep
12.	Risk behavior	The donor shall be free from any disease transmissible by blood transfusion, as far as can be determined by history and examination The donor shall not be a person considered "at risk" for HIV, hepatitis B or C infections (transgender, men who have sex with men, female sex workers, injecting drug users, persons with multiple sexual partners or any other high risk as determined by the medical officer deciding fitness to donate blood)
13.	Travel and residence	The donor shall not be a person with history of residence or travel in a geographical area, which is endemic for diseases that can be transmitted by blood transfusion and for which screening is not mandated or there is no guidance in India
14.	Donor skin	The donor shall be free from any skin diseases at the site of phlebotomy. The arms and forearms of the donor shall be free of skin punctures of scars indicative of professional blood donors or addiction of self-injected narcotics
Physiological status for women		
15.	Pregnancy or recently delivered	Defer for 12 months after delivery
16.	Abortion	Defer for 6 months after abortion
17.	Breastfeeding	Defer for total period of lactation
18.	Menstruation	Defer for the period of menstruation

Contd...

Contd...

Sl. No.	Condition	Criteria
Nonspecific illness		
19.	Minor nonspecific symptoms including but not limited to general malaise, pain, headache	Defer until all symptoms subside and donor is afebrile
Respiratory (lung) diseases		
20.	Cold, flu, cough, sore throat, or acute sinusitis	Defer until all symptoms subside and donor is afebrile
21.	Chronic sinusitis	Accept unless on antibiotics
22.	Asthmatic attack	Permanently defer
23.	Asthmatics on steroids	Permanently defer
Surgical procedures		
24.	Major surgery	Defer for 12 months after recovery (Major surgery being defined as that requiring hospitalization, anesthesia (general/spinal) had blood transfusion and/or had significant blood loss)
25.	Minor surgery	Defer for 6 months after recovery
26.	Received blood transfusion	Defer for 12 months
27.	Open heart surgery including bypass surgery	Permanently defer
28.	Cancer surgery	Permanently defer
29.	Tooth extraction	Defer for 6 months after tooth extraction
30.	Dental surgery under anesthesia	Defer for 6 months after recovery
Cardiovascular diseases (heart disease)		
31.	Has any active symptom (chest pain, shortness of breath, and swelling of feet)	Permanently defer
32.	Myocardial infarction (heart attack)	Permanently defer
33.	Cardiac medication (digitalis, nitroglycerine)	Permanently defer
34.	Hypertensive heart disease	Permanently defer
35.	Coronary artery disease	Permanently defer
36.	Angina pectoris	Permanently defer
37.	Rheumatic heart disease with residual damage	Permanently defer
Central nervous system/psychiatric diseases		
38.	Migraine	Accept if not severe and occurs at a frequency of less than once a week

Contd...

Contd...

Sl. No.	Condition	Criteria
39.	Convulsions and epilepsy	Permanently defer
40.	Schizophrenia	Permanently defer
41.	Anxiety and mood disorders	Accept person having anxiety and mood (affective) disorders like depression or bipolar disorder, but is stable and feeling well on the day regardless of medication

Endocrine disorders

Sl. No.	Condition	Criteria
42.	Diabetes	• Accept person with diabetes mellitus well controlled by diet or oral hypoglycemic medication, with no history of orthostatic hypotension and no evidence of infection, neuropathy, or vascular disease (in particular peripheral ulceration) • Permanently defer person requiring insulin and/or complications of diabetes with multiorgan involvement • Defer, if oral hypoglycemic medication has been altered/dosage adjusted in last 4 weeks
43.	Thyroid disorders	Accept donations from individuals with Benign thyroid disorders if euthyroid (asymptomatic goiter, history of viral thyroiditis, autoimmune hypothyroidism). Defer if under investigation for thyroid disease or thyroid status is not known. Permanently defer, if: 1. Thyrotoxicosis due to Graves' disease 2. Hyper-/hypothyroid 3. History of malignant thyroid tumors
44.	Other endocrine disorders	Permanently defer

Liver diseases and hepatitis infection

Sl. No.	Condition	Criteria
45.	Hepatitis	• Known hepatitis B, C—permanently defer • Unknown hepatitis—permanently defer • Known hepatitis A or E—defer for 12 months
46.	Spouse/partner/close contact of individual suffering with hepatitis	Defer for 12 months
47.	At risk for hepatitis by tattoos, acupuncture or body piercing, scarification and any other invasive cosmetic procedure by self or spouse/partner	Defer for 12 months
48.	Spouse/partner of individual receiving transfusion of blood/components	Defer for 12 months
49.	Jaundice	Accept donor with history of jaundice that was attributed to gallstones, Rh disease, mononucleosis or in neonatal period
50.	Chronic liver disease/liver failure	Permanently defer

HIV infection/AIDS

Sl. No.	Condition	Criteria
51.	At risk for HIV infection (transgender, men who have sex with men, female sex workers, injecting drug users, persons with multiple sex partners)	Permanently defer

Contd...

Contd...

Sl. No.	Condition	Criteria
52.	Known HIV positive person or spouse/partner of PLHA (person living with HIV AIDS)	Permanently defer
53.	Persons having symptoms suggestive of AIDS	Permanently defer person having lymphadenopathy, prolonged and repeated fever, prolonged and repeated diarrhea irrespective of HIV risk or status
Sexually transmitted infections		
54	Syphilis (genital sore, or generalized skin rashes)	Permanently defer
55.	Gonorrhea	Permanently defer
Other infectious diseases		
56.	History of measles, mumps, chickenpox	Defer for 2 weeks following full recovery
57.	Malaria	Defer for 3 months following full recovery
58.	Typhoid	Defer for 12 months following full recovery
59.	Dengue/chikungunya	• In case of history of dengue/chikungunya: Defer for 6 months following full recovery. • Following visit to dengue/chikungunya endemic areas: 4 weeks following return from visit to dengue endemic area, if no, febrile illness is noted
60.	Zika virus/West Nile virus	• In case of zika infection: Defer for 4 months following recovery • In case of history of travel to West Nile virus, endemic area or Zika virus outbreak zone: Defer for 4 months
61.	Tuberculosis	Defer for 2 years following confirmation of cure
62.	Leishmaniasis	Permanently defer
63.	Leprosy	Permanently defer
Other infections		
64.	Conjunctivitis	Defer for the period of illness and continuation of local medication
65.	Osteomyelitis	Defer for 2 years following completion of treatment and cure
Kidney disease		
66.	Acute infection of kidney (pyelonephritis)	Defer for 6 months after complete recovery and last dose of medication
67	Acute infection of bladder (cystitis)/UTI	Defer for 2 weeks after complete recovery and last dose of medication
68.	Chronic infection of kidney/kidney disease/renal failure	Permanently defer
Digestive system		
69.	Diarrhea	• Person having history of diarrhea in preceding week • Particularly if associated with fever: Defer for 2 weeks after complete recovery and last dose of medication
70.	GI endoscopy	Defer for 12 months
71.	Acid peptic disease	• Accept person with acid reflux, mild gastroesophageal reflux, mild hiatus hernia, gastroesophageal reflux disorder (GERD), hiatus hernia: Permanently defer person with stomach ulcer with symptoms or with recurrent bleeding

Contd...

Contd...

Sl. No.	Condition	Criteria
Other diseases/disorders		
72.	Autoimmune disorders like systemic lupus erythematosus, scleroderma, dermatomyositis, ankylosing spondylitis, or severe rheumatoid arthritis	Permanently defer
73.	Polycythemia vera	Permanently defer
74.	Bleeding disorders and unexplained bleeding tendency	Permanently defer
75.	Malignancy	Permanently defer
76.	Severe allergic disorders	Permanently defer
77.	Hemoglobinopathies and red cell enzyme deficiencies with known history of hemolysis	Permanently defer
Vaccination and inoculation		
78.	**Nonlive vaccines and toxoids:** Typhoid, cholera, papillomavirus, influenza, meningococcal, pertussis, pneumococcal, polio injectable, diphtheria, tetanus, plague	Defer for 14 days
79.	**Live-attenuated vaccines:** Polio (oral), measles (rubella) mumps, yellow fever, Japanese encephalitis, influenza, typhoid, cholera, hepatitis A	Defer for 28 days
80.	Antitetanus serum, antivenom serum, antidiphtheria serum, and antigas gangrene serum	Defer for 28 days
81.	Antirabies vaccination following animal bite, hepatitis B Immunoglobulin, immunoglobulins	Defer for 1 year
82.	Swine flu	Defer for 15 days
Medications taken by prospective blood donor		
83.	Oral contraceptive	Accept
84.	Analgesics	Accept

Contd...

Contd...

Sl. No.	Condition	Criteria
85.	Vitamins	Accept
86.	Mild sedative and tranquillizers	Accept
87.	Allopurinol	Accept
88.	Cholesterol lowering medication	Accept
89.	Salicylates (aspirin), other NSAIDs	Defer for 3 days, if blood is to be used for platelet preparation
90.	Ketoconazole, antihelminthic drugs including mebendazole	Defer for 7 days after last dose if donor is well
91.	Antibiotics	Defer for 2 weeks after last dose, if donor is well
92.	Ticlopidine, clopidogrel	Defer for 2 weeks after last dose
93.	Piroxicam, dipyridamole	Defer for 2 weeks after last dose
94.	Etretinate, acitretin or isotretinoin. (used for acne)	Defer for 1 month after the last dose
95.	Finasteride used to treat Benign prostatic hyperplasia	Defer for 1 month after the last dose
96.	Radioactive contrast material	8 weeks deferral
97.	Dutasteride used to treat Benign prostatic hyperplasia	Defer for 6 months after the last dose
98.	Any medication of unknown nature	Defer till details are available
99.	Oral antidiabetic drugs	Accept, if there is no alteration in dose within last 4 weeks
100.	Insulin	Permanently defer
101.	Antiarrhythmic, anticonvulsions, anticoagulant, antithyroid drugs, cytotoxic drugs, cardiac failure Drugs (digitalis)	Permanently defer
Other conditions requiring permanent deferral		
102.	Recipients of organ, stem cell and tissue transplants. Donors who have had an unexplained delayed faint or delayed faint with injury or two consecutive faints following a blood donation	Permanently defer
Residents of other countries		
103.	Residents of other countries	Accept only after stay in India for three continuous years

3. Under the heading "II. BLOOD DONATION CAMPS":
   i. Under "Notes", at serial number (i), after the words "constituted by a State Government" the following words shall be inserted, namely—"in accordance with procedure laid down by the National Blood Transfusion Council in this regard".
   ii. Under the subheading "(B) Personnel for Outdoor Blood Donation Camp", for serial number (ii), the following shall be substituted, namely—
   "(ii) two counselors or medical social workers"
   iii. Under subheading "C. Equipment", for item (12), the following shall be substituted, namely—
   "12. Portable Hb meter or copper sulfate method or any quantitative method can be used for determination of hemoglobin estimation."
4. Under the heading "III. PROCESSING OF BLOOD COMPONENTS FROM WHOLE BLOOD BY A BLOOD CENTER":
   i. Under subheading "(B) Equipment"—
   (a) For item (iv) and item (xi), the following shall be substituted, namely—
   "(iv) Plasma Expresser or automated extractor or multihead tube sealer;
   (xi) Deep freezer or snap freezer maintaining a temperature between -30–$40°C$ and -75–$80°C$."
   (b) After item (xiii), the following shall be inserted, namely—"(xiv) Cryobath and any better equipment or technology."
   ii. Under subheading "(E) CATEGORIES OF BLOOD COMPONENTS"—
   a. In clause (1), for the portion beginning with the words "The product shall be" and ending with the words "from human blood.", the following shall be substituted, namely—
   "The product shall be known as "Packed Red Blood Cells" that is packed red blood cells remaining after separating plasma from human blood, which also include modified packed red blood cells including semipacked red blood cells, washed red blood cells, leukoreduced red blood cells, irradiated red blood cells and frozen red blood cells.
   Types of red cell components:
   i. Saline-washed red cells: Red cells washed with sterile normal saline by centrifugation at 2-8°.
   ii. Leukodepleted red cells: Red cells shall be prepared by a method known to reduce leukocytes in the final component to less than 5×10^8 when intended to prevent febrile reactions and to less than 5×10^6 when required to prevent alloimmunization or *Cytomegalovirus* infection. For achieving a level of less than 5×10^6 leukocyte filters are necessary.
   iii. Irradiated red cells: These are prepared by gamma cell or X-ray irradiation at 25 Gy to prevent graft-versus-host disease due to proliferation of lymphocytes.
   iv. Frozen packed red blood cells: Cryoprotective substance may be added to the packed red blood cells for extended storage between $-80°C$ and $-196°C$.
   The quality control criteria for validation of the processes should be as follows:
   1% of packed red cells may be tested of which atleast 75% of the packed red cells shall conform to following quality control criteria—
   a. **Volume:**
   250 mL ± 10% from 450 mL bag
   150 mL ± 10% from 350 mL bag

b. **Hematocrit:**
65–70% when stored in CPDA1 solution
50–60% when stored in SAGM solution
c. **Culture:**
Sterile

b. In clause (2), after first paragraph, the following shall be inserted, namely—
"Types of platelets:
i. Platelet-rich plasma: Plasma which is rich in platelets and separated from whole blood
ii. Random donor platelet concentrates:
   a. Prepared from platelet-rich plasma
   b. Prepared from buffy coat
iii. Pooled platelets:
   a. Prepared by pooling of 6 units of random donor platelets, preferably ABO or Rh type matched, are pooled into one bag of "Pooled Platelets."

c. In clause (2), after subclause (v), the following shall be inserted, namely—
"Preparation of pooled platelet concentrate:
One single unit of random donor platelets is not enough to provide adequate hemostatic dose in an adult patient. Therefore, up to 6 units of random donor platelets, preferably ABO or Rh type matched, are pooled into one bag of "Pooled Platelet Concentrate". The pooled platelets may be prepared by pooling buffy coats and then processed into one unit of pooled buffy coats—pooled platelet concentrate. Alternatively, pooling can be done after preparation of random donor platelets by platelet-rich plasma method or buffy coat method. If the pooling is done in an open system (using spikes for pooling), the shelf life of the pooled platelets will be 6 hours, while for closed system (using sterile connecting device) the expiry date will be that of the platelet unit having the shortest expiry date. The labeling requirements for the final pooled product shall remain same as any other platelet product except that the final pack should have a unique pool number or donation numbers of all contributing units. The platelet content in the pooled product should be $\geq 2 \times 10^{12}$/unit. Modified platelet component includes: leukodepleted, irradiated, washed platelets, or platelets suspended in additive solution."

d. In clause (3), for subclause (i) and (ii), the following subclauses shall respectively be substituted, namely—
"(i) Granulocyte concentrates are prepared either by pooling multiple units of buffy coat or by apheresis as described under apheresis section. The same shall be stored at 20–24°C and used within a maximum period of 24 hours.
(ii) Pooled granulocytes shall meet the same Quality Control requirements as that for apheresis granulocytes (at least 1×10 raised to the power 10)."

e. In clause (4), after first paragraph, the following shall be inserted, namely—
"The quality control criteria for validation of the processes should be as follows:
Volume:
180–220 mL from 350 mL bag
220–300 mL from 450 mL bag
Factor VIII: At least 70 IU/bag
Excess and expired plasma may be issued for fractionation to the licensed fractionation center in the country with justification to be recorded in writing."

f. In the said rules, in Schedule F, in Part XII B under the heading

"III. PROCESSING OF BLOOD COMPONENTS FROM WHOLE BLOOD BY A BLOOD BANK", under subheading "(E) CATEGORIES OF BLOOD COMPONENTS", in clause (5), for the portion beginning with the words "Concentrate of antihemophilic" and ending with the words "–30°C", the following shall be substituted, namely—
"Concentrate of antihemophiliac factor shall be prepared by thawing fresh frozen plasma (FFP) at 4°C in a cold room or blood bank refrigerator or 4–10°C in a cryobath. –80°C deep freezer should be used for faster freezing of plasma for preparation of cryoprecipitate.

The quality control criteria for validation of the processes should be as follows:

Volume: 15–20 mL
Fibrinogen: At least 150 mg/bag
Factor VIII: At least 80 IU/bag

Preparation of pooled cryoprecipitate:
One single unit of cryoprecipitate is not enough to provide adequate hemostatic dose in an adult patient. Therefore, multiple units of cryoprecipitate may be pooled in one bag. If the pooling is done in an open system (using spikes for pooling), the shelf life of the pooled cryoprecipitate will be 6 hours.

The labeling requirements for the final pooled product shall remain same as any other cryoprecipitate product except that the final pack should have a unique pool number or donation numbers of all contributing units."

5. For subheading "F. PLASMAPHERESIS, PLATELETPHERESIS, LEUKAPHERESIS USING A CELL SEPARATOR", the following shall be substituted, namely—
"**F. Apheresis using a cell separator**
General requirements:

a. **Accommodation:** An air-conditioned area of 10 square meters shall be provided for apheresis/therapeutic procedures in the blood center.
b. **Equipment:**
   i. Cell separator
   ii. Dielectric tube sealer
   iii. Other emergency equipment/items:
      - Oxygen cylinder with mask, gauge, and pressure regulator. 5% glucose or normal saline.
      - Disposable sterile syringes and needles of various sizes.
      - Disposable sterile IV infusion sets.
      - Ampoules of adrenaline, noradrenaline, mephentine, betamethasone or
      - dexamethasone, metoclopramide injections.
      - Aspirin.
c. **Criteria for selection of donors:**
   At least 48 hours must elapse between successive apheresis and not more than twice in a week. For hematopoietic stem cells, the procedures can be done daily.
   Types of apheresis:
   1. Plasmapheresis
   2. Plateletpheresis for harvesting platelet concentrate (single donor platelets)
   3. Leukapheresis for harvesting:
      - Granulocyte concentrate
      - Lymphocytes
      - Mononuclear cells
   4. Erythrocytapheresis: Red cell apheresis including double unit red cell collection
   5. Hematopoietic stem cells (peripheral blood stem cells).

1. **Plasmapheresis:**
   The total serum protein shall be 6 g/dL before the first plasmapheresis procedure.
   In repeated plasmapheresis:
   a. It should be tested before the third procedure, if done within 4 weeks, and it shall be 6 g/dL.

b. The quantity of plasma separated from the blood of donor shall not exceed 500 mL per sitting and once in a fortnight or shall not exceed 1,000 mL per month.

2. **Plateletpheresis (single donor platelets):**
   i. Plateletpheresis shall not be carried out on donors who have taken medication containing aspirin within 3 days prior to donation.
   ii. Platelet count, WBC counts; differential count may be carried out.

   The term plateletpheresis includes platelets collected by apheresis, using a cell separator and the product is called single donor platelets and includes washed single donor platelets, modified single donor platelets (with replacement of compatible plasma), leukoreduced single donor platelets, and double-single donor platelets collected from single donor. Single donor platelets should have a platelet count of $\geq 3 \times 10^{11}$/unit.

   i. Storage: Shall be kept up to 5 days between 20°C and 24°C with continuous agitation.
   ii. Apheresis platelet concentrates should contain minimum of 3×1011 platelets in 75% of the units tested among 1% of monthly production or 4 platelet concentrates per month, whichever is higher.
   iii. The pH must be 6 or higher at the end of permissible storage period.

3. **Leukapheresis:**
   This procedure includes collection of granulocytes (granulocytopheresis), lymphocytes or peripheral blood stem cells or hematopoietic stem cells for treatment of traditional conditions followed by their preservation.

4. **Erythropheresis**
   This is the collection of 2 units of red cells from a single donor meeting specified requirements.

   Therapeutic plasmapheresis and cytapheresis:
   Therapeutic apheresis activity is allowed in the blood center attached to the hospital having apheresis facilities under the responsibility of Registered Medical Practitioner (RMP) who has obtained the consent of patient and record of which shall be maintained and signed by the RMP and blood bank medical officer.

   This shall be done only at the written request of the patient's physician. Patient's informed consent shall be taken. Records of the procedure shall be maintained. Provisions for emergency care shall be available by the patient's physician."

9. In the said rules, in Schedule K, in Serial Number 5B and in Serial Number 30, for the words **"Blood Bank", the words "Blood Center" wherever they occur shall be substituted**.

Chapter XIII: Guidelines for Opening and Licensing of Blood Bank

1301. Blood Bank

Blood center/bank: Blood bank means, a center within an organization or an institution for collection, grouping, cross-matching, storage, processing, and distribution of whole human blood or human blood products from selected human donors.

1302. Licensing Policy and Legal Framework for Blood Banks

An adequate legal framework has been provided in Schedule X B of the Drugs and Cosmetics

Act/Rules published in The Gazette of India: Extraordinary [Part II-Section 3 (i)], which stipulates mandatory testing of blood for blood transmissible diseases, including HIV. The rules provide for adequate testing procedures, quality control, standard qualifications, and experience for blood bank personnel, maintenance of complete and accurate records, etc. The Drugs Controller General (India) is the Central License Approving Authority whereas the regulatory control remains under the dual authority of the State and the Central Government. The blood banks under the Act require a manufacturing license.

1303. Application for Grant or Renewal of License

Application for grant or renewal of license for operation of blood bank shall be made to the Licensing Authority in Form 27-C and shall be accompanied by license fee of Rs. Six hundred (₹ 600/-) and inspection fee of Rs. Two hundred (₹ 200/-) in the case of renewal of license.

Provided that if the applicant applies for renewal of license after its expiry but within 6 months of such expiry, the fee payable for the renewal of the license shall be ₹ 600/- plus an additional fee at the rate of ₹ 200 per month or a part thereof in addition to the inspection fee.

A fee of ₹ 100/- shall be paid for a duplicate copy of a license issued, if the original is defaced, damaged, or lost.

The forms required to be filled up for application for grant or renewal of license, original license, and renewal of license is given at the end of this chapter.

1304. Prerequisite for Grant of License for Blood Bank (Rule 122G)

1. The operation of the blood bank or processing of whole human blood for components and/or manufacture of blood products shall be carried out under the active direction and personal supervision of competent technical staff consisting of at least one person who is whole time employee, a Medical Officer who is a Graduate in Medicine of a University recognized by the Central Government having experience in blood bank for 6 months during regular service. He shall also have adequate knowledge and experience in blood group serology, blood group methodology, and medical principles involved in the procurement of blood.
2. The applicant shall provide adequate space, plant and equipment for any or all the operations of blood collection or blood processing. The space and equipment required for various operations are given later on in the chapter.
3. The applicant shall provide and maintain adequate technical staff.
4. The applicant shall provide adequate arrangements for storage of whole human blood, human blood components, and blood products.
5. The applicant shall furnish to the licensing authority, if required to do so, data on the stability of whole human blood, its components, or blood products which are likely to deteriorate for fixing the date of expiry, which shall be printed on the labels of such products on the basis of the data so furnished.

1305. Inspection

Before a license in Form 28-C is granted, the licensing authority, as the case may be, shall cause the establishment in which blood bank is proposed to be operated to be inspected by one or more inspectors, appointed under the Act, and/or along with the expert in the concerned field. The Inspector or Inspectors shall examine all portions of the premises and appliances/equipment and inspect the process of manufacture intended to be employed or being employed along with the means to be employed or being employed for operation of blood bank together with their testing facilities and also enquire into the professional qualification of the expert staff and other technical staff to be employed.

If within a period of 6 months from the rejection of application for a license, the applicant informs the licensing authority that the conditions laid down have been satisfied and deposits an inspection fee of ₹ 50/-, the licensing authority may, if after causing further inspection to be made, is satisfied that the conditions for the grant of a license have been complied with, shall grant a license in Form 28-C.

Any person who is aggrieved by the order passed by the licensing authority or central license approving authority, as the case may be, may within 30 days from the date of receipt of such order, appeal to the State Government or Central Government, as the case may be, after such enquiry into the matter, as it considers necessary and after giving the said person, an opportunity for representing his view in the matter may pass such order in relation thereto as it thinks fit.

1306. Duration of License

An original license in Form 28-C or a renewed license in Form 26-G, unless suspended or cancelled, shall be valid up to the 31st December of the year, following the year in which it is granted or renewed.

1307. Cancellation and Suspension of Licenses

1. The licensing authority or central license approving authority may, for such licenses granted or renewed by him after giving the licensee an opportunity to show cause why such an order should not be passed by an order in writing stating the reasons thereof, cancel a license issued under this part or suspend it for such period as he thinks fit, either wholly or in respect of some of the substances to which it relates, if in his opinion, the licensee has failed to comply with any of the conditions of the license or with any provision of the Act or Rules there under.
2. A licensee whose license has been suspended or cancelled may, within 3 months of the date of the order under sub-rule (1), prefer an appeal against that order to the State Govt. or Central Govt., which shall decide the same.

1308. Conditions of License

A license in Form 28-C shall be subject to the special conditions set out in Schedule F, Part XII-B and Part XII-C, as the case may be, which relate to the substance in respect of which the license is granted to the following general conditions:

i. a. The licensee shall provide and maintain adequate staff, plan and premises for the proper operation of a blood bank for processing whole human blood, its components and/or manufacture of blood products.
 b. The licensee shall maintain staff, premises and equipment as specified in Rule 122-G. The licensee shall maintain necessary records and registers as specified in Schedule F, Part XII-B and XII-C.
 c. The licensee shall test in his own laboratory whole human blood, its components and blood products and registers in respect of such tests as specified in Schedule F, Part XII-B and XII-C. The records and registers shall be maintained for a period of 5 years from the date of manufacture.
 d. The licensee shall maintain/preserve reference sample and supply to the Inspector, the reference sample of the whole human blood collected by him in an adequate quantity to conduct all the prescribed tests. The licensee shall supply to the Inspector the reference sample for the purpose of testing.
ii. The licensee shall allow an Inspector appointed under the act to enter, with or without prior notice, any premises where the activities of the blood bank are being carried out, for processing of whole human blood and/or blood products, to inspect the premises and plant and the process of manufacture and the means employed for standardizing and testing the substance.
iii. The licensee shall allow an Inspector appointed under the Act to inspect all registers and records maintained under these rules and to take samples of the manufactured product and shall supply to Inspector such information as he may

require for the purpose of ascertaining whether the provisions of the Act and Rules thereunder have been observed.
iv. The licensee shall from time to time report to the licensing authority about any changes in the expert staff responsible for the operation of a blood bank/processing of whole human blood for components and/or manufacture of blood products and any material alterations in the premises or plant used for the purpose which have been made since the date of last inspection made on behalf of the licensing authority before the grant of license.
v. The licensee shall maintain an Inspection Book in Form 35 to enable an Inspector to record his impression and defects noticed.

1309. Space, Equipment and Supplies Required for a Blood Bank (PART XIIB of Schedule F)

A. Accommodation for a blood bank
(refer page 545 under Part XIIB, B)
Minimum total area shall be 100 square meters having appropriate lighting and ventilation with washable floors and shall consist of following rooms namely:
1. Registration and Medical Examination room with adequate furniture and facilities for registration and selection of donors.
2. Blood Collection Room (This shall be air-conditioned).
3. Room for Laboratory for blood group serology. (This shall be air-conditioned).
4. Room for Laboratory for Transmissible diseases like hepatitis, syphilis, malaria, and HIV antibodies, etc. (This shall be air-conditioned).
5. Sterilization and washing room.
6. Refreshment room.
7. Store and Records Room.

Note: The Laboratories of the blood bank shall be used exclusively for blood bank work.

B. Equipment
I. For blood collection room, the following would be needed (refer Box 25.2).
II. Hemoglobin determination (refer Box 25.3).
III. Temperature and pulse determination (refer Box 25.4)
IV. Blood containers
a. Disposable plastic packs (closed system) as per the specification of USP.
b. Blood collection bottles: 540 mL with graduated capacity of up to 500 mL graduation mark provided with two rows in opposite direction indicating intervals of 50 mL from 0 to 500 mL.
c. Anticoagulants: Anticoagulant solution shall be sterile, pyrogen free and of composition that will ensure satisfactory safety and efficacy of the whole human blood and all the separate human blood components.
  i. Citrate phosphate dextrose solution (CPD) or citrate phosphate dextrose adenine-I (CPDA-I) 14 mL. Solution shall be required for 100 mL of blood. In case of double/triple blood collection bags used for blood components preparation, CPDA, blood collection bags may be used.
  ii. Acid Citrate Dextrose Solution (ACD. and Formula-A) IP Grade 15 mL. solution shall be required for 100 mL of blood.

Note: The licensee shall ensure that the anticoagulant solution bottles/packs conform to the standard laid down in IP/USP. Disposable sterile bleeding sets shall only be used.

V. Disposable sterile bleeding sets shall only be used
VI. Blood transfusion sets
Sterile disposable sets with filters and plastic spike shall only be used.
VII. Emergency equipment (refer Box 25.5)
VIII. Accessories. (refer Box 25.6)

C. Refreshment services
Provision for serving refreshments to the donor after phlebotomy shall be made so that he/she may be kept for observation in the blood bank for any untoward reactions.

D. Laboratory equipment (refer Box 25.7)
E. Reagents
1. Standard blood grouping sera Anti-A and Anti-B and Anti-AB: All in double quantity

and each of different brand or if from the same supplier then each supply should be of different lot numbers.
2. Rh typing sera: All in double quantity and each of different brand or if from the same supplier then each supply should be of different lot numbers.
3. Reagents for serological tests for syphilis and positive sera for controls.
4. Antihuman globulin serum (Coomb's serum).
5. Albumin: 20–30% for tests/enzymes.
6. 0.9% saline.
7. Culture media and tubes.
8. Wax pencils and tables.
9. RPHA/ELISA kits for hepatitis.
10. Detergents and other agents for cleaning laboratory glasswares.
11. ELISA kits/rapid diagnostic kits in case the licensee opts for HIV antibodies testing.

F. General supplies
Autoclave with temperature and pressure recording device.

G. Personnel
Every blood bank shall have following categories of full time technical staff and their number shall depend upon the quantum of work:
1. Doctor: Degree in Medicine of a University recognized by the Central Government having experience in blood bank for 6 months during regular services. He shall have adequate knowledge and experience in Blood Group serology. Blood Group Methodology and medical principles involved in procurement of blood.
2. Registered nurse.
3. Blood bank technician with MLT qualification or its equivalent having adequate experience in blood grouping and serology work.
4. Laboratory assistant with MLT qualifications or its equivalent.
5. Laboratory attendant.

H. Testing of whole human blood
1. It shall be the responsibility of the licensee to ensure that the whole human blood supplied conforms to the standards laid down in the current edition of Indian Pharmacopoeia and for all other tests published by the Central Government from time to time.
2. Every licensee shall get samples of every blood unit tested before use for freedom from HIV antibodies either from such laboratories specified for the purpose by the Central Government or in his own laboratory. The results of testing shall be recorded on the label of the container also.

Note:
1. Blood samples of donors in pilot tube and the blood samples of the recipient shall be preserved for 72 hours after transfusion.
2. The blood intended for transfusion shall not be frozen at any stage.
3. Blood containers shall not come directly in contact with ice at any stage.

I. Expiry date
The date on which the blood is drawn and the date of expiry which shall be as prescribed under Schedule P to the said Rules.

J. Records and labels
The permanent records which the licensee is required to maintain are:
1. Blood donor register: Indicating serial number, date of bleeding, name of donor with particulars, age, weight, hemoglobin, blood pressure, medical examination, signature of Medical Officer bleeding the donor, bottle bag number and patient's detail for whom donated in case of recipient donation, remarks on donation (voluntary/replacement/professional). Disposal record.
2. Blood stock register: indicating bottle bag number, date of collection, date of expiry, quantity in milliliters, ABO/Rh Group, results for testing of HIV antibodies, malaria, VDRL, hepatitis B surface antigen, irregular antibodies (if any), name of donor with particulars, utilization issue number, components prepared or

discarded, certified by Medical Officer In-charge).

Note: Similar records shall be made for blood components. Groupwise stock register shall be maintained.

3. Issue register: Indicating serial number, date and time of issue, bottle number, ABO/Rh group, total quantity in mL, name of the recipient, group of recipient, unit/institution, details of cross-matching report, and indication for transfusion. Particulars of product supplied (whole human blood, red cell/platelet concentrates, cryoprecipitates, etc.), quantity supplied, compatibility report, and signature of issuing persons.
4. Register for ACD/CPD/CPD-A: Bottles/packs giving details of firm, batch number, date of supply, and results of testing.
5. Register for diagnostic reagents used.
6. Blood bank must issue the cross-matching report of the blood of the patient along with the blood bottle.
7. Transfusion adverse reaction records.
8. Records of purchase, use and stock in hand of disposable needles, syringes, plastic bags, sets shall be maintained.

K. Labels

The label on the blood container shall contain the following particulars namely:
1. The serial number of the bottle.
2. The date on which the blood is drawn and the date of expiry as prescribed under Schedule P to the said Rules.
3. The ABO groups with the corresponding color; the following color scheme for labels shall be used for different groups. (refer Table 25.6)
4. The results of the tests for hepatitis, syphilis, freedom from HIV antibodies.
5. The Rh group.
6. Total volume of fluid, the preparation of blood, nature and percentage of anticoagulant.
7. Name and address of Blood Bank.
8. License number.
9. Instruction to keep continuously at 4–6°C.

The label should also include the following inscriptions:

10. Disposable transfusion sets with filter must be used in administration equipment.
11. Appropriate compatible cross-matched blood without a typical antibody in recipient should be used.

Caution: The contents should not be used if there is any visible evidence of deterioration like hemolysis, clotting or discoloration.

Note: The above requirements of blood bank are subject to modifications at the discretion of the Licensing Authority or the Central License Approving Authority if he is of the opinion that having regard to the extent of manufacturing operations it is necessary to relax or alter them in the circumstances of a particular case.

Part XII C of Schedule F deals with minimum requirements for grant of license to process blood components from whole blood.

LICENSING PROCEDURE

License from Food and Drugs Control Administration (FDCA) is a must for operating a blood bank as per legal provisions laid down in of Drugs and Cosmetics Act, 1940.

In India, the regulatory body is Central Drugs Standard Control Organization (CDSCO), which is headed by the Drugs Controller General (India) (DCGI). The DCGI is the Central License Approving Authority (CLAA), whereas the regulatory control remains under the dual authority of the State and the Central Government.

- **Application** (Box 25.9) for grant (first time) or renewal of license for operation

Box 25.9: Fresh application for grant of license and the accompanying documents required.

- Application Form 27-C (Fig. 25.1)
- License fee and inspection fee (in the case of renewal of license)
- Submit the floor plan of the blood bank to the provincial (state) FDCA and a copy to the CDSCO office at zonal level

> **Form 27-C**
> (See rule 122-F)
> **(Application for grant or renewal of licence)**
>
> Application for grant or renewal of licence for the Operation of Blood bank processing of Whole Human Blood for components and or manufacture of blood products
>
> 1. I/We _____ of M/s _____ hereby apply for the grant of licence / renewal of licence number _____ dated _____ to operate a Blood Bank, for processing of whole Human blood and/or* for preparation of its components and/or manufacture of blood products on the premises situated at _____.
>
> Names of the Human Blood Components intended to be processed shall be specified
>
> 2. Name(s) of the item(s):
>   1.
>   2.
>   3.
>
> 3. The name(s), qualification and experience of competent Technical Staff are as under:
>
>   (a) Name(s) of Medical Officer.
>   (b) Name(s) of Technical Supervisor.
>   (c) Name(s) of Registered Nurse.
>   (d) Name(s) of Blood Bank Technician.
>
> 4. The premises and plant are ready for inspection/will be ready for inspection on _____.
>
> 5. A licence fee of rupees _____ and an inspection fee of rupees _____ has been credited to the Government under the Head of Account _____ (receipt enclosed).
>
> Signature _____
>
> Dated _____   Name and Designation _____
>
> * delete, whichever is not applicable.
>
> Note:
> 1. The application shall be accompanied by a plan of the premises, list of machinery and equipment for collection, processing, storage and testing of whole blood and its components, memorandum of association/constitution of the firm, copies of certificate relating to educational qualifications and experience of the competent technical staff and documents relating to ownership or tenancy of the premises.
> 2. A copy of the application together with the relevant enclosures shall also be sent to the Central Licence Approving Authority and to the concerned Zonal/Sub-Zonal Officers of the Central Drugs Standard Control Organization.

Fig. 25.1: Application for blood bank Form 27-C.

of a blood bank should be submitted to the Licensing Authority in Form 27-C
- Once FDCA approves the floor plan, the management should **submit the application in Form 27-C along with requisite fees**. The application form **should accompany** multiple documents:
  – **Legal status of the organization**
  – **No objection certificate (NOC) from local municipality**
  – **Clinical license** (in case of hospital-based blood bank)
  – **List of competent personnel**
  – **List of equipment**
  – **Standard operating procedures** for all major technical and nontechnical

Transfusion Regulation and Legislation

areas, and samples of all stationeries to be used in the blood banks.
- **Inspection**: Once the application is in order, a joint **inspection is conducted** by the provincial **FDCA and CDSCO** officials. During onsite inspection, the inspectors examine all sections of the premises, infrastructure, and equipment and also inspect the process of manufacture proposed to be used or being used along as well as testing facilities, personnel, SOPs, and calibration of equipment.
- **State licensing authority:** After completion of joint inspection and favorable recommendation by the team of inspecting officers, the state licensing authority examines the suitability and eligibility of the applicant with respect to the facilities provided. If the applicant is able to fulfill the conditions of license, rules, regulations, and provisions of the act, recommendation to grant the license is forwarded to the CLAA, New Delhi for approval.
- **Approval by CLAA:** The power of CLAA has been designated to DCGI, New Delhi. Once the license has been duly approved and signed (Fig. 25.2) by CLAA, it is handed over to the applicant to allow blood bank activities.
- **Validity:** Every blood bank license is valid for a period of 5 years. After approval of license, the state licensing authority may carry out surprise inspections any time in addition to regular yearly surveillance. During this visit, if any noncompliance is observed, the blood bank has to correct the deficiency to continue to have the license for operations. The renewal is done using Form 26-G (Fig. 25.3).

Form 28-C
(See rule 122-G)
(Original Licence)

Licence to operate a blood bank for collection, storage and processing of whole human blood and/or* its components for Sale or distribution

Number of Licence _____   Date of Issue _____

1. _____ is hereby licensed to operate a Blood Bank to process Whole Human Blood for components and/or manufacture of blood products as the premises situated at the _____.
2. Name of the Product(s) _____.
3. Name of approved expert staff _____
   1. _____
   2. _____
   3. _____
4. The licence authorise the distribution and the sale and storage for distribution or for sale by the licensee of Whole Human Blood, Human Blood Components and/or blood product under this Licence subject to the conditions applicable to licence for sale.
5. The licence shall be in force from _____ to _____.
6. The licence shall be subject to the conditions stated below and to such other conditions as may. (xi) The licensee shall destroy the stocks of batch unit, which does not comply with Standard tests in such a way that it would not spread any disease/infection by way of proper disinfection method.

Dated _____   Signature _____

  Name and Designation _____

  Licensing Authority

  _____
  Central Licence Approving Authority

*delete, whichever is not applicable

Fig. 25.2: Original licence.

```
                            Form 26-G
                          (See Rule 122-F)
                          (Renewal Licence)
Certificate of Renewal of Licence to Operate A Blood Bank For Processing of Whole Human Blood for
components and/or Manufacture of Blood Products and/or Manufacture of Blood Products

1. Certified that licence number_____granted on _____ to
   M/s _____ for the operation of a Blood Bank for processing of whole
   blood and/or for preparation of its components at the premises situated at _____
   is hereby renewed with effect from _____ to _____.

2. Name (s) of Items/Product(s):
   1.
   2.
   3.

3. Name(s) of competent Technical Staff:
   1.
   2.
   3.
   4.
   5.
   6.

   Dated_____                           Signature_____

                                               Name and Designation _____

                                               Licensing Authority

                                               _____
                                               Central Licence Approving Authority
```

Fig. 25.3: Renewal of licence.

EVOLUTION OF BLOOD SAFETY PROGRAM IN INDIA

In 1987, the National AIDS Control Program began to take shape in the Directorate of Health Services, Ministry of Health and Family Welfare, Government of India, with three major components: (i) surveillance; (ii) health education and information; and (iii) screening of blood and blood products. During 1989–90, a program was commenced on "prevention of infection and modernization of blood banking services". It emphasized the following:

1. **Modernization of blood banks:** Financial assistance was given for purchase of equipment to upscale and modernize 138 blood banks generating over 2,000 units of blood per annum. It was made mandatory (1988), to screen blood for HIV under the amended Drug and Cosmetic Rules, 1945.
2. **HIV testing facilities:** HIV testing facilities were identified in 154 Zonal Blood Testing Centres (ZBTC) with functional linkages to blood banks that did not have the facilities to screen blood for HIV. These ZBTC were equipped with the enzyme-linked immunosorbent assay (ELISA) readers and HIV testing kits for detecting both HIV I and HIV II strains. All blood banks in India sent blood samples to the ZBTC for HIV testing. The results were reported to the respective blood banks, often on the same day either as seronegative (blood units may be utilized for blood transfusion) or seroreactive in respect of HIV antibodies (unit to be discarded with the appropriate measures for biosafety). This strategy put in place systems for the testing of blood units rather than blood donors to ensure recipient safety.
3. **Training:** Every year, and on a regular basis, laboratory technicians working in ZBTC were provided "hands-on" training in respect of the protocols to be followed for testing of blood.

1992-1999: Implemented by the National AIDS Control Organization (NACO)

The Drug Controller General of India, in accordance with the Drugs and Cosmetics Act, licences blood banks in India. Standards in respect of blood banks differ from state-to-state, and policing of violations was initially limited, though on the increase. In 1992, a writ petition was filed in the Supreme Court of India, against the Union of India and others to address the deficiencies and shortcomings in the collection, storage, and supply of blood in the country. In 1996, Supreme Court of India passed an order in Common Cause vs Union of India and others directing government to improve the blood transfusion service. As a result, the National and State Blood transfusion Councils (NBTC/SBTC) were created to develop policies and programs for bringing about improvements in blood centers.

Guidelines for Testing for HIV

By 1992, the spread of HIV/AIDS in India had begun to raise issues well beyond the purely medical aspects. These related to privacy, confidentiality and ethics. National Guidelines were formulated, in line with the WHO guidelines, in respect of testing for HIV. The view prevailed that testing for HIV would have the following objectives:
  i. **Surveillance:** In order to evaluate trends in the spread and prevalence of disease within a given segment of population. In turn, this would facilitate an appropriate intervention. This objective was best achieved by an unlinked anonymous ELISA test for HIV on two different antigen preparations. A unit of blood testing positive by one ELISA is tested with a second ELISA having a different test protocol/antigen system.
  ii. **Protection** from transfusion-transmitted infections: In order to minimize the risk of transfusion-transmitted infections, blood being utilized for transfusion would mandatorily be screened and tested for hepatitis B and C, syphilis, malaria, and HIV. For HIV a single ELISA test was perceived as sufficient to ensure protection in the event of transfusion. In the event that a unit of blood tested seropositive for HIV, then the sample was to be discarded and destroyed and not to be deployed in transfusion.
  Provisioning for adequate numbers of testing facilities for pretest and post-test counseling to prepare persons to access voluntary testing for HIV (on account of asymptomatic/symptomatic HIV-related infections).

Modernization of Blood Banks

The National AIDS Control Organization launched a scheme providing central government assistance to states to upgrade and provide minimum facilities to blood banks in the public sector, as well as those run by charitable organizations. This assistance facilitated the purchase of equipment, consumables, test kits, chemicals, glassware, blood bags, and reagents. NACO has supported the modernizing of 815 blood banks (282 major blood banks and 533 district level blood banks). 40 blood component separation facilities were set up between 1992 and 1997 to promote the rational use of blood.

1999-2004: Implemented by the National AIDS Control Organization

The blood safety program begins to build upon and consolidate the initiatives of phase I (1992-99). NACO has already strengthened/modernized 815 blood banks and 40 component separation units. During Phase II, NACO plans to set up an additional 20 major blood banks, 40 blood component separation units, and to augment and strengthen blood banks at district levels. Voluntary blood collection has improved.

Highlights

1. **Establishing model blood banks:** In underserved states, in terms of quality

transfusion services in the government sector, National AIDS Control Organization supports the establishment of model blood banks. Sites for setting up these blood banks have been identified and the procurement process for equipment has been initiated. NACO would assist them in operating the project for the initial 3 years, after which it will be handed over to the state government. During this period, the staff will be fully trained in respect of standardized protocols and management of transfusion services. For other states, NACO would provide logistic and technical support for upgrading services of the existing blood banks. In order to enhance supply of blood and blood products, these blood banks would be linked to existing blood banks in the vicinity. These blood banks will function as demonstration projects in the states or regions where they are set up. They are also expected to function as nodal blood banks, which look after training and quality control requirements of transfusion services in the region.

2. **HCV testing facilities:** Testing of blood for hepatitis C virus (HCV) antibodies was made mandatory with effect from June 1, 2001. Training was provided by the National Institute of Biologicals, Government of India, at different regional blood banks. Mandatory testing for hepatitis C, hepatitis B, HIV, syphilis, and malaria is being implemented in respect of all donated blood units.

3. **Upgrading training:** With a view to improving standards of service delivery in blood banks, NACO facilitates frequent workshops (with WHO assistance), for training of blood banking personnel and sensitization of program officers from states.

4. **Blood storage centers:** In order to enhance access to safe blood, particularly in rural areas where it may be infeasible to establish full-fledged blood banks, government has facilitated the setting up of blood storage centers. These will be affiliated to larger blood banks, and will store screened blood for transfusion. The blood storage centers will be invaluable in the event of emergency obstetric care (EOC) and other emergent requirements as in road/rail accidents.

5. **Technical resource group (TRG):** NACO constituted a TRG on Blood Safety in 1994. This TRG has been deliberating the best practices in the clinical use of blood. National guidelines on the rational use of blood were circulated during 1995. More recently, in 2002, the WHO Guidelines on the Clinical Use of Blood have been adopted by NACO, and are being widely circulated to all stakeholders, in order to disseminate the protocol, and inter alia, to encourage and promote the rational use of blood.

6. **Role of the nongovernment, armed forces, and the private sector:**
   - A significant portion of the blood banking activity in India is carried out in the nongovernment sector, for instance, through the Indian Red Cross Society (IRCS), other NGOs, as well as private, for-profit hospitals, and so on. The IRCS is already well known in the field of donor recruitment and has several well-known blood centers in the country. It has recently embarked on an ambitious project to develop its blood service on the principles of voluntary blood donation, screening blood, quality management and good transfusion practice. Initially, linkages were provided to these blood banks with a view to ensuring that (a) all units of blood used for purposes of transfusion, without exception, is appropriately screened and tested and further (b) to bring on board all stakeholders in a movement for blood safety. When the ELISA equipment and HIV testing kits became readily available in the market, the blood banks outside of the public sector started investing in testing, autonomous of government. The private and the nongovernment sectors have made a remarkable contribution to the

blood banking industry in India. It is a recognized fact that the private health care industry will play a major role in the overall health care sector and therefore the private/nongovernment blood banks should be deemed eligible for facilities extended to government blood banks (not for profit facilities in particular). This will provide due encouragement and incentive to improve performance and service delivery.
- In order to improve the blood transfusion services and to have "good manufacturing practices (GMP)", it is imperative that this activity of blood banking be adequately modernized. All blood banks should be equipped with the state-of-the-art equipment and reagents. Similarly, any evaluation of the demand for blood and blood products cannot overlook the requirements of the nongovernment sectors.
- Armed Forces Transfusion Services (AFTS): The AFTS with 52 hospital blood banks is a well-organized network providing life-saving blood and blood components to armed forces personnel and their dependents. The AFTS also provides support for civilian emergencies, natural disasters and to populations in remote and inaccessible areas.

SUMMARY

- Increased awareness about transfusion transmitted diseases has necessitated the enforcement of stricter control over the quality of blood and its components.
- Regulatory affairs in the Indian blood banking system are controlled by central and provincial Drug Control authority under Drug Controller General of India.
- Human blood is covered under the definition of "Drug" under Section 3(b) of Drugs and Cosmetics Act 1940. Hence, it is imperative that blood centers (Banks) need to be regulated under the Drugs and Cosmetics Act and rules thereunder. The Central Government amends the rules from time-to-time.
- Part XB of the act deals with requirements for the collection, storage, processing, and distribution of whole human blood, human blood components by blood banks, and manufacture of blood products.
- Part XIIB of the act deals with requirements for the functioning and operation of a blood bank and/or for preparation of blood components.

SELF-ASSESSMENT EXERCISE

Write short essays/notes on:
- Discuss the essentials required for a new blood center/bank
- Discuss the regulatory authorities in India concerned with blood center/bank and transfusion
- Discuss blood banking requirements for licensing authorities
- Discuss evolution of blood safety program in India
- Discuss organization and legal concerns of blood banking

Bibliography

1. AABB. Standards for Blood Banks and Transfusion Services, 27th edition. Bethesda, MA: AABB Press; 2011.
2. An Action Plan for Blood Safety. National AIDS Control Organisation. Ministry of Health and Family Welfare. Government of India, 2007. Available from http://www.naco.gov.in/sites/default/files/An%20Action%20Plan%20for%20blood%20safety_2.pdf. [Last accessed on 2019 September 07].
3. Bain BJ, Bates I, Laffan MA. Dacie and Lewis Practical Hematology, 12th edition. London: Churchill Livingstone; 2017.
4. Barnes BC, Chiasera JM, Cook S, et al. Elsevier's Medical Laboratory Science Examination, Missouri: St Louis; 2015.
5. Bio-Medical Waste Management (Amendment) Rules, 2019. Available from http://www.indiaenvironmentportal.org.in/files/file/Bio%20medical%20waste%20management%20(amendment)183847.pdf. [Last accessed on 2019 September 10].
6. Blood transfusion safety. Available from https://www.who.int/bloodsafety/en/Blood_Transfusion_Safety.pdf. [Last accessed on 2019 September 08].
7. Choudhury N, Desai P. Blood bank regulations in India. Clin Lab Med. 2012;32(2):293-9.
8. Drugs and Cosmetics Act, 1940 and its amendments. Available from http://legislative.gov.in/sites/default/files/A1940-23.pdf. [Last accessed on 2019 September 08].
9. Harmening DM. Modern Blood Banking and Transfusion Practices, 6th edition. Philadelphia, PA: FA Davis Company, 2012.
10. Hemovigilance. Available from https://www.who.int/bloodsafety/haemovigilance/en/. [Last accessed on 2019 September 08].
11. Hillyer CD, Shaz BH, Zimring JC, Abshire TC. Transfusion Medicine and Hemostasis: Clinical and Laboratory Aspects, 1st edition. Elsevier: New York; 2009.
12. Howard PR. Basic and Applied Concepts of Blood Banking and Transfusion Practices, 4th edition. Elsevier Inc: Missouri; 2017.
13. Jaspreet Kaur Boparai, Surjit Singh. Hemovigilance: A new beginning in India. Int J Appl Basic Med Res. 2015;5(3):200-2.
14. Johns GS, Gockel-Blessing EA, Zundel W, Denesiuk L. Clinical Laboratory Blood Banking and Transfusion Medicine: Principles and Practices, 2nd edition. Pearson Education, Inc: New Jersey; 2015.
15. Klein HG, Anstee DJ. Mollison's Blood Transfusion in Clinical Medicine, 12th edition. West Sussex: John Wiley and Sons, Ltd; 2014.
16. Makroo RN. Compendium of Transfusion Medicine, 2nd edition. New Delhi: Kongposh Publications Pvt Ltd; 2009.
17. McCullough J. Transfusion Medicine, 4th edition. West Sussex: Wiley-Blackwell; 2017.
18. McPherson RA, Pincus MR. Henry's Clinical Diagnosis and Management by Laboratory Methods, 23rd edition. Philadelphia: WB Saunders; 2016.
19. Ministry of Environment, Forest and Climate Change Notification. Available from http://www.indiaenvironmentportal.org.in/files/file/Bio%20

medical%20waste%20management%20(amendment)183847.pdf. [Last accessed on 2019 September 08].
20. Ministry of Health and Family Welfare (department of health and family welfare) Notification, New Delhi, the 29th November, 2018. Available from https://cdsco.gov.in/opencms/opencms/system/modules/CDSCO.WEB/elements/download_file_division.jsp?num_id=MjE3OQ== [Last accessed on 2019 September 08].
21. Murphy MF, Roberts DJ, Yazer MH. Practical Transfusion Medicine, 5th edition. West Sussex; John Wiley and Sons Ltd; 2017.
22. National Blood Policy. Available from http://www.naco.gov.in/sites/default/files/National%20Blood%20Policy_0.pdf. [Last accessed on 2019 September 07]).
23. National standards for blood transfusion service. Available from https://www.who.int/bloodsafety/transfusion_services/BhutanNationalStandardsBTServices.pdf. [Last accessed on 2019 September 08].
24. Published in the Gazette of India, Extraordinary, Part II, Section 3, Sub-section (i)] Government of India, Ministry of Environment, Forest and Climate Change Notification. Available from http://www.indiaenvironmentportal.org.in/files/file/BMW%20Rules,%202016.pdf. [Last accessed on 2019 September 08].
25. Quinley ED. Immunohematology: Principles and Practice, 3rd edition. Baltimore: Lippincott Williams and Wilkins; 2012.
26. Regulatory Requirements of Blood and/or its Components Including Blood Products. Available from http://www.cfdamp.nic.in/pdf/guidelines_for_blood_bank.pdf [Last accessed on 2019 September 07].
27. Revised Guidelines for Common Bio-medical Waste Treatment and Disposal Facilities. Available from http://www.ppcb.gov.in/Attachments/Bio%20Medical%20Waste/CBMWTF.pdf. [Last accessed on 2019 September 08].
28. Safe management of wastes from health-care activities. Available from https://apps.who.int/iris/bitstream/handle/10665/85349/9789241548564_eng.pdf;jsessionid=6589784E37E1F963546FCAF7A585B6D0?sequence=1. [Last accessed on 2019 September 10].
29. Saran RK. Transfusion Medicine Technical Manual: World Health Organization, 2nd edition. New Delhi: Mehta Offset Pvt Ltd; 2003.
30. Screening donated blood for transfusion-WHO recommendations. Available from http://www.who.int/bloodsafety/Screening Donated Blood for Transfusion.pdf. [Last accessed on 2019 September 08].
31. Simon TL, McCullough J, Solheim BJ, Strauss RG. Rossi's Principles of Transfusion Medicine, 5th Edition. West Sussex: John Wiley and Sons, Ltd; 2016.
32. Standards for Blood Banks and Blood Transfusion Services. Available from http://www.naco.gov.in/sites/default/files/Standards%20for%20Blood%20Banks%20and%20Blood%20Transfusion%20Services.pdf. [Last accessed on 2019 September 07].
33. The Bio-Medical Waste Management (Amendment) Rules, 2018. Available from http://www.indiaenvironmentportal.org.in/content/453336/the-bio-medical-waste-management-amendment-rules-2018 [Last assessed on 2019 September 08].
34. The Gazette of India: Extraordinary, Ministry of Health and Family Welfare, Notification GSR 218(e). 28 Mar, 2001. Available from: http://www.cdsco.nic.in/writereaddata/GSR_218(E).pdf [Last accessed on 2019 September 08].
35. Turgeon ML. Linne and Ringsrud's Clinical Laboratory Science, 7th edition. Missouri: Elsevier Mosby; 2016.
36. Voluntary Blood Donation Programme-An Operational Guideline, National AIDS Control Organization Ministry of Health and Family Welfare, Government of India, 2007. Available from http://naco.gov.in/upload/Policies%20 and %20Guidelines/29,%20voluntary%20blood%20donation.pdf. [Last accessed on 2019 September 08]

Index

Page numbers followed by *b* refer to box, *f* refer to figure, *fc* refer to flowchart, and *t* refer to table.

A

A antigens 45
   common structure for 42
   formation of 42
A genes 54
A_1 and B red cells 75
A_2 red cells 48
ABO 41, 55, 59, 60, 235, 258, 387
   agglutinins, reduced titer of 172
   and D grouping, controls for 85
   antibody
      acquired 58
      less common 57
      monoclonal 70
      titers 56*b*
   antigens 47, 57, 57*f*, 59
      and antibodies, clinical
         significance of 58
      characteristics of 41
      poor development of 399
      typing 70
   blood group 33, 61, 70*t*, 72, 72*b*, 73*f*, 399
      alleles of 54
      antigen and phenotype 75
      production of 52*f*
      red cells 71
      system 33*t*, 38, 41, 45*fc*, 54*t*, 98, 99, 190
   compatibility 265
      agglutination indicates 227
   compatible blood 233
   discrepancies 86, 86*b*, 87, 87*b*, 88*fc*, 89*t*, 90, 90*t*, 91, 91*t*, 92*t*, 94*t*, 95*fc*
      resolution of 86, 93
      summary of 94
   expression, anomalous 50
   genes 44
   genetic loci controlling
      expression of 43
   group 69, 72, 76, 224, 225, 233, 235, 390, 393, 400
      blood selection 393*t*
      determination 335
      interpretation of 72*t*
      methods of 71
      system, genetic features of 53
   hemolytic disease of fetus and newborn 234, 397
   incompatibility 228, 296, 380, 399, 531, 531*t*
      minor 531
   incompatible
      antibodies, transfusion of 303
      organ, transplantation of minor 320
      red cells, transfusion of 303
   phenotypes 45
   reagents 469
   serum testing 75, 75*t*
   subgroups 90
   system 40, 59
      inheritance patterns 55*f*
   type 75, 282
Abortions 550
Accelerate graft rejection 510
Accreditation 488
Acetylglucosamine 46
Acid elution test 397*f*
Acid-base
   disorders 239
   disturbances 292
Acid-citrate-dextrose 163, 169, 288
Acquired immunodeficiency syndrome 23, 141, 346, 349, 445, 571
   transfusion-transmitted 443
Activate complement system 297
Activated partial thromboplastin time 268
Acute graft-versus-host disease 516
Acute hemolytic transfusion reaction 302, 303, 304*fc*, 321, 333, 337, 337*b*, 341*fc*
   signs of immune-mediated 303*b*
   symptoms of immune-mediated 303*b*
Acute immune mediated transfusion reactions 328
Acute intravascular hemolytic transfusion reaction 337*f*
Acute lung injury
   immune transfusion-associated 309
   transfusion-related 252, 303, 309, 312*t*, 340, 481, 494, 517
Acute nonhemolytic transfusion reactions 302, 306
Acute normovolemic hemodilution 413
Acute respiratory
   disease 569
   distress syndrome 309, 311
Acute transfusion reaction 302, 303*fc*, 317*t*
   evaluation of 339*fc*, 340*fc*
   nonimmunological 312
   type of 317
Acute transplant rejection 119
Adaptive immune cells 2
   response 2, 5
      components of 5
Additive solutions 169, 270
   composition of 166*t*
Additive system 165, 248
   advantages of 166
Adenine 26, 165, 166
Adenosine triphosphate 513
   binding cassette 135
Adhesion molecules, interactions of 287
Adipocytes 520
Adoptive cell transfer 536
Adsorption 211
   allogeneic 212
   commercial reagents for 212
   homologous 212
   technique, uses of 213*b*
Adverse reaction 333*b*, 532
Adverse transfusion
   incident 439
   reaction 300, 330
      recognizing of 333
Agammaglobulinemia
   acquired 56
   congenital 56
Agarose gel electrophoresis 375
Agglutination 11, 68, 194, 198, 225, 228, 229
   based methods 17
   first stage of 66
   grading system 187*t*

reactions 77
   grading of 183
   strengths of 87
   second stage of 66
   stages of 11
   temperature of 13
   weaker 86
Aggressive immunotherapy 324
   classification system 561t
   embolism 239
   pollution of 445
Albumin 245
   infusion 327
   reagents 232
Alcohol, denatured 367
Alleles 31, 37, 41, 505
   multiple 31, 33
   types of 31, 31f
Allelic antigens 100, 129
   five sets of 125
Allergic reaction 292, 308, 309, 338
   following transfusion 308b
   mild 308, 310
Allergic transfusion 331
   reaction 307, 310t, 340
Alloadsorption 201
Alloantibody 20, 91, 127, 190, 231, 400, 508
   clinically significant 206
   detection of 10
   formation of 117
Allogeneic donation 139
Allogeneic hematopoietic progenitor cell
   harvest 523
   transplantation 527
Allogeneic stem cell transplantation 533, 533f
Allografts 495
   rejection of 515
Alloimmunization 104, 381, 535
   factors influencing rate of 327
Alpha numeric terminology 100
American Association of Blood Bank 226, 451, 489
American Society for Apheresis Categorization of Apheresis Indications 287t
Amino acid 7
Aminophylline 293
Amniocentesis 104, 389
   indications for 389
Amorph 46
Amorphic gene 43
Amplicon, production of 502
Amplification 372
Amplifier molecule 376
Anamnestic immune response 9
Anaphylactic reactions 292, 293, 307, 308, 332
Anaphylactic response 308, 310
Anaphylactoid 308, 310

Anaplasma phagocytophilum 428
Anemia 146, 250, 381, 405
   acute 409
   alloimmune hemolytic 410
   aplastic 527, 530
   chronic 325
   requiring transfusion support 409
   risk for 36
   severe 250
Angioedema 308
   localized 308
Angiotensin converting enzyme 314
   inhibitors 327
Anguilla anguilla 69
Animal anatomical waste 447
Animal immune system 175
Antecubital veins 148f
Anti-A and anti-B 58
   A and B group 56
   in O group 56
Anti-A reagents, commercial 49
Anti-A_1 57
   lectin 71, 71f
Antibiotic therapy 316
Antibody 3, 5, 12, 41, 57, 69, 71, 82, 114, 122, 128, 203, 210, 218, 225, 350, 353, 387, 515
   absence of 21
   acquired 20, 85, 103
   additional 91
   against
      additives 232
      Rh antigens 103
   anticomplement 175
   antigen reaction 83
   circulating 207
   classification 79
   clinically significant 190
   complete 7
   concentration levels 215
   dependent cell-mediated cytotoxicity test 388
   detection 114, 188, 191, 514
   and identification 68
   methods 190, 193
   purpose of 188b
   reagents for 191
   development of 56, 327
   dose-dependent 189
   enhancement of 116
   excessive 12
   exclude presence of 399
   exclusion 206
   formation 4
   forming B lymphocytes 64
   high prevalence 205
   high-titer 58
   identification 188, 198, 199b, 200b, 207, 208b, 215, 218
   panel sheet 202f

   preanalytic phases of 200
   reagents for 198
   red cell panels, features of initial 198
   results of 203
   IgG type of 383
   immune complex 11
   incomplete 7, 11, 173, 179
   Indian 132
   interactions 79
   layers of 361
   low prevalence 205
   mediated graft rejection 516
   molecule 64, 67
   naturally occurring 190, 201
   nature of 104
   original 98
   passive 201
   plasma for 211
   potentiators 66
      mechanism of 69t
      type of 69
   private 509
   producing cells 105
   production of 5, 379
   reactions in vitro 10
   reactive 225t
   reagents, commercial 62
   resolution 188
   responses
      primary 10f
      secondary 10f
   salient features of 9t
   screening 94, 188, 197t, 225, 236, 387, 405, 426, 427, 510f
   gel method for 195f
   indications for 191b
   purpose of 191
   test 10, 188, 231
   separating multiple 215
   serum for 211
   significance of 114, 219
   sources of neutralization substances for 210t
   specificity of 188, 386
   temperature for 217
   testing 565
   titration 215, 387
   types of 56, 354, 379, 510
   warm 201
   weak 85
   weakly reactive 12, 191
Anticoagulant 521, 551
   acid citrate dextrose A 166
   citrate dextrose 278
      solution 282f
   preservative
      amount of 243
      solutions 163, 165t
Anticoagulation 276
Anti-Cromer antibodies 131

Index

Anti-D
  monoclonal reagents 105, 106*b*
  production of 99
Anti-Dombrock antibodies 127, 128
Antifibrinolytic agents 239
Antigen 3, 49, 67, 99, 120, 135, 350, 353, 386, 492
  antibody 21
    binding 15
    complex 11, 49
    ratio 12, 17
    reaction 14, 15, 58, 61, 205
  antithetical 124
  authenticated 101
  binding fragment, formation of 6*f*
  characteristics of 3
  dosage 204
  endogenous 495
  excessive 12
  exogenous 22, 496
  expression 113, 118, 121, 125, 127, 128, 130, 189, 189*t*
  functions 495, 496
  gradient of 49*f*
  heterozygous 189
  high-frequency 203
  high-prevalence 193, 218
  identification red cell panels 198
  in common, presence of 217
  interactions 79
  low-frequency 203
  low-prevalence 218
  mixtures 365
  negative
    blood donors 36
    red blood cells 234
  number of 498*t*
  per cell 42
    normal 102
  phenotypes 192
  positive reagent red cells 203
  presentation 495, 496
  processing of 5
  specific
    dendritic cells, autologous 536
    T-cells 493
  systems, dozen of 19
  typing, methods of 208
Antigenic
  determinant 3
  exposure 380, 383
Antiglobulin 83
  crossmatch 229
    method of 229
    requirements 226*f*
  drops of 108, 182
  phase 228
  reagents 61, 183, 192
    conventional polyspecific 175
  quality control of 185
  serum, addition of 102
  techniques, applications for indirect 184*t*
  test 96, 104, 105, 127, 173, 178, 180*f*, 181, 182, 183*f*, 185, 186*t*, 187, 426*f*
    advantages of 186*t*
    direct methods of 180*f*
    disadvantages of 186*t*
    history of 173
    indirect 67, 79, 102, 114, 179, 181, 183*t*, 184, 227, 228
    interpreting positive direct 205*t*
    materials required indirect 182
    principles of 179*b*
    procedure, indirect 185*t*
    quality control for 185
    sources of error in 185
    technique indirect 182
    types of 178
    uses of direct 181
    uses of indirect 182
Antigram 192
Anti-H 57
  reagents 71*f*
Antihemophilic factor 264, 420
  concentrate of 557
Antihuman globulin 7, 102, 173-175, 190, 225
  cards 78
  preparation of 175
  reagent 15, 63, 174, 174*f*, 469
  serum 551, 582
  technique, indirect 229
  test 173, 178, 427
    sensitivity of 187
Antihuman leukocyte antigen antibody 513
Anti-Kell autoantibodies 117
Anti-Rh antibodies, reactivity of 104
Antiseptic solution 148
Antisera 61, 62, 72
  commercial 69, 71
Antiserum 11, 83, 500, 501
  against human 11
Anti-trypanosoma cruzi 481
Anuria 332
Anxiety 332
Apheresis 274, 276, 277*f*, 281, 281*b*, 284, 521
  adverse effects of 292*b*
  basic principles of 275*f*
  blood components 294*t*
  donation 140
  donors 293
  general requirements for 280*b*
  granulocytes 168
  indications for 275, 275*b*
  licensing 444
  machine 276, 277
  methods of 276
  monitoring for 558
  physiology of 276
  procedures 292
  red blood cells 254
  time needed for 284
  types of 274, 577
Apnea 328
Apoptosis 527
Armed forces transfusion services 589
Arrhythmia, cardiac 306
Artery
  accidental puncture of 154
  disease, coronary 570
  forceps and scissors 148
Artificial oxygen carriers, potential benefits of 415*b*
Aseptic precautions 316
Autoadsorption 201, 212*f*
Autoantibody 3, 20, 92, 124, 127, 190, 196, 201, 508
  warm 68
Autoanti-P 123
Autoclaving 448
Autoimmune diseases 494
Autoimmune hemolytic anemia 35, 84, 104, 117, 179, 181, 239, 342, 410
  diagnosis of 184
  severe 130
Autologous blood 412*b*, 539
  donation 411
  preoperative 240
  transfusion 328, 411
    advantages of 411*b*
    contraindications for 412*b*
    disadvantages of 412*b*
Autologous control
  positive 196
  result of 205
Autologous donation, preoperative 328
Autologous hematopoietic progenitor cell transplant 533, 534
  indications for 532*b*
Autologous red cell phenotype 200, 207, 216
Autologous transfusion 240
  types of 412, 413*b*
Automation 422
  advantages of 422
  use of 423
Auto-Rh antibody 104

Autosomal dominant and X-linked recessive 121
Autosomal recessive 119
　phenotype 121
Avidin-linked detection system 505
Azide methemoglobin 157
Azurophilic granules 5

B

B antigen 45
　acquired 85, 88, 89t
　acquisition of 50
　common structure for 42
　formation of 42
B cell 4, 63
　functions of 5
　isolation of 502
　lymphomas 536
　malignancies 535
B genes 54
B lymphocytes 3, 5, 64, 495, 512
　stimulation of 515
B phenotype
　acquired 50
　inherited 50
Babesia microti 357
Babesiosis 288, 443
Bacteria 243
　gram-negative 172
　gram-positive 172
　retaining filters 559
Bacterial contamination 307, 331, 472
　sources of 314
　suspected 481
Band aids 148
Bandeiraea simplicifolia 50
Barcode label system 423
Basic immunoglobulin structure 6f
Basic test procedure 364
Bead-chip technology 35
Bilirubin
　conjugated 381
　metabolism of 382f
Bind oxygen 403
Biologic false positives 355
Biomedical waste 436, 444, 445
　categories of 447t
　containers/bags, label for 448f
　disposal option for 447t, 448b
　generation of 445
　management 446
　scientific management of 446, 446fc
Biotechnology 447
Birth canal 347
Bleeding 259
　disorder, diagnosis of 268fc
Blood 346
　acute loss of 244
　agitator 547

and blood products
　in blood bank, quality control of 473t
　quality control of 472
artificial 414
bacterial contamination of 314b
bags 162
　primary 162
　quality of 162
　selection of 434
　system 162
　traceability of 434
　types of 163, 163t
bank 20, 61t, 138, 369, 422, 425, 425b, 426b, 428, 429, 429t, 433, 468b, 475b, 538, 539, 545, 553, 555, 558, 578
　accommodation for 545, 581
　audits in 488
　by drugs controller, licensing of 443
　document control system in 477
　enzyme used in 115
　equipment used in 471t
　information systems 424
　license for operation of 541
　licensing of 443, 545t, 578
　licensing policy and legal framework for 578
　modernization of 586, 587
　policy 336
　prerequisite for grant of license for 579
　quality control of reagents in 469t
　quality management system for 452f
　reagents, licensing of 61
　registers in 475
　regulations and legal framework 538
　renewal of license for operation of 542
　requirements for operation of 545
　safety for 488
　size of 444
　staff requirement in 546t
　supplies required for 581
　system 538
　technician 546
　technology 567
banking
　and transfusion services 442
　applications of molecular genetics to 34, 370

　challenges in 441
　genetic principles in 30
　historical overview of 22
　recent advances in 425
basic principles in 138
borne disease 445, 470, 486
brain barrier 383
cell 43
　ex vivo generation of 417
　lineages of 520
　processor 253
　serology 138
center 138, 538, 539
　operation of 539
　policy 336
　staff requirement in 546t
　well equipped 441
clinical use of 442
collecting container 548
collection 138, 141, 147, 148b, 159b, 434, 468
　bag 148, 162
　equipment 149
　for components 246
　monitor 150f
　of whole blood, process of 148
　perioperative 413
　process of 149f
　room 545, 550, 581
　set 242, 243f
　technique of 472
　triple plastic bag for 163f
compatible 188
component 140, 242, 245, 269, 269t, 270f, 275, 281, 306, 316, 475, 539, 545, 553, 555, 558
　availability of 441
　categories of 555, 577
　expiration of 168t
　issue register 476
　preparation of 246, 246f, 248b, 545
　processing of 554, 577
　quality control of 472
　remove particular 275
　separation of 434
　transfusion of 347, 405, 517
　uses of 245t
container 581, 583
　weighing device 547
derivative 418
donation 155t, 438, 549
　adverse reactions to 152
　camps 444, 554, 555b
　criteria for 549
　deferment of 550t
　program 443
　types of 139
donor 36, 350fc, 359, 367, 438

prospective 573
record 552
register 582
registration 475
selection 431, 568
errors during collection
    of 222
establishments 138
functions of 414, 414b
genotyping, advantages of 84
group 19, 33, 38, 70, 79, 101,
    112b, 209, 304, 427, 553t,
    565
  A 45
  AB 47
  alloantibodies 20
  and compatibility testing
    431
  and labeling 431
  antibodies 76
  antigen 3, 17, 19, 399
  autoantibodies 20
  B 45
  chimera 85
  effect on 209t
  genetics 25
  infant's 393
  interpretation of 73f
  O 46, 52
  reagents 468
  secretors 47t
  selection for transfusion
    405
  serology 1
  serums 548
  slide method interpretation
    of 73f
  system 38, 39t, 40, 41, 42f,
    44, 54, 79, 112, 115, 122,
    122t, 135, 191
hematocrit of 394
in cold room, storing of 167
in refrigerator, storing of 167
issue of 434
loss 250
  acute 139
  iatrogenic 404
massive transfusion of 312
mixers 148
preservation 162
  aims of 162b
pressure 147, 311
processing 468
production of 473
products 138, 251, 284b, 419,
    431, 539, 543
  bacterially contaminated
    305
  manufacture of 539, 540,
    542, 544, 561

requirements for
    manufacture of 558, 559,
    563
  testing of 562
quality control in collection of
    467
rapid transfusion of 312
rational use of 431
recovery, perioperative 328
safe administration of 432
safety
  elements of 444
  program, evolution of 586
sample 179, 186, 221, 222b, 390,
    432
  depicting location of cellular
    components 9f
  large number of 76
selected for exchange
    transfusion 393
selection of 393, 577
separation, flow pathway of
    278f
shield statutes 443
specimen, acceptability of 222
stock register 582
storage of 162, 166
substitutes 414
transfusion 138, 296, 338t, 347,
    353, 387, 392, 400, 414b,
    436, 437, 516
  adverse effects of 296
  complications of 302b
  crossmatching for 182
  history of 386, 550
  process similar to 531
  reactions 300
  service 22, 538
  sets 581
  therapy 138
  transmissible by 569
transmissible
  diseases 545
  infections, testing 470
transport of 162, 432
type 40
unit 393, 405
  arrangement of 167
  utilization monitoring 485
  vending machine 430
vessels 347
volume of 150, 165, 394, 412
whole blood, staff requirement
    in 546t
within hospital, transport of
    167
Body's own antigens 3
Bombay blood group 51, 94, 95t
Bombay phenotype, salient features
    of 53b

Bone marrow 59, 132
  autologous 526
  collection 522b
  derived hematopoietic
    progenitor cells 520
  examination 323
  transplant 56
Bovine albumin 14, 65, 68, 548
Brain 134
  natriuretic peptide 311, 313,
    340
  assay of 313
Breastfeeding 146, 550
Breath sounds, abnormal 311
Bromelain 68
Bronchospasm 308
Buffy coat 528
  concentration 528
  method 257, 257fc
  pooling set 258
  reinfusion of 289
  removal method 257

C

Calcium hypochlorite 367
Campylobacter jejuni 60
Cancer 59, 146, 530
  immunotherapy 535
Candida vaginitis 114
Carbohydrate
  antigens 13, 40
  chains 42
Carbon dioxide 103
Card before test 367f
Card test 355
Cardiac arrest 531
Cardiac disease 311
Cardiac surgery
  bleeding during 402b
  previous history of 402
Cardiovascular diseases 570
Cardiovascular support 340
Cartwright antibodies 126
Cartwright antigens 125
Cartwright blood group system 125
Catadromous fish 69
CD59
  antibodies 136
  antigen 136
  blood group system 136
Cell
  abnormal 64
  allogeneic 495
  cycle 27
    major phases of 27, 27f
  dehydration 529
  depletion 528
  division 25, 27
    types of 27
  dual populations of 80

effector 4
enrichment 529
expansion 529
free hemoglobin solutions 415
free plasma 247
mediated immunity 5
membrane 4, 41, 42
    shape 169
mixed 80
panel
    preservation of 192
    selected 209
populations 530
purging 529
    and reduction 529
selection systems 528
surface 492
to-serum ratio 12
transfusions 492
Cellular
    antigen systems 429
    blood components 323*f*
        concentration of 309
        irradiation of 324*b*
    elements, effect on 169
    immunity 5
    immunodeficiency 322
        congenital 324
    loss 276
    therapeutics 430
    therapy 430, 519
Centers for Disease Control and
        Prevention 312
Central nervous system 383, 409,
        570
Central venous
    access 523
    catheter 314
Centrifugation 246, 248, 254, 279,
        423, 500, 527
    duration of 247
    methods of 277
    speed of 247
Centrifuge 470
    blood bags 255
    bowl, cross-section of 278*f*
    post-transfusion 335
Cerebral artery peak systolic
        velocity, middle 388,
        391
Cervical secretions 47
Chagas disease 145, 481
Chemical
    cryoprotective 529
    removal 36
    waste 447
Chemiluminescent immunoassay
        369, 444
Chemotherapy, high-dose 324
Chest X-ray 311
Chido/Rodgers

antibodies 130
antigens 129
blood group system 129
Chills 306, 532
Chimera, artificial 85
Chimeric antigen receptors 536
Chimerism 530
    artificially induced 90
Chlamydia trachomatis 378
Chlorine 367
Chloroform 210
Cholera 146, 550
Choriocarcinoma 125
Chromatography, affinity 279, 280*f*
Chromosome 25, 493
    autosomal 19, 25
    components of 25
    homologous 29
    number of 28, 29
    structure of 26*f*
Chymotrypsin 117, 128
Circulatory disorders 146
Cirrhosis, alcoholic 125
Cis-Ab phenotype 50
Citrate 164, 165
    anticoagulants 189
    phosphate-dextrose 163, 169
        adenine 163, 169, 551
        dextrose 163
        solution 581
    phosphate-double dextrose 169
    toxicity 238, 292, 326, 523
Citric acid 164, 166
Closed system bag 148
Clostridium 300
Coagulation 60, 239
    abnormalities 239
    cascade, activation of 300
    disorder 269
    factor
        concentrate, disadvantages
            of 411
        reduced levels of 239
Coagulopathy 294
    transfusion treatment of 267
Coding region 30
Codons 30
Cold
    agglutinin 57
    alloantibodies 91, 92*t*, 93*t*, 203
    antibodies 81, 91
    autoantibodies 91, 92*t*, 93*t*, 217
    hemagglutinin disease 342
Collected sample, appearance of
        223
Colloids 419, 420
    advantages of 420*t*
    artificial 419
    disadvantages of 420*t*
    solutions 419
Colon cancer 536

Colony stimulating factors 418
Color codes 468
Color Doppler middle cerebral
        artery peak systolic
        velocity 388
Colorectal carcinoma 89
Colored band indicating test 356*f*,
        367*f*
Colton antibodies 128
Colton antigen 128
Colton blood group system 128
Colton system 112
Column agglutination 78
    system, uses of 79, 79*b*
    technology 17, 78, 78*f*, 80, 81*f*,
        108, 183*f*, 195, 230*f*, 426*f*
    systems 426
    test 78
Communicable disease 445
Community acquired hemolytic-
        uremic syndrome 124
Compatibility 431
    test 183, 220, 235
        components of 220
        record 476
Compatible plasma, replacement
        of 578
Complement activation,
        consequences of 297
Complement system 20, 497
    activation, pathways of 21
    functions of 21*f*
Complete blood count 527
Complex antibody
    identification 216
    problems 68
Compliment activation releases
        vasoactive amines 298*f*
Component separation, principle
        of 275
Computer crossmatch 229
    advantages of 230*b*
Computer system validation 464
Conjugation 417
Continuous medical education 455
Conventional tube testing 186
Coombs antiglobulin test 179
Coombs control cells 178, 187, 194
Coombs crossmatches 339
Coombs phase tests 79
Coombs reagent 179
Coombs serum 551, 582
Coombs test 23, 104, 173, 180
    history of 173
Copper sulfate 468
    solution, preparation of 156
    specific gravity method 156
Cord blood 516, 532
    bilirubin 390
    collection 524
    product, processing 525

Cord cells 124
Cord hemoglobin value 390
Cord red blood cells 189, 189*t*
Cordocentesis 388
Corticosteroids 282, 309
Cotton wool swabs 148
Creutzfeldt-Jakob disease 366
Cromer antibodies 131
Cromer antigens 130
Cromer blood group 136
  system 130
Crossmatch 431
  interpretation of 226*t*, 229
  procedures 226
  techniques 226, 226*b*
  testing 220, 225
    limitations of 230
    purposes of 226
    types of 226
Cryo-poor plasma 245
Cryoprecipitate 245, 247, 269, 271, 369, 406, 557
  bag of 265*t*
  indications for 265, 265*b*
  pooling of 266
  production of 266*f*
  salient features of 264*b*
  thawing of 265
Cryoprecipitated antihemophilic factor 264, 266, 267, 270, 411, 472
Crystalloid 419, 420
  advantages of 420*t*
  disadvantages of 420*t*
  solutions 419
Cyanmethemoglobin method 157, 159*f*
Cyanosis 328
Cylinder enzyme-linked immunosorbent assay 363
Cytapheresis 274, 280
Cytokine 4, 5, 306, 497, 529
  production 514
  release of 307
  side effects of 523
Cytomegalovirus 251, 252, 320, 357, 393, 420, 525, 535
  infection 404, 575
  status 141
  transmission 535
Cytopenia 331
Cytosine 27
Cytotoxic reactions 495
Cytotoxicity
  complement-dependent 501*t*

D

D antigen 98, 101, 102, 386
  absence of 99
  detection of 102
  partial 103

D phenotype 102
Dane particle 350
Data handling, automation of 424*b*
Deep freezer 267*f*
Delated nonimmunological iron overload 325
Delayed transfusion reaction 302, 318, 326*t*
  etiology of 318*fc*
Dendritic cell 2, 4, 5, 495, 519, 535, 536
  use of 535
  vaccine 536*b*
Dengue fever 443
Deoxyribonucleic acid 25, 26, 26*f*, 37, 370
  based molecular typing 502
  based techniques, advantages of 502
  duplex, denaturation of 373
  isolation of 503
  location of 26
  preparation and amplification of 503
  synthesis 513
  virus, hepatotropic 349
Deoxyribose sugar moiety 27
Detect weak antibodies 305
Dextrose 164-166
D-galactosyltransferase 45
Diabetes 146, 571
Diagnostic kits and reagents, register for 553
Dichloromethane 214
Dideoxyribonucleoside triphosphate 506
Diego antibodies 125
Diego antigens 125
Diego blood group system 125
Diego system 112, 137
Diffuse intravascular coagulopathy 318
Digestive system 572
Dimethyl sulfoxide 529
Diphtheria 79, 146, 550
Direct antiglobulin techniques, applications for 184*t*
Direct antiglobulin test 79, 102, 178, 179, 184, 194, 195, 214, 318, 335, 337, 340, 341, 344, 379, 390, 400, 429
  procedure 178*t*, 185*t*
Direct solid phase test systems 83
Disinfection 487
Disposable blood collection bags, types of 150, 151*t*
Disposable sterile bleeding sets 581
Disseminated intravascular coagulation 268, 300, 341, 406, 411

Document
  control 477
    elements of 477*b*
    maintenance 478
Documentation control system, pyramid of 477*f*
Dolichos biflorus 48, 50
Dombrock antibodies 128
Dombrock antigens 127
Dombrock blood group system 112, 127, 127*t*, 128
Donath-Landsteiner test 123, 123*f*
Donation, autologous 139
Donor
  ABO group selection 233*t*
  additional qualifications of 550
  adverse
    events 479
    reactions, number of 484
  and blood unit records, retention of 474
  and donation, types of 139
  apheresis 275, 279
  autologous 523, 526
  blood
    collection, record of 475
    processing of 160
    product, antibody in 517
    product, T cells in 517
    repeat testing of 224
    screening of 431
  commercial paid 139
  counseling of 431
  cytapheresis 275, 280
  eligibility 147
  erythrocytapheresis 283
  granulocytoapheresis 281
  hemoglobin estimation of 156
  hemovigilance 438
  human leukocyte antigen antigens 517
  leukocytapheresis 281
  leukocyte infusion 534
  lymphocyte 254
    infusion 534
  physical assessment of 146
  plasmapheresis 275, 285
  plateletapheresis 281
  post-donation
    instructions to 153
    management of 152
  preparation of 254
  professional 139, 540
  recipient crossmatch 507
  record 475
    number of incomplete 484
  red cells 87, 228*f*, 337
  registration of 141
  sample 338
  screening 140, 140*f*

selection 138, 140, 144, 280-282, 434, 467
   and registration 475
   criteria for 283
   requires 141
specific antibody 513
suitability of 556
testing 357
treatment of 282
types of 139
units, selection of appropriate 233
Dopamine 293
Dot blot assay 363
Double red blood cell collections
   advantages of 284b
   disadvantages of 284b
Double red cell
   collection 283
      automated 283
   donation 283
Drabkin solution 159
   constituents of 158t
   detergent-modified 158
Drug-induced hemolysis, investigation of 184
Drugs and Cosmetics
   Act 444, 538, 565
      and Rules 538
   Amendment Rules 565
   Rules 539, 566
Dry heat sterilisation 448
Duffy antigens 118
Duffy blood group system 118, 137
Duffy glycoprotein 119
Duffy system 112
   phenotypes in 118t
Dysfibrinogenemia 269
Dyspnea 310, 331

E

Edema, conjunctival 308
Electrolytes 292
   effect on 170
Electronic crossmatch 229
Electrophoretic separation 375
Elevated lactate dehydrogenase 337
Elution 208, 210, 390
   partial 211
   technique
      principle of 210f
      uses of 210b
   total 211
Emergency drugs 148, 153
Empty satellite bag 269
Encapsulation 417, 448
Encoding genes 118
Encountering during donation, problems 153
Endocrine disorders 571
Endogenous pyrogens, release of 306

Endothelial cells 59, 119, 515, 520
Endothelium 310
Endotoxins 315
Endotracheal intubation 293
Enzyme 15, 68, 209, 548
   enhance cold 68
   immunoabsorbent assays 369
   immunoassay 17, 350fc, 357, 358, 365, 368, 369
      advantages of 358b
   labeled anti-human immunoglobulin antibody 364
   linked antiglobulin test 359
   linked fluorescence assay 444
   linked immunosorbent assay 17, 19, 350, 359, 363, 428, 508, 551, 552
      applications of 359, 359b
      competitive 362, 363f
      indirect 360
      procedures, advantages of 359b
      technique, advantages of 511
      test 511
      types of 359
      uses of 359
   linked immunosorbent crossmatch assays 508, 511
   spot 514
   substrate 511
   test method, one-stage 209
   treatment 209t, 216
   reactivity with 209
Epidermis 135
Epilepsy 146
Epinephrine 293, 309
Epithelial membrane 59
Epitope 3
Epstein-Barr virus 64, 251, 357
   infections 125
Equipment
   maintenance of 470
   quality control of 470
   selection of 457
   validation for new 457
Erythema 308
Erythroblastosis fetalis 324, 385fc
Erythroblasts 381
Erythrocyt apheresis 566
Erythrocytapheresis 274
   benefits of 283
Erythrocyte magnetized technology 427
Erythroid membrane associated protein 127
Erythro-magnetic technology 427
Erythropheresis 578
Erythropoiesis, accelerated 381
Erythropoietin 403, 404, 418

   low 403
   response 403
Escherichia coli 123, 315
Ethanol 367
Ether 210]
Ethyl alcohol 367
Ethylenediaminetetraacetic acid 552
Ex utero collection 524
Exchange transfusion 234, 244, 341, 392-394, 400
   advantages of 393b
   criteria for 392
Exons 30
Exotic disease 443
External proficiency exercise 470
External quality assessment 489
   scheme 442
   benefits of 490b
External quality assurance 472
Extravascular hemolysis 22, 300
   consequences of 301f
Extrinsic pathway, activation of 300

F

Fab fragments 7
Faint muscular twitching/spasms 155
False reactions 227
False-negative
   reactions 94, 96
   test, causes of 185, 338
False-positive
   reactions 94, 197
   causes of 197b
   tests, causes of 185
Fascioliasis 122
Febrile nonhemolytic transfusion reaction 252, 303, 306, 307b, 307t, 494, 517
Febrile reaction 307, 332
Fetal
   antigen 383
   circulations 380
   deoxyribonucleic acid testing 388
   genotyping 389
   hemoglobin 397f
   maturity 389
   red blood cells 403
      premature destruction of 379
   red cells, immune destruction of 381
   Rh hemolytic disease, pathogenesis of 384f
   spleen 382f
Fetomaternal hemorrhage 380, 395, 396
   amount of 385
   detection of 396f

Fever 303f, 304, 306, 331, 532
  development of 320
Fibrin
  degradation products 268
  sealant 267
Fibrinogen 245
  level 268
  replacement of 269
Ficin 68, 134, 209
Filtration 279
Fisher-race
  DCE terminology 110
  haplotype 100
  notations 100
Flow centrifugation, continuous 278
Flow cytometry 19, 507, 508, 511
Fludarabine therapy 324
Fluid
  phase assays 17fc
  shifts 276
Fluorescein isothiocyanate 511
Fluorescent
  caps 502
  treponemal antibody 19, 356
  test 356
Flushing 532
Food and Drug Administration 369, 457, 489
Foreign antigen 1
Foreign red cells 200
Forensic investigations 493, 494
Formalin 501
Fraction antigen binding 7
Fragmented blood transfusion service 444
Free hemoglobin, false-positive test for 337
Free plasma hemoglobin 337
Freezing hematopoietic progenitor cells, preparation for 529
Fresh blood 179
Fresh frozen plasma 168, 242, 245, 260, 261f, 266f, 269, 271, 285, 406, 420, 432, 436, 557, 577
  indications for 261, 262b
Fresh whole blood 244
Frozen red blood cells 252
Fucosyltransferase 43, 48
Fully automated
  immunohematology analyzer 426f
  transfusion-transmitted infection system 428f
Fungal infection 406

G

Galactose 46
Gamma
  globulin 146, 550
  irradiation 324

Gastric juice 47
Gastrointestinal cell cancers 114
Gastrointestinal symptoms 308
Gastrointestinal tract 4, 47
  lower 89
Gel based testing 17
Gel card 78, 426
  features of 78
  method 183
  technology 78, 108
    interpretation of 81f
Gel filled microtube 79
Gel low-ionic antiglobulin test 185
Gel method 186, 195f
Gel test 183
  antibody screen 195f
  specific 185
  types of 183
Genes 25, 30, 37
  activation 514
  alleles of 32
  block of 99
  groups of 514
  location of 126, 497f
  loci of 493
  regions of 30
  structure of 30
Genetic code 30
Genetic disease 527
Genetic forms 347
Genetic locus 31, 37
Genital fluids 347
Genitourinary tract 47
Genotype 32, 36, 41, 44, 99, 101
  determination of 54
  types of 32
Gerbich antigens 130
Gerbich blood group system 130
Gerbich null phenotype 130
Germ cell division 27
GIL antibodies 135
GIL antigens 134
GIL blood group system 134
Glass bead
  matrix 80f, 81f
  technology 426
Glass microbead
  matrix 78, 79, 183f, 229
    appearance of 78f
  technology 17
Glass slide 35
Glassware 447
Globoside blood group system 122
Glucose 166
Glutaraldehyde 367
Glycan 42
Glycerol 253
  cryoprotectant, process of removal of 253
Glycine 67
  acid 131, 210
Glycolipid 40, 42

Glycophorin A 115
Glycophorin B 115
Glycoprotein 40, 494
  acetylcholinesterase 125
  molecules 42
  primarily 42
Glycosylphosphatidylinositol 40, 125
Glycosyltransferase 44, 113
  enzymes 45, 48t
Gonads, germ cell of 28
Good manufacturing practices 548, 589
Graft
  alloantigens 515
  autologous 534
  cells, killing of 515
  disease, risk of 529
  rejection 534
  versus-host disease 251, 406, 408, 534
Gram stain and culture 316
Granulocyte 169, 324, 406, 519, 532
  collection 406
  colony-stimulating factor 520, 521
  components 324
  concentrate 245, 270, 271, 557, 576
    preparation of 271b
    volume of 282
  macrophage colony stimulating factor 271, 520
  stimulation 284
  transfusion 281, 324
    complications of 271, 272b
    indications for 271, 271b
  yield, increase 282
Granulocytopheresis 280
Graves' disease 571
Gravity leukopheresis 271
Group B red cells 70
Group O
  cells 46
  donors 191
  reagent screen cells 71
  red blood cells 198
  Rh-negative packed cells 235
Group red blood cells antigens 70
Guanine 26
Guinea pigs 98

H

H antigen 44-46
  amount of 53
  common structure for 42
  concentration of 44, 44f
  formation of 42, 43
H blood group system antigens 41
H gene 43, 51
H influenzae type B 132
H transferase 51

Hairy cell leukemia 286, 288
Haploid cells 29
Haplotype 101
Haptens 3
Haptoglobin 298, 299
   levels 320
   low 337
Headache 523
Heart
   disease 146, 570
      coronary 60
      hypertensive 570
   lung transplants 407
   surgery 139
   transplants 407
Heat freeze-thaw 210
Heavy chain, types of 7t
Heavy spin 247, 248
   centrifugation 254
Helicobacter pylori 60, 114
Hemagglutination 11, 17, 81, 203
   assays 425
      uses of 425b
   grading of 15t
   indirect 356
   reaction 79
   reversed passive 552
   scoring of 15t
   testing 34
Hemapheresis 274
Hematocrit 394
   centrifuge 547
   level 147
Hematologic cells, ex vivo
      manipulation of 535
Hematologic malignancy 251, 311, 324, 536
Hematological parameters 400
Hematological tests 79
Hematoma 153, 155
Hematopoietic cells 495
Hematopoietic graft
   cryopreservation of 529
   recipients 530
Hematopoietic growth factors 283, 417
Hematopoietic progenitor cell 59, 140, 284, 370, 429, 519, 520, 526, 526t, 533
   advantages of collection of 522b
   by bone marrow collection, risks of 521
   collection 284, 520
      benefits of 521
      procedure 523
   disadvantages of collection of 522b
   donor concerns 523
   dose 521
   mobilization 522
      side effects of 523
   processing methods, specialized 528
   products 520b
      processing 527
   reinfusion of 531
   terminology of 520
   transplant, types of 525
   transplantation 324, 407, 494, 519
      goals of 520b
      indications for 525, 526b
      purpose of 520b
      transfusion therapy for 535
   washing of 528
Hematopoietic stem cell 519, 520, 526, 578
   transplantation 96, 502, 516, 520
      complications of 533
   sources of 520b
Hematuria 332
Hemiglobincyanide 159t
Hemo-cue blood hemoglobin
   apparatus 157f
   system 157
Hemoglobin 147, 156, 157, 300, 337, 381, 414, 415
   based oxygen carriers 415, 416, 416b
   concentration 159, 159f
   content 565
   determination 550, 551b, 581
   estimation
      methods of 156
      sources of errors in 157
   into plasma 299
   level after transfusion 244
   types of 415
Hemoglobinemia 298, 300, 306, 337
Hemoglobinometer 547
Hemoglobinopathy, test for 525
Hemoglobinuria 298, 300, 306, 332, 337
   asymptomatic 305
Hemolysin 16
Hemolysis 15, 58, 59, 194, 196, 198, 203, 225, 228, 229, 294, 296, 319, 320, 331, 381, 531
   absence of 227
   acute 337f
   after birth 382
   alloantibody-induced 342
   elevated liver enzymes, low platelet count 342
   types of 296
Hemolytic anemia 250
   drug-induced 410
Hemolytic disease 58
   of fetus and newborn 7, 59, 98, 104, 114, 181, 182, 188, 225, 379, 382f, 383, 387t, 398t, 393, 400, 429
      cause of 110
      classification of 379, 380b
      diagnosis of 184
      risk of 84
Hemolytic properties 57
Hemolytic reaction 98
   serious 531
   symptoms of 298f
Hemolytic transfusion reactions 14, 58, 104, 218, 335, 338, 341fc, 342b
   control 305b
   delayed 117, 318, 319, 320b, 321, 321t
   investigation of 181, 184
Hemolytic uremic syndrome 342, 409, 420
Hemolyzed plasma 334f
Hemophilia 139, 411
   A 411
   B 411
Hemostatic abnormalities 239
Hemostatic disorders 410, 411
Hemovigilance 436, 438
   goal of 436
   reporting 483
   system 438
      terminology in 438
Hepa filters 559
Heparin 171
   effect of 402
Hepatitis 352f, 366
   A 146
   acute 352f, 353f
   B 146, 244, 370, 445, 582
      acute 353
      infection 145
      positive test for 145
      surface antigen 565
      virus 349, 352f, 357, 437, 525
   C 244, 445
      antibody 565
      virus 352, 357, 437, 486
   chronic 352f, 353f
   infection 571
Heteroantibodies 3
Heterohybridomas 64
Heterozygotes
      hypercholesterolemia 292
Hexose molecule, basic structure of 42f
Highly decentralized blood banks 441
Hinge region 6

Histocompatibility complex 3
  gene
    major 493
    polymorphism of major 493, 497
  major 497f, 536
  molecules, major 492
  restriction, major 493, 495
Histocompatibility testing 502, 515
  and matching, techniques of 498
Histone 26
Hodgkin's disease 534
Hodgkin's lymphoma 324, 532
Homologous chromosomes, pair of 29, 37
Homozygous 32, 33, 45, 51, 189
  antigen 189
  expression 189, 198
Hook effect 362
Hospital blood bank 450
  activities of 451b
Hospital transfusion committee 472, 487
  goals of 487b
Host disease, risk of 529
Host factors 386
Human alloantisera 501
Human anatomical waste 447
Human antibody molecules 175
Human B lymphocytes 64, 511
Human blood 538, 543
  components 539
  for components of blood products, processing of whole 540, 541
  for manufacture or blood products, processing of whole 540, 541
  group 38
    system 98
  operation of whole 564
  processing of whole 542
  testing of whole 582
Human cell cultures 511
Human derived coagulation factor concentrates, infusion of 328
Human embryonic stem cells 417
Human erythrocyte antigen 35
Human globulins 173
Human immunodeficiency virus 123, 141, 244, 346, 347, 350fc, 357, 437, 486, 525, 548
  1 antibody tests 349
  antibodies tests 552
  antigen testing 349
  infected whole blood 347
  infection 349f, 350b, 571
    transmission of 347
  isolation 349
  properties of 347
  related infections 587
  structure of 348f
  testing facilities 586
Human immunoglobulin molecules 177
Human leukocyte antigen 140, 251, 310, 340, 342, 503, 514, 516, 517, 524, 525
  allele 505, 506
  alloimmunization 535
  and sex, mismatched for 534
  antibody 517
    detection of 511
    formation of 509
    identification of 510
    methods of detecting 510
    screen 512
    specific 501
    techniques for detection of 509
  classification of 494
  codominant expression of 497
  complex 493, 496f, 497f
  detection 499
  evaluation 508
  haplotype 493, 497
  identical siblings 516
  inheritance 497
  matched platelet 324
    concentrates 324
  molecular techniques 502
  nomenclature for 497, 498
  specific antibodies
    after immunization 509
    in pregnancy 509
    in transfusion 509
    in transplantation 509
  system 492
  techniques for detection of 498
  testing to identify 499
  types of donor 514
  typing 498, 515
    method for 500
    procedures 503
    sera trays 501
Human major histocompatibility complex 493
Human mesenchymal stem cells 125
Human neutrophil antigen 310, 340
  antibodies 517
Human peripheral lymphoid cells 5
Human platelet antigen 324, 517
Human polyclonal origin, high-protein reagents of 105
Human proteins, family of 173
Human red blood corpuscles 555
Human resources 454
Human retrovirus, nontransforming 347
Humoral immunity 5
Humoral rejection 516
Hybrid cells 64
Hybridoma 64, 64f, 70, 176
  cell line 64
  technology 63, 177f
Hydatid cyst disease 122
Hydroclaving 448
Hydrogen
  bonds 27
  peroxide 367
Hydrolysis 448
Hydrops fetalis 381, 382
Hydroxyethyl starch 280, 283, 290, 293, 419
  solution 271
Hyperactive immune system 2
Hyperbilirubinemia 298, 320, 337, 381, 382
Hyperkalemia 238, 306
Hyperleukocytosis 287
Hyperparasitemia 288
Hypersensitivity reaction, stimulation of delayed 515
Hypertriglyceridemia 159
Hyperventilation 155
Hypocalcemia 238, 292
  risk of 523
Hypochlorite solution 486
Hypofibrinogenemia 239, 406
Hypogammaglobulinemia
  acquired 56
  congenital 56
Hypokalemia 238, 523
Hypomagnesemia 523
Hypoplastic anemia 250
Hypotension 293, 308, 331, 531
  treatment of 293
Hypotensive transfusion reaction 439
Hypothermia 238, 239, 402, 404
Hypotonia 328
Hypovolemia 244, 250, 293
Hypoxemia 310

I

I blood group
  antigens 124
  system 124
Iberis amara 50
Immature dendritic cells 135
Immune
  alloantibodies 190
  reconstitution 532
  serum globulin 242
  thrombocytopenic purpura 268
Immune hemolytic
  anemias 410
  reaction 336

Immune-mediated
  acute hemolytic transfusion reaction, causes of 304
  hemolytic transfusion reaction 343
Immune response 493, 495
  primary 8, 10t, 319
  secondary 9, 10t, 319
Immune system 2, 3
  cell of 4
  components of 4
  role of 2
  types 2
Immunity 1
Immunization 146, 147, 550
  active 397
  passive 397
Immunoadsorption 280
Immunoblot 364
Immunocompromised state 324
Immunodominant sugars 43, 44
Immunoelectroblot 364
Immunoelectrophoresis 16
Immunofluorescence assay 350
Immunogen 3
Immunogenicity 3, 19
Immunoglobulin 3, 6, 9t, 12, 17, 69, 245
  A antibodies 8, 173
  class 56, 386
  digestion of 7
  molecule 7t
  structure of 6
  types of 6, 7, 386
Immunoglobulin G 340
  antibodies 7, 66, 83
  weak 203
  isotype 130
  monoclonal anti-D 107
  sensitized red cells 178
  preparation of 178
Immunoglobulin M
  antibody 7, 66, 173
  molecules 66
  anti-D monoclonal reagent 105
  anti-HbC indicates recent infection 352
  isotype 116
  monoclonal anti-D/saline agglutination test 107
Immunohematology 1, 10, 434
  automation in 422
  transfusion therapy 138
Immunologic status 403
Immunological disorders 20, 526
Immunology, basic concepts of 1
Immunomagnetic beads 501
Immunomagnetic selection 528
Immunosuppressive therapy 56
Immunotherapy 535
In utero collection 524

In vitro
  bacterial contamination 96
  serologic reactions 56
  technique 502
Incompatible fluids 342
Incubation time, increased 213
Infections 534
  bacterial 50, 406, 481
  chronic 353
  markers tests, record of 476
Infectious agents 461
  risk of exposure to 461
Infectious disease 145, 355, 434, 446, 460, 490, 572
  markers 280
  test kits 460, 470
  testing for 468, 526
Inflammatory reaction 515
Inflate blood pressure cuff 149
Influenza 146
Innate immune cells 2
Intermittent flow centrifugation 277, 278f
International Hemovigilance Network 437
  functions of 437b
International Society of Blood Transfusion 101, 112, 437, 439b, 489
Intestinal obstruction 89
Intracellular infections 495
Intracellular pathogens 5
Intracellular red cell parasite 320
Intraoperative collection 413
Intraoperative hemodilution 328
Intrauterine transfusion 235, 324, 391
  indications for 391b
Intravascular hemolysis 22, 119, 296, 297, 302t
  causes of 296b, 300b
  consequences of 299f
Intravenous
  antihistamines 309
  drug abusers 347
  fluid infusion 223
  immune globulin 325, 391, 392
Intrinsic pathway, activation of 300
Ionic strength 14
  saline
    low 104, 193, 548
    normal 193
  solution, low 66, 228
Iron overload 410
Irradiated blood components, indications for 254, 254b
Irradiation, method of 254
Isoantibody 69
Isopropyl alcohol 367
Itching 308, 332

J
Jaundice 320, 571
John Milton Hagen
  antibodies 134
  antigens 134
  blood group system 134
  protein 134
Jr antibodies 135
Jr antigen 135
Jr blood group system 135
Jumbo plasma 285

K
K and K antigens 117
K antigens 117
Kell and Kx blood group systems 116
Kell antibodies 117, 118
Kell antigens 116, 117, 386
Kell blood group antigens 137
Kell glycoprotein 117
Kell phenotypes 116b
Kell system 112
Keratinocytes 323
Kernicterus 383
Kidd antibodies 120
Kidd antigen 119
  expression of 119
Kidd blood group 23
  system 119, 137
Kidd system 112, 119
  phenotypes in 119t
Kidney disease 146, 572
  severe 171
Kits, quality control of 470
Kleihauer-Betke acid-elution test 395
Kleihauer-Betke test 396
Knops antibodies 131
Knops antigens 131
Knops blood group system 131
Knops resides 131
KX antigen 117

L
Labels and label control 478
Labile coagulation factors, amount of 243
Labor, premature induction of 391
Laboratory centrifuge 471
Laboratory information management systems 424
Lactate dehydrogenase 320, 337, 340
Lactic dehydrogenase 318, 340, 341
Lan antibodies 135
Lan antigen 135
Lan blood group system 135
Landsteiner's rule 69

Index

Landsteiner-Eiener blood group system 129
Landsteiner-Wiener blood group system phenotypes 129*b*
Langerhans cells 495
Lattice formation 11
Lectin 68, 548
 pathway 21
Leishmaniasis 79
Leptospira 300
Lethargy 328
Leukapheresis 282, 521, 523, 540, 558, 577, 578
 products 532
Leukemia 90, 91, 129, 523, 534
 acute
  lymphoblastic 287, 535
  myelogenous 287, 532, 534
 chronic lymphocytic 56, 535
 relapse of 534
Leukemogenesis 289
Leuko reduced blood components, transfusion of 251*b*
Leukocytapheresis 288
Leukocyte 132, 140, 251, 332, 492
 and tissue 492
 antibody 510
 concentrates 540
 filter, modified 473
 functions, maintain 139
 poor red cells 473
 reduced components 251, 472
 reduction 251
  categories of 252
  disadvantages of poststorage 252*b*
  filter 251, 408
  poststorage 252
  prestorage 252, 307
Leukodepleted red cells 575
Leukodepletion 251
 benefits of prestorage 252*b*
Leukoreduced single donor platelets 578
Leukoreduction 251, 323
 method of 251
  poststorage 252
  prestorage 252
Levy-jennings chart 444
Lewis antibodies 113
Lewis antigens 113, 114
Lewis blood group 137
 biological role of 114
 system 113
Lewis system 112
 antigens 16
 phenotypes of 113*b*
L-fucose 43
L-fucosyltransferase enzyme 43
Licenses, cancellation and suspension of 543, 580

Licensing procedure 583
Light spin 247, 255
 centrifugation 254
Lipid envelope 348
Lipoprotein
 apheresis, selective removal of low-density 292
 high-density 292
 low-density 60
Liposome-encapsulated hemoglobin, advantages of 417*b*
Lips, edema of 308
Liquid plasma 169, 263
Liquid-phase techniques 193
 tubes and microplates 193
Live attenuated vaccines 573
Liver
 biopsy 323
 disease 571
  chronic 237, 571
 failure 571
 fluke 122
 transplant, complications of 407
 transplantation 407
Locus 37, 41
Low-ionic strength solution, disadvantages of 67
Luminex 504
 analyzer 513
 based technique 510
 single antigen 513
 technique 508
Lung disease 146, 570
Lutheran antibodies 121
Lutheran antigens 120, 121
Lutheran blood group system 120, 137
Lutheran system 112, 120
 phenotypes in 120*t*
Lymphocytapheresis 274, 289
Lymphocyte 4, 5, 169, 274, 501-503, 515, 519
 antibody secreting 64
 culture, mixed 513
 indicates 501
 lysis of 501
 microcytotoxicity test 499
 preparation 499
  amount of 514
 reaction, mixed 513
 separation 500*f*
 use of 512
Lymphocytotoxic human leukocyte antigen antibodies 510
Lymphocytotoxicity 499
Lymphoid
 line 519
 tissue, mucosa-associated 4
Lymphoma 129
 relapse of 534

Lymphotoxin 497
Lyophilized synthetic platelets 417

M

M and N antigens 115
Macroglobulin 494
Macrophages 3-5, 495
Macroscopic tests 367
Maculopapular rash 308, 323
Magnetic beads 500
Malaria 60, 119, 147, 244, 288, 357
 antigen test 367, 367*f*
 detection of 367
 history of 550
 infection 135
Malarial adhesion protein 133
Malarial antibody, tests for 367
Malarial parasite 565
Malignant cells 519
Mandatory screening tests 369
Mannitol 165, 166
Mannose-binding lectin 21
Manual tube testing 17
Massive bleeding, management of 237
Massive blood transfusions 262
Massive fetomaternal hemorrhage 395
Massive intravascular hemolysis 297
Massive transfusion 35, 234, 236, 237, 238*t*
 complications of 237
Master formula records 563
Maternal antibody, effect of 385
Maternal circulations 380
Maternal liver 381, 382*f*
Mature lymphocytes 4
McLeod syndrome 117, 137
Measles 79, 146
Mechanical mixing device 150*f*
Medical laboratory technology, postgraduate diploma in 568
Medical termination of pregnancy 386
Meiosis 28
 sites of 28
 stages of 29, 29*f*
Melanoma, advanced 536
Membrane attack complex 16, 22*f*, 297, 298*f*
Membrane filtration 279
Memory cells 4
Mendelian dominant fashion 40
Meningitis, bacterial 130
Menstrual bleeding, excessive 146
Mesenchymal stem 520
 cells 123
Metabolic alkalosis 239, 523
Metabolic complications 238, 328

Metabolism, inborn error of 526
Metabolize citrate 404
Metallic body implants 447
Methemalbumin 157, 339
Methylated spirit 367
Methylene chloride 210
Microangiopathic hemolytic anemia 409
Microbial pathogens 123
Microbiological tests, separate room for 486
Microbiology 447
Microchimerism 535
Microglobulin polypeptide 494
Microhemagglutination assay 356
Microlymphocytotoxicity 499, 500*f*
  complement-dependent 507, 507*f*, 510, 510*f*
  typing, complement-dependent 499
Micropinocytosis 135
Micropipette 107*f*
Microplate
  method 76, 77*f*, 78*f*
  technique 108
Microtiter 501
  plate wells 361
Microtyping system 78, 426
Microvascular bleeding 239
Microvascular hemorrhage 238
Ministry of Health and Family Welfare 538, 563
Miscarriage 386
Mislabeling errors 478
Missed antibody, causes of 231*b*
Mitochondrial deoxyribonucleic acid 26
Mitosis 25, 27
  phases of 28, 28*f*
  sites of 28
Mitotic phase 27
Mixed-field
  agglutination 196, 202
  appearance 96
  reactions 90, 208
  causes of 90
Molecular blood grouping 72, 84, 85
  applications of 84
Molecular forces, types of 27
Molecular genetics 33
Molecular immunohematology 33
Molecular methods 208
Molecular techniques 428
Molecular testing
  applications of 34, 34*t*, 429*t*
  clinical applications of 35
Molecule 4, 175
Monoclonal antibody 62-65, 65*t*, 64*f*, 175, 361
  products 62

reagents 63
  disadvantages of 65
  use of 65
Monoclonal anti-D
  antibodies 105
  reagents 105, 106
Monoclonal antihuman globulin production 175
Monoclonal antisera 105
Monoclonal blends 106
Monoclonal murine antibody 64*f*
Monocytes 519
Monohydrate 166
Mononuclear cell
  component suspension, preparation of 288
  count 522
Mononuclear phagocyte system, macrophages of 300
Mononuclear phagocytic system 179
Mononucleosis, infectious 125
Monospecific antihuman globulin 176
  reagents 175
Mother's blood group 393
Multicomponent apheresis donation 284
Multiple antibody 196, 203, 216
  resolution 216
Multiple component systems 278
Multiple myeloma 56, 93, 159, 523, 532, 534
Multiple platelet apheresis products 281
Multiplex immunoassay (luminex) 512
Mumps 146
Murine monoclonal blends 49
Muscle pain 523
Mutilation 448
Myalgia 523
Mycoplasma pneumoniae 124, 201
Myeloablative transplants 530
Myelodysplastic syndrome 526
Myeloid line 519
Myeloma cells 63, 64

N

N-acetyl-D-galactosamine sugar 45
N-acetylgalactosamine 45, 89
N-acetylgalactosaminyltransferase 45
Naïve lymphocytes 4
National AIDS Control Organization 538, 587
  role of 442
National Blood Policy 436, 441-444, 538

National Blood Transfusion Council 442, 539
National Institute of Virology 539
Natural killer cells 5, 519
Nausea 154, 523, 532
Needle-related injuries 153, 154
Negative cells 501
Negative control cells 208
Negative indirect test 83
Negative test 228
Neisseria gonorrhoeae 378
Neocytopheresis 284
Neonatal transfusion 236, 328, 403, 407*b*
Nephrotic syndrome 133
Nephrotoxic free hemoglobin 528
Neuroblastoma 324
Neurologic ischemia 531
Neurologic toxicity 531
Neutral gel 185
Neutralization 16
  techniques 209
Neutropenia, severe 406
Neutrophils 310
  engraftment of 532
Newborn transfusions 392
Nonagglutinating antibody 83, 173
Noncoding region 30
Nonconformance management 479
Nonconformance reporting 481
Nonconformance type 480*t*
Nonexpressed genes 36
Non-governmental Organizations 538
Nonhematologic malignancies 536
Nonhemolytic transfusion reaction 343
Non-Hodgkin's lymphoma 523, 532, 534, 535
Non-human leukocyte antigen antibodies 508
Nonimmune hemolysis 342
Nonimmune mediated
  hemolysis 305
  hemolytic transfusion reaction 343
  red cell hemolysis, causes of 305
Noninfectious
  complications 302
  conditions 355
Noninfectious waste 445
Non-ionic detergent 158
Nonlive vaccines 573
Nonmyeloablative
  conditioning 530
  transplant 534
Nonremunerated donors 467
Nonsecretors 47, 60
Nonself antigen 8

Index

Non-serological crossmatch 226, 229, 230
Nontreponemal antibody-screening tests 354
Nucleated cell 494
   total 525
Nucleic acid 368, 370
   amplification
      test 23, 349, 350*fc*, 350*fc*, 369, 370, 372*f*, 428
      techniques of 372*b*
   extraction of 372
   probe 502
   sequence 506
      based amplification 372, 377
   types of 26
Nucleic acid test 34, 370, 371, 378, 429, 444, 525
   advantages of 371*b*
   applications of 371, 372*b*
   benefits of 371*b*
   techniques of 372
Nucleocapsid protein 348
Nucleotide
   chain of 26
   sequence 504
   unit, structure of 26, 27*f*

O

O gene 32, 43, 46
Occupational hazard 445
OK antigens 133
OK blood group system 133
Oligonucleotide 504
   probes 504
      reverse sequence-specific 504
      sequence-specific 503
Oligosaccharide 42
   chains, type 1 43
Oliguria 332
Oncofetal antigens 125
Oncology 408
Opsonization 297
Oral polio vaccine 146
Organ systems 308
Organ transplantation 493, 498, 514
Organic solvents 214
Original licence 585*f*
Oropharyngeal airway 153
Osmotic fragility 169
Osteoblasts 520
Osteogenic progenitor cells 520
Ovalocytosis 130
Ovarian cyst fluid 47
Oxygen 293
   and mask 153
   carriers, artificial 414
   delivery, immediate restoration of 416
   exchange for 380
   saturation 311
   therapeutics 414
Oxygenating pump, time of 402

P

P blood group 122, 137
   antibodies 122
   antigen 122
      expression 122
   biological role 123
   physiologic role of 123
Packed cells 256*f*
Packed red blood cell 138, 245, 247, 271, 318
   features of 251*b*
   frozen 556
Packed red cells 255*f*
Pain 332
Pancreatic cancer 59
Pancytopenia 535
Panel reactive antibody 508, 511
Papain 11, 68, 134, 209
Para-Bombay blood group 52
Paraglobeside 42
Parasite 172
   causing 481
Parenteral transmission 347
Paresthesias 328
Paroxysmal cold hemoglobinuria 123
Paroxysmal nocturnal hemoglobinuria 79
   detection of 82
Particle agglutination assays 364
   advantages of 364*t*
   disadvantages of 364*t*
Particle gel immunoassay 82
   test 357
Parvovirus
   B_{19}, receptor for 123
   infection 79
Passenger lymphocyte syndrome 531, 532
Paternal samples, testing of 36
Pathogen reduction technology 428
Pathologenic humoral factors, removal of 289
Pediatric transfusion 236, 403
Pedigree chart 55*f*
Peptic ulcer, chronic 146
Percutaneous umbilical blood sampling 388
Perfluorocarbon emulsions 415
Perfluorocarbons
   advantages of 416*b*
   disadvantages of 416*b*
Perfluorochemical emulsions 415
Performing test, time period of 387
Perinatal period 380
Perinatal spread 347
Perinatal transmission 347
Periodic competency assessment 456
Periorbital area, edema of 308
Peripheral blood 5, 520, 522, 526
   lymphocytes 499, 500
   progenitor cells 520, 521
   smears, microscopic examination of 367
   stem cells 284, 577
Peripheral lymphoid organs, T cell zones of 4
   tissues 5
Peripheral organs 4
Permanent chimera 85
Permanent deferral 144
Pertussis 146
pH 214
   effect of 13, 170
   reduction of 214
Pharmacogenomic applications 493, 494
Phenotype 32, 36, 41, 72, 99, 101, 114, 125, 202
   weak 50
Phlebitis and cellulitis, mild 153
Phlebotomy 148, 149, 153, 166, 169, 269
   donor care after 152
   inspection of site of 147
Phosphate
   buffered saline 548
   diester bonds 27
   molecule 27
Photoactivable drug 289
Photoactivation by ultraviolet A light 289
Photochemotherapy, extracorporeal 288
Photometric devices 78
Photopheresis 288
   extracorporeal 288, 288*t*
Phototherapy 392, 400
Phycoerythrin 505
Physical examination requirements 147*t*
Phytohemagglutinin 513
Pilot samples 556
Pilot tubes 148
Placenta 59, 114, 134
   during pregnancy, role of 380
   umbilical cords 524
Placental trophoblasts 131
Plague 146, 550
Plasma 12, 53, 168, 172, 198, 263, 334, 369, 557, 560
   antibody in 99
   by additive solution, replacement of 172
   cells 3, 5, 515
   citrate level 238

cold insoluble portion of 264
collection of 558
components 260
　selective removal of 291
containing blood components 58
cryoprecipitate reduced 265
derivative 245, 245t
　infusion of 327
　products 260
dextrose 170
double 284
excess 289
exchange 275, 285
　mechanisms of action of 289
expanders 232
expresser 248, 249f
from blood, separation of 165
frozen 169, 269
individual 560
K⁺ 170
less 250
normal 334f
products 285
　transfusion of 235
protein fraction 245
pyrolysis 448
regain, rapid 354, 355
removal 307
significant volumes of 332
substitutes 419
testing 87, 91, 94
transfusion 407
triple 284
Plasmapheresis 274, 275, 391, 540, 558, 577
　donors, criteria for 285
Plasmodium
　falciparum 60
　　infection 130
　vivax 119
Plastic bags, types of 171, 171t
Plastic closed bag system 246f
Plastic collection bag 242
Plasticized polyvinyl chloride 162
Platelet 59, 167, 168, 170, 245, 258, 269, 274, 284, 369, 406, 432, 494, 519
　additive solutions 171, 172b
　　advantages of 171, 172b
　advantages of 281b
　alloimmunization 327
　apheresis of 258, 558
　collection of 140, 278, 282f
　components 254
　concentrate 170, 245, 247, 251, 255, 256f, 257, 258, 271, 473, 556
　　advantages of 257
　　indications for 259, 259b

preparation of 256fc, 257, 257fc
production of 256f
transfusions 315
count 239, 259
　minimum 281
disorders 139
dysfunctional 269
engraftment of 532
　delayed 535
functions of 254b, 402
irradiated 168
leukocytes 260
pooled 259
poor plasma 256f
　removal of 254
preservation 171
refractoriness 494, 517
　causes of 259b
rich plasma 245, 247, 255f, 256f, 270
　centrifugation of 254
　method 256fc
selection for refractory 493
shelf life of 171, 171t
sources of 254
substitutes 417
therapy 251
transfusion 259b, 407, 510, 535
　efficacy of 259
　poor response to 492
　refractoriness 327
　salient features of 260b
units 472
　platelet count in 472
Plateletpheresis 274, 280, 281, 540, 558, 577, 578
Poisonous diluents 159
Polar body 29
Policies and process documents 474, 478
Policy document 477
Polyacrylamide gel electrophoresis 375
Polyagglutination 94
Polybrene 15, 193
Polyclonal antibody 62, 65, 65t, 175
　blends 105
　products 62
　reagents 63, 65
Polyclonal antihuman
　globulin
　　production 175
　　reagents 176f
　　immunoglobulin G 63
Polyclonal antiserum 63
Polyclonal immune response 63, 63f
Polycythemia vera 121
Polyethylene glycol 15, 67, 104, 417
Polygonal anti-D reagents 106

Polymerase chain reaction 35, 358, 371, 372, 374f, 502, 503
　components of 374t
　primer 502
　products
　　analysis of 375
　　detection of 375
　sequence-specific
　　oligonucleotides
　　　hybridization 503
　　primers typing 505
　testing 502
Polymerization 417
Polymorphism 493, 506
Polymorphonuclear neutrophils 2
Polyspecific antihuman globulin 175
　reagents 174
Polyspecific reagent 192
Pooled buffy coat, platelet extraction from 257
Pooled platelet concentrate,
　advantages of 257
Population genetics 33
Positive cells 501
Positive control cells 208
Positive direct antiglobulin test,
　causes of 181t
Positive indirect test 83
Positive reaction 18, 77, 79, 199, 203
　reaction strength of 203
Positive test 228
Positivet lymphocytes 513
Postcentrifugation 423
Post-donation care 152
Postnatal management of infant 392
Post-transfusion
　blood sample 334, 335, 338
　purpura 318, 324, 327
　reaction blood and urine
　　samples 334
　serum hemoglobin 336
　urine sample 335, 338
Post-transplant immunological
　monitoring 513
Postzone effect 12, 17
Potassium 404
　cyanide 158
　dihydrogen phosphate 158
　ferricyanide 158
Potency 61
Potent hemolysin 123
Potential phenotype exclusion 217
Povidone iodine 367
Preamplifier molecule 376
Preanalytic information 200
Preanalytical modules 423
Precentrifugation 423
Preexisting disease 312
Prematurity, anemia of 403
Presyncope 153

Index

Pre-transfusion
  antibody screen 201
  blood sample 335
  compatibility testing 79
  sample 335
  testing 220, 224t, 234, 412, 428
    protocol 221b
Primer extension 374
Prion disease 366
Procedure documents 477
Process document 477
Process validation 463
Professional antigen-presenting
    cells 495
Proficiency testing 485
  program 472
Progenitor cell 524
  collection 521
  cryopreserved 531
  lineage-restricted 519
  product 408
Prolymphocytic leukemia 286, 288
Pronase 128
Protease enzyme 128
Proteasomes 495
Protein 26
  antigens 13
  chains 494
  complement 174, 175
  concentration of 65
  increased precipitation of 67
  molecules 68
  reagent
    control, low 65
    low 105
  synthesis 30
Proteolytic enzyme 11, 68, 83
Prothrombin time 268
Prozone 12
  phenomenon 17
Pruritus 308
Psychiatric diseases 570
Public health hazard 446
Pulmonary capillaries 118
Pulmonary edema 310, 311
Pulmonary wedge pressure 313
Pulse 147
Punnett square 54, 55f
Purified human immunoglobulin
    175
Purines 26
Purkinje cells 118
Pyridoxylated hemoglobin
    polyoxyethylene 417
Pyrimidines 27
Pyrogenic reaction 338
Pyrogens 306
Pyruvate kinase deficiency 300

Q

Quality assurance 451, 464
  audits 488
  components of 465t
  elements of 465b
Quality control 62, 247, 250, 258,
    265, 451, 466, 470, 487,
    562
  documentation, components of
      467b
  internal 467
  tests 475
  type and frequency of 466
  versus validation 466
Quality incidents and exceptions
    488
Quality indicators 484
Quality management 451
  system 451, 452, 453b
Quality manager 482
Quality manual 474, 478
Quality program 451
Quality system 451
  scheme 442
Quantitative method 283
Quick-fix solution, initial 482

R

Rabies vaccination 550
Radiation therapy 324
Radioimmunoassay 365
Radioimmunoprecipitation assay
    358
Random donor 260
  platelets 258, 498
RAPH blood group system 133
Rash 331
Reaction
  negative 18, 77, 199, 203
  phase of positive 204
  severe 308, 310
  strength and phase of 196
Reagent anti-D 102
Reagent cells, antigenic profile of
    192
Reagent control 65
Reagent group O red cells 191
Reagent product insert 61
Reagent red blood cell 70
Reagent red cell 61, 62, 65, 76, 79,
    82, 198, 200b, 201, 218
Reagin antibodies 354
Reagin test, automated 355
Recipient adverse events 480
Recipient blood sample 221
Recipient hemovigilance 438
Recipient leukocyte antibodies
    306
Recipient red cells 222
Recombinant coagulation factors
    430
Recombinant immunoblot assay
    358
Record, protection of 474
Records management 478

Red blood cell 1, 13, 32, 40, 66, 98,
    102, 164, 166, 168, 220,
    246, 253, 270, 274, 284,
    379, 403, 420
  alloimmunization 327
  and plasma 166
  components 247
  deglycerolized 253
  disorders 526
  engraftment 532
    delayed 531
  exchange 274
  groups 38
  hematocrit 472
  low volume 165
  membrane 14
    loss of lipid in 169
  phenotype 101
  sensitization of 11f
  separation of 248
  transfusion 315, 405, 407, 410
    indications for 405
Red cell 7, 41, 49, 71, 75, 77, 82, 101,
    102, 105, 135, 179, 211,
    252, 369, 432
  additive solutions 165
  adherence 78
  agglutination of 11
  antibody 41, 49, 91, 190, 198
    detection 79
    identification panels 198
    identification studies 337
  antigen 10, 19, 35t, 38, 40, 42,
      58, 68, 69, 198, 319
    and antibody 9f
    detection of 183
    expression 189
    inheritance of 40
    phenotyping of 183
  apheresis 283, 286
  clumping of 12f
  components, types of 575
  concentrate 245, 247, 473
  crossmatching of 282
  defect, intrinsic 305
  destruction of 305
  during storage 165
  exchange 288, 341, 410
  exposure of 305
  genotype analysis 429
  grouping 70
  ionic charge 13
  irradiated 575
  lysis 22f, 297, 298f
  membrane 38, 66, 68
    contains antigen 9f
  panel 104
  phenotype 59
    prediction of 35
  population of 96
  preparations 76
  procedure in 211

rapid destruction of 303
reagent panel 199
reduction 527, 528
sample 198
significant number of 332
storage of 163
substitute 414, 415, 415b
testing 87
transfusion of incompatible 58
typing 34
washed 253, 473
Red Cross Society 538
Refrigerated centrifuge 247, 249f, 471, 547
Regulatory regions 30
Rejuvenation solution 167
Remedial action 482
Renal damage 532
Renal disease
  chronic 408, 408t
  end-stage 133
Renal dysfunction 294, 409
Renal failure 304, 306, 332, 531
  prevention of 341
Renal graft rejection 114
Renal injury develops 337
Renal medulla 119
Renal transplant 407
Renewal of licence 586f
Repeat compatibility test 337
Replacement donors 139
Replacement fluid 269, 285, 289, 291
Residual leukocyte counts 472
Respiratory
  diseases 570
  distress 308
  epithelium 134
  symptoms 308, 331
Restarting transfusion 309
Retention, record 474
Reticulocyte typing 208
Reticuloendothelial system 22
Reverse-transcriptase polymerase chain reaction 375
Rh antibodies 103
  characteristics of 103
  production, causes of 103
Rh antigen 101, 103, 379
Rh antisera 469
Rh blood group 102f
  system 98, 99, 100, 101
Rh compatibility 258
Rh deficiency syndrome 103
Rh genes 98
Rh group 235, 387
Rh grouping
  controls for 106
  methods of 106b
  techniques 106
Rh haplotype 100

Rh hemolytic disease of fetus and newborn 234
Rh immunization, antenatal management of 391
Rh immunoglobulin 201, 379, 394
  injection 258
  prophylaxis of 104
Rh inheritance, normal pattern of 99f
Rh negative 99, 101, 102
  blood 233
  phenotype 103
Rh positive
  blood 98, 234
  cells, normal 102
Rh system 110
  basic genetics of 98
  biochemistry 103
  discovery of 98
Rh terminologies 101
Rh types 224, 225, 233, 390, 400
  sera 582
Rh typing reagents, types of 105
Rhesus monkeys into rabbits 98
Rhesus system 40, 98
Rheumatic heart disease 570
Ribonucleic acid 30f, 370, 375
  small amount of 26
  viruses 347
Rigors 306
Room temperature, reactive at 124
Root cause analysis 440, 454
Rosenfield nomenclature 101
Rosette technique 395
Rouleaux 93, 197
  characteristics of 197
Rouleaux formation 85, 93t, 228, 231
  causes of 197
Routine antigen typing 208
Routine blood bank 101, 136
  quality control procedures 466
R-phycoerythrin 511
Rubber ball 149
Rubella 146
Rule out hemolysis 315
Rule out hemolytic transfusion reaction 307

S

Safe blood transfusion 430
  ethical issues in 443
Safe transfusion, no standards for 444
Saline
  equal volume of 93
  normal 306f, 469
  room temperature technique 74
  washed red cells 575
Saliva 47

Salk polio 146
Salt-poor albumin 67
Sample collection
  errors 327
  test tubes for 148
  tubes 222
Sample tubes 147
Sandwich enzyme linked immunoassay 361
  technique 361f
Scianna antigens 126, 127
Scianna blood group system 126
Screen cell sample, number of 196
Screening assays, principles of 358
Screening cells 65
  pooled 192
Screening method 357
Sealing blood collection bag 152f
Sedimentation agents, using 527
Sedimentation method 250
Sedimented blood sample 247
Self-antigens 207
Semiautomated immunohematology analyzer 426f
Seminal fluid 47
Sensitization, risk of 394
Sensitized cells 173
Separate sterile room 524
Septicemia, gram-negative 89
Seroconversion window 370
Serologic crossmatch 231
Serologic cross-matching 17
Serologic rotators 547
Serologic screening test, presumptive 355
Serologic testing 342, 386, 412
Serological crossmatch 226
  techniques 227
Serological test 357
  principles of 227
Serological typing 499
Serum 12, 69, 87
  bilirubin 400
  concentration 392
  cell ratio 12, 13
  proteins, group of 6
  reactivity, matching of 204
  testing 87
Settle method 364
Severity of disease 399
Sex chromosomes 25
Sexual contact 353
Sexual transmission 347
Sexually transmitted
  disease 353
  infections 572
Sézary cell syndrome 286, 288
Shiga toxins, receptors for 123
Shock 304
  causes of 309
  prevent 139

Index

Short tandem repeats 506
Shredding 448
Sialic acid 13
Sialic acid rich glycoprotein 115
Sialoglycoprotein 115
Sickle cell 79
    anemia 121, 325, 409, 530
    disease 288, 409b
Simply transfusion reactions 300
Single antibody 196
    specificity 203
Single donor
    apheresis platelets 260
    plasma 245, 264
Single donor platelet 140, 258, 281, 578
    collection of 282f
    kit 282f
    modified 578
Single nontraumatic venepuncture 255
Single nucleotide polymorphisms 34
Single unit leukopheresis 271
Single-nucleotide polymorphisms 208, 502
Skin biopsy 323
Slide technique 72, 106
Small blood volumes 278
Smallpox 146
Society of blood transfusion 437
Sodium
    azide 157
    biphosphate 165
    chloride 67, 166
    deoxycholate 157
    dihydrogen monophosphate 166
    hypochlorite 367
    nitrite 157
Soil, pollution of 445
Soiled waste 447
Solid organ transplantation 407
Solid phase
    adherence tests 185, 195
    assays 17, 18, 18f
    immunoassay 358
    immunosorbent assays 358
    red cell adherence
        assay 82
        assays technology 84f
        methods 228
    technology, advantages of 82
    test systems, types of 82
Solid support nitrocellulose membrane 365
Solid tumors 324
Solvent-detergent plasma 263
Somatic cell 25
    division 27
Sophisticated thermocyclers 377

Spermatozoa 29, 29f
Spherocytes 103
Sphygmomanometer 148
    cuff 152
Spillage 487
Spin
    crossmatch, immediate 227, 228f, 425
    phase, immediate 193
    technique, immediate 74
    types of 247, 247t
Spirochete 172
    treponema pallidum 353
Spleen 134
Spontaneous agglutination 65
Stable cyanmethemoglobin 157
Stacked coin appearance 197
Stacked coins 93
Standard basic immunohematology testing 320
Standard blood grouping 551
Standard numerical nomenclature 40
Standard operating procedure 62, 461, 432, 474, 478, 548
    advantages of 463b
    system 482
    usual contents of 463b
State licensing authority 585
Stem cell 519b
    transplantation, autologous 533b
Sterile connecting device 245
Sterile products, manufacture of 561t
Sterilization-cum-washing 545
Stethoscope 148
Stimulate immunocompetent 513
Stock solution, preparation of 156
Stomatocytes 103
Stomatocytosis, hereditary 300
Stop transfusion immediately 333
Storage area 560
Storage equipment 458
Storage lesion 169
Storage of blood, refrigerator for 470
Strand displacement assay 372
Streptococcus
    pyogenes 132
    suis 124
Stromal cells 520
Stronger reaction 204
Subsequent pregnancy 385
Sulfhydryl reducing agents 128, 129, 131
Supplier qualifications 459
Supportive therapy 333
Surgery, cardiac 402
Surgical procedures 570
Suspension array technology 19

Syngeneic hematopoietic progenitor cell transplantation 526
Syphilis 244, 353, 357
    diagnosis of 79
    laboratory diagnosis of 353
    serology reagents 548
Systemic inflammatory response syndrome 531
Systemic reactions 154

T

T cytotoxic cells 4
T helper cells 4
T lymphocytes 4, 496, 512
    subsets of 4
T pallidum hemagglutination assay 356, 356f
T pallidum particle agglutination test 357
Table top centrifuge 75f
Tachycardia 310, 331
Target antigen 82, 211
Target cell 495
Tattoo 550
T-cell
    activation of 517
    depleted marrow and leukemia, use of 516
    depletion 530
        disadvantages of 530
    mediated graft rejection 515
    sensitization in vivo or ex vivo of 535
Technical resource group 588
Technical supervisor 546
Techniques targeting T-cells 530
Telomere 26
Temperature and humidity 560
Temperature and pulse determination 550, 581
Temperature dependent methods 214
Temporary central storage 448
Temporary donor deferral 145t
Test method validation 464
Test plasma 96
Test tube racks 148
Tetanic spasms 155
Tetanus 146, 550
Thalassemia 325, 410
Thawed fresh frozen plasma, appearance of 263f
Thawed plasma 169, 263
Thawing 266, 528, 530
    bath 262f
Therapeutic apheresis 275, 279, 286, 293, 328
    indications of 286
Therapeutic cytapheresis 275, 286, 578
    indications of 286b

Therapeutic erythrocytapheresis 288
Therapeutic leukapheresis 286
Therapeutic leukocytapheresis 287
Therapeutic plasma
   exchange 269, 274, 289, 290*t*, 291*t*, 409
      complications of 291, 291*b*
   pheresis 275, 578
Therapeutic platelet apheresis 286
Therapeutic procedures 444
Thrombocythemia 287
Thrombocytoapheresis 274
Thrombocytopenia 239, 409
   heparin-induced 79
Thrombocytosis 286, 287
   reactive 286
Thromboplastin time, partial 294
Thrombotic thrombocytopenic purpura 285, 342, 409, 420
Thymine 27, 134
Thyroid
   disease 571
   disorders 571
   tumors, malignant 571
Tile technique 72, 106
Tissue
   injury 239
   transplantation 493
   typing 515
Titer level 215
   uses of 215
Tongue
   depressor 153
   edema of 308
Total-body irradiation 530
Toxic reactions 495
Toxoids 146, 573
Traditional tube method 224
Trained healthcare professionals, shortage of 441
Training and competency testing 487
Transcription mediated amplification 372, 377
   assay 372
Transcription-based amplification 377
Transfected human leukocyte antigen deficient human lymphoid cells 511
Transferring blood, process of 138
Transfused donor red cells, acute intravascular destruction of 303
Transfused red cells 51, 57
Transfusing blood products 234
Transfusion 96, 208, 409
   chronic 35
   discontinuation of 340

   duration, extension of 312
   hazards 436
   hemosiderosis 325
   history of 223*b*
   laboratory, quality assurance in 487
   practice, quality control in 472
   procedures, clinical 432
   recipient 316
   regulation and legislation 538
   related acute lung injury 311, 340
      diagnosis of 311*b*
   services 138
   strategies 240
   support 420*t*
   therapy 402
   transmitted infections, screening blood donors for 357
Transfusion associated
   acute lung injury, pathogenesis of 309
   circulatory overload 303, 311, 312, 313*t*, 340
   graft versus host disease 318, 322, 325*t*, 535
   hypotension 313
   infection 481
   mortality 311
   sepsis 303, 314, 316*b*, 314, 340
Transfusion medicine 1, 1*f*, 58, 138, 296, 300, 314*b*, 425, 450, 567
   branches of 138
   common antibodies in 204*t*
   quality control in 467
   requirements in 458
   types of antibodies in 190
Transfusion reaction 129, 181, 205, 302*b*, 326, 330, 331*b*, 335, 335*b*, 336*b*, 344*fc*, 492
   immediate 331
   recognition of 331
   record of 476
   reporting form 438
   summary of 343*t*
   types of 307, 333, 517
Transfusion-transmitted
   disease 302, 346, 357, 443, 464, 472
   risk for 140
   infections 172
   relevant 141
   infectious agents 346*t*
   viral disease 320
Transmissible spongiform encephalopathies 366
Transmission
   congenital 351

   mode of 351, 353
   route of 347
Transplacental transmission 353
Transplan*t*
   preparing products for 530
   rejection of 515
   related complications 532
Transplantation 407, 408
   allogeneic 140, 535
   autologous 140, 532
   fresh products 529
Transplanted organs, rejection of 492
Treponema pallidum immobilization 356
Treponemal antibodies 356
Treponemal tests 356
Trichomonas vaginalis 378
Trisodium citrate 166
True agglutination and rouleaux formation 197
Trypan blue 501
Trypanosoma cruzi 357
   infection 145
Trypsin 128
Tube
   antibody screen test 194*f*
   method 73, 74*f*
      procedure of 193
   techniques 106
   test 76, 107, 183
      protocols 199
      techniques 193
Tumor 495
   cells 530, 536
   lysis syndrome 287
   necrosis factor 497
Two-stage enzyme 193
   test method 209
Typhoid 146, 550

U

Ultraviolet A 288
Umbilical cord blood 520, 525*b*, 526
   collection, features of 524*b*
   derived hematopoietic progenitor cell 524
   processing 525
Umbilical cord hematopoietic progenitor cells, advantages of 524*b*
Unacceptable Quality control 467
Unconjugated bilirubin 381
Unique equipment identification 457
Unique sequences, specific for 505
Unit using sterile technique 312
Universal donor 23
   high-titer 58
Universal leukocyte reduction 251

Index

Universal precautions in blood bank 486*b*
Universal recipient 23
Universal red cells 16
Unrelated donors 527
Upper airway involvement 309
Urinary tract infection 114
Uroepithelial cell cancers 114
Urticaria 293, 308
Urticarial reactions
   mild 309
   severe 309
Urticarial response 308, 310
Uvula, edema of 308

V

Vaccination 146, 147
   and inoculation 573
   approach 536
Vaginal secretions 47
Validation, type of 457
Vasoactive amines 297
Vasovagal
   reaction 293
   syncope 154
Venepuncture 468
   site of 155
Venereal disease research laboratory 16, 246, 354, 552
Venipuncture 149
Vibrio cholerae 60
Vicia graminea 50
Viral core 348
Viral inactivation process 561
Viral infections 5, 201, 481
Viral load tests 378
Viral replication, active 352
Viral transmission 347
Virtual blood bank 429
Virus, direct inoculation of 347
Visible agglutination 11
Visual check for hemolysis 335
Visual hemolysis 336
Vital staining 501
Vital stains 501
Volume expansion 293
Voluntary blood donor 431, 566
Voluntary donors 467
Voluntary nonremunerated donors 139, 431
Vomiting 154, 523, 531
von Willebrand disease 268, 410
von Willebrand factor 245, 269

W

Waldenström's macroglobulinemia 93, 159
Waste
   and infectious materials, disposal of 558
   chemicals 445
   sharps 447
   types of 447
Water
   bath
      and incubator 471
      thawing in 262
   pollution of 445
West Nile virus 525
Western blot 350, 358, 364, 365
Wharton's jelly 85
White blood cell 1, 246
   disorders 526
Whole blood 243, 473, 557
   by blood bank 577
   collection 524
   donation 139
   indications for 244*b*
   testing of 552
   transfusion of 139
Whole human blood 540, 543
Wiener haplotype, modified 100
Wiener terminology 100
   modified 100
Working solution, preparation of 156
World Health Organization 437

X

X chromosomes 25
Xenoantibodies 3
Xylene 214

Y

Y chromosome 25
Yellow fever 146
Yt system 112

Z

Zygosity 34